G. G. Jackson · H. D. Schlumberger · H. J. Zeiler (Editors)

Perspectives in Antiinfective Therapy

Current Topics in Infectious Diseases and Clinical Microbiology

Edited by I. Braveny

Vol. 1 **Ciprofloxacin**
Microbiology – Pharmacokinetics – Clinical Experience

Vol. 2 **Perspectives in Antiinfective Therapy**

Bayer AG Centenary Symposium

Perspectives in Antiinfective Therapy

Washington, D. C., Aug. 31–Sept. 3, 1988

Editors: G. G. Jackson
H. D. Schlumberger
H. J. Zeiler

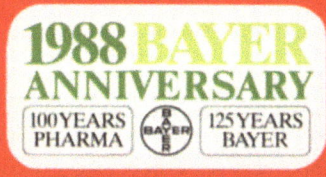

Springer Fachmedien Wiesbaden GmbH

The use of general descriptive names, trade names, trademarks, etc., in this publication, even if the former are not especially identified, is not to be taken as a sign that such names, as understood by the Trade Marks and Merchandise Marks Act, may accordingly be used freely by anyone.

While the advice and information of this book is believed to be true and accurate at the date of going to press, neither the authors nor the editors nor the publisher can accept any legal responsibility for any errors or omissions that may be made. The publisher makes no warranty, express or implied, with respect to the material contained herein.

All rights reserved

© Springer Fachmedien Wiesbaden 1989

Originally published by Friedr. Vieweg & Sohn Verlagsgesellschaft mbH, Braunschweig in 1989.

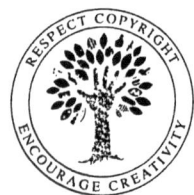

No part of this publication may be reproduced, stored in a retrieval system or transmitted in any form or by any means, mechanical, photocopying, recording or otherwise, without prior permission of the copyright holder.

ISBN 978-3-528-07979-6   ISBN 978-3-322-86064-4 (eBook)
DOI 10.1007/978-3-322-86064-4

Foreword

Pharmaceutical research has a long-standing tradition in Bayer since the establishment of a Pharmaceutical Department 25 years after the foundation of the Farbenfabriken of Friedrich Bayer & Co. in the city of Elberfeld, Germany. In 1888 one of the first antipyretic drugs, phenacetin, was synthesized. A milestone was marked by the discovery and launch of Aspirin^{TM} in 1899, the most widely used and appreciated drug since then.

The success of Bayer 205 (Germanin^{TM}) in the treatment of sleeping sickness led not only to the worldwide recognition of Bayer as a pharmaceutical company but also to intense research into anti-infective therapy. The antimalarial drugs Atebrin^{TM}, Plasmochin^{TM} and Resochin^{TM} were the first of a whole series of significant contributions and even breakthroughs in the therapy of infections. The advances and the success of antibacterial therapy was heralded by the discovery of the antibacterial activity of the sulfonamides by Domagk, Klarer and Mietsch. The first drug of this class of compounds, Prontosil^{TM}, opened the new era of therapeutic control of bacterial infections. In 1939 Domagk received the Nobel Prize for Medicine for this breakthrough. A further breakthrough in the chemotherapy of the scourge of tuberculosis was achieved in 1946 by Domagk and his colleagues Behnisch, Mietzsch and Schmidt with the development of Conteben^{TM}, followed shortly afterwards by the discovery of isoniazid (Neoteben^{TM}) by Domagk, Offe and Siefken. The discovery of the antimycotic activity of azoles marked another significant achievement in the pharmacotherapy of infectious diseases. The first antimycotic drug of this new class of compounds, clotrimazole, has set new standards in the treatment of mycoses.

The tradition of the company in the chemotherapy of tropical diseases was continued by the development, together with E. Merck, Darmstadt, Germany, of praziquantel for the therapy of schistosomiasis. The cure of schistosomiasis, a disease that affects 200 to 300 million patients, by a single-dose treatment was regarded as such a significant therapeutic achievement that it was honoured by the renowned Prix Gallien in 1987. Recently, progress in antibacterial chemotherapy has been achieved by the development of broad-spectrum antimicrobial agents such as mezlocillin and azlocillin, and of ciprofloxacin, a gyrase inhibitor. This quinolone derivative is effective by both oral and parenteral routes.

This tradition of pharmaceutical research, especially in the field of anti-infective therapy, is certainly an obligation to continue the scientific endeavours of Bayer into the future. Consequently, it was clear that the Bayer Health Care Sector, into which the tiny Pharmaceutical Department of 1888 has now grown, would celebrate its centenary with a series of scientific symposia in different parts of the world. One of these symposia was held in Washington, DC, and was dedicated to "Perspectives in Antiinfective Therapy."

The aim of this centenary symposium was to review the state of anti-infective therapy and discuss opportunities and possibilities for new or improved therapies with leading scientists of different disciplines and different areas of interest. The scope of the topics addressed in this symposium was intentionally broad so that there could be an exchange of experience, practical and intellectual, across the interdisciplinary barriers. It was clear that the broad spectrum of topics could not be dealt with in depth; the lectures of the symposium are therefore to be regarded as representative of a particular research area. The symposium addressed, for example, the mechanisms of action of anti-infective drugs and microbial pathogenic mechanisms that are susceptible to drug intervention as well as mechanisms of microbial drug resistance and problems of drug delivery. Further topics were dedicated to the interaction of the host with the infectious agent, new diseases and disease epidemiology, the application of new technologies in the development of anti-infectious agents, and drug design. It was concluded that there are new opportunities for the development of better drugs for many infectious diseases. This is possible because of new understanding and capabilities resulting from new technology in molecular biology. It is needed not only because of the profound changes in the demographic structure of the populations of the developed countries but also because of the changes and new developments in diseases and modes of therapy. The symposium closed with statements on the future development and use of anti-infective chemotherapy with special emphasis on the regulation of new drugs, the barriers to effective use of anti-infective drugs and the optimal clinical use of anti-infective therapy. We are pleased to present the results of this symposium in this volume.

We would like to express our sincerest thanks and our gratitude to the authors of this volume for their contributions and their cooperation. We are also indebted to all who helped and contributed to the success of the symposium and to the preparation of this volume.

G. G. Jackson   H. D. Schlumberger   H. J. Zeiler

Contents

Foreword
G. G. Jackson*, H. D. Schlumberger, H. J. Zeiler V

The Challenge of Perspective
G. G. Jackson 1

On Bacteriological Research
R. Koch 3

Background to Robert Koch's Lecture at the International Congress in Berlin, 1890
J. Parascandola 6

Classical Mechanisms of Antibacterial Drugs

Multiple Penicillin Binding Protein Profiles in Penicillin Resistant Pneumococci:
Evidence for the Clonal Nature of Resistance Among Clinical Isolates
A. Tomasz*, D. Jabes, Z. Markiewicz, J. García-Bustos, S. Nachmann 11

Antibiotic Uptake into Gram-Negative Bacteria
R. E. W. Hancock*, A. Bell 21

Inhibition of Protein Biosynthesis by Antibiotics
K. H. Nierhaus*, R. Brimacombe, H. G. Wittmann 29

Inhibition of DNA Gyrase: Bacterial Sensitivity and Clinical Resistance to 4-Quinolones
M. E. Cullen, A. W. Wyke, F. McEachern, C. A. Austin, L. M. Fisher* 41

Mechanisms of Nonbacterial Anti-Infective Drugs

Mechanisms of Antiretroviral Compounds in Inhibition of Viral and Cellular
DNA Polymerase
K. Ono 51

Effects of Drugs on Lipids and Membrane Integrity of Fungi
N. H. Georgopapadakou 60

Membrane Changes Induced by Praziquantel
P. Andrews*, A. Harder 68

Mechanisms of Action of Antimalarial Drugs
W. Peters 76

Pathogenic Microbial Mechanisms Susceptible to Drug Application

Bacterial Adherence in Pathogenicity
   S. Normark*, S. Hultgren, B.-I. Marklund, G. Nyberg, A. Olsén, N. Strömberg, J. Tennent 89

Haemophilus influenzae Gene Expression and Bacterial Invasion
   E. R. Moxon*, J. S. Kroll, J. N. Weiser 95

Coordinate Regulation of Bacterial Virulence Genes
   W. Goebel*, J. Hacker 99

Microbial Drug Resistance

Transposon Transfer of Drug Resistance
   F. H. Kayser*, B. Berger-Bächi 109

Bacterial Proteins Involved in Antimicrobial Drug Resistance
   C. C. Sanders 115

Persistent Herpes Simplex Virus Infection and Mechanisms of Virus Drug Resistance
   H. J. Field 122

Pharmacology and Drug Delivery

Antiviral Therapy with Small Particle Aerosols
   V. Knight*, B. Gilbert 135

Liposomes and Lipid Structures as Carriers of Amphotericin B
   A. S. Janoff 146

Targeted Liposomes Bearing Sendai for Influenza Envelope Glycoproteins as a Potential Carrier for Protein Molecules and Genes
   A. Loyter 152

Host Determinants in Anti-Infective Chemotherapy

Cell Mediated Immunity, Immunodeficiency and Microbial Infections
   S. H. E. Kaufmann*, I. E. A. Flesch 165

Neutropenia: Antibiotic Combinations for Empiric Therapy
   L. S. Young 174

Modulation of the Host Flora
   R. van Furth*, H. F. L. Guiot 179

Enhancement of Host Resistance by Control of Fungal Growth
   D. Pappagianis 186

Nonvaccine Immunoalteration of the Host

Passive Immunotherapy of Infectious Diseases: Lessons from the Past, Directions for the Future
J. E. Pennington 197

T-Cell Mediated Immunopathology in Viral Infections
R. M. Zinkernagel 202

New Diseases and Disease Epidemiology

Adherence and Proliferation of Bacteria on Artificial Surfaces
G. Peters 209

Current Knowledge of *Chlamydia* TWAR, an Important Cause of Pneumonia and Other Acute Respiratory Diseases
J. T. Grayston*, S. P. Wang, C. C. Kuo 216

Current Status of Antiviral Chemotherapy for Genital Herpes Simplex Virus Infection: Its Impact on Disease Control
L. Corey 229

Induction and Maintenance Therapy for Opportunistic Infections in Patients with AIDS
M. A. Sande 235

New Technology and Drug Design

Nucleic Acid Hybridization: A Rapid Method for the Diagnosis of Infectious Diseases
N. Dattagupta, E. Huguenel, P. Rae, D. Crothers* 241

New Technology and Immunospecific Reactions in Helminthic Diseases
B. Gottstein 248

Molecular Targets of Chemotherapeutic Agents Against the Human Immunodeficiency Virus
E. De Clercq 255

Modern Strategies in the Design of Antimicrobial Agents
J. K. Seydel 268

Future Development and Use of Anti-Infective Chemotherapy

The Future Challenge of Infectious Disease
F. E. Young 281

Barriers to Effective Anti-Infective Therapy: The Perspectives of a Clinical Pharmacologist
L. Lasagna 284

Optimal Use of Antimicrobial Agents
H. C. Neu 288

Views of Future Anti-Infective Therapy (Panel Discussion)
W. Goebel, E. R. Moxon, L. Young 295

* Denotes person to whom inquiries and requests for reprints should be addressed.

The Challenge of Perspective

G. G. Jackson

The Centenary of Bayer AG being celebrated in 1988 marks a century in which the firm has contributed to the discovery and production of medicines for the relief of disease and promotion of health. All mankind has benefitted. We add a new round of congratulations to the generations of scientists who have made the record so distinguished and commend the company for generating the philosophy of research that produced the successes. We are confident in our hope and wish that the years ahead will extend the success and build the record with new achievements. It is a thoughtful gesture on Bayer's part to celebrate the important event in their history by sponsoring scientific symposia to assess concurrent advances in science and health. Few, if any, disciplines exceed antiinfective therapy in these accomplishments.

A symposium oriented around a landmark rather than a scientific topic, a disease, or a product permits us to pause, ponder our state of knowledge and develop a perspective of the field. With scientific and social revelry we can celebrate the gains and anticipate the future. Participants in the symposium are small in number and broad in the diversity of disciplines of interest. Thousands of involved scientists and clinical investigators could be recognized for their contributions to the development, understanding, and use of antiinfective therapy. The representative essayists at this time come from universities, industry, research laboratories and clinics. Their responsibilities include the direction of basic research, health policy programs, drug development, drug regulation and patient care. The cumulative experience provides the breadth essential for a perspective having social and clinical relevance built on the scientific foundations of a century.

The venue of the meeting is also historical. The first Antibiotic Annual meetings were held at the Willard Hotel under the sponsorship of the commissioner of the U.S. Food and Drug Administration. The FDA brought together representatives from university, industry and government, as we have done, to discuss antibiotic agents and chemotherapy. The preceding discoveries, the stimulus of those meetings and the course of development of antiinfective therapy have had an inestimable impact on multiple disciplines in science, industry and medicine during the last half-century. Virtually all people in all nations have been exposed to some measure of antiinfective therapy. The sociology of the world has been changed.

No field marches alone. In the period we are commemorating, rapid growth in technology has been a key instrument. New techniques have put us into full gallop of speed and capability in probing biologic secrets previously withheld. Parallel advances by pioneers in clinical investigation established standards for objective and quantifiable clinical assessment of antiinfective drugs. Concerns for social equity with genuine empathy for individuals has given focus and definition to ethical and moral values in the development and application of drugs as is necessary to realize full satisfaction in the advances.

In the broad perspective of conquest of infectious diseases, antiinfective therapy is focussed principally on treatment among seven identifiable steps from recognition to eradication of a disease (Figure 1). Development of knowledge does not necessarily follow the sequence of the steps, but it tends to do so. As we gain information from one of them, it opens new horizons and opportunities for development of the others. The first four steps are descriptive and depend on the genius of astute original observations by individuals. Intellectual curiosity and academic pursuit elicit the epidemiology, pathophysiology and etiology of each disease. On the basis of that understanding, antiinfective therapy can be applied to alter the course by cure, prevention, and even eradication of some infections. Success in applied intervention is the result of effective integration of professional relationships, the productivity of industry, and social acceptance of the products.

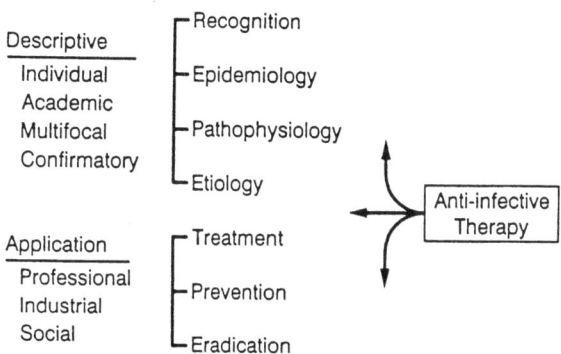

Figure 1: Seven steps in the conquest of infectious diseases through description and application of knowledge, noting the focus of anti-infective therapy in altering the course.

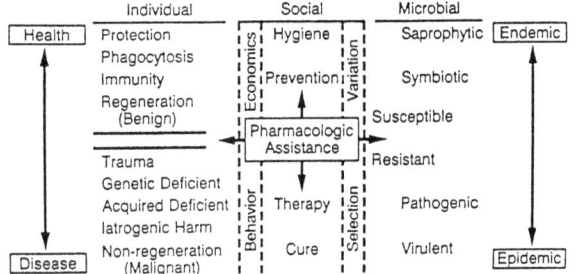

Figure 2: Pivotal roles of anti-infective drugs (pharmacologic assistance) affecting interactive components in the occurrence and characteristics of infection.

	Malaria	Tuberculosis	Variola	AIDS
Recognition	400 BC / 1624	1000 BC / 1689	1677	1981
Epidemiology	1897 (Ross)	1846 (Klencke)	1685 (Sydenham)	1982
Pathophysiology	1850 (Drake)	1916 (Ghon)	1766 (Rhages)	1983
Etiology	1880 (Lavaron)	1882 (Koch)	1715 / 1926	1984
Treatment	1632 Bark / 1926 Plasmaquine / 1946 Chloroquine	1945 SM / 1952 INH	1960 (Methisazone)	1985
Prevention	1940s / 1990s	1924 (Calmette)	1798 (Jenner)	Future
Eradication	No Decrease	Diminished	1980	Future

Figure 3: Perspective of present (AIDS) and historical performance in developing understanding of essential steps in the conquest of some classical infectious diseases.

A proper perspective of antiinfective therapy recognizes the interaction of individual host defense mechanisms, social and environmental events, and characteristics of the microbial universe (Figure 2). With antiinfective therapy the aim is to use pharmacological assistance of the patient to tilt the balance from disease toward health and away from virulent epidemics toward a saprophytic endemic relationship with microbes. In this equation social behaviour can become overriding and the selective effect of drug use itself can sometimes be adverse.

Time is a critical component of perspective. Examination of the rate of progress in three classic diseases and the current epidemic of AIDS indicates that centuries have literally been collapsed into years in obtaining the results of inquiry (Figure 3). Even with the exclusion of hippocratic and biblical references, the time from medical description to determination of etiology of these classic diseases required about two centuries. Usually another century or more was required to find specific treatment. The track of progress in understanding AIDS, which shows the same accomplishments in years, is exemplary of the scientific resources and capabilities we have. The challenge before us is to develop a perspective that will make this capability most productive for the future. If we are successful, it would mean that within the lifetime of a single individual a major effect could be exerted on some of the principal infectious diseases that afflict the people of the world.

The symposium will begin with molecular, chemical and cellular knowledge of how illustrative antiinfective drugs work. This understanding must be complemented by knowledge of the pathogenesis of infections and the effect of treatment then integrated with the pharmacologic behavior of drugs. The specificity required in diagnosis and manifested in drug action presents challenges for the development of new rapid sensitive tests and new drugs with unique target sites of action. On that basis of knowledge a perspective and plans for future action can emerge. The publication of the proceedings is a display of the skills and capabilities that can be used in addressing the problems of infections and the opportunities for enhancing antiinfective therapy. The record and perceptions should serve initially as a useful reference and stimulus for new research with application. After another century we would like it to remain as a historical landmark to be read with amusement and may be amazement. Then, as now, readers may be surprised by how much we know and can do. The challenge is to gather the resources into a perspective that will serve the future.

G. G. Jackson

Professor of Medicine (Emeritus), University of Illinois College of Medicine, Chicago, Illinois, and Professor of Clinical Virology, Department of Medical Microbiology, The London Hospital Medical College, London, UK.

On Bacteriological Research*

R. Koch

When I was given the honourable task of presenting one of the lectures for this international congress, I was offered the choice of taking for my subject that science with which I have now been principally occupied, namely that of hygiene, or bacteriology, to which I was at one time able to dedicate myself almost exclusively for many years.

Bacteriology is, at least as far as we doctors are concerned, a very young science. As recently as 15 years ago we knew little more than the fact that in anthrax and relapsing fever, strange, exotic structures were produced in the blood, and that occasionally, so-called "vibrios" occurred in wound infections. Proof that these objects were the cause of those diseases had not at that time been obtained, and with the exception of a few researchers who were considered to be dreamers, such structures were viewed more as curiosities than pathogens. In fact, one could hardly have thought otherwise at the time, since it had not once been proved that these were independent organisms that were specific to those diseases. Bacteria that seemed to be not different from the anthrax bacilli had been found in putrescent fluids, particularly in the blood of asphyxiated animals. Some researchers did not consider them to be living particles at all, but rather crystal-like structures. Bacteria identical to the spirilla of relapsing fever were found to occur in bog water and dental mucus, and bacteria similar to the micrococci observed in wound infections were found in supposedly healthy blood and tissues.

No further progress was possible in view of the optical and laboratory equipment then available, and the situation would have remained thus for some considerable time had not new research methods come into being which, at a stroke, led to the discovery of completely new relationships and opened up the way toward unlocking the closed doors of unknown areas. Using improved optical systems that were specially adapted for the purpose, and, with the help of aniline dyes, even the smallest bacteria were easily visible and were able to be differentiated from other microorganisms by their morphology. At the same time, by using nutrient media, either in liquid or solid form as required, it became possible to separate the individual organisms and obtain therefrom pure cultures from which the characteristics peculiar to each individual type could be ascertained beyond all doubt.

The potential of these new methods and equipment soon became apparent. A number of well-characterised types of pathogenic microorganisms were discovered, and, of even greater importance, the causal relationship between these organisms and the corresponding diseases was established. Since the pathogens observed all belonged to the class of bacteria, the impression must have been given that the actual infections were caused exclusively by certain types of bacteria which were separate from one another, and it was hoped that in the not too distant future, the corresponding pathogens would be found for all the infectious diseases.

This expectation has not, in fact, been fulfilled and the further development of bacterial research in other respects has repeatedly followed an unexpected course. Moreover, in another important matter, namely as regards proving the causal connection between the pathogenic bacteria and the corresponding infectious diseases, certain relationships have become much clearer and more simplified than they previously were.

The idea that microorganisms must have been the *cause* of the infections was expressed at an early stage by certain distinguished individuals, although general opinion could not become accustomed to the idea and was consequently very sceptical about the initial discoveries in this area. It was all the more important, from the first, to provide incontrovertible evidence supporting the fact that the microorganisms observed in an infectious disease were actually the cause of that disease. At that time the objection was made, quite legitimately, that the combined appearance of disease and microorganisms was a random event and that the latter were not, therefore, dangerous in any way, but rather harmless parasites which discovered conditions necessary for their existence only in the diseased organs and not in the healthy body.

Some scientists did indeed acknowledge the pathogenic properties of bacteria, but they considered it possible that the bacteria were originally harmless microorganisms, occurring by chance or in some regular pattern, that only became pathogenic under the influence of the disease process. However, once the following had been proved – firstly, that the

---

*Translated excerpt taken from the Proceedings of the Xth International Medical Congress, 1890, In: Schwalbe, J., Gaffky, G. und Pfuhl, E. (ed.): Gesammelte Werke von Robert Koch. Volume 1. Verlag von Georg Thieme, Leipzig, 1912, p. 650 ("Über bakteriologische Forschung").

parasite was found in every individual case of the relevant illness and, moreover, in a manner which corresponded to the pathological changes and the clinical course of the diseases; secondly, that the parasite was not observed in any other illness as a chance, non-pathogenic organism; and thirdly, that in complete isolation from the body and when cultured in sufficient quantities in pure cultures, it was in a position to reproduce the disease-once these had all been proved, then the parasite could no longer be considered as a chance by-product of the illness, and the only relationship between parasite and illness that could subsequently be inferred was that the parasite was the cause of the illness.

I should just like to mention the results of investigations into bacteria regarding their metabolites. Certain of these metabolites possess strange, toxic effects and may possibly affect the symptoms, perhaps even the most important ones, of an infectious illness. Of particular note in this regard are the recently discovered toxic proteins, the so-called toxalbumins, which can be obtained from cultures of anthrax, diphtheria and tetanus bacteria.

There is currently much enthusiasm regarding research into the pertinent question of the nature of *immunity*, a problem that can only be solved with the help of bacteriology. No actual conclusions have been drawn as yet, but increasingly it appears that the idea which has been uppermost in people's minds for some considerable time now is losing ground, namely, that immunity involves merely cellular processes, a kind of struggle between the invading parasites and the phagocytes acting as the body's defence mechanism. It is extremely probable that here too, chemical processes play the major role.

Concerning the *etiology* of infections, it is particularly important to point out that bacteria can only multiply in moist conditions, either in the presence of water or other suitable fluids, and that they are unable by their own impetus to transport themselves into the air from moist surfaces. Consequently, pathogenic bacteria can only be carried in the air in the form of dust or dust particles, and only those which can survive for an extended period in the dry state are able to be transported by air currents. However, they are never capable of multiplying in the air as had once been supposed of miasmatic material.

In several areas, admittedly in those areas where little was expected, bacteriological research has let us down completely. I refer to the research that has been carried out on a number of infectious diseases that seemed to offer an easy target for research in view of their marked infectivity. Primarily involved is the whole group of exanthematous infections, namely measles, scarlet fever, smallpox and exanthematic typhus. We have been unable to discover even the slightest indication of what might be the type of pathogen in any one of these diseases. Even vaccinia, which is so readily available and so easily tested in experimental animals, has stubbornly resisted all attempts to determine the actual agent of these illnesses. The same applies to rabies canina.

Furthermore, we still do not know anything about the pathogens of influenza, pertussis, trachoma, yellow fever, cattle plague, pneumonic plague and many other diseases which are undoubtedly infectious. In researching most of these diseases we have shown no lack of skill or perseverance in employing all the methods that are currently avaible to us, and we can only conclude from the negative results produced by the attempts of numerous scientists that the methods of investigation which so far have proved themselves worthy in so many cases are now no longer adequate for these tasks.

I am disposed towards the opinion that the aforementioned diseases do not involve bacteria, but rather organised pathogens belonging to completely different groups of microorganisms. This theory is supported particularly by the fact that strange parasites belonging to the lowest category of the animal kingdom, protozoa, have recently been found in the blood of many animals and humans suffering from malaria. We have thus far been unable to progress from the simple detection of these remarkable and very important parasites, and the situation is likely to remain thus until these protozoa have been cultured outside the body, in a fashion similar to that for bacteria, in artificial nutrient media or in some other way, preferably in natural conditions. We also need to study their living conditions and how they develop. If this task is accomplished, and there seems no reason to think otherwise, then it is very likely that another branch of science will emerge alongside bacteriological research which will involve the investigation of pathogenic protozoa and related microorganisms. It is hoped that this research will enlighten us as regards the previously mentioned infectious diseases, the etiology of which has not yet been investigated.

Hitherto, I have intentionally left untouched one particular question, even though it is one that is most frequently and, it must be admitted, not without reproach, directed towards the bacteriologists. I refer to the question which seeks to know the *purpose* of all thus arduous research into bacteria which has been carried out so far. As a matter of fact such a question should not be asked, since genuine research pursues its own course, unhampered by the consideration as to whether the work is of immediate benefit or not; however, I do not consider this question to be so unwarranted in this particular case, since even those who are only marginally involved in bacteriological research have not completely ignored the practical aims.

In no way, however, can those results of bacteriological research that have so far been practically evaluated be considered meager, as those questioners suppose. I would remind you of what has been achieved in the area of *disinfection*. In the early stages there was a complete absence of any clues. People were working completely in the dark and large sums of money were wasted on useless disinfection, not to mention the indirect harm which can result from the inappropriate use of hygienic measures. We now have reliable markers available, with the help of which we shall be in a position to determine the efficacy of the disinfectants. Although there is yet much to be done in this area, we can still say that inasmuch as they have passed the tests, the currently used disinfectants do actually fulfill their purpose.

Although bacteriological research in this area has produced such insignificant results in spite of the intense efforts made, I am nevertheless not of the opinion that such will always be the case. On the contrary, I am convinced that bacteriology will also be of the *greatest significance in therapy*. However, I do not expect that there will be as much success in the treatment of diseases that have a short incubation period and a rapid course. With these diseases, for example, with cholera, the main emphasis will always be on prophylaxis. I am thinking rather of those diseases that do not progress so rapidly and that consequently present possible targets for therapeutic intervention at a much earlier stage. Indeed, there is hardly any other disease which, partly for this reason and partly owing to its overwhelming importance compared with all other infectious diseases, requires bacteriological research as urgently as does tuberculosis.

Impelled by such thoughts, and following the discovery of the tubercle bacilli, I soon began the search for substances which could be used in the treatment of tuberculosis. I have, hitherto, pursued these experiments unceasingly, although interrupted many times by professional matters. I am certainly not alone in my conviction that there must be a cure for tuberculosis.

Proceeding along these lines, I have, in the course of time, tested a very large number of substances to see what influence they exert on tubercle bacilli that have been grown in pure cultures. The results indicate that quite a number of substances are in a position, at very low dosages, to *inhibit the growth* of tubercle bacilli. Of course, a drug need achieve no more than that. It is not necessary, as is often mistakenly assumed, for the bacteria to be killed in the body; it is sufficient merely to prevent their growth, their multiplication, in order to render them harmless to the body.

Despite my lack of success, I was not deterred from continuing the search for inhibiting agents, and I eventually discovered substances that were capable of preventing the growth of the tubercle bacilli not only in the test tube but also in animals. As those who have carried out serious experiments on the disease know, investigations into tuberculosis are very lengthy affairs. Consequently, many experiments on these substances have still not been completed, although they have already taken almost a year of my time. I can therefore merely state that guinea pigs, which are known to be particularly susceptible to tuberculosis, no longer react to inoculation with tuberculous virus when exposed to the action of one of these substances, and that in guinea pigs already suffering from high-grade generalised tuberculosis, the disease process can be brought to a halt without the body being adversely affected by the agent.

And so I should like to conclude my lecture with the hope that the *powers of the nations may join forces* in the fight against the smallest, though most dangerous, enemies of humankind, and that in this struggle for the well-being of all humanity, one nation may continually surpass another in its success.

Background to Robert Koch's Lecture at the International Congress in Berlin, 1890

J. Parascandola

It is appropriate at this conference on antiinfective therapy, commemorating the centennial of the pharmaceutical division at Bayer, that we should turn back the hands of time just about 100 years to hear a lecture on bacteriological research delivered by Robert Koch at the International Medical Congress in Berlin in 1890. Koch was certainly the right choice to deliver such a lecture to that distinguished audience, for he was one of the principal founders of bacteriology as a modern science. At the time, he was perhaps at the peak of his career, and was one of the most respected figures in medicine worldwide.

Yet success did not come early or easy to Robert Koch. He was born in Clausthal, Germany, on December 11, 1843, to a family of mining officials. Early in life he developed an interest in natural history, stimulated by his mother and his maternal grandfather. At Göttingen University he studied medicine, receiving his medical degree in 1866. Among his teachers was the anatomist Jacob Henle, whose own interest in bacteria may have influenced the young Koch, although Koch was not to embark upon research on microorganisms for some time to come.

For the next half a dozen years Koch led a rather unsettled existence, earning a living through private practice or through various hospital posts. He also served for a time as a field hospital physician in the Franco-Prussian War. In 1872, he became a district medical officer at Wollstein, where he began microscopic research on bacteria. Koch was 40 years of age, and essentially unknown as a medical scientist, when he began his work on anthrax, work that was to start him on the road to fame.

Bacteriology hardly existed as a science at the time, and the idea that microbes could cause disease was still a highly controversial one. Ever since microorganisms were first observed under the microscope by van Leeuwenhoek in the 17th century, there was speculation that these organisms might be the cause of infectious disease. The work of Louis Pasteur in 1860s on the spoilage of wine and beer by microorganisms and on silk worm disease, which Pasteur showed was also caused by microbes, stimulated interest in microbiology and provided evidence in support of the germ theory of disease. Convinced by Pasteur's work that microbes were the likely cause of infections in wounds, the Scottish physician Joseph Lister introduced antiseptic surgery (using phenol as a germicide) in 1865.

Koch himself favored the germ theory of disease. In his study of anthrax, he developed new bacteriological techniques, including the suspended drop method for studying cultures. Using this latter method he was able to trace for the first time the life cycle of the anthrax bacillus. He discovered that it could form spores that remained viable for long periods of time in unfavorable environments, explaining why blood that contained no observable anthrax bacilli could sometimes cause the disease. His classic paper of 1876 on anthrax lent support to the idea that the bacillus caused the disease and helped to bring his name to the scientific community (Pasteur, for example, commented favorably on the paper).

Time does not permit me to discuss all of Koch's contributions to bacteriology, including the development of the postulates associated with his name. His most spectacular success, of course, was the isolation of the tubercle bacillus in 1882 and the demonstration that it was the causative agent in the terrible disease tuberculosis. This work ensured him a place among the immortals in the history of medicine and gave a great boost to the germ theory of disease.

In 1885, Koch was appointed to a new chair of hygiene at Berlin University. Once he had discovered the cause of tuberculosis, Koch began searching for a cure. The lecture that follows, delivered at the International Congress in 1890, was basically an overview of bacteriological research, but it created a sensation because of a few paragraphs at the end. Here Koch indicated that he had at last "discovered substances which were capable of preventing the growth of the tubercle bacilli not only in the test tube, but also in animals."

Injection of a substance which Koch later called "tuberculin" into guinea pigs rendered healthy animals resistant to tuberculosis and arrested the disease in animals already suffering from it. Although Koch offered some words of caution about how much more work needed to be done, hopes were raised that he had indeed discovered a cure for tuberculosis. This optimistic outlook was further stimulated by early results in clinical trials. Suddenly Koch's name became almost a household word, and physicians and patients made pilgrimages to Berlin, clamoring for his "cure".

Although the future seemed bright, Koch was actually entering upon a most difficult period in his life.

As further studies were done, tuberculin did not live up to its early promise. Serious doubts were raised about its efficacy as a therapeutic agent. Koch had yielded to political and social pressures in making optimistic claims for tuberculin too soon. Although tuberculin was an important contribution to medical science in that it became a useful diagnostic agent for the disease, as a remedy it was a failure and a disappointment. In the meantime, Koch, who had been having marital problems, divorced his wife and married an attractive actress 30 years younger than he was. Koch then found his personal life as well as his scientific work being criticized, but he soon rebounded from these domestic and professional troubles.

A new Institute for Infectious Disease was built for him by the German government, with a budget equaling the total research funds for all of the scientific departments at Berlin University. Important work was carried out in this Institute by Koch and his coworkers over the next two decades. It was here, for example, that Emil von Behring, with assistance from Paul Ehrlich, developed and made available the diphtheria antitoxin in 1894.

Koch himself spent much time traveling around the world, investigating and developing public health measures to combat diseases such as bubonic plague and cholera (a disease for which he had isolated the causative organism in 1884). His interest in controlling tuberculosis also never ceased. In 1905, he was awarded the Nobel Prize in Medicine and Physiology for his work on tuberculosis.

In closing, I would like to quote the following tribute to Koch from Paul DeKruif's popular classic, "Microbe Hunters" (1926): "I beg leave to remove my hat and make bows of respect to Koch — the man who really *proved* that microbes are our most deadly enemies, who brought microbe hunting near to being a science, the man who is now the partly forgotten captain of an obscure heroic age."

J. Parascandola

History of Medicine Division, National Library of Medicine, Bethesda, Maryland 20894, USA.

References

1. **Dolman, C. E.:** Heinrich Hermann Robert Koch. In: Gillespie, C., (ed.): Dictionary of scientific biography. Volume VII. Charles Scribner, New York, 1973, p. 420–435.
2. **Carter, K. C.:** Koch's postulates in relation to the work of Jacob Henle and Edwin Klebs, Medical History 1985, 29: 353–374.
3. **Carter, K. C.:** The Koch-Pasteur debate on establishing the cause of anthrax. Bulletin of the History of Medicine 1988, 62: 42–57.
4. **Coleman, W.:** Koch's comma bacillus: the first year. Bulletin of the History of Medicine 1987, 61: 315–342.

**Classical Mechanisms
of Antibacterial Drugs**

Multiple Penicillin Binding Protein Profiles in Penicillin Resistant Pneumococci: Evidence for the Clonal Nature of Resistance Among Clinical Isolates

A. Tomasz, D. Jabes, Z. Markiewicz, J. Garcia-Bustos, S. Nachman

Previous studies have shown that penicillin resistance in pneumococci is a multigenic property that involves the accumulation of chromosomal mutations in the structural genes of penicillin binding proteins (PBPs), resulting in the greatly decreased reactivity of these proteins for beta-lactam antibiotics. We examined the patterns and affinities of PBPs in 160 clinical isolates representing a wide range of MICs (from 0.005–16 µg/ml), serotypes, isolation dates and sites. The vast majority of penicillin-susceptible isolates showed a common, predictable pattern of five PBPs with high affinities for benzylpenicillin in the relative order of $3 > 1A > 2A > 1B > 2B$. In contrast, the PBP profiles became variable in strains for which MICs were > 0.1 µg/ml and PBPs 1A, 2A and 2B of these strains showed decreased penicillin affinity parallel to the increasing levels of antibiotic resistance. While resistant strains exhibited a variety of distinct PBP profiles, these were stable for each particular strain and it is suggested that clinical isolates sharing a common PBP profile may represent the progeny of a distinct mutant clone. Penicillin-resistant clinical isolates and genetic transformants showed profoundly altered cell wall stem peptides. Our data suggest that the decreased penicillin affinity of mutationally altered PBPs results in such a distortion of the active sites that these PBPs also become altered in their reactivity toward their normal natural substrates. Successful expression of high level penicillin resistance in pneumococci may require the acquisition of auxiliary mutation(s) that assure a sufficient supply of the chemically unusual wall precursors needed for the synthesis of the cell wall in penicillin-resistant pneumococci.

In celebrating 100 years of success in the design and use of antibacterial agents, it is interesting to look at the other side of the coin, too: how the targets of those agents, the microbial pathogens, "learn" to evade the inhibitory action of an initially powerful antibiotic. Identification of the molecular basis of drug resistance is, of course, essential for the development of new antibiotics of improved design. In addition, understanding the mechanism of drug resistance often provides insights into the mechanism of action of the same drug in the sensitive bacteria as well. Presented here is an overview of penicillin resistance in pneumococci.

The appropriate backdrop for this topic is the history of "coexistence" between penicillin and *Streptococcus pneumoniae*, a major human pathogen that exists in its ecological habitat, the human nasopharynx, in distinct "families" differentiated by 83 stable capsular types. Upon deployment of penicillin into chemotherapeutic practice in the mid-1940s, pneumococci was found to be an easy prey: MICs for natural isolates of this bacterium were very low, in the range of a few nanograms per milliliter. Furthermore, penicillin treatment caused irreversible damage to these bacteria: massive lysis, cell wall degradation, and rapid loss of viability have been the hallmarks of pneumococcal response to penicillin. Penicillin chemotherapy caused a dramatic decline in the mortality of pneumococcal disease, but attack rates have probably remained unchanged.

The first report of decreased susceptibility to penicillin in a clinical isolate dates back to 1967 (1), but the true picture of pneumococcal penicillin resistance was first revealed by a series of reports from South Africa describing epidemics caused by penicillin-resistant and multiply drug-resistant pneumococcal isolates in 1977 (2).

Penicillin Binding Protein Alterations as the Basis of Penicillin Resistance

Soon after the epidemiological reports from South Africa, studies in our laboratory determined that the general mechanistic basis of pneumococcal penicillin resistance in two of the highly resistant South African

The Rockefeller University, 1230 York Avenue, New York, New York 10021–6399, USA.

strains (8249 and D20) involved the restructuring of the target enzymes of penicillin action in the bacteria, the PBPs (3, 4), in such a way that their reactivity with penicillin had decreased. The process involved multiple steps of gradually decreasing the affinity of at least three if not four of the pneumococcal PBPs, and each one of these steps could be identified as a distinct upward change in MIC transferable by genetic transformation as a set of distinct, genetic determinants.

The most useful tool in these early studies of the mechanism of pneumococcal penicillin resistance was genetic transformation. Most likely, the gradually increasing MICs and the gradually shifting PBP patterns obtained in the laboratory for the stepwise transformants reconstructed the mutational steps that originally led to the emergence of the highly penicillin-resistant strain 8249 in South Africa. If this interpretation is correct, then the number of mutations that have accumulated in this strain is remarkable indeed, considering the low incidence (10^{-6} or less) of spontaneous mutations even to low levels of penicillin resistance (5).

Analysis of the PBPs of genetic transformants constructed with DNA from the resistant donor strains 8249 and D20 led to a model of the mechanism of penicillin resistance in pneumococci. The order of penicillin reactivity of the relevant PBPs in susceptible pneumococci is 1a > 2a > 1b > 2b. Thus, one would expect the MIC increase at the lowest level of resistance to be due to the introduction of a lower-affinity form of PBP 1a. This in fact appears to be the case, at least in the instance of genetic transformants constructed with the DNA of strain 8249. However, the next higher levels of resistance appear to involve simultaneous changes (lower reactivity) in more than one PBP, and this may partially explain why transformation frequencies were found to decline rapidly with increasing levels of resistance, in spite of the fact that the recipients used in each round of transformation were always transformants with the nearest lower level of penicillin resistance isolated in the previous cross (3).

It should be emphasized, however, that these speculations cannot fully explain the apparent sequential order of PBP alterations observed in the series of isogenic transformants that span the range of MICs from that obtained for the recipient cell to the nearly 1,000 times higher MIC obtained for the DNA donor cells. The basic question that remains unanswered is why the most extensively changed forms of a given PBP would appear only in transformants for which MICs were above certain critical levels. For instance, PBP 1a was shown to undergo multiple stepwise changes in penicillin affinity up to its most extensively changed form (which is PBP 1c). It was not clear why PBP 1c has never been detected in low-level transformants as well. Perhaps recombinants that have integrated the most extensively changed form of the PBP 1a gene (which carries multiple point mutations and codes for PBP 1c) do actually form, even in the first genetic crosses, but such recombinants may not be viable. One reason for this may be that the extensively modified low-affinity form of PBP 1a cannot perform its physiological function in cell wall synthesis in a cell in which the other PBPs are still present in unaltered, highly reactive forms. This proposal assumes that a PBP with lower reactivity to the penicillin molecule (which is a structural analog of the cell wall building blocks) will also show abnormalities in its physiological function in catalyzing the incorporation of wall building blocks during cell wall synthesis. This is indicated by experimental evidence obtained recently in our laboratory (see below).

This proposition leads to the interesting prediction that PBPs in pneumococci, and perhaps in other bacteria as well, function in a cooperative manner as a kind of assembly line in the synthesis of the cell wall. In this model the relative catalytic activities of individual PBPs must be coordinated with one another, and extensive alterations in only a single PBP (without an appropriate parallel decrease in the reactivities of other PBPs) may make cooperative functioning impossible. Figure 1 shows a model in which the donor DNA prepared from the highly resistant strain 8249 contains DNA molecules carrying the genetic determinant of PBP 1a in a form that is assumed to have several point mutations. When fully expressed, this DNA codes for the lowest affinity form of PBP 1a (= PBP 1c). This model assumes that both kinds of recombinants (1 and 2) actually form between the donor DNA and its allelic determinant present in the penicillin-susceptible recipient cell. Both recombinants 1 and 2 are formed already in the first round of transformation, which yields only low-level penicillin-resistant transformants. The fact that such transformants do not contain the highly mutated form of PBP 1a is explained by assuming that such a low-affinity protein could not perform its normal physiological function in the company of unaltered PBPs 2a, 1b, and 2b, implying a cooperative functioning of PBPs.

All these previous studies were done with two highly resistant South African strains — 8249 and D 20. In view of the continued geographic spread of penicillin-resistant pneumococci and the apparent increase in resistance levels of isolates in at least some areas of the world, we felt it was important to test a larger number of clinical isolates to determine if the conclusions drawn from the studies of the two South African strains have general validity. (A. Markiewicz, 88th Annual Meeting of the American Society for Microbiology, Miami Beach, Fla., 1988, Abstract no. A63; and A. Markiewicz and A. Tomasz, unpublished data.)

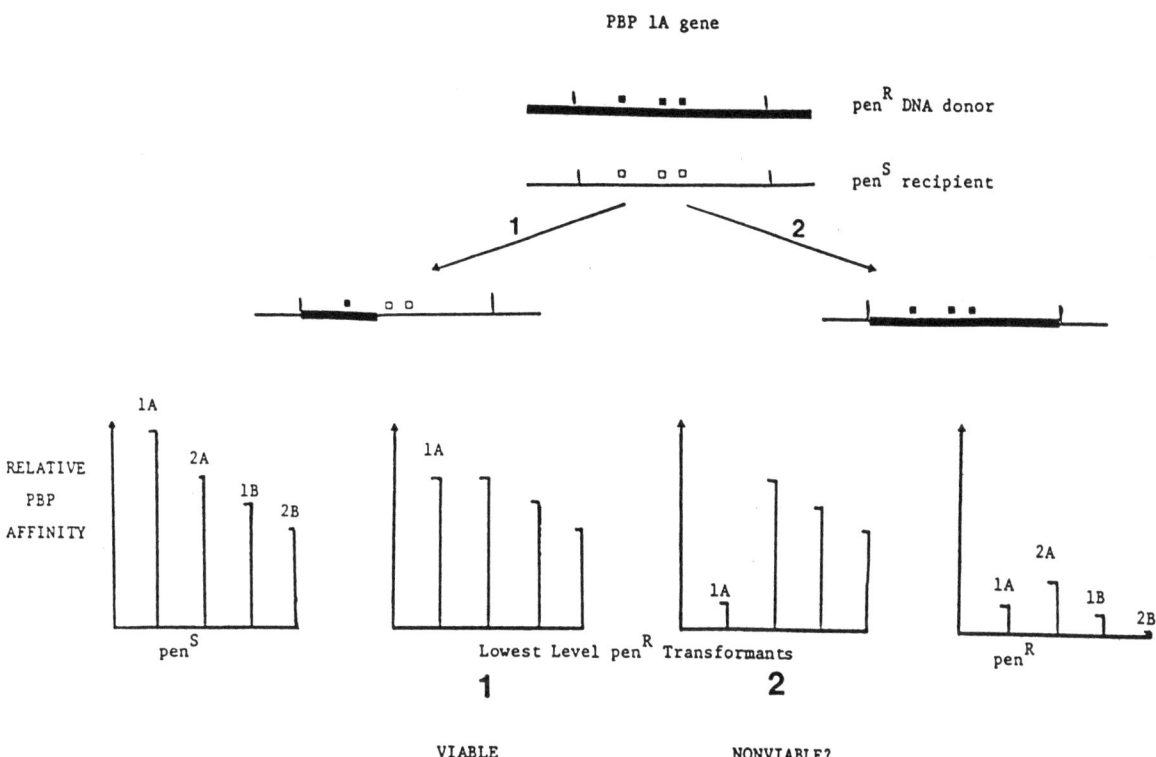

Figure 1: Model for the apparent orderliness of PBP alterations in genetic transformants to penicillin resistance. ■ = sites of mutation. □ = sites corresponding to the mutated sites in the donor DNA. The different connotations for donor and recipient DNA (heavy versus thin lines) do not imply lack of homology but serve strictly as illustrative devices. The lower portion of the figure depicts the relative drug affinities (and presumed substrate affinities) of four pneumococcal PBPs in the penicillin susceptible recipient (left-side barogram, pen^S) and in the two low-level transformants (1 and 2), of which transformant 2 is assumed to be nonviable, and the relative PBP affinities in the DNA donor strain (right-side barogram, pen^R). Reproduced with permission of the American Society for Microbiology.

PBP Affinities and Patterns in 160 Clinical Isolates

We undertook to determine the PBP patterns and affinities of over 160 clinical isolates, and this work has allowed us not only to confirm most of the conclusions drawn from earlier studies, but also to recognize an unanticipated feature of resistance: the existence of multiple and yet genetically stable PBP profiles among resistant strains of different origins. These new observations provide evidence for the remarkable genetic plasticity of the PBP structural genes and have also allowed us to identify the clonal nature of resistance.

The screening of clinical isolates for reactivity with a series of concentrations of penicillin showed quite clearly that the gradual decrease in penicillin affinities of PBP 1A, 2A and 2B in clinical isolates was a global occurrence in resistance development. Figure 2 shows the results of a large number of affinity titrations in which individual PBP reactivities of over 160 isolates were tested. For 40 of the strains examined, MICs were ⩾ 1.0 μg/ml; MICs for 80 strains were between 0.003 and 0.03 μg/ml. For semiquantitative screen of affinity changes that may accompany an increase in the MIC of the isolates, live bacteria were exposed for 10 min to a single low concentration of ^{3}H-penicillin (10 ng/ml) and the detectability of PBPs 1A, 2A and 3 was determined after a standard time of exposure of the fluorograms. For the evaluation of affinity change in the PBP 2B component of isolates, the concentration of ^{3}H-penicillin was increased to 1 μg/ml. The results clearly indicate that with few exceptions a great majority of isolates had decreased PBP affinities. One PBP, PBP 3, remained unchanged in affinity throughout the entire broad range of MICs represented by the collection of strains (D. Jabes, S. Nachman and A. Tomasz, unpublished data).

When high concentrations of radioactive penicillin were used in the same isolates in order to recognize all the PBPs present, the surprising observation was made that bacteria with comparable high levels of resistance showed not a single common PBP pattern,

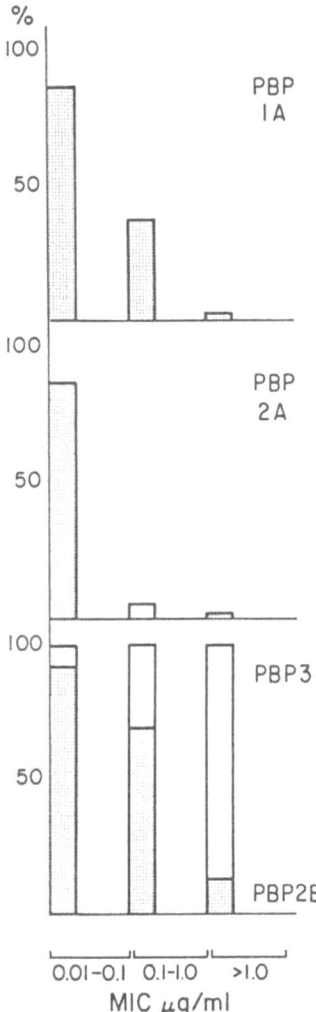

Figure 2: Decreasing penicillin affinities of PBPs 1A, 2A and 2B in penicillin recipient clinical isolates of pneumococci. Affinities of PBPs for penicillin were evaluated in 160 clinical isolates of pneumococci with a variety of different serotypes, geographic sources and MIC values. Bars represent the percentage of strains in which a given PBP was detectable under the conditions described in the text.

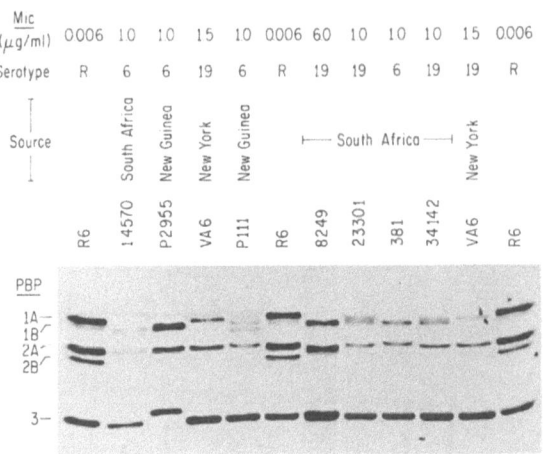

Figure 3: Multiplicity of PBP patterns in penicillin resistant clinical isolates of pneumococci.

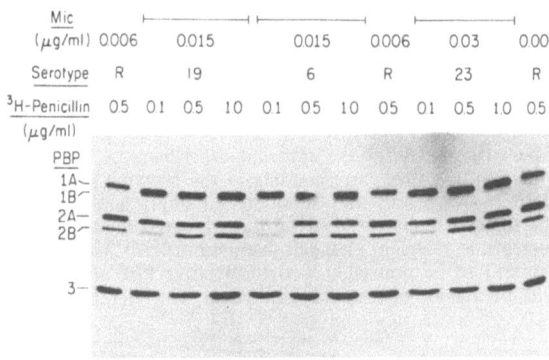

Figure 4: Common PBP patterns of high-affinity binding proteins in penicillin susceptible strains of pneumococci.

but rather a whole series of multiple PBP profiles reproducible for the particular strain (Figure 3) (A. Markiewicz, 88th Annual Meeting of the American Society for Microbiology, Miami Beach, Fla., 1988, Abstract no. A63; and A. Markiewicz and A. Tomasz, unpublished data). This multiplicity of profiles was clearly related to the MIC value, since most penicillin susceptible strains (MIC 0.003–0.05 µg/ml) showed a common, predictable profile of five PBPs of similar relative penicillin affinities (Figure 4). The multiplicity of PBP profiles in resistant strains was surprising at first. Clearly, not all highly resistant strains shared the PBP profiles identified in the two extensively analyzed South African strains 8249 and D20 (MICs of penicillin were 6 and 12 µg/ml, respectively) that were used in most of the early studies.

PBP Families: Clonal Nature of Penicillin Resistance in Pneumococci

For any interpretation of the multiple PBP profiles in penicillin-resistant isolates it was critical to establish the stability of each one of these profiles. In order to test this the following experiments were done. Nineteen penicillin-resistant isolates representing 11 different PBP profiles were each grown in antibiotic-free medium through serial passage that involved as many as 100 cell generations. The PBP profiles were then determined in the original isolate and in its passaged derivative. No differences could be observed: the unique numbers and molecular sizes of PBPs were precisely reproduced in each one of the cultures.

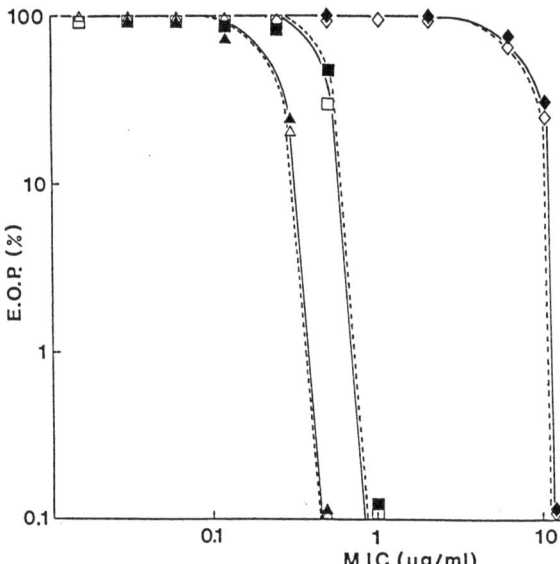

Figure 5: Population analysis of three penicillin resistant isolates of pneumococci. Three resistant strains were analyzed to determine precise MICs of penicillin: strain 29044 (origin: Czechoslovakia; ◊ and ♦), strain P111 (origin: Papua New Guinea; □ and ■), and strain P3003 (origin: Papua New Guinea; △ and ▲). The fraction of cells capable of forming colonies on agar containing various concentrations of penicillin was determined. Empty symbols refer to the original isolate; solid symbols represent the same strain after 100 generations of serial passage in drug-free medium.

It was also important to establish the stability of not only the PBP profiles but the penicillin resistance levels of the strains as well. Therefore, the MICs of penicillin for the strains were determined before and after the 100 cell generation passage, using the method of population analysis on selective agar. Various dilutions of the cultures were plated on agar containing different concentrations of penicillin, and the fraction of total viable cells capable of giving rise to colonies was determined. Figure 5 shows the results of such a test for three strains, one from Czechoslovakia and two from Papua New Guinea. Each isolate was made up of homogeneous populations of cells for which MICs were sharply defined. There was no evidence for the presence of multiple populations analogous to the phenomenon of heterogeneity in the methicillin-resistant *Staphylococcus aureus* (6). Each of the 19 strains retained both homogeneity and the precise MIC values during nonselective passage.

Our earlier studies of the genetic transformation of resistance in two highly penicillin-resistant South African strains (strains 8249 and D 20) showed that the introduction of even relatively small incremental increases in resistance (e. g. increase in MIC by 10–50 μg/ml) were difficult and occurred with low frequency only. In the interpretation of the multiplicity of PBP profiles of various resistant clinical strains, the possibility remained that the binding proteins differences were actually related to small but significant MIC differences undetectable by the large margin of error of the tube dilution MIC determination. This error may be very substantial in the range of high penicillin concentrations. In order to test this possibility we chose nine penicillin-resistant isolates carrying six different PBP profiles for which MICs were 1–4 μg/ml penicillin. About 1,000 colonies of each strain were replica-plated from drug-free agar to a series of agar plates containing a very closely spaced series of concentrations of penicillin which differed from one another not by a factor of two but by 20 to 50 % only. From such agar plates single colonies were selected for which MICs of penicillin were homogeneous and very sharply defined. For instance, colonies selected for an MIC of 1.5 μg/ml were made up of bacteria in which all cells were able to give rise to normal size colonies on agar containing 1.2 μg/ml penicillin, while no cells grew (< 1/1,000) on agar with 1.5 μg/ml penicillin (Table 1). Determination of the PBP profiles of three such subselected clones showed that these strains retained their original, unique PBP patterns. Thus, the different set of PBPs could not be explained by small differences in MICs.

Pneumococcal clinical isolates may be classified on the basis of 83 distinct capsular types which, in the absence of genetic exchange, appear to be highly conserved. Penicillin resistance has been identified in pneumococci belonging to a wide variety of serotypes, but resistance was most frequently associated with a rather limited number of serotypes. It was therefore conceivable that differences in PBP profiles may be related to differences in capsular type. However, this was clearly not the case, because the great majority of penicillin-susceptible isolates (MIC values for benzylpenicillin in the range of 0.003–0.01 μg/ml) shared a common PBP profile of five PBPs showing a common relative order of penicillin affinities of PBP 3 > 1A ≥ 2A > 1B > 2B, and this was irrespective of serotype or geographic origin. Furthermore, identical PBP profiles could be shared by resistant pneumococcal isolates belonging to different serological groups. Finally, strains of the same serogroup could exhibit different PBP profiles. There was no absolute correlation immediately evident between the geographic source of a strain and its PBP profile. For instance, several South Africa strains that shared PBP profiles (but not serotypes) with resistant isolates were identified, most of which came from Europe.

Recently we had the opportunity of examining clinical isolates from three epidemiological clusters of resistant pneumococci in Europe and in the USA. Twenty-four isolates originating in Europe could be clearly divided into two groups on the basis of PBP profiles. One group included 16 strains, all of which

Table 1: Selection of clones from resistant strains as indicated by sharply defined MICs of penicillin. Maximum concentration allowing growth produced the same number of colonies as seen on drug-free plates (2×10^3). Minimum concentration preventing growth showed less than one colony per plate.

Strain	PBP pattern[a]	Maximum penicillin concentration (μg/ml)[b] allowing growth on agar	Minimum penicillin concentration (μg/ml)[b] preventing growth on agar
66147	1	3.5	4
CO 7	1	3	3.5
34142	2	1.2	1.5
23301	2	2.5	3
140	2	3.5	4
VA 2	5	1.5	2
VA 6	5	1.2	1.5
P 2955	6	0.5	1
14750	8	0.5	1
P 111	10	0.5	1

[a] Numbers refer to the particular PBP profile characteristic for this strain.
[b] 100 μg portion of an overnight culture diluted and plated (2×10^3 CFU/plate).

were of serotype 23, MICs of penicillin for all strains were 1–1.5 μg/ml and all strains were resistant to tetracycline and chloramphenicol as well. The other group of eight isolates sharing a second, distinct PBP profile all belonged to serotype 6, and most strains were also resistant to both tetracycline and chloramphenicol. A third group of six strains from New York (7) again had a distinct PBP profile different from those of the two European groups; all strains were of serotype 19A and they were also tetracycline-resistant.

The clustering of PBP profiles in isolates that also share other epidemiologically useful properties may be considered additional evidence that indicates the stability and truly strain-specific nature of PBP patterns. Taking all the arguments together, it seems reasonable to suggest that resistant bacteria sharing a particular PBP profile belong to the progeny of an independently arisen penicillin-resistant mutant clone. The multiplicity of PBP profiles among resistant strains also suggests that pneumococci must have developed resistance-related PBP alterations on a worldwide scale more than once.

Molecular Basis of PBP Alterations

The data reviewed above strongly suggest that identical physiological resistance levels could be attained by the bacteria through more than one mechanism of remodeling the PBPs. On a molecular level, the resistance-related PBP alterations in pneumococci seem to involve three kinds of distinguishable features: a gradual decrease in the PBP affinity for penicillin, the actual "disappearance" of PBPs from the fluorograms, and the appearance of PBPs of anomalous molecular size in the fluorograms of resistant cells. While methodologically distinguisable, these three features are nevertheless most likely interrelated.

The disappearance of a PBP from the gels is most likely the result of affinity change of such a degree that the penicillin binding technique can no longer recognize the protein. This has been demonstrated using antiserum prepared against PBP 2B of susceptible pneumococci. When SDS-PAGE preparations of resistant strains were developed (by Western blotting) with an anti-PBP 2B serum, all strains showed the presence of a strongly reactive band in the position that corresponded to the position of PBP 2B in susceptible cells (8). In resistant pneumococci for which MICs of penicillin are $\geqslant 1$ μg/ml, PBP 2B is seldom detectable by the binding technique. Regarding the appearance of one or more PBPs with unusual molecular size in resistant strains, we suggest that the anomalous size of these proteins was the consequence of the same molecular restructuring of PBPs that results in decreased penicillin affinity.

The basic mechanism of PBP-linked resistance seems to be the replacement of amino acid residues in these proteins (due to mutational base changes in the structural genes of PBPs) with the consequence of altered reactivity to the antibiotic molecule. We suggest that if these amino acid substitutions occur within certain domains of the protein, a conformational change may also be brought about (in addition to lower drug affinity) and the apparent "newness" of such a PBP on the fluorogram is simply a consequence of a retention of this conformation (and/or an altered detergent binding capacity) under the conditions of SDS-PAGE. This type of phenomenon has already been described. Disproportionately large changes in apparent molecular size have been shown to accompany single amino acid replacements in some bacterial proteins

(9, 10). It is important to stress that all the "novel" PBPs seen in the fluorograms of resistant pneumococci also have low penicillin binding capacities. Thus, while the molecular size changes are quite helpful as identifying features of strains, the underlying molecular mechanisms need not involve alterations as drastic as suggested by the degree of apparent size change. In other words, the novel PBPs seen in some resistant strains may be the remodeled versions of one of the original PBPs. Experiments are in progress to identify the original PBPs that may be the progenitor proteins of the various anomalous binding proteins.

Recently, direct experimental evidence has been obtained indicating that at least some of the resistance-linked molecular rearrangements may occur close to the beta-lactam binding site (i.e. enzymic active center) of PBPs. The highest molecular size PBPs of three resistant strains and a susceptible strain were compared by peptide mapping. The binding proteins were labeled with radioactive penicillin, separated in the first dimension by the usual technique and then the highest molecular size PBPs were treated with a protease and the partial proteolytic digests were separated by gel electrophoresis. While the radioactive peptide patterns were clearly related to one another in all four strains, each one of the patterns was also distinct. Thus, each resistant PBP differed not only from the susceptible progenitor PBP but from one another as well (8). This is direct experimental proof of the existence of alternative molecular PBP restructuring mechanisms which lower penicillin affinities of these proteins and increase the degree of penicillin resistance of the bacterial cells.

Biological Price of Penicillin Resistance

Perhaps the most intriguing aspect of PBP-linked beta-lactam antibiotic resistance is the fact that such mutants exist at all. If the beta-lactam ring is indeed an active site-directed acylating agent with structural analogy to the D-alanyl-D-alanine carboxy terminus of cell wall building blocks, then decreased affinity for the substrate analog (as seen in resistant mutants) should also lower catalytic efficiency in the physiologically important reactions catalyzed by these proteins. Thus, mutants of this type could be expected to have abnormalities in wall assembly and growth, yet this is clearly not the case.

We tested 39 penicillin-resistant isolates (MIC $\geqslant$ 1 μg/ml), belonging to several serotypes and from a variety of geographic sites and infection sites, for the ability to grow in an enriched but chemically defined medium. All strains grew. We also tested the growth rate of the strains in the same basic medium enriched by 0.2 % yeast extract. All strains grew with reasonable generation times between 30 and 100 minutes (Table 2). Table 2 shows the stability of PBP profiles in the strains tested. Thus, by these simple laboratory criteria, the presence of altered PBPs in these pneumococcal isolates caused no apparent problems in growth. Epidemiological surveys indicate the stability of these strains under in vivo conditions as well, and the presence of normal virulence factors is indicated by the ability of resistant strains to colonize the nasopharynx in healthy carriers (11). Table 2 also shows that with the exception of two resistant strains, all of the remaining isolates listed were also resistant to penicillin-induced lysis, a trait recently identified in natural populations of pneumococci (12, 13).

While the presence of low-affinity PBPs in the resistant strains caused no detectable abnormality in growth and survival, a careful analysis of the cell walls of these bacteria revealed a remarkable degree of structural alterations. Recently we developed a technique that allows the resolution of cell wall stem peptides of pneumococci to over 30 reproducible components that can be separated by reverse phase high performance liquid chromatography (HPLC) (14). The complete chemical structure of the ten major peptide components was determined using chemical analysis, sequencing and mass spectrometry. Application of this technique to the analysis of cell walls prepared from ten clinical and laboratory isolates for which MICs of penicillin were low (0.003–0.01 μg/m) showed a reproducible common pattern. On the other hand, walls of penicillin-resistant strains showed a wall peptide pattern with a dramatic shift toward the more hydrophobic set of peptides (15). The shift in wall composition was clearly related to penicillin resistance, since the same change in wall peptide composition could also be reproduced when the cell walls of penicillin-resistant genetic transformants were analyzed.

Clearly, in addition to the anomalous PBPs inherited from the DNA donor South African strain 8249, the anomalous wall peptide pattern of the resistant DNA donor strain was also inherited (Figure 6). Analytical work led to the identification of new, anomalous peptide components that were the most prominent peptides in the walls of resistant strains. The common feature of these anomalous peptides was the presence of a short dipeptide branch on the epsilon amino groups of the lysine residues of the wall peptides. In contrast, most of the lysine epsilon amino groups were free in penicillin-susceptible cells, and in these bacteria neighboring peptides were crosslinked directly. In the resistant cells, neighboring peptides were most frequently crosslinked via dipeptide bridges (Figure 7).

The wall peptide change in resistant bacteria may be interpreted in the following manner. Under the penicillin pressure, pneumococci remodel the struc-

Table 2: Biological properties of strains for which the MIC of penicillin was ⩾ 1 µg/ml.

Strain	MIC of penicillin (µg/ml)	Mass doubling time (min)	Growth in synthetic medium	penicillin-induced lysis	Stability of PBP type (no. of generations)
64147	4	50	+	−	56
10760	4	65	+	−	44
CO 7	4	63	+	−	46
34142	1	63	+	−	46
23301	1	51	+	−	56
140	3	45	+	−	64
M 11126	1.5	57	+	−	ND
95210	2	100	+	−	ND
Straus	2	ND	+	−	ND
M 4352	1.5	60	+	−	ND
VA 1	1.5	78	+	−	37
VA 2	2	40	+	−	72
VA 3	2	32	+	−	90
VA 6	1.5	42	+	−	70
VA 9	2	33	+	−	87
P 2955	1	42	+	−	68
M 1827	1.5	42	+	−	ND
M 3070	1.5	51	+	−	ND
M 4364	1.5	30	+	−	ND
M 2990	1.5	33	+	−	ND
M 3409	1.5	39	+	−	ND
M 9300	1.5	38	+	−	ND
M 3875	1.5	32	+	−	ND
381	1	54	+	−	53
14750	1	57	+	−	ND
M 5229	1	115	+	ND	ND
M 5367	1.2	38	+	−	ND
M 11125	1.5	38	+	−	ND
M 10788	2	45	+	−	ND
M 11128	2	43	+	−	ND
M 5224	1.5	39	+	−	ND
M 8792	1.5	36	+	−	ND
M 5219	1.5	33	+	−	ND
M 9890	1.5	26	+	−	ND
29044	16	45	+	+	64
29055	8	36	+	+	80
P 111	1	48	+	−	60
D 20	12	40	+	−	72
8249	6	40	+	−	100

ND = not determined.

ture of several of their PBPs so that the reactivity of these proteins toward penicillin decreases. This remodeling apparently affects the natural function(s) of these proteins, too. It seems that the distorted active sites can no longer maintain the normal wall precursors containing linear stem peptides; rather, the deformed active sites prefer an alternative (more hydrophobic?) family of wall precursors which contain branched stem peptides. It is quite possible that the maintenance of an adequate supply of these new types of precursors requires the resistant cells to acquire another mutation in addition to the mutations in PBP structure. A mutation of this type should occur in the early stages of wall precursor synthesis. Difficulties encountered in the transformation of high level penicillin resistance may be the result of a need for this auxiliary mutation. It is intriguing that in staphylococcal methicillin resistance a formally analogous situation seems to exist: expression of resistance requires not only the presence of a new low-affinity PBP (PBP 2a), but in addition, an auxiliary mutation coding for a hypothetical "Factor X" as well (13).

A tentative scenario for the emergence of penicillin-resistant pneumococcal strains may now be drawn. The frequent association of a lysis defect with resistance suggests that these strains have been selected by the dual antibiotic pressure characteristic of the in vivo generated cyclic fluctuation in drug concentration (12). The result of this would be the widespread appearance of a survival trait among natural isolates, and it may be assumed that resistant strains would tend to be recruited from this pool of lysis-defective

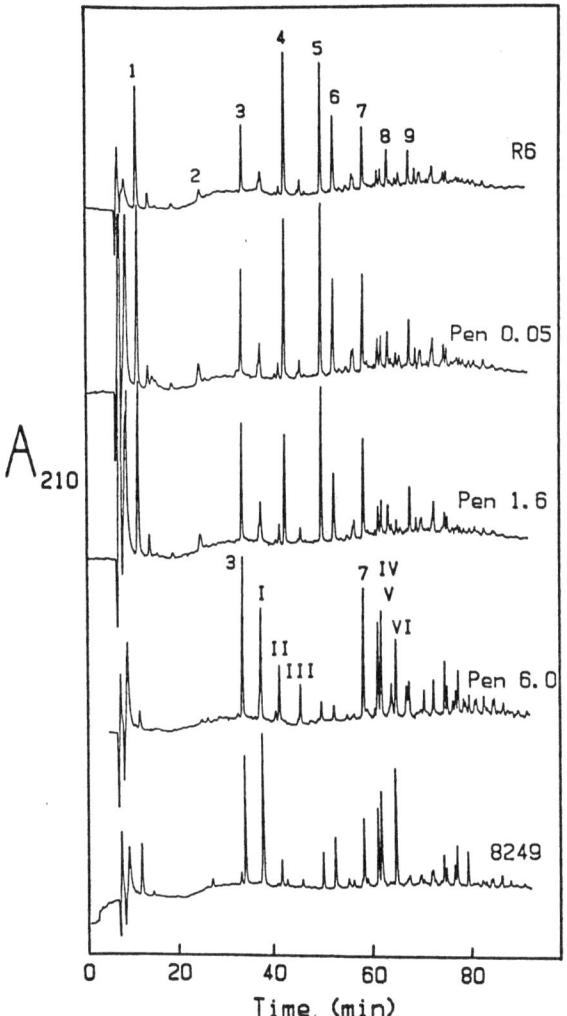

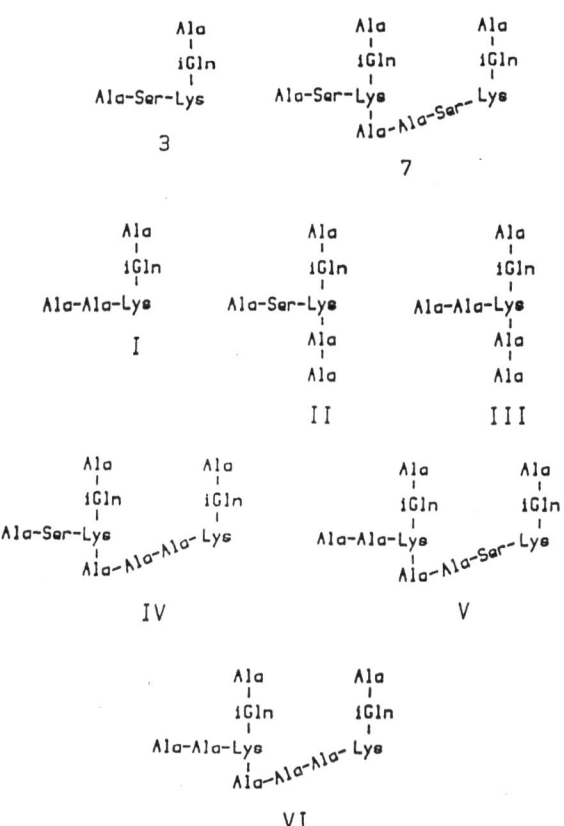

Figure 6: HPLC chromatograms of cell wall stem peptides from the pneumococcal strains listed in Table 1.

Approximately 15 nmol of stem peptides from strain R6 and 20 nmol from the other strains were applied to the column and eluted as described in the text. The individual strains are indicated at the end of the corresponding chromatograms. Peaks 1 to 9 represent peptides whose structures have been previously described; peaks I to VI are characteristic of the highly resistant strains and are described in the text. These peptide patterns were completely reproducible, and the same results were obtained with two independent cell wall preparations from strain Pen 6.0 (more than ten analyses) and five independent preparations from strain R6 (more than 15 analyses). Reproduced with permission of the Journal of Bacteriology.

Figure 7: Proposed structures for the main wall peptides of strain Pen 6.0. Peptides 3 and 7 have already been described for strain R6; peptides I to VI have nobel structures. Reproduced with permission of the Journal of Bacteriology.

strains. The increase of the MIC value is achieved by the accumulation of point mutations in the chromosomal determinants of the structures of three or possibly four of the five pneumococcal PBPs detectable by the method currently used in our laboratory. These mutations cause amino acid substitutions in the molecular domain(s) of the PBPs such that the rate of binding and/or acylation by the antibiotic molecule decreases.

Our new findings with a large number of clinical isolates suggest that such a gradual, resistance-related decrease in the affinities of PBPs 1A, 2A and 2B is a global occurrence with most if not all pneumococci. At least some of the resistance-related amino acid substitutions occur in the vicinity of the active site of PBPs, and in some but not all cases, this structural rearrangement also seems to affect the conformation of the PBP, resulting in the alteration of apparent molecular size in SDS-PAGE. These size changes have allowed us to identify a multiplicity of heritable PBP patterns characteristic of a given resistant strain. These molecular size changes have also become fortuitously helpful markers by which the progeny of a particular resistant mutant can be identified, and using this method we have suggested that at least some groups of clinical isolates are most likely of clonal nature. From all this it follows that pneumococci must have developed penicillin resistant more than once and that these bacteria can attain identical, high levels of resistance by more than one alternative molecular restructuring of their PBPs. Eventually, definitive answers to these points will come from the molecular cloning of pneumococcal PBPs.

A remarkable consequence of the PBP alterations appears to be a distortion of the catalytic activity of these proteins with their endogenous normal substrates, since the low-affinity PBPs of resistant pneumococci build an abnormal wall of profoundly altered peptide composition. This may be the "biological price" of penicillin resistance. However, this price is clearly affordable, since resistant pneumococci grow with normal rates, show no new nutritional needs, and the high level of penicillin resistance is a stable trait compatible with all physiological and ecological functions of these bacteria.

Conclusion

Our findings suggest that the particular kind of penicillin pressure used in the clinical environment and the particular protective mechanisms developed by pneumococci to survive this antibiotic pressure have resulted in the selection of pneumococcal strains that differ from penicillin-susceptible pneumococci in so many properties that they may very well be considered new pathogens that present a radically altered surface to an infected host. Penicillin-resistant pneumococci posses not only remodelled penicillin binding proteins but remodelled peptidoglycan as well. An overwhelming majority of resistant strains belong to a few (four to six) of the 83 existing serotypes. A great majority of resistant strains also have altered autolysin control, which prevents lysis of the cells during penicillin treatment. Some new observations suggest that pneumococci equipped with this lysis-defective trait may also cause disease of altered course (13).

References

1. Hansman, D., Andrews, G.: Hospital infection with pneumococci resistant to tetracycline. Medical Journal of Australia 1967, 1: 498–501.
2. Ward, J.: Antibiotic-resistant *Streptococcus pneumoniae*: clinical and epidemiologic aspects. Reviews of Infectious Diseases 1981, 3: 254–266.
3. Zighelboim, S., Tomasz, A.: Penicillin binding proteins of the multiply antibiotic resistant South African strains of pneumococci. Antimicrobial Agents and Chemotherapy 1980, 17: 434–442.
4. Handwerger, S., Tomasz, A.: Alterations in kinetic properties of penicillin-binding proteins of penicillin-resistant *Streptococcus pneumoniae*. Antimicrobial Agents and Chemotherapy 1986, 30: 57–63.
5. Handwerger, S., Tomasz, A.: Alterations in penicillin-binding proteins of clinical and laboratory isolates of pathogenic *Streptococcus pneumoniae* with low levels of penicillin-resistance. Journal of Infectious Diseases 1986, 153: 83–89.
6. Hartman, B. J., Tomasz, A.: Expression of methicillin resistance in heterogeneous strains of *Staphylococcus aureus*. Antimicrobial Agents and Chemotherapy 1986, 29: 85–92.
7. Simberkoff, M. S., Lukaszewski, M., Cross, A., Al-Ibrahim, M., Baltch, A. L., Smith, R. P., Geiseler, P. J., Nadler, J., Richmond, A. S.: Antibiotic-resistant isolates of *Streptococcus pneumoniae* from clinical specimens: a cluster of serotype 19A organisms in Brooklyn, New York. Journal of Infectious Diseases 1986, 153: 78–92.
8. Hakenbeck, R., Ellerbrok, H., Briese, T., Handwerger, S., Tomasz, A.: Penicillin binding proteins of penicillin susceptible and resistant pneumococci: immunological relatedness of altered proteins and changes in peptides carrying the beta lactam site. Antimicrobial Agents and Chemotherapy 1986, 30: 553–558.
9. Kendall, D. A., Bock, S. C., Kaiser, E. T.: Idealization of the hydrophobic segment of the alkaline phosphatase signal peptide. Nature 1986, 321: 706–708.
10. Vlasuk, G. P., Inouye, S., Inouye, M.: Effects of relacing serine and threonine residues within the signal peptide on the secretion of the major outer membrane lipoprotein of *Escherichia coli*. Journal of Biological Chemistry 1984, 259: 6195–6200.
11. Klugman, K. P., Koornhof, H. J., Wasas, A., Storey, K., Gilbertson, I.: Carriage of penicillin resistant pneumococci. Archives of Diseases of Children 1986, 61: 377–381.
12. Moreillon, P., Tomasz, A.: Penicillin resistance and defective lysis in clinical isolates of pneumococci: evidence for two kinds of antibiotic pressure operating in the clinical environment. Journal of Infectious Diseases 1988, 157: 1150–1157.
13. Tuomanen, E., Pollack, H., Parkinson, A., Davidson, M., Facklam, R., Rich, R., Zak, O.: Microbiological and clinical significance of a new property of defective lysis in clinical strains of pneumococci. Journal of Infectious Diseases 1988, 158: 36–43.
14. Garcia-Bustos, J. F., Chait, B. T., Tomasz, A.: Structure of the peptide network of pneumococcal peptidoglycan. Journal of Biological Chemistry 1987, 262: 15400–15405.
15. Garcia-Bustos, J. F., Chait, B. T., Tomasz, A.: Altered peptidoglycan structure in a pneumococcal transformant resistant to penicillin. Journal of Bacteriology 1988, 170: 2143–2147.

Antibiotic Uptake into Gram-Negative Bacteria

R. E. W. Hancock*, A. Bell

Antibiotics taken up into gram-negative bacteria face two major diffusion barriers, the outer and cytoplasmic membranes. Of these, the former has been most studied and is discussed in detail here. Evidence from antibiotic MIC studies on porin-deficient mutants compared with their porin-sufficient parent strains has provided strong support for the proposal that some antibiotics, particularly β-lactams, pass across the outer membrane through the water-filled channels of a class of proteins called porins. Nevertheless substantial evidence has accumulated for the importance of non-porin pathways of antibiotic uptake across the outer membranes of gram-negative bacteria. Examples discussed include the uptake of polycationic antibiotics via the self-promoted pathway, the uptake of hydrophobic antibiotics in some bacterial species and in mutants of others via the hydrophobic pathway, and the possible importance of poorly understood non-porin pathways of uptake of a variety of antibiotics. Other potential barriers to diffusion, including the cytoplasmic membrane, are briefly discussed.

Since the initiation of the modern era of antibiotic usage in the 1940s, considerable research effort has been expended in determining the mechanism of uptake and mode of action of all groups of antibiotics. In many cases the mode of action of individual antibiotics is quite well understood, however antibiotic uptake mechanisms have remained more elusive. This is perhaps best illustrated by the aminoglycosides which have been studied in enormous detail. Despite this, the mechanism of aminoglycoside uptake across the cytoplasmic membrane of bacteria remains controversial. It is of little assistance that all known aminoglycoside resistant mutants influence antibiotic uptake (1), since it is difficult to differentiate mutants that exclusively affect uptake from those that additionally influence mode of action. As a result of this and similar problems, this brief review will concentrate on an area of antibiotic uptake which has become increasingly well understood, that is uptake across the outer membranes of gram-negative bacteria. Brief mentions will be made of other cell layers which might be considered to be influential in antibiotic uptake into cells.

The outer membranes of gram-negative bacteria vary somewhat in composition, but may generally considered to be lipopolysaccharide (LPS): phospholipid bilayers (in the outer and inner monolayers respectively) studded with proteins (Figure 1). The outer membrane, where studied, is in direct physical contact with the underlying peptidoglycan by means of strong non-covalent or sometimes covalent interactions. The structure of the outer membrane has been described in some detail recently (2, 3) and only two concepts of direct relevance to antibiotic uptake will be discussed here. Firstly, the outer membrane is usually described as a semi-permeable barrier (or molecular sieve), in which those hydrophilic molecules of sizes below a given exclusion limit can pass through the channels of proteins called porins (2, 3). In contrast the remainder of the outer membrane has been considered to exclude uptake of hydrophilic and, in all except a few cases, hydrophobic molecules. As described below, this generalization is probably an oversimplification. Secondly, the pioneering work of Leive (4) on the mode of interaction of EDTA with *Escherichia coli* demonstrated that the interactions of divalent cations with LPS molecules were important determinants of outer membrane structural stability and barrier function. Because of space limitations, review articles have been extensively utilized as references rather than original manuscripts.

Porin-Mediated Antibiotic Uptake Across the Outer Membrane

General Porin Properties

The structure, genetics and in vitro model membrane properties of porins have been reviewed in some detail elsewhere (2, 3, 5). In general, porins comprise

---

Department of Microbiology, University of British Columbia, 6174 University Boulevard No. 300, Vancouver, British Columbia V6T 1W5, Canada.

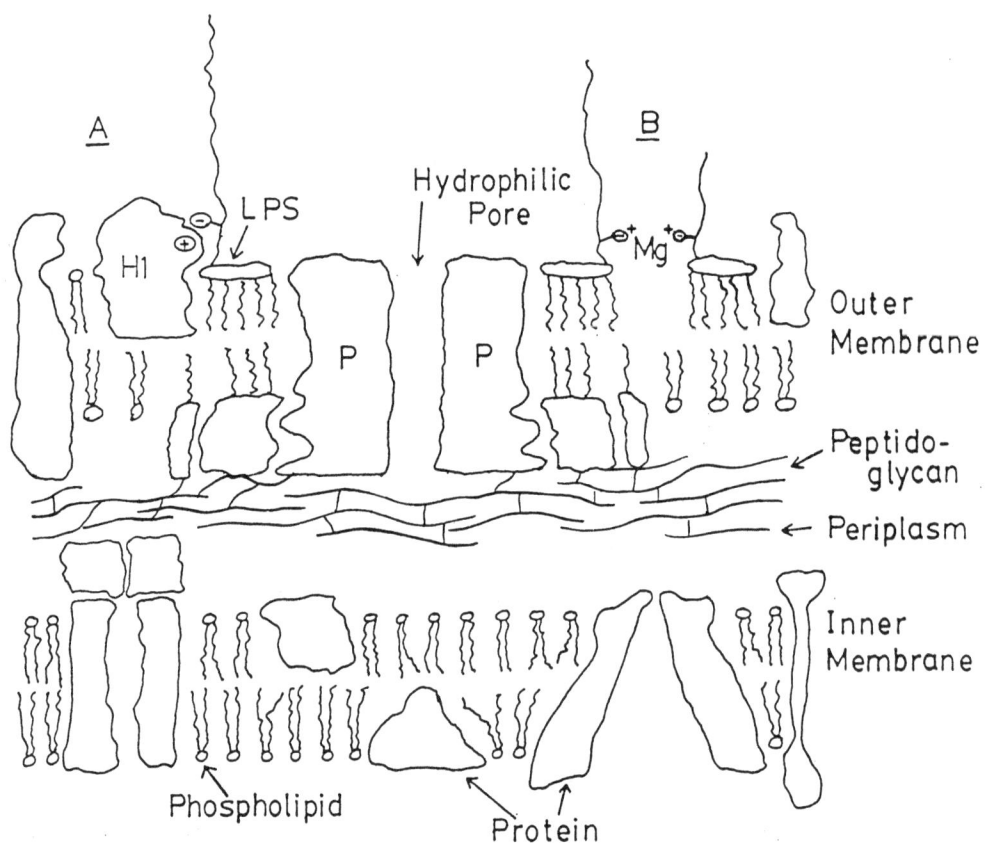

Figure 1: Schematic representation of a cross section of the cell envelope of gram-negative bacteria. P = porin protein involved in uptake of hydrophilic antibiotics, LPS = lipopolysaccharide. H1 = other membrane protein H1. A represents sites at which self-promoted uptake is blocked by protein H1 in *Pseudomonas aeruginosa* (see text). B represents sites at which polycations and chelators can displace divalent cations from LPS, resulting in self-promoted uptake. Alteration in the nature of the B sites (e.g. reduction in the affinity of LPS for divalent cations) might result in a non-porin pathway of uptake for antibiotics that are not polycations (including hydrophobic antibiotics).

oligomeric aggregates (usually trimers) of monomer molecular weights in the range of 28,000 to 48,000. Where studied they have a high content of β-sheet structure which confers extraordinary structural stability on many porins such that they often resist denaturation upon heating in sodium dodecyl sulphate. Porins are tightly but non-covalently associated with the underlying peptidoglycan and with LPS. However, porins often vary from this general scheme in one or more properties (5).

Nakae first demonstrated by liposome reconstitution experiments that porins contained water-filled channels capable of allowing size-dependent uptake of saccharides (6). Subsequently, a variety of model membrane studies (5) have demonstrated that porin channels have the following intrinsic properties. They are large (diameter 0.6–2.3 nm), water-filled channels, the dimensions of which apparently determine their exclusion limits for hydrophilic molecules. Most porins demonstrate little chemical selectivity, although exceptions exist. The interior of a porin channel contains charged amino acids. The number and positioning of these charged amino acids relative to the most constricted portion of the channel apparently determines the ion selectivity of porin channels (which are usually weakly selective for small ions). Generally, model membrane studies have suggested that porin molecules contain passive diffusion channels which can influence uptake of β-lactams by virtue of their channel size relative to the permeating β-lactam, and by their intrinsic ion selectivity relative to the charge on the β-lactam. Thus these studies predict that β-lactam passage through porins should be definable in terms of general channel theory as described by specific equations (5). In many cases this has been proven to be correct.

Role of Porins in Beta-Lactam Uptake

Zimmermann and Rosselet (7) first described outer membrane permeability to β-lactams in terms of

Fick's first law of diffusion. Thus Vd = C (So−Si) in which Vd is the rate of diffusion across the outer membrane, So is the external and Si the periplasmic concentration of β-lactam, and C is a permeability parameter dependent on the total area of porin channels per outer membrane, the inverse of the length of porin channels and the diffusivity coefficient (5). This theoretical treatment of outer membranes, which assumes a semi-permeable membrane perforated by porins, makes three testable predictions. Firstly, the rate of diffusion Vd should increase proportionally as the concentration gradient (So−Si) across the outer membrane increases, a concept that has been tested in *Escherichia coli* (7) and *Pseudomonas aeruginosa* (8) (note that since So ≫ Si, Vd is approximately proportional to So). Secondly, the total area of channels per outer membrane should influence antibiotic uptake, a concept that has been used to explain the greater intrinsic resistance to antibiotics of *Pseudomonas aeruginosa* compared to *Escherichia coli* (8). Thirdly, the diffusivity coefficient should be strongly influenced by the physico-chemical nature of the β-lactam antibiotic and the channel properties. In agreement with this, Nikaido and colleagues have shown that small differences in channel size (e.g. comparing the OmpF and OmpC channels of *Escherichia coli*) and differences in the nature of individual β-lactams can influence the penetration rates of β-lactams in model membrane studies (2).

Nevertheless, the strongest data favouring an in vivo role for porins in uptake of some β-lactam antibiotics across the outer membrane comes from comparisons of porin-deficient mutants with their isogenic wild type strains. Such mutants have significant increases in MIC for some but not all β-lactams (Table 1) (8−13), as well as measurable decreases in the uptake rates of given β-lactams (14). However, the increased MICs occur for only a subset of β-lactams (12). Indeed in constructed mutants, e.g. oprF::Ω of *Pseudomonas aeruginosa* lacking the proposed porin protein F, Woodruff and Hancock (12) were unable to measure large increases in MIC compared to wild-type for any β-lactam (Table 1). There are several potential explanations for these data. For example, it has been suggested that the amount and kinetics of periplasmic β-lactamase and the kinetics of its action on substrates are influential in determining MICs and in overriding differences in outer membrane penetration rates due to altered porin content (2). Alternatively, Woodruff and Hancock (12) demonstrated increased hydrophobic permeability of *Pseudomonas aeruginosa* protein F-deficient mutants and suggested that this might reflect counteractive uptake of β-lactams via non-porin pathways (see below) caused by the loss of a major outer membrane structural component. Consistent with this latter proposal, Godfrey and Bryan (13) isolated a putative protein F-altered mutant with substantial increases in antibiotic MICs [cf. a protein F-deficient mutant (12)]. In addition, Siden and Boman (15) observed increased uptake of hydrophobic substances in several *Escherichia coli* OmpC (porin deficient) mutants but not in others. Similarly, Then and Angehrn (11) observed two types of mutants with drastic reductions in the amounts of two outer membrane proteins probably corresponding to *Enterobacter cloacae* porins. One, AZT-R, was supersusceptible to hydrophobic agents including acridine orange, trimethoprim and SDS, and demonstrated no decrease in antibiotic susceptibility to two β-lactams (ampicillin and piperacillin) but large changes in susceptibility to many others. The

Table 1: Influence of porin deficiencies on antibiotic resistance in various bacteria. Data from references No. 9, 10, 11, 12, and 13.

Antibiotic	Ratio of MICs of porin-deficient mutant/porin-sufficient parent									
	Escherichia coli	*Proteus mirabilis*	*Proteus vulgaris*	*Morganella morganii*	*Providencia rettgeri*	*Providencia alcalifaciens*	*Enterobacter cloacae*		*Pseudomonas aeruginosa*	
							AMA-R	AZT-R	oprF::Ω	PCC-23
Ampicillin	4−16	2	2	2	2	2	16	0.5	−	−
Piperacillin	2	1	1	1	1	1	16	1	1.4	83
Cefotaxime	2	−	−	−	−	−	−	−	3.2	333
Ceftazidime	2	−	−	−	−	−	16	16	1.6	21
Cefoxitin	16−32	16	16	32	32	16	−	−	−	−
Cefazolin	8−16	32	4	16	8	32	−	−	−	−
Aztreonam	4	−	−	−	−	−	128	64	1.7	−
Imipenem	1	−	−	−	−	−	4	4	0.8	4
Tetracycline	3	4	4	4	4	4	−	−	−	0.5
Chloramphenicol	1.5	1	1	1	1	1	4	0.25	−	−
Norfloxacin	4	−	−	−	−	−	32	1	1	0.25
Minocycline	1.5	1	1	1	1	1	−	−	−	−

other, AMA-R, showed normal resistance to hydrophobic agents and resistance to all β-lactams including piperacillin and ampicillin. One explanation for these phenomena is that porin-deficient mutants are normally more susceptible to hydrophobic agents (due to the loss of a major outer membrane component and consequent increase in lipidic components) (12), but can undergo adaptive changes causing structural alterations and loss of supersusceptibility to such hydrophobic agents.

Role of Porins in Uptake of Other Antibiotics

The discovery of the role of porins in uptake of other antibiotics stems largely from examination of the antibiotic MICs of porin-deficient mutant compared with wild type strains. On this basis chloramphenicol, tetracycline, and some quinolones may be taken up by porin pathways (2, 16). Nevertheless, porin-deficient mutants demonstrate substantial residual uptake of these antibiotics, suggesting the possibility of additional significant uptake systems. In contrast, porin-deficient mutants are usually not more resistant to aminoglycosides and we consider the role of porins in uptake of aminoglycosides in any bacterium to be unresolved.

Other Porin-Like Pathways

There is as yet little definitive evidence for the involvement, in uptake of specific antibiotics, of porins other than the major diffusion channels of gram-negative outer membranes. However, certain possibilities have recently come to light. Iron transport in gram-negative bacteria often involves chelation of ferric iron by siderophores. Such chelates bind to specific outer membrane receptor proteins and are subsequently translocated across the cell envelope of *Escherichia coli* in a *tonB*-protein dependent step (2). It is as yet unknown how the ferric-siderophore complex is translocated across the outer membrane but it may involve the outer membrane receptor functioning as a specific porin. Recently, a potent anti-pseudomonal cephalosporin, E-0702, was developed and it apparently utilizes one of the *tonB*-dependent iron transport systems of *Escherichia coli* (17). Similarly, the semi-synthetic rifamycin derivative CGP4832 is taken up across the outer membrane via the *tonB*-dependent ferrichrome uptake system of *Escherichia coli* (18). *Pseudomonas aeruginosa* mutants resistant to the broad-spectrum carbapenem β-lactam antibiotic, imipenem, lack a specific 45 kDa outer membrane protein (19). It has been suggested that this protein serves as an imipenem-specific porin since mutants lacking this protein retain susceptibility to other antibiotics.

Non-Porin Pathways of Antibiotic Uptake Across the Outer Membrane

Self-Promoted Uptake

Certain antibiotics appear to cross the outer membrane by pathways other than diffusion through porins. One such pathway is known as self-promoted uptake. It was named on the basis of studies of the mechanism of uptake of polycationic antibiotics in *Pseudomonas aeruginosa* (3, 20). However, the earlier studies on EDTA interaction with the *Escherichia coli* outer membrane by Leive and colleagues, and on polymyxin uptake in a variety of bacteria were suggestive that such a mechanism of uptake is more widely distributed (2, 3, 20).

The initial stages of self-promoted uptake seem to occur at negatively-charged sites (phosphate and/or carboxyl groups) on LPS, which bind divalent cations such as Mg^{2+} and Ca^{2+} strongly. The non-covalent association between LPS and divalent cations is an essential component of outer membrane integrity (4). Its disruption by the chelator ethylenediaminetetra-acetate (EDTA) results in the release of large quantities of LPS from *Escherichia coli* and *Pseudomonas aeruginosa*, and increased susceptibility to various hydrophobic and hydrophilic compounds. EDTA is one of a class of compounds, known as permeabilizers, that can enhance outer membrane permeability to other agents in a number of gram-negative bacteria (20). The mode of action of permeabilizers has been investigated by using hydrophobic (e.g. N-phenylnaphthylamine) and hydrophilic (e.g. nitrocefin) probes of outer membrane permeability, measuring release of LPS and periplasmic enzymes, and examining outer membrane morphological changes. Compounds that can act as outer membrane permeabilizers include polymyxin B and related compounds, other polycations, monovalent organic cations, divalent cation chelators and host defense factors. The polycations are presumed to act by displacing divalent cations from binding sites on LPS, and the kinetics of this process have been investigated using a fluorescently-labeled polymyxin derivative and a cationic spin label probe (21). The actions of these permeabilizers are generally antagonized by added divalent cations including Mg^{2+} and Ca^{2+}.

Mutants of *Pseudomonas aeruginosa* cross-resistant to EDTA/Tris, polymyxin B and aminoglycosides were isolated (3, 20) and found to constitutively overproduce an outer membrane protein, Hl. Wild type cells grown in media deficient in certain divalent cations had similar resistance properties and were induced for protein Hl expression. Cells with mutational overproduction of protein Hl displayed altered kinetics of streptomycin uptake and had reduced Mg^{2+} levels in their cell envelopes. There was no change, however, in susceptibility to other antibiotics such as β-lactams and tetracyclines (20), or in the outer membrane permeability to the β-lactam nitrocefin (8). It was concluded that protein Hl probably inhibited a common uptake pathway that was essential to the bactericidal action of polycations and EDTA/Tris (1, 3, 20). Since these compounds were known to disrupt LPS-divalent cation interactions and permeabilize the outer membrane, they could presumably enhance their own uptake. Protein Hl was hypothesized to inhibit self-promoted uptake by replacing divalent cations at negatively charged sites on LPS (1). The protein, being stably anchored in the membrane, could not be displaced by the permeabilizers, and thus could prevent membrane disruption and consequent uptake of the disrupting polycation. Figure 1 illustrates how the overproduction of protein Hl could lead to decreased self-promoted uptake. The exact nature of the protein Hl binding site on LPS is unknown, but several LPS mutations abolished protein Hl-mediated polymyxin B resistance in *Pseudomonas aeruginosa* (unpublished data).

Protein Hl-mediated resistance affected all aminoglycoside antibiotics tested, although these compounds had previously been assumed to cross the outer membrane through porins in *Escherichia coli* (1). Nevertheless, the above data strongly suggests that self-promoted pathway is a plausible mechanism of uptake of aminoglycosides, at least in *Pseudomonas aeruginosa*.

A somewhat similar type of mutation has been described in *Salmonella typhimurium* (2). The *pmr*A mutant was resistant to polymyxin B and EDTA/Tris killing and permeabilization, apparently owing to alterations which reduced the negative charges on LPS. In addition, polymyxin B and its deacylated derivative polymyxin B nonapeptide have been demonstrated to bind to *Escherichia coli* LPS, and to permeabilize the outer membranes of *Escherichia coli* and other bacterial species. Thus, we conclude that self-promoted uptake of polymyxin also occurs in a variety of bacteria including *Escherichia coli*. *Pseudomonas cepacia*, closely related to *Pesudomonas aeruginosa*, was apparently resistant to self-promoted uptake even without induction of any protein analogous to Hl (22). However, serious investigation into the possibility that self-promoted uptake operates widely in gram-negative bacteria has yet to be undertaken.

The precise molecular nature of the uptake process following disruption of LPS-cation interactions remains obscure, and its elucidation probably depends on a better understanding of abnormal structures in LPS-containing membranes. There is electron microscopic evidence for the accumulation of transient holes in gentamicin-treated outer membranes (23). Analysis of the effects of polycations on LPS using a cationic spin probe has led to the proposal that displacement of cations causes rigidification of LPS-aggregates and allows antibiotics to rearrange LPS packing, causing "cracks" in the structure (21). In any event, a better understanding of the nature of self-promoted uptake would assist in the design of agents capable of crossing outer membranes.

Hydrophobic Uptake

Most wild type gram-negative bacteria exclude moderately hydrophobic substances (2). For example, the hydrophobic fluorescent probe 1-N-phenylnaphthylamine is excluded from wild type *Escherichia coli* and *Pseudomonas aeruginosa* cells (3, 20). The reason for this impermeability to hydrophobic substances seems to be that the external surface of the outer membrane prevents or resists the partitioning of moderately hydrophobic substances into the interior of the membrane. Permeabilization to hydrophobic substances can be achieved by addition of compounds which remove, be chelation (e.g. EDTA), or competively displace (e.g. polycations) divalent cations from their LPS binding sites at the cell surface (3, 20). Thus the stabilizing influence of divalent cations and LPS at the cell surface is a primary factor in exclusion of moderately hydrophobic substances. Some antibiotics can be considered moderately hydrophobic in that they will partition into organic solvents in two phase partitioning experiments. Nevertheless, most of these antibiotics are water-soluble at therapeuticallyrelevant concentrations. The high MICs of bacterial species for such antibiotics (e.g. Table 2) are probably indicative of the barrier effect of the outer membrane. In agreement with this, alteration of this barrier by treatment with permeabilizers or by specific outer membrane mutations affecting LPS (20, 25) will decrease MICs for these antibiotics (Table 2). In some bacterial species (e.g. *Neisseria* and *Haemophilus*), MICs for moderately hydrophobic antibiotics are substantially decreased (Table 2) and it can be assumed that these bacteria present outer surfaces to the environment that are less effectively stabilized.

Other Non-Porin Pathways

Hinma and colleagues (26) have demonstrated that certain β-lactam antibiotics have substantial permeation rates across reconstituted lipid bilayers. These include the moderately hydrophilic antibiotics, ampicillin and benzyl penicillin, although almost all β-lactams measured had some degree of permeability. The authors suggested that such permeation across lipid bilayers is regulated by lipopolysaccharide and can explain differential susceptibility to β-lactams of certain mutants. In vivo data with at least two classes of mutants suggest that this is true. The *Pseudomonas aeruginosa* antibiotic supersusceptible mutant Z61 contains at least two separate mutations which cause

Table 2: MICs for moderately hydrophobic antibiotics in various gram-negative bacteria. Data from references No. 20 and 24.

Antibiotic	MIC (µg/ml)						
	Pseudomonas aeruginosa		Salmonella typhimurium		Neisseria gonorrhoeae	Neisseria meningitidis	Haemophilus influenzae
	Wild type	Mutant (Z61)	Wild type	Mutant (Deep rough)	Wild type	Wild type	Wild type
Erythromycin	200	–	75	2	< 0.5	< 2	0.5– 8
Novobicin	> 128	0.05	500	5	4	< 4	0.2– 0.8
Fusidic acid	300	–	300	–	< 1	< 0.25	–
Clindamycin	> 64	–	> 64	–	< 4	–	0.5–16
Rifampicin	50	0.2	10	< 1	0.5	–	–
Minocycline	100	–	–	–	0.4	1.6	1.6

different changes in LPS (25). One of these, the *absA* mutation, causes substantial increases in susceptibility to hydrophobic agents, in addition to a wide range of β-lactams and aminoglycosides. The other, the *absB* mutation, has an apparent alteration in LPS-divalent cation binding and an increase in susceptibility to many β-lactams and to aminoglycosides but not to hydrophobic agents. Studies from two laboratories (2, 25) have failed to identify any changes in porin function in the mutant Z61. Similarly, the *Escherichia coli* antibiotic supersusceptible mutant DC2 has an alteration in LPS that alters divalent cation binding (27), but no porin alterations (2). These mutants are 16-fold more susceptible to ampicillin, as well as several more hydrophobic antibiotics.

Based on these findings, we feel that the case for the existence of non-porin pathways of antibiotic uptake is strong, at least in mutants. One might predict that in organisms with a less effective porin-mediated uptake pathway, like *Pseudomonas aeruginosa* and *Pseudomonas cepacia*, these non-porin pathways might become more important.

Influence of Other Cell Layers on Antibiotic Uptake

Cytoplasmic Membrane

Beta-lactam antibiotics act upon a series of penicillin binding proteins located in the periplasm and thus do not need to cross the cytoplasmic membrane. Others, including a variety of hydrophobic antibiotics (see below), apparently cross the cytoplasmic membrane by passive diffusion.

In the case of aminoglycosides, transport across the cytoplasmic membrane is apparently tightly coupled to the bactericidal action of these antibiotics (1). Despite 40 years of research, there is little concensus concerning either the mode of action or transport mechanism of aminoglycosides (1, 28, 29). Nevertheless, some generalizations can be made. Most researchers agree that streptomycin uptake across the cytoplasmic membrane is energized by the protonmotive force (1). Transport is unidirectional (i.e. inwards) and substantially irreversible. Bryan and colleagues (28) have suggested that respiratory quinones are involved in transport, but this is controversial (29). Streptomycin uptake involves two energized phases, a slow phase EDPI, followed by a more rapid phase EDPII, which appears to be initiated at the same time as or subsequent to the lethal event (1, 28). Thus one way of rationalizing the two points of view expressed in the literature is that quinone-dependency is restricted to EDPI, whereas the bulk of energy dependent uptake (represented by EDPII) is not absolutely dependent on quinones.

Tetracycline can be taken up across the cytoplasmic membrane of *Escherichia coli* via two systems, an initial rapid passive diffusion system which is followed by a slower energized system (28). The driving force for energy-dependent transport of tetracycline appears to be the protonmotive force. Apparently, the tetracycline variant, minocycline, can be taken up by passive diffusion but does not serve as a substrate for energized transport.

It is generally accepted that hydrophobic antibiotics can cross the cytoplasmic membrane of bacteria (as well as phospholipid membranes of host cells) by passive diffusion. Whereas transport across the outer membrane of many bacteria is a problem for hydrophobic antibiotics, the inner membrane is assumed to offer no permeability barrier. However, not all authors agree on which drugs can be called hydrophobic and thus can be assumed to penetrate in this way. Trimethoprim, fusidic acid, rifampicin, novobicin and by some accounts sulphonamides, clindamycin, lincomycin and macrolides are assumed to enter by passive diffusion (28). Chloramphenicol is lipophilic enough to diffuse across the cytoplasmic membrane, however some authors suggest it may enter by active transport. The 4-quinolones represent an unusual case, and are discussed separately below.

Experimentally, the rates of passive diffusion of lipophilic molecules below about 250 Da correlate reasonably well with their lipid/water partition coefficients (2, 28). Partition coefficients in octanol/phosphate buffer are generally used as a measure of hydrophobicity of antibiotics, but high solubility in octanol is not necessarily a reliable index of ability to passively penetrate phospholipid bilayers. Detailed study of hydrophobic uptake was been largely avoided, probably because the experiments are difficult and often inconclusive. For example, Chopra (30) was unable to demonstrate decreased uptake of fusidic acid across the cytoplasmic membrane of *Staphylococcus aureus* strains with plasmid-mediated resistance to the drug, even though changes in phospholipid composition were found and other mechanisms of resistance had been ruled out.

Some hydrophobic antibiotics exert their bactericidal action by inserting into the cytoplasmic membrane. They may cause major disorganization of the membrane (e.g. polymyxin B), break down membrane integrity by pore formation (e.g. gramicidins) or act as ionophores (28). Antibiotics with targets inside the cytoplasmic membrane may also disrupt the membrane during penetration and/or indirectly.

Nalixidic acid is fairly hydrophobic and has been assumed to penetrate the cytoplasmic membrane by passive diffusion (28). The newer 4-quinolones such as norfloxacin and enoxacin have a similar mode of action (28) and are more active on the whole, but appear to be considerably less hydrophobic (16).

The mechanism of enoxacin uptake across the cytoplasmic membranes of *Escherichia coli* and *Bacillus subtilis* was studied by Bryan and colleagues (16). All of the kinetic data favoured the passive diffusion mechanism, and inhibitors of energized uptake had no effect. The pharmacokinetic properties of the 4-quinolones suggest that they readily traverse eukaryotic membranes. On the limited information available, it seems that low hydrophobicity as measured by oil/water partition need not necessarily be a barrier to passive diffusion across the membrane. More detailed experimental evidence is needed before assumptions about the passive diffusion of drugs of different degrees of hydrophobicity can be confirmed.

Peptidoglycan

Most bacteria contain peptidoglycan as an essential component of the cell wall. The peptidoglycan network is assumed to have no sieving effect on molecules in the size range of antibiotics (31).

Periplasm

The aqueous space between the outer and inner membranes of gram-negative bacteria, the periplasm, is not known to act as a barrier to antibiotics. Compounds which are sufficiently hydrophilic to diffuse through outer membrane porins would presumably continue until reaching the surface of the inner membrane. However, alteration of antibiotics during passage through the periplasm by protonation, binding to macromolecules, or alteration by enzymes (30) may affect the compound's subsequent penetration of the cytoplasmic membrane.

Extracellular Polymers

Many bacteria possess extracellular polymers, usually polysaccharides. If the polymer is present in a discrete layer around the cell it is usually called a capsule, whereas material casually associated with the cell is referred to as slime. In addition, the term "surface arrays" has been used for extracellular polymers with repeating subunit structures.

Theoretically, extracellular polymeric layers could act as a barrier to diffusion of antibiotics from the extracellular medium to the cell surface. This possibility has been studied seriously only in *Pseudomonas aeruginosa*. This organism is notoriously resistant to antibiotics and can be isolated in mucoid form, especially from the lungs of patients with cystic fibrosis (32). The mucoid exopolysaccharide (MEP) of these strains is chemically heterogeneous and distinct from the slime associated with non-mucoid isolates. Several studies, summarized by Slack and Nichols (32), have compared antibiotic susceptibilities of mucoid and non-mucoid isolates. In some cases the mucoid strains have been more resistant to certain antibiotics but in others they have been equally or more susceptible. This lack of concensus may be the result of inconsistent test conditions and the diversity of MEP chemotypes.

Purified MEP has been shown to retard diffusion of aminoglycosides, but not β-lactams, in vitro. The anionic uronic acid groups of the MEP were thought to act as cation exchangers for the positively charged aminoglycoside molecules. However, Slack and Nichols concluded that inhibition of aminoglycoside diffusion by MEP was unlikely to be the rate-limiting step of uptake (32). It is difficult to say at present whether extracellular polymers can present a significant barrier to antibiotic uptake.

Acknowledgements

The authors wish to acknowledge the financial assistance of the Canadian Cystic Fibrosis Foundation and the Natural Sciences and Engineering Research Council of Canada for their own research. A.B. is a recipient of a CCFF Studentship.

References

1. Hancock, R. E. W.: Aminoglycoside uptake and mode of action – with special reference to streptomycin and gentamicin. Journal of Antimicrobial Chemotherapy 1981, 8: 249–276, 429–445.
2. Nikaido, H., Vaara, M.: Molecular basis of bacterial outer membrane permeability. Microbiological Reviews 1985, 49: 1–32.
3. Nikaido, H., Hancock, R. E. W.: Outer membrane permeability of *Pseudomonas aeruginosa*. In: Sokatch, J. R. (ed.): The bacteria: a treatise on structure and function, Volume 10. Academic Press, New York, 1985, p. 145–193.
4. Leive, L.: The barrier function of the gram-negative cell envelope. Annals of the New York Academy of Sciences 1974, 235: 109–127.
5. Hancock, R. E. W.: Model membrane studies of porin function. In: Inouye, M. (ed.): Bacterial outer membranes as model systems. John Wiley, New York, 1986, p. 187–225.
6. Nakae, T.: Identification of the major outer membrane protein of *Escherichia coli* that produces transmembrane channels in reconstituted vesicle membranes. Biochimica et Biophysica Acta 1976, 71: 877–884.
7. Zimmermann, W., Rosselet, A.: Function of the outer membrane of *Escherichia coli* as a permeability barrier to β-lactam antibiotics. Antimicrobial Agents and Chemotherapy 1977, 12: 368–372.
8. Nicas, T. I., Hancock, R. E. W.: *Pseudomonas aeruginosa* outer membrane permeability: isolation of a porin protein F-deficient mutant. Journal of Bacteriology 1983, 153: 281–285.
9. Mitsuyama, J., Hiruma, R., Yamaguchi, A., Sawai, T.: Identification of porins in outer membrane of *Proteus*, *Morganella* and *Providencia* spp. and their role in outer membrane permeation of β-lactams. Antimicrobial Agents and Chemotherapy 1987, 31: 379–384.
10. Harder, K. J., Nikaido, H., Matsuhashi, M.: Mutants of *Escherichia coli* that are resistant to certain β-lactam compounds lack the OmpF porin. Antimicrobial Agents and Chemotherapy 1981, 20: 549–552.
11. Then, R. L., Angehrn, P.: Multiply resistant mutants of *Enterobacter cloacae* selected by β-lactam antibiotics. Antimicrobial Agents and Chemotherapy 1986, 30: 684–688.
12. Woodruff, W. A., Hancock, R. E. W.: Construction and characterization of *Pseudomonas aeruginosa* protein F-deficient mutants after in vitro and in vivo insertion mutagenesis of the cloned gene. Journal of Bacteriology 1988, 170: 2592–2598.
13. Godfrey, A. J., Bryan, L. E.: Penetration of β-lactams through *Pseudomonas aeruginosa* porin channels. Antimicrobial Agents and Chemotherapy 1987, 31: 1216–1221.
14. Hancock, R. E. W.: Role of porins in outer membrane permeability. Journal of Bacteriology 1987, 169: 929–933.
15. Siden, I., Boman, H.: *Escherichia coli* mutants with altered sensitivity to cecropin D. Journal of Bacteriology 1983, 154: 170–176.
16. Bedard, J., Wong, S., Bryan, L. E.: Accumulation of enoxacin by *Escherichia coli* and *Bacillus subtilis*. Antimicrobial Agents and Chemotherapy 1987, 31: 1348–1354.
17. Watanabe, N.-A., Nagasu, T., Katsu, K., Kitoh, K.: E-0702, a new cephalosporin, is incorporated into *Escherichia coli* cells via the *tonB*-dependent iron transport system. Antimicrobial Agents and Chemotherapy 1987, 31: 497–504.
18. Pugsley, A. P., Zimmermann, W., Wehri, W.: Highly efficient uptake of a rifampycin derivative via the FhuA-tonB-dependent uptake route in *Escherichia coli*. Journal of General Microbiology 1987, 133: 3505–3511.
19. Quinn, J. P., Dudek, E. J., DiVincenzo, C. A., Lucks, D. A., Lerner, S. A.: Emergence of resistance to imipenem during therapy for *Pseudomonas aeruginosa* infections. Journal of Infectious Diseases 1986, 289–294.
20. Hancock, R. E. W.: Alterations in outer membrane permeability. Annual Reviews of Microbiology 1984, 38: 237–264.
21. Rivera, M., Hancock, R. E. W., Sawyer, J. G., Haug, A., McGroarty, G. J.: Enhanced binding of polycationic antibiotics to lipopolysaccharide from an aminoglycoside-supersusceptible *tolA* mutant strain of *Pseudomonas aeruginosa*. Antimicrobial Agents and Chemotherapy 1988, 32: 649–655.
22. Moore, R. A., Hancock, R. E. W.: Involvement of outer membrane of *Pseudomonas cepacia* in aminoglycoside and polymyxin resistance. Antimicrobial Agents and Chemotherapy 1986, 30: 923–926.
23. Martin, N. L., Beveridge, T. J.: Gentamicin interaction with *Pseudomonas aeruginosa* cell envelope. Antimicrobial Agents and Chemotherapy 1986, 29: 1079–1087.
24. Garrod, L. P., Lambert H. P., O'Grady, F.: Antibiotic and chemotherapy. Churchill Livingstone, Edinburgh, 1981.
25. Angus, B. L., Fyfe, J. A. M., Hancock, R. E. W.: Mapping and characterization of two mutations to antibiotic supersusceptibility in *Pseudomonas aeruginosa*. Journal of General Microbiology 1987, 133: 2905–2914.
26. Hinma, R., Yamaguchi, A., Sawai, T.: The effect of lipopolysaccharide on lipid bilayer permeability of β-lactam antibiotics. FEBS Letters 1984, 170: 268–272.
27. Rocque, W. J., Fesik, S. W., Haug, A., McGroarty, E. J.: Polycation binding to isolated lipopolysaccharide from antibiotic-hypersusceptible mutant strains of *Escherichia coli*. Antimicrobial Agents and Chemotherapy 1988, 32: 308–313.
28. Bryan, L. E.: Bacterial resistance and susceptibility to chemotherapeutic agents. Cambridge University Press, Cambridge, 1982.
29. Nichols, W. W.: On the mechanism of translocation of dihydrostreptomycin across the bacterial cytoplasmic membrane. Biochimica et Biophysica Acta 1987, 895: 11–23.
30. Chopra, I., Ball, P.: Transport of antibiotics into bacteria. Advances in Microbial Physiology 1982, 23: 183–240.
31. Scherrer, R., Gerhardt, P.: Molecular sieving by the *Bacillus megaterium* cell wall and protoplast. Journal of Bacteriology 1971, 107: 718–735.
32. Slack, M. P. E., Nichols, W. W.: Antibiotic penetration through bacterial capsules and exopolysaccharides. Journal of Antimicrobial Chemotherapy 1982, 10: 368–372.

Inhibition of Protein Biosynthesis by Antibiotics

K. H. Nierhaus*, R. Brimacombe, H. G. Wittmann

Many antibiotics interfere with the protein biosynthetic process, which means their site of action is the ribosome. The first part of this article briefly surveys the current knowledge of ribosomal structure and function. The second part discusses the inhibition mechanisms of various antibiotics at the ribosomal level, and describes the strategies which the cell has developed in order to acquire resistance against antibiotics.

The term "antibiotic" describes a heterogeneous group of compounds, synthesized and secreted by certain bacteria and fungi, which inhibit the growth of other organisms. The synthesis occurs preferentially in situations where impaired growth conditions trigger an alteration in the producer; in bacteria this is the transition from rapid logarithmic growth to the stationary phase. The antibiotics excreted under unfavourable growth conditions impair the growth of competing organisms, prevent the further exploitation of food resources, and thus offer a selective advantage which improves the survival chance of the antibiotic-producing microorganism. When the microorganism shifts to the stationary phase, DNA and protein synthesis (as well as most other metabolic activities) become reduced, with the result that the antibiotic can do little harm to its producer. Furthermore, the producer is in many cases specifically resistant to its own product.

The only common features of antibiotics are that they are synthesized by microorganisms and usually have a molecular mass of less than 2,000 daltons. However, with regard to their structure and mechanism of inhibition, antibiotics are extremely heterogeneous. In some cases (e.g. chloramphenicol), a particular reaction is inhibited in prokaryotes, whereas the corresponding reaction in higher organisms is not. Alternatively, an antibiotic (e.g. tetracycline) may inhibit a reaction equally well in both pro- and eukaryotes, but may pass more easily through the membrane of bacteria than through the eukaryotic cell wall. These two properties form the basis of the vital importance of antibiotics as therapeutic tools in medicine.

Antibiotics can inhibit replication (e.g. nalidixic acid), transcription (e.g. rifampycin), translation (e.g. tetracycline), synthesis or function of the bacterial cell membrane (e.g. penicillin), or they can interfere with cell metabolism (e.g. trimethoprim). However, most of the known antibiotics operate at the level of translation, probably as a result of the great complexity of the translational machine – the ribosome – which offers many possible points of obstruction. This focus on the inhibition of translation is on the other hand not reflected in the spectrum of industrially produced antibiotics, since other criteria such as lack of side effects or low production costs play a decisive role. For example, a single substance – trimethoprim – represented about 30% of the West German antibiotic production in 1985. This drug inhibits the synthesis of N^{10}-formyl-tetrahydrofolate and thus disturbs the C_1 metabolism.

In this brief survey, we confine our attention to those inhibitors of protein synthesis which on the one hand are of therapeutical importance, and on the other hand play a role as specific inhibitors of particular ribosomal functions. The structure and function of the ribosome itself is first described, followed by a discussion of the inhibition mechanisms of some antibiotics within this framework. Finally, the various mechanisms of resistance which have been developed by the prokaryotes in response to antibiotics are explained.

Flux of Genetic Information

The central importance of proteins in living processes rests on the fact that enzymes are almost exclusively proteins, and that the enzyme pattern of a cell defines its metabolism. It follows that the genetic information stored in the DNA, which is transmitted by replication during cell division, is primarily directed toward the synthesis of proteins and the components of the protein-synthesizing apparatus, the

---

Max-Planck-Institut für Molekulare Genetik, Ihnestraße 73, D-1000 Berlin 33 (Dahlem), FRG.

ribosome. The proteins are synthesized according to the prescription carried in the DNA. The ribosome does not read the information directly from the DNA, but instead uses another nucleic acid — "messenger" or mRNA — which is a copy of one strand of the chromosomal double-stranded DNA. The copying process (DNA producing mRNA) is termed transcription, and each mRNA molecule carries the genetic information for at least one polypeptide (protein) chain.

Nucleic acids are linear polymers constructed from four "building blocks" (nucleotides): A, C, G and T in the case of DNA, and A, C, G, and U in RNA. The nucleotides have the important property of being able to form complementary base pairs with one another, G pairing with C, and A with U or T, with the pairs held together by hydrogen bonds. This property forms the basis of the chain copying process which takes place in both replication and transcription (Figure 1). Proteins are also linear unbranched polymers, but here there are 20 different "building blocks", which in this case are the amino acids. It is thus self-evident that a single nucleotide in mRNA does not contain enough information to code for an amino acid during translation, and in fact a sequence of three nucleotides (triplet or codon) is required to direct the incorporation of a single amino acid into a protein chain. The ribosome cannot read the triplet "words" of the mRNA on its own, but makes use of adaptor molecules during the translation. These adaptors are small L-shaped RNA molecules (tRNA), which at one end carry a triplet (anticodon) complementary to the mRNA codon and which at the other end are covalently attached to the corresponding amino acid. There exists an enzyme for each of the 20 amino acids, which guarantees the specificity of the coupling between each tRNA molecule and its amino acid. This coupling is a vital step in the translation process, as it forms the bridge between the information stored in the nucleic acids (via the anticodon) and the end-product (the amino acid in the protein). The task of the ribosome is to transfer the information in the mRNA one triplet at a time by accurately aligning the corresponding aminoacyl-tRNA molecules in the ribosomal decoding site. The amino acids from the successive aminoacyl tRNA molecules become linked together one after another at this site, forming the polypeptide chain.

Structure of Ribosomes

The most well-known organism in biology is the eubacterium *Escherichia coli*. The following section describes primarily the ribosomes from this organism, and briefly surveys the current state of knowledge, with emphasis on recent developments. A collection of reviews on all aspects of ribosome research has been published previously (1).

All ribosomes can dissociate into a small and a large subunit. In the case of the *Escherichia coli* ribosome (sedimentation coefficient 70S), the small subunit (30S) contains 21 different ribosomal proteins (Figure 2) named S1 to S21, together with a single RNA molecule (16S RNA). The RNA is 1542 nucleotides in length and comprises two-thirds of the molecular mass. Similarly, the large ribosomal subunit (50S) contains 33 different proteins, named L1 to L36; the discrepancy in these numbers results from the fact that two proteins (L7 and L12) were found to be identical (with the exception of an acetyl group at the terminus of protein L7), a further protein, L8, was found to be a complex between other ribosomal proteins, and a third protein, L26, is identical to S20, sometimes appearing associated with the 50S subunit, sometimes with the 30S subunit. All the proteins are present in a single copy per ribosome, with the exception of L7 and L12 (see above), which are present in four copies. Again, the ribosomal RNA accounts for two-thirds of the mass of the 50S subunit, and consists of two molecules, one (23S RNA) being 2904 nucleotides long and the other (5S RNA) 120 nucleotides long. The primary sequences of all the ribosomal protein and RNA molecules are known. Despite the large number and complexity of the components, it is important to note that in the case of *Escherichia coli*, fully active ribosomal subunits can be reconstituted from isolated ribosomal proteins and RNAs (2, 3).

In addition to the ribosomal RNA from *Escherichia coli*, ribosomal RNA sequences from many other organisms have now been determined, and these sequences have played an important part in elucidating the secondary structures of the 16S and 23S mole-

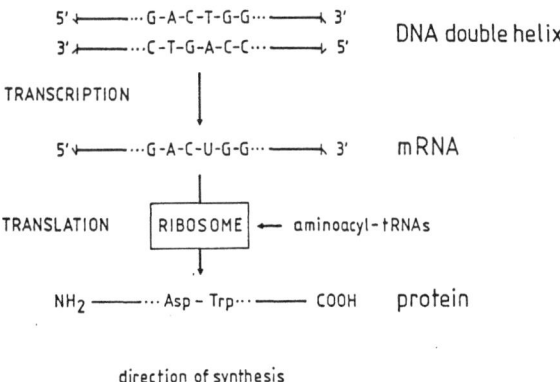

Figure 1: The flow of information during gene expression, from DNA to protein.

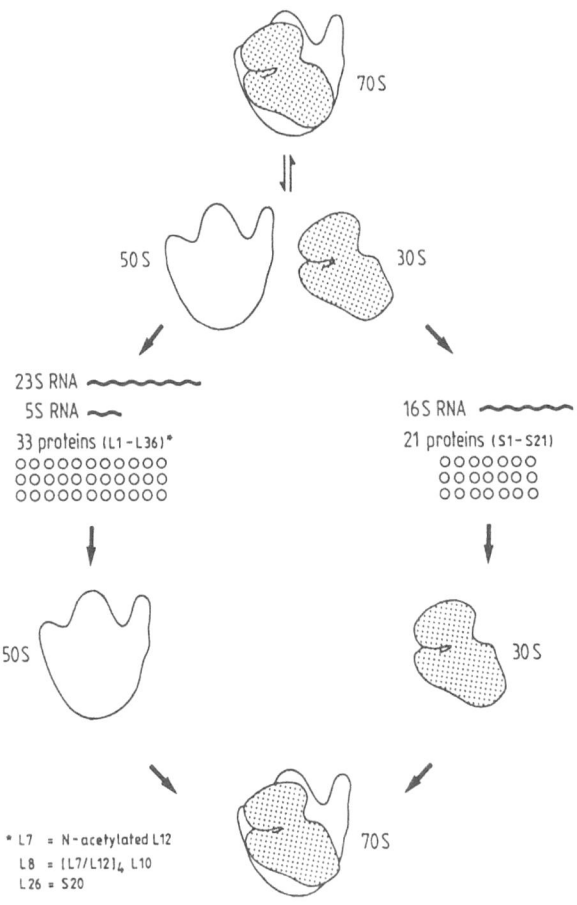

Figure 2: The components and the reconstitution of the ribosomal subunits from *Escherichia coli*. The shapes of the 70S, 50S and 30S particles are those observed electron microscopically.

cules. RNA molecules can fold back on themselves, forming double-helical hairpin loop structures which obey the same A-U, G-C base-pairing rules that apply to DNA. By comparing sequences from similar but not identical organisms, the plausibility of a proposed hairpin-loop structure can be tested. Thus, if an A residue in a double-helix is replaced by a G in the corresponding double-helix from another organism, then the U residue paired to that A must change to a C in order to preserve the integrity of the helix. Many thousands of such compensatory base changes have now been observed, with the result that — in combination with experimental methods — the secondary folding of the RNA molecules is now well established. Furthermore, the application of this principle has strikingly documented the fact that ribosomes from all sources, whether pro- or eukaryotic, have a basic structural identity.

Considerable progess has been made in understanding the quaternary structure of the ribosome (i.e., how the RNA and proteins are arranged in the subunits), mainly by application of the four following methods: (A) The ribosome is large enough (diameter ca 250 Å) for its shape to be determined by electron microscopes and for the positions of epitopes from ribosomal proteins to be located on the subunit surfaces (4). (B) Two-dimensional ribosomal crystals have also been examined electron microscopically with a view to three-dimensional image reconstruction. These studies have revealed interesting features, such as a tunnel about 120 Å in length and 20 Å in diameter within the 50S subunit (5). (C) The internal topography of the ribosomal proteins can be revealed by neutron scattering experiments. This technique allows the three-dimensional locations of the mass centres of individual ribosomal proteins to be triangulated, and a study of the 30S subunit has recently been completed (6). (D) The analysis of cross-links between various regions of the RNA as well as between the RNA and individual proteins allows the RNA to be folded into three dimensions and to be positioned relative to the proteins. The various data just mentioned have been merged into a detailed model of the 30S subunit (7), which is illustrated in Figure 3.

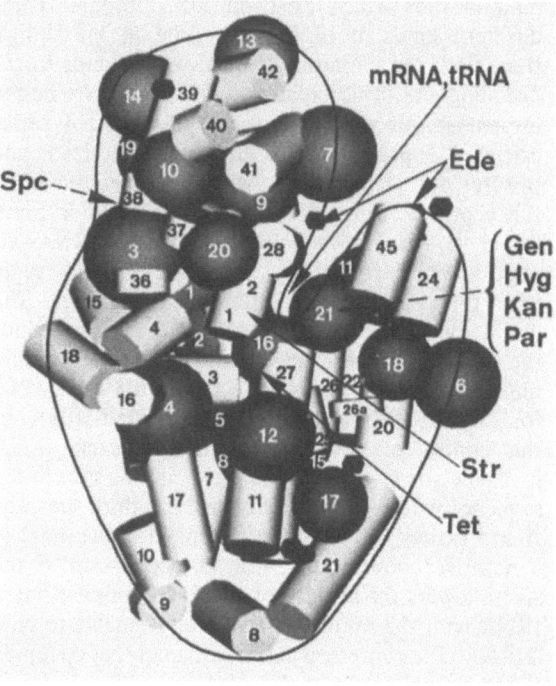

Figure 3: A computer-generated model of the *Escherichia coli* 30S ribosomal subunit. The spheres represent the proteins, and the cylinders the double-helical regions of the RNA. The silhouette indicates the electron microscopically observed shape of the subunit. Sites of interaction with mRNA, tRNA and various antibiotics are indicated (a dotted line denotes that the site concerned is at the rear of the particle in the position shown).

Ribosomal Function

Protein synthesis on ribosomes takes place in three phases: the initiation phase, the elongation cycle (in which the already existing peptide chain is lengthened by one amino acid at a time), and the termination phase. All three stages are regulated by distinct protein factors, correspondingly named initiation, elongation and termination factors, and these factors bind only transiently to the ribosome. In the initiation phase, the small ribosomal subunit finds the start signal on the mRNA. In prokaryotes this start signal consists of an AUG codon together with a defined sequence of 4–12 nucleotides "upstream" of the AUG. The latter sequence is able to base-pair with the 3′-terminus of the 16S RNA, and can thus increase the probability that the starter AUG lies close to the 30S decoding site. A specific initiator tRNA — the fMet-tRNA — binds to the AUG codon on the 30S subunit, and this complex binds a 50S subunit forming the so-called 70S initiation complex, which can then enter the next phase, the elongation cycle.

Before describing the mechanism of the elongation, it is necessary to enumerate the various kinds of tRNA derivatives that are present on the ribosome during protein biosynthesis and the various tRNA binding sites which exist on the ribosome. Three different kinds of tRNA participate in the elongation; first, the aminoacyl tRNA, which binds to the decoding site in accordance with the mRNA codon present at this site; next, the peptidyl tRNA which carries the peptide chain already synthesized; and thirdly, deacylated tRNA, which is generated when the peptidyl residue of the peptidyl tRNA is transferred to the newly-bound aminoacyl tRNA via peptide bond formation. These three tRNA types have three corresponding tRNA binding sites. The A-site, being the decoding site, preferentially binds the aminoacyl tRNA, the adjacent P-site preferentially binds the peptidyl tRNA, and finally the E-site ("E" for exit) exclusively binds the deacylated tRNA. In the course of protein biosynthesis, each tRNA molecule passes through the three binding sites in the sequence A to P to E. The first and the third sites, the A and E sites, are allosterically linked in the sense of a negative cooperativity; that is, occupation of the A-site lowers the affinity of the E-site for deacylated tRNA with the result that the latter is unable to bind a tRNA. The converse is also true; namely, an occupied E-site strongly reduces the capacity of the A-site to bind an aminoacyl tRNA. Consequently, there are always two tRNA sites (A and P, or P and E) during the elongation cycle which have a high affinity for tRNA. In each case, both high affinity sites are occupied by tRNA, and both adjacent tRNA molecules are connected to the mRNA via codon-anticodon interaction (8–10), see Figure 4A.

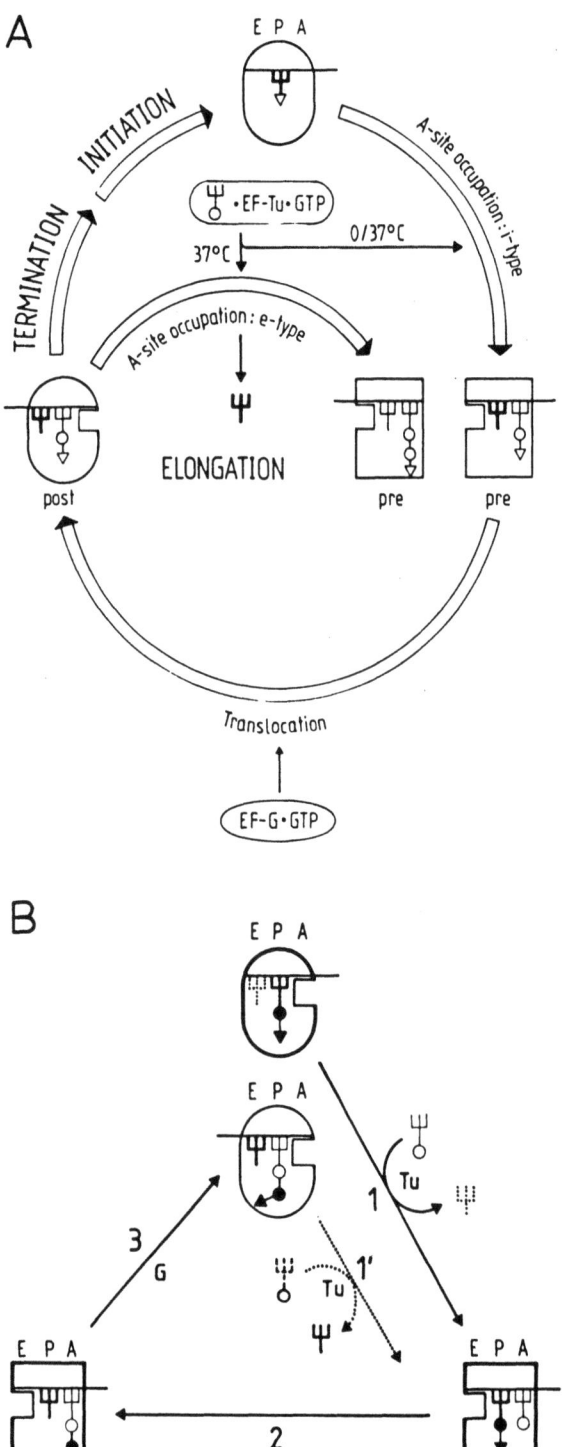

Figure 4: The ribosomal elongation cycle. (A) The two types of A-site occupation during elongation: the i-type ("i" for initiation) with free E-site, and the e-type ("e" for elongation) with occupied E-site (Reference No. 18). (B) The three essential reactions of the elongation cycle, according to the allosteric three-site model: 1. aminoacyl tRNA binding to the A-site; 2. peptidyl transfer; 3. translocation. Tu and G are the elongation factors EF-Tu and EF-G. The pretranslocational ribosome is drawn as a rectangle, the post-translocational ribosome as an oval.

In Figure 4B the description of the elongation cycle is simplified to three basic reactions. The starting point is a ribosome carrying a deacylated tRNA in the E-site and a peptidyl tRNA in the P-site. The first reaction is the occupation of the A-site with the next aminoacyl tRNA; codon-anticodon interaction at this site presumably triggers a transition of the ribosomal functional state, so that the A-site becomes the high-affinity site, the deacylated tRNA being therefore simultaneously released from the E-site. The second reaction is the peptidyl transfer, in which the peptide residue is transferred from the P-site bound peptidyl tRNA to the amino acid residue of the A-site bound aminoacyl tRNA. The result is that a deacylated tRNA is present at the P-site, and the peptidyl tRNA (lengthened by one amino acid residue) is at the A-site. The enzymatic centre of the peptidyl transferase is an integral part of the 50S subunit. Note that the peptidyl transfer does not change the tRNA occupation state of the ribosome, i.e. the A and P sites each still carry a tRNA as before. The tRNA occupation state, however, is changed during the third reaction, namely the translocation step, in which the tRNA-mRNA complex is moved relative to the ribosome by one codon length. The result of this reaction is a state which is equivalent to the starting point (above), but with a new codon at the A-site. The functional transitions from the pre- to the post-translocational state (the translocation reaction itself) and from the post- to the pretranslocational state (triggered by A-site occupation) both require considerable activation energy. This energy barrier is overcome with the help of the elongation factors, combined with the hydrolysis of GTP. The transition from the post- to the pre-translocational state is aided by the elongation factor EF-Tu, which forms a ternary complex with the aminoacyl tRNA and a GTP molecule, and binds as such to the ribosomal A-site. When binding has taken place, the GTP is enzymatically cleaved by the factor, resulting in a conformational change on the factor which then drops off the ribosome and allows the peptidyl transfer to occur. In an analogous manner the elongation factor EF-G (together with the cleavage of a second molecule of GTP) aids the transition from the pre- to the post-translocational state. As with EF-Tu, the factor dependent GTP cleavage triggers the dissociation of the factor from the ribosome.

Inhibition of Ribosomal Functions by Antibiotics

The allosteric three-site model of tRNA binding just described has a special feature which is of particular importance in explaining the inhibition characteristics of some antibiotics. Namely, the model distinguishes two types of A-site occupation (Figure 4A). Immediately following initiation, where the initiator tRNA (fMet-tRNA) is located at the P-site, the A-site becomes occupied for the first time without there being any tRNA molecule at the E-site. Thus, no energy-consuming release of tRNA from the E-site is involved, and this type of A-site occupation is referred to as i-type occupation ("i" for initiation). In contrast, after the first elongation cycle the E-site is occupied, and it follows that all subsequent occupations of the A-site must generate the costly transition from the post- to the pre-translocational state, with concomitant release of tRNA from the E-site. This is referred to as e-type A-site occupation ("e" for elongation). Some antibiotics completely block A-site occupation of the e-type, but surprisingly hardly influence that of the i-type. The order in which the antibiotics are discussed is determined by the chain of reactions describing the ribosomal functions (Figure 5). Initiation is divided into six steps (I1 to I6), the elongation cycle into five steps (E1 to E5), and the termination into three steps (T1 to T3). The essential features of the antibiotics are summarized in Table 1, and have been reviewed previously (11–13).

Inhibitors of Ribosomal Initiation

Since initiation is a functional property of the small ribosomal subunit, all initiation-inhibiting antibiotics bind to the small subunit, whereas elongation inhibitors can bind either to the 30S or 50S subunit (Table 1).

Aurintricarboxylic acid (ATA) inhibits the mRNA binding to the 30S subunit, as well as to the isolated ribosomal protein S1. It does not affect intact cells, because it is unable to permeate through the membranes. At higher concentrations (above 80 μM) other ribosomal reactions are non-specifically impaired as well.

Edeine. The antibiotic complex edeine consists of four components, named A_1, A_2, B_1 and B_2. Only A_1 and B_1 show antibiotic activity. Edeine A_1 inhibits the binding of mRNA to the small subunit (Figure 5, I3) and thus also the binding of fMet-tRNA. However, edeine A_1 is not a specific inhibitor of tRNA binding to the P-site, as is often erroneously assumed. The binding site of edeine A_1 is shown in Figure 3.

Kasugamycin. Formerly, kasugamycin was assigned to the large and important group of aminoglycosides (see below). However, this drug is no longer regarded as an aminoglycoside for the following reasons. It deviates structurally, i.e. it is not a derivative of 2-deoxystreptamine as are the gentamicin, the kanamycin and the neomycin groups, nor is it related to streptamine as are the streptomycins. Furthermore, the inhibition pattern is not typical for an amino-

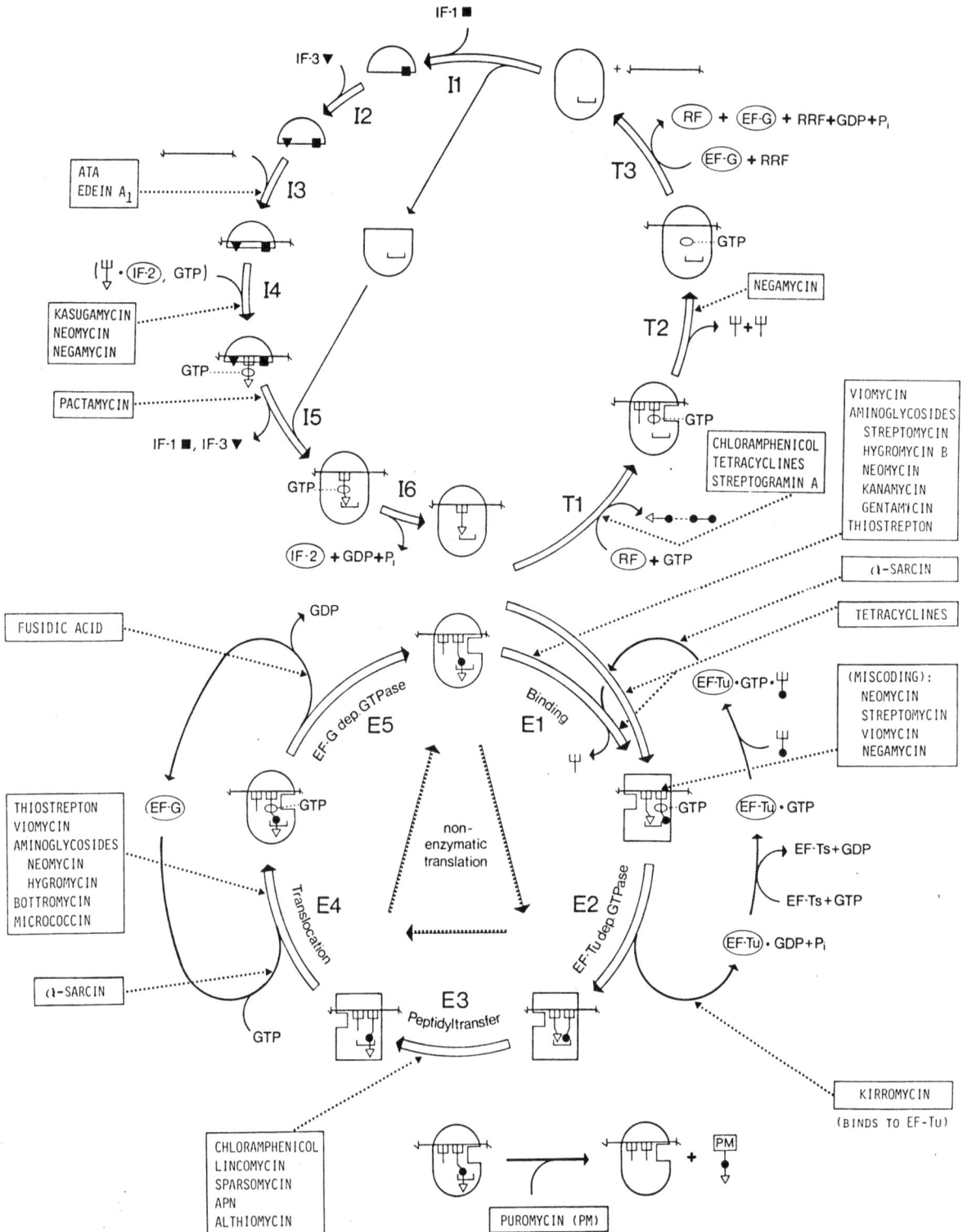

Figure 5: Scheme of ribosomal function, showing the points of attack of a number of antibiotics, modified from Reference No. 25.

Table 1: Features of antibiotics which inhibit protein synthesis.

Antibiotic	Producer	Inhibited Function[a]	Specificity[a] P/E 30S/50S	Component involved in binding or adjacent to the binding site	Component altered in resistant strain	Remarks
Aurintricarboxylic acid		I3: mRNA binding	P.E. 30S	S1		active only in cell free extracts
Edeine A1	*Bacillus brevis*	I4: fMet-tRNA binding	P.E. 30S (50S)	16S rRNA: G693, G926, A794, C795		
Kasugamycin	*Streptomyces kasugaensis*	I3: mRNA bindung	P. 30S	16S rRNA: A1518, A1519	mutation in ksgA (methylase of 16S rRNA) and/or ksgB (membrane permeability)	aminoglycoside with uncommon structure
		I4: fMet-tRNA binding, no miscoding				
Pactamycin	*Streptomyces pactum*	I5: 50S association	P.E. 30S	unknown		
Tetracycline	*Streptomyces aureofaciens*	E1: A-site occupation (i- and e-type)	P.E. 30S	16S rRNA: A892		inhibits the IF-dependent binding of fMet-tRNA to the P-site
α-Sarcin	*Aspergillus giganteus*	E1 + E4: elongation factor binding	P.E. 50S	23S rRNA: G2661		cleaves phosphodiester bond after G2661 of the 23S rRNA
Aminoglycosides Streptomycin	*Streptomyces griseus*	E1: A-site occupation (e-type), miscoding	P. 30S	S3, S5, 16S rRNA (913-5)	modified S12, 16S rRNA: C912→U	streptomycin dependence
Gentamicin	*Micromonospora purpurea*			16S rRNA: A1408, G1494 (C525)		
Kanamycin	*Streptomyces kanamyceticus*				L6 16S rRNA: methylation of G1405 or A1408	
Neomycin	*Streptomyces fradiae*	Neo.: E1 + E4: change of the allosteric conformation				Pararomycin (Neo. Group); resist. 16S rRNA C1409→G G1491
Negamycin	*Streptomyces purpeofuscus*	E1: miscoding	P. (E) 30S	unknown		no aminoglycoside
Kirromycin	*Streptomyces collinus*	E2: dissociation of EF-Tu from ribosome	P. —	EF-Tu	mutation in tufA and tufB	
Chloramphenicol	*Streptomyces venezuelae*	E3: peptidyltransfer	P. 50S	L16	mutations in the 23S rRNA: G2057→A, G2447→A, A2451→U, C2452, A2503→C, U2504→C	
Puromycin	*Streptomyces alboniger*	E3: peptidyltransfer to puromycin causes chain termination	P.E. 50S	L23		presumably disturbs polypeptide positioning at the exit channel
Viomycin	*Streptomyces puniceus*	E1 (only e-type) + E4: change of the allosteric conformation	P. 30S (50S)	unknown	modified 16S- or 23S rRNA	
Thiostrepton	*Streptomyces aureus*	E1 (only e-tyoe) + E4: change of the allostreic conformation	P.E. 50S	L11	absence of L11; methylation of A1067 in the 23S rRNA	
Fusidic acid	*Fusidium coccineum*	E5: dissociation of EF-G from ribosome	P.E. —	EF-G	modified EF-G	
Erythromycin	*Streptomyces erythreus*	see 'Remarks'	P. 50S	L15, L16	modifications in L4, L22; methylation of A2058 in the 23S rRNA, G2057→A	presumably disturbs polypeptide positioning at the exit channel

[a]P.E.: Antibiotic inhibits ribosomes of the 70S type (P, prokaryotes) or 80S type (E, eukaryotes). 30S, 50S: Antibiotic binds to the small subunit (30S, in eukaryotes 40S) or to the large subunit (50S, in eukaryotes 60S). I3–I5 and E1–E5 correspond to the reactions shown in Figure 5.

glycoside. Kasugamycin does not increase the error in the selection process of aminoacyl-tRNA (leading to incorporation of incorrect amino acids); rather, this drug seems to prevent the binding of fMet–tRNA to the small ribosomal subunit (14). In regard to resistance against kasugamycin, at least two mechanisms must be distinguished. In one case, the 16S RNA is undermethylated, lacking four methyl groups at the adjacent positions A-1518 and A-1519 of the 16S RNA. Here a mutation in the gene ksgA inactivates a specific methylase. Alternatively, resistance can be caused by a mutation in the gene ksgB, which alters the membrane permeability. In this case, however, the ribosomes are still kasugamycin-sensitive.

Pactamycin blocks the association of the large ribosomal subunit (Figure 5, I5) and thus leads to an accumulation of the initiation complex fMet-tRNA*mRNA*30S.

Inhibitors of the Elongation Cycle

Tetracyclines inhibit A-site occupation of both the i- and the e-type, but this inhibition is not exclusive, because tetracyclines also prevent the initiation factor-dependent binding of fMet-tRNA to the P-site in the presence of natural mRNA. A likely explanation is that tetracycline blocks A-site binding of ribosomes in the pre-translocational state and P-site binding of those in the post-translocational state (14). The binding site of the tetracyclines is shown in Figure 3. Tetracycline inhibition is universal, i.e. it occurs with all classes of ribosomes. The more or less specific inhibition of prokaryotes (and thus the great importance of this group of antibiotics in medicine) results from the fact that the net transport through the bacterial membrane is more efficient than that through the walls of animal cells. Interestingly, tetracycline prevents binding of the ternary complex aminoacyl-tRNA*EF-Tu*GTP to the A-site, but not the EF-Tu dependent GTP hydrolysis (15). This was the first hint that A-site binding occurs in two steps, the first being formation of a "loose" contact between the ternary complex and the A-site, and the second being GTP hydrolysis, which "tightens" the binding and simultaneously causes release of the binary complex EF-Tu*GDP from the ribosome. Clearly, tetracycline exclusively prevents this "tight" binding of aminoacyl-tRNA to the A-site. No *Escherichia coli* cells containing tetracycline-resistant ribosomes have so far been found.

α-*Sarcin*. The antibiotic α-sarcin is an interesting case of a nuclease which causes cleavage of a single phosphodiester bond in the large subunit, namely at position G-2661 in the 23S RNA. This nucleotide is located in a 12-base sequence which is universally conserved in ribosomes of all organisms, and is thus obviously important. The consequence of the cleavage is a loss of the capacity to bind the elongation factors EF-Tu (as the ternary complex) and EF-G, whereas all EF-independent ribosomal functions remain unimpaired (16). Both elongation factors have overlapping binding sites on the ribosome, and it is probable that the 23S RNA region around G-2661 is part of the overlapping area.

Aminoglycosides. The members of the large group comprising the aminoglycosides (the streptomycins, and the gentamicin, kanamycin and neomycin families) are all structurally related, have identical or adjacent binding sites (17) (Figure 3) and show a similar pattern of resistance. Recently, these antibiotics were assigned a common inhibition pattern (18): they block the occupation of the A-site, but the blockage is exclusively of the e-type occupation (see above). In addition, they increase misreading effects, a property which was accepted for a long time as a criterion for aminoglycoside inhibition, but which is not in fact the cause of their bactericidal effects. The members of the neomycin group furthermore inhibit translocation (Figure 5, E4).

Negamycin. The peptide antibiotic negamycin, in contrast to the aminoglycosides, does inhibit protein synthesis primarily by strongly increasing the misincorporation of amino acids.

Kirromycin does not bind to the ribosome, but rather to the elongation factor Tu. In the presence of the antibiotic the ternary complex EF-Tu*aminoacyl-tRNA*GTP is able to bind to the A-site, and GTP is cleaved, but the next step — the dissociation of the binary complex EF-Tu*GDP from the ribosome — is prevented. Thus, the EF-Tu remains on the ribosome and in turn prevents the subsequent peptidyl transfer and binding of EF-G. Kirromycin is able to trigger the cleavage of GTP in a binary complex containing just EF-Tu and GTP, and this was the first proof that the GTPase centre resides on the factor rather than on the ribosome. It has taken many years to find mutants that are resistant to kirromycin, because there are two almost identical genes for EF-Tu (tufA and tufB), which together produce a large amount of the factor. EF-Tu accounts for 10% of the total protein mass in *Escherichia coli*, and is the most abundant protein in this organism, there being statistically one EF-Tu molecule for every tRNA molecule in the cell. To generate resistant mutants, either both EF-Tu genes must be altered in the same way (a very rare event), or alternatively one of the genes has to be inactivated before selecting for resistance mutations. In this context it is worth noting that all other ribosomal factors as well as the ribosomal proteins themselves are encoded in each case by a single gene on the *Escherichia coli* chromosome. In contrast, there are seven genes for the ribosomal RNA. This explains why it is practically impossible to obtain resistant mutants in which the resistance is conferred by an altered ribosomal RNA without resorting to the techniques of genetic manipulation.

Chloramphenicol. The best known inhibitor of bacterial peptidyl transferase activity (Figure 5, E3) is chloramphenicol, which has been chemically synthesized since 1950. It probably disturbs the ribosomal location of the CCA-region at the 3'- end of an A-site bound aminoacyl-tRNA, and thus also disrupts the positioning of the aminoacyl residue in the peptidyl transferase centre. As a consequence, blockage of the peptidyl transferase activity is observed in simple model systems. In more physiological systems, however, another effect seems to prevail, namely the release of short oligopeptidyl-tRNAs. The abortive release of such oligopeptidyl-tRNAs (in particular dipeptidyl-tRNAs) from the ribosome is by no means a rare event, and chloramphenicol further destabilizes these products, thus amplifying their release (unpublished results). Reconstitution and affinity labelling experiments have revealed that ribosomal protein L16 is involved in the binding of chloramphenicol, and this protein is essential for the assembly of the peptidyl transferase centre. Chloramphenicol-resistant ribosomes have been found in mitochondrial mutants of yeast and mammalian cells, the cause of the resistance being alterations in the large subunit RNA at locations corresponding to positions 2447, 2451, 2503 or 2504 in the *Escherichia coli* 23S RNA (19).

Puromycin. The antibiotic puromycin also interferes with reaction E3 (Figure 5), and was the first antibiotic for which the inhibition mechanism could be elucidated at the molecular level. Figure 6A illustrates that puromycin is an analogue of the 3'-end of an aminoacyl-tRNA, but with the essential distinction that the aminoacyl residue is linked to the ribose by an amide bridge instead of an ester bond. This amide bond cannot be cleaved by the peptidyl transferase.

The similarity to the 3'-end of aminoacyl-tRNA enables the puromycin to bind to the A-site region of the peptidyl transferase centre, and to accept the peptidyl residue from the neighbouring P-site bound peptidyl-tRNA. At this stage the peptidyl-puromycin is likely to fall off the ribosome, since the antibiotic lacks the rest of the tRNA structure. However, even if this does not occur and the peptidyl-puromycin complex is translocated to the P-site, no further rounds of peptidyl transfer can take place, due to the amide bridge already mentioned. Thus, puromycin does not actually inhibit the peptidyl transferase, but rather allows a single peptide bond to form, resulting in the unusable side-product peptidyl-puromycin. This makes the antibiotic an important tool for the study of the peptidyl transferase reaction, and the operational definition of the ribosomal P- and A-sites is based on the ability or inability, respectively, of a ribosome-bound peptidyl tRNA to undergo reaction with puromycin. Puromycin binds to the large ribosomal subunit, near to protein L23 (20). No mutants resistant to puromycin have so far been found.

Viomycin, Thiostrepton. The next step in the elongation cycle is the translocation reaction. This allosteric transition is totally blocked by two structurally unrelated antibiotics, viomycin and thiostrepton At the same time, both antibiotics block the reverse allosteric transition from the post- to the pre-translocational state as well (corresponding to A-site occupation of the e-type; see above). It follows that the action of the antibiotics is to freeze the actual state of the ribosome and thus to block the allosteric transitions in each direction. A-site occupation of the i-type is not hampered by either antibiotic, but thiostrepton shows an additional effect, namely the impairment of EF-G binding to the ribosome. Resistance against viomycin is peculiar in that it can be

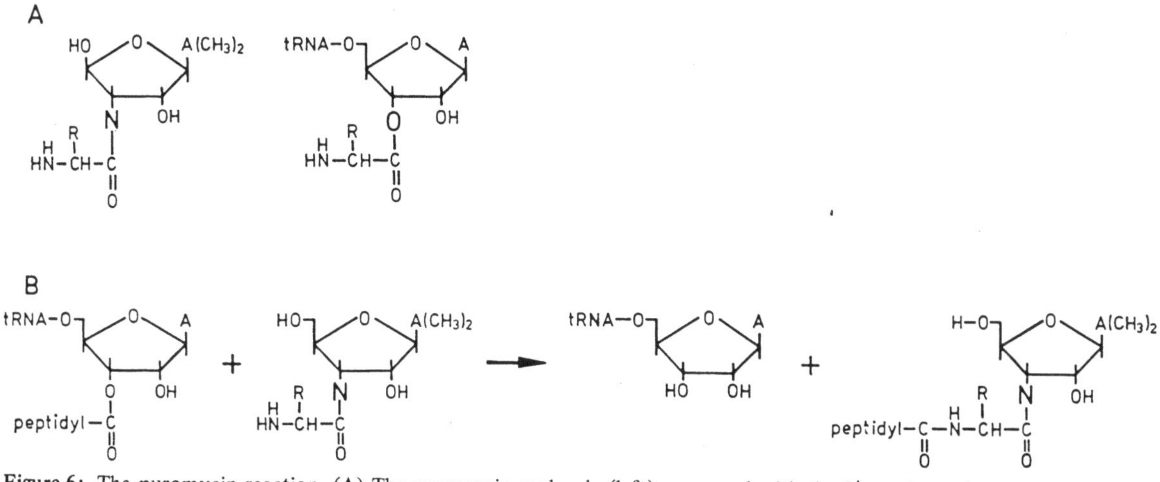

Figure 6: The puromycin reaction. (A) The puromycin molecule (left) compared with the 3'-terminus of an aminoacyl-tRNA (right). (B) Scheme of reaction. A peptidyl-tRNA at the P-site reacts with puromycin at the A-site leading to formation of peptidyl puromycin (right). See text for details.

caused by alterations in the RNA of either the small or the large subunit. Resistance against thiostrepton is conveyed either by a lack of protein L11 or by a 2'-OH methylation at position A-1067 of the 23S RNA (19).

Fusidic acid is the counterpart to kirromycin, since this drug does not bind to the ribosome, but rather to the elongation factor EF-G. Fusidic acid does not interfere with the EF-G binding to the ribosome, nor with the translocation reaction, nor with the EF-G dependent GTP cleavage, but instead appears to block the conformational change in the EF-G which is concomitant with the GTPase reaction. This prevents the dissociation of the factor from the ribosome, and hence the next step in the elongation cycle — the binding of the ternary complex with EF-Tu — is blocked, since the binding of both elongation factors is mutually exclusive.

Erythromycin. Although erythromycin is the most well known representative of the macrolides, there is some controversy surrounding its mechanism of inhibition. It is possible that the effects of the antibiotic are too subtle to be resolved by currently available tests. The following explanation accounts for most of the apparently contradictory reports. As mentioned in the structure section, the 50S ribosomal subunit contains a tunnel (5) for the growing polypeptide chain, and it is possible that erythromycin inhibits the initial "threading" of the polypeptide chain into this tunnel. This would explain the observations that the antibiotic does not impair either initiation, peptidyl transfer or translocation, but rather triggers the release of small oligopeptides shortly after initiation. This is reminiscent of the effects of chloramphenicol already mentioned, and indeed one and the same mutation in the 23S RNA (at position G-2057 (21)) confers resistance against both antibiotics. Furthermore, erythromycin blocks the binding of chloramphenicol to the 50S subunit. As in the case with streptomycin (Table 1) resistance to erythromycin can be caused either by an altered ribosomal protein (L4 or L22) or by an altered RNA (in this case the 23S). The alteration in the RNA is the introduction of N^6, N^6-dimethyladenine at position 2058, a methylation which is not normally found in 23S RNA.

Inhibitors of Termination

No specific inhibitor of the termination process has yet been described. One reason for this is that the precise sequence of events during termination is not known, and suitable test systems are lacking. A second reason is that some of the reactions of the elongation cycle also play a role in termination. It is therefore not surprising that inhibitory effects on termination have been described for tetracycline, negamycin, thiostrepton and chloramphenicol. In the case of chloramphenicol, for example, the optimal positioning of the aminoacyl residue of the aminoacyl-tRNA is disturbed, so that the amino group (as the acceptor for the peptide bond) is not in its usual position, thus impairing both peptidyl transfer and the threading of the peptidyl residue into the tunnel. During termination, an OH-group from a water molecule is the acceptor rather than the amino group of an aminoacyl-tRNA, and if the reacting OH-group is similarly displaced from its normal position by the chloramphenicol, then the consequence would be an inhibition of the hydrolysis of the peptidyl-tRNA at termination.

Mechanisms of Bacterial Resistance

At least five different mechanisms of resistance against antibiotics can be distinguished, some of which have already been mentioned in the preceding section (or reviewed previously (22)).

1. Modification of the Antibiotic. This mechanism inactivates the compound or alternatively inhibits its transport into the cell. Examples of such inactivations are the acetylation of chloramphenicol and the ring cleavage of penicillin, the corresponding enzymes (acetyl transferase and β-lactamase, respectively) being encoded by plasmids. Examples of antibiotics with transport inhibition activity are the aminoglycosides, which can be acetylated, phosphorylated or adenylated by enzymes located in the periplasmatic space (between the inner and outer membranes), thus rendering the transport of the antibiotic into the cell more difficult. These modifying enzymes are also plasmid-encoded.

2. Blockage of Antibiotic Transport without Modification. The tetracyclines are an example of antibiotics with this mechanism. Their transport is inhibited by the inducible, plasmid-encoded "tet"-proteins via a mechanism which is not yet clear. Another case is that of fusidic acid, resistance to which can be caused by an impermeability of the cell.

3. Alteration of the Target Site of the Antibiotic. In most cases the cause of resistance is a strongly reduced binding of the antibiotic. The simplest situation is an alteration in the binding component, as is seen with EF-Tu and EF-G (resistance against kirromycin or fusidic acid, respectively). Another possibility is the loss of a component important for the binding of the antibiotic, as in the case of protein L11 and thiostrepton resistance. Not only altered proteins but also alterations in the RNA can confer resistance, several examples of which have already been mentioned, e.g. the mutations causing chloramphenicol resistance, the undermethylation in the case of kasugamycin, and the overmethylation with erythromycin.

Indirect changes of the binding site, i.e., cooperative effects via a change in a ribosomal component which is not itself part of the binding site, are more common than direct changes. One example is the resistance against streptomycin, where an alteration in protein S12 strongly reduces the binding capacity of the drug although the antibiotic does not bind to S12 but probably to proteins S3 and S5 in the small subunit. The existence of such cooperative effects is clearly demonstrated by resistance against one and the same antibiotic conferred by alterations in different components. Examples already mentioned are the resistance against erythromycin, which can be generated by alterations in proteins L4 and L22 or by overmethylation of 23S RNA, or resistance against viomycin, which can be conferred by an altered RNA in either subunit. An extreme example, which illustrates the extent to which the ribosome must be regarded as a dynamic reactor rather than a rigid matrix, is provided by the case of a streptomycin-dependent mutant (i.e. a cell that can grow only in the presence of the drug). This mutant contains both an altered protein S12 and an altered S8, and the phenotype can be changed to one of streptomycin independence by a third alteration in the ribosome. Astonishingly, the third alteration can reside in a large number of the 50 ribosomal proteins, regardless whether they are from the small or the large subunit. This observation played an important role in the genetic mapping of some ribosomal protein loci on the *Escherichia coli* chromosome (23).

4. Bypassing or Replacement of the Inhibited Reaction. Trimethoprim and the sulfonamides are known examples of antibiotics possessing this mechanism and a special case is the a priori resistance of species which do not carry out the inhibited reaction at all. The penicillins, which inhibit the synthesis of the bacterial cell wall by disturbing a late reaction during the biosynthesis of peptidoglycan, are another important example. A resistance against penicillin, which could not be traced back to any β-lactamase activity, is probably due to the incorporation of another component into the cell wall instead of peptidoglycan, thus bypassing the synthesis of peptidoglycans.

5. Overproduction of the Inhibited Substrate. This represents a "titration" of the antibiotic, and again trimethoprim is an example of an antibiotic with this mechanism. This drug inhibits folic acid metabolism by inhibiting the dihydrofolate reductase, which is essential for the cell. The affinity of the bacterial enzyme for the drug is about 60,000-fold larger than that of the mammalian enzyme, and this selective toxicity is the basis of the successful application of the antibiotic in medicine. In some cases resistance against trimethoprim was found to be due to a strong overproduction of the dihydrofolate reductase (24).

Conclusions

The elucidation of the structure, the analysis of the function, and the study of the inhibition patterns of antibiotics support and complement each other. A detailed knowledge of ribosome structure is a prerequisite for a molecular explanation of its function. An analysis of the function helps in understanding which parts of the structure are more or less important and is in turn a prerequisite for understanding the inhibition mechanisms of the antibiotics. Finally, the antibiotics themselves are not only the objects of functional analyses, but are themselves useful tools for functional analysis.

Acknowledgements

We thank J. Belart and E. Philippi for help and support and Dr. T. P. Hausner for discussions and advice.

References

1. **Hardesty, B., Kramer, G.** (ed.): Structure, function and genetics of ribosomes. Springer-Verlag, Heidelberg, 1986.
2. **Held, W. A., Ballou, B., Mizushima, S., Nomura, M.:** Assembly mapping of 30S ribosomal proteins from *Escherichia coli*: further studies. Journal of Biological Chemistry 1974, 249: 3103–3111.
3. **Herold, M., Nierhaus, K. H.:** Incorporation of six additional proteins to complete the assembly map of 50S subunit from *Escherichia coli* ribosomes. Journal of Biological Chemistry 1987, 262: 8826–8833.
4. **Stöffler, G., Stöffler-Meilicke, M.:** Immuno electron microscopy on *Escherichia coli* ribosomes. In: Hardesty, B., Kramer, G. (ed.): Structure, function, and genetics of ribosomes. Springer-Verlag, Heidelberg 1986, p. 28–46.
5. **Yonath, A., Leonard, K. R., Wittmann, H. G.:** A tunnel in the large ribosomal subunit revealed by three-dimensional image reconstruction. Science 1987, 236: 813–816.
6. **Capel, M. S., Engelman, D. M., Freeborn, B. R., Kjeldgaard, M., Langer, J. A., Ramakrishnan, V., Schindler, D. G., Schneider, D. K., Schoenborn, B. P., Sillers, I.-Y., Yabuki, S., Moore, P. B.:** A complete mapping of the proteins in the small ribosomal subunit of *Escherichia coli*. Science 1987, 238: 1403–1406.
7. **Schüler, D., Brimacombe, R.:** The *Escherichia coli* 30S ribosomal subunit; an optimized three-dimensional fit between the ribosomal proteins and the 16S RNA. EMBO Journal 1988, 7: 1509–1513.
8. **Nierhaus, K. H., Rheinberger, H.-J.:** An alternative model for the elongation cycle of protein biosynthesis. Trends in Biochemical Sciences 1984, 9: 428–432.
9. **Rheinberger, H.-J., Nierhaus, K. H.:** Allosteric interactions between the ribosomal transfer RNA-binding sites A and E. Journal of Biological Chemistry 1986, 261: 9133–9139.
10. **Rheinberger, H.-J., Sternbach, H., Nierhaus, K. H.:** Codon-anticodon interaction at the ribosomal E site. Journal of Biological Chemistry 1986, 261: 9140–9143.

11. Vazquez, D.: Inhibition of protein biosynthesis. Springer-Verlag, Berlin, 1979.
12. Gale, E. F., Cundliffe, E., Reynolds, P. E., Richmond, M. H., Waring, M. J.: The molecular basis of antibiotic action. Wiley, New York, 1981, p. 402–547.
13. Nierhaus, K. H., Wittmann, H. G.: Ribosomal function and its inhibition by antibiotics in prokaryotes. Naturwissenschaften 1980, 67: 234–250.
14. Geigenmüller, U., Nierhaus, K. H.: Tetracycline can inhibit tRNA binding to the ribosomal P-site as well as to the A-site. European Journal of Biochemistry 1986, 161: 723–726.
15. Modolell, J., Cabrer, B., Parmeggiani, A., Vazquez, D.: Inhibition by viomycin and thiostrepton of both aminoacyl-tRNA and factor G binding to ribosomes. Proceedings of the National Academy of Sciences of USA 1971, 68: 1796–1800.
16. Hausner, T.-P., Atmadja, J., Nierhaus, K. H.: Evidence that the G2661 region of 23S rRNA is located at the ribosomal binding sites of both elongation factors. Biochimie 1987, 69: 911–923.
17. Moazed, D., Noller, H. F.: Interaction of antibiotics with functional sites in 16S ribosomal RNA. Nature 1987, 327: 389–394.
18. Hausner, T.-P., Geigenmüller, U., Nierhaus, K. H.: The allosteric three-site model for the ribosomal elongation cycle: New insights into the inhibition mechanism of aminoglycosides, thiostrepton, and viomycin. Journal of Biological Chemistry 1988, in press.
19. Cundliffe, E.: On the nature of antibiotic binding sites in ribosomes. Biochimie 1987, 69: 863–869.
20. Nicholson, A. W., Hall, C. C., Strycharz, W. A., Cooperman, B. S.: Photoaffinity labelling of *Escherichia coli* ribosomes by an aryl azide analogue of puromycin. On the identification of the major covalently labelled ribosomal proteins and on the mechanism of photo-incorporation. Biochemistry 1982, 21: 3797–3808.
21. Ettayebi, M., Prasad, S. M., Morgan, E. A.: Chloramphenicol-erythromycin resistance mutations in a 23S rRNA gene of *Escherichia coli*. Journal of Bacteriology 1985, 162: 551–557.
22. Davies, J., Smith, D. I.: Plasmid-determined resistance to antimicrobial agents. Annual Reviews in Microbiology 1978, 32: 469–518.
23. Dabbs, E. R.: Mutational alterations in 50S proteins of the *Escherichia coli* ribosome. Molecular and General Genetics 1978, 165: 73–78.
24. McCuen, R. W., Sirotnak, F. M.: Hyperproduction of dihydrofolate reductase in *Diplococcus pneumoniae* by mutation in the structural gene. Biochimica et Biophysica Acta 1974, 338: 540–544.

Inhibition of DNA Gyrase: Bacterial Sensitivity and Clinical Resistance to 4-Quinolones

M. E. Cullen[1], A. W. Wyke[2], F. McEachern[1], C. A. Austin[1], L. M. Fisher[1]*

DNA gyrase catalyzes ATP-dependent supercoiling of DNA and is essential for bacterial DNA replication and other DNA transactions. Synthetic antibacterial 4-quinolones inhibit DNA gyrase in vitro and rapidly block DNA synthesis in vivo. Mechanistic studies on *Escherichia coli* gyrase indicate that quinolones interrupt DNA breakage and reunion via the A subunits of the tetrameric A_2B_2 gyrase complex. To gain deeper insight into quinolone action in the clinical setting, clinical isolates of *Escherichia coli* highly resistant to nalidixic acid and the new fluoroquinolones were studied. Gyrase A protein purified from several of these uropathogenic isolates was shown to generate a quinolone-resistant DNA supercoiling activity when reconstituted with purified gyrase B subunit. Drug-resistant gyrase A protein examined from one clinical strain was the same size as its quinolone sensitive gyrase A counterpart. These observations suggest that point mutation of the gyrase A protein may often be implicated in high level clinical resistance to 4-quinolones. The nature of these drug-resistant mutations is discussed with regard to current knowledge of quinolone action.

Recent interest in inhibitors of bacterial DNA replication as anti-infective agents has centered on the so called 4-quinolones (Figure 1a), and to a lesser degree, on the coumarin class of drugs (Figure 1b) (1, 2). The prototypic agents, nalidixic acid and novobiocin, were known inhibitors of DNA synthesis and were used clinically before their putative target, the bacterial enzyme DNA gyrase, was discovered by M. Gellert and colleagues in 1976 (3). Development of yet more potent and wider spectrum derivatives has continued apace with the introduction of the new fluoroquinolones such as ofloxacin, norfloxacin and ciprofloxacin. In contrast to nalidixic acid, originally used for urinary tract infections, the newer agents hold promise for treating systemic infections. Whereas oxolinic acid, norfloxacin and ciprofloxacin are true quinolones in the chemical sense, other derivatives are not; for example, nalidixic acid and enoxacin are strictly naphthyridines (Figure 1). However, for the sake of simplicity the collective term 4-quinolones is used in this report. Despite structural differences, 4-quinolones are all thought to act by blocking DNA snythesis through the inhibition of DNA gyrase (4-6).

Gyrase, bacterial toposiomerase II, catalyzes ATP-dependent negative supercoiling of DNA (3). The enzyme acts in concert with the DNA relaxing enzyme, DNA topoisomerase I, to maintain the supercoiled state of the bacterial chromosome (7). Gyrase is essential for bacterial growth and through DNA supercoiling plays a key role in DNA replication, recombination, transcription and repair, and in the differential control of gene expression (8, 9). Mechanistic studies have shown that gyrase acts by introducing a transient double-stranded DNA break within a 120–150 base pair DNA segment wrapped on the outside of the enzyme, and passing a second DNA segment through the break which is then resealed (10–15). The two A subunits of the A_2B_2 gyrase complex catalyze DNA breakage and reunion whereas the B subunits bind and hydrolyze ATP (16, 17). The presence of both subunits is required for enzyme activity.

The functional difference between the A and B subunits is highlighted in their interaction with gyrase inhibitors. Coumarins, e.g. novobiocin, inhibit ATP hydrolysis and act on the B subunit (18, 19). Quinolones interfere with enzymatic DNA breakage-reunion and act on the A subunit (4). Addition of detergent to DNA gyrase-DNA complexes formed in the presence of a quinolone, e.g. oxolinic acid, generates site-specific double-stranded DNA breaks, each 5′ DNA end of which becomes covalently linked to an A subunit via tyrosine 122 (4, 12, 20, 21). These sites are putative locations on DNA where

---

[1] Department of Biochemistry, St. George's Hospital Medical School, University of London, Cranmer Terrace, London SW17 0RE, UK.
[2] Department of Microbial Biochemistry, Glaxo Group Research, Greenford Road, Greenford, Middlesex UB6 0HE, UK.

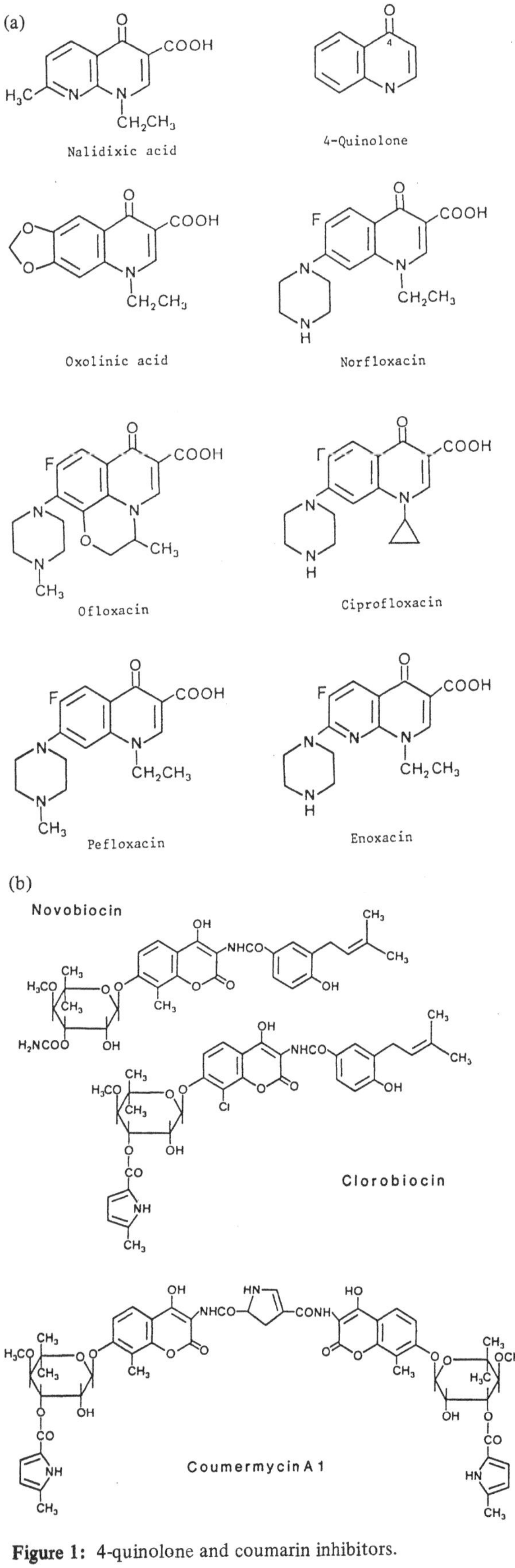

Figure 1: 4-quinolone and coumarin inhibitors.

gyrase catalyzes DNA supercoiling. Consequently they have been intensively studied by DNA sequencing, DNase I footprinting and site-directed mutagenesis approaches (12–15, 20, 22, 23). The molecular mechanism by which quinolones inhibit DNA supercoiling and promote DNA cleavage by gyrase is poorly understood.

Exposure of *Escherichia coli* to either the coumarins or the quinolone oxolinic acid causes rapid inhibition of DNA synthesis (24–26). For coumermycin A_1, this is accompanied by a concommitant loss of chromosomal DNA supercoiling and pleoitropic biological effects (27). Moderate levels of oxolinic acid, however, do not induce chromosomal relaxation and the hypothesis has been advanced that inhibition of DNA synthesis arises from the trapping of gyrase complexes ahead of DNA replication forks (28). Consistent with this view is the fact that inhibition of DNA synthesis was not observed in an *Escherichia coli* strain carrying the *nal* A (*gyr* A) mutation conferring high level resistance to nalidixic acid and oxolinic acid (24, 25). It is not clear how inhibition of DNA replication results in the bactericidal effects of quinolones. Possible mechanisms include the production of double-strand DNA breaks and/or the induction of DNA repair pathways such as the SOS response (29). Indeed, for some derivatives, cell killing appears to require active protein synthesis (1).

One approach to elucidating the mechanism of quinolones at both the cellular and the local molecular level is to study quinolone resistance. For laboratory strains of *Escherichia coli* (30–35) and other bacterial strains (36–39), resistance has been mapped to a large number of different chromosomal loci. However, comparatively little clinically relevant work has been reported (40). Here we describe biochemical, enzymological and genetic studies on DNA gyrase in uropathogenic *Escherichia coli* strains resistant to nalidixic acid and other quinolones.

Materials and Methods

Strains. Nalidixic acid resistant clinical isolates of *Escherichia coli* from patients with urinary tract infections were very kindly provided by Dr. Laura Piddock (41). Quinolone-sensitive *Escherichia coli* strains RW1053 [*rec* AΔ (*bio att gal*)], N4186 and MK47 were from Dr. Martin Gellert. Strain N4186 is RW1053 containing the quinolone-sensitive *gyr* A gene cloned in a expression plasmid (42). MICs were determined by the broth dilution method using microtitre plates with an inoculum of 2×10^4 cells per well. Cultures were scored for turbidity either visually or by using a Titertek Multiskan (Flow Laboratories, UK) microtitre plate reader. Similar results were obtained with both methods.

Purification of Escherichia coli Gyrase A and B Subunits. Gyrase A protein was partially purified from clinical isolates or N4186 by a modification of the method of Mizuuchi et al. (42). Ten litre batches of cells were grown in L-broth to late log phase ($OD_{600} \sim 1.5$). The cells were harvested by centrifugation, washed in 50 mM Tris-HCl, pH 8, 10 % glycerol, 1 mM dithiothreitol, resuspended in 50 mM Tris-HCl, pH 7.5, containing 10 % (w/v) sucrose (0.4–0.5 g of wet cells per ml) and frozen in liquid nitrogen prior to storage at $-70\,°C$. Cells were thawed, lysed with lysozyme, and gyrase A protein was isolated by fractionation on Polymin P, ammonium sulphate precipitation and ion exchange chromatography on DEAE-Sepharose essentially as described (42). Two minor modifications from the Mizuuchi procedure were (a) the Polymin P precipitate was washed twice with 0.45 M NaCl to release bound gyrase A protein, and (b) Polymin P pellets were resuspended in one-tenth of the suggested volumes (42). For DNA cleavage experiments, gyrase A protein was purified as follows. Crude cell lysates prepared as above were loaded onto a 500 µl novobiocin-Sepharose column (43). Gyrase A protein was eluted with 1 M KCl in 50 mM Tris-HCl, pH 7.5, 10 % glycerol, 1 mM EDTA and 5 mM dithiothreitol. The resulting A subunit was > 90 % pure and was free from endonuclease activity. Gyrase B protein was purified from the overproducing strain MK47 (42).

DNA Supercoiling by Gyrase: Inhibition by 4-Quinolones. DNA supercoiling activity was assayed by the method of Gellert et al. (3). Fractions containing partially purified gyrase A protein (1–2 units) were preincubated with excess gyrase B subunit and assayed using relaxed plasmid pBR322 DNA as substrate in the absence or presence of serial dilutions of quinolone drugs. One unit of gyrase activity resulted in supercoiling of 50 % of the relaxed pBR322 substrate in 30 min under the assay conditions. For inhibition studies, peak fractions from the DEAE-Sepharose columns were used (see preceding section). Reactions were stopped by the addition of 0.25 volumes of loading dye (0.025 % bromophenol blue, 5 % sodium dodecyl sulphate, 25 % glycerol). Samples were electrophoresed in 0.8 % agarose gels at 40 V overnight in electrophoresis buffer containing 89 mM Tris, 89 mM boric acid and 2.5 mM Na_3EDTA. Gels were stained for one hour with ethidium bromide (1 µg/ml of electrophoresis buffer) and photographed under UV light using Polaroid film.

DNA Cleavage by DNA Gyrase. The ability of gyrase A subunit preparations to mediate quinolone-dependent DNA cleavage when complemented with gyrase B protein was assayed according to Fisher et al. (23). Reactions contained 25 units each of the gyrase A and B subunits, and 600 ng of supercoiled pBR322 DNA in a 35 µl final assay volume. DNA breakage was induced by addition of sodium dodecyl sulphate, and following proteinase K treatment, DNA samples were electrophoresed and analysed on 0.8 % agarose gels as described for the DNA supercoiling assay (23).

Immunological Characterization of Gyrase A Protein. Western blot analysis of gyrase A protein purified from clinical strains was carried out as follows. Proteins were electrophoresed on duplicate 10 % polyacrylamide/sodium dodecyl sulphate gels. One gel was stained with Coomassie Brilliant Blue while proteins on the second gel were transferred onto nitrocellulose (Schleicher and Schuell) using a semi-dry electro-blotter (Sartorius Sartoblot II, Sartorius Instruments, UK) according to the manufacturer's instructions. Immunostaining was performed at room temperature using a rabbit polyclonal antiserum raised against *Escherichia coli* gyrase A protein and a goat (antirabbit IgG)-horseradish peroxidase conjugate (BioRad Immuno-Blot, GAR-HRP, Biorad Laboratories, UK) according to the manufacturer's instructions.

Results

Quinolone-Resistant Clinical Isolates of Escherichia coli

Eight nalidixic acid resistant clinical isolates of *Escherichia coli* (41) were examined for susceptibility to various quinolones (Table 1). The isolates exhibited a range of nalidixic acid resistance when compared to the sensitive *Escherichia coli* K12 strain RW1053. Strains 218 and 227 showed particularly high nalidixic acid resistance. Interestingly, all eight uropathogenic strains were cross-resistant to the other quinolones that were tested (Table 1). In contrast, when sensitivities to gentamycin or ceftazidime were examined, most of the strains exhibited wild-type sensitivity. As gentamycin and ceftazidime have killing mechanisms different from quinolones, it seems likely that the observed resistance to quinolones was not due to permeability changes. These results suggest the possibility that high level quinolone resistance might arise from mutations in the *gyr* A gene for DNA gyrase.

Table 1: Drug sensitivity profiles for eight nalidixic acid resistant clinical isolates of *Escherichia coli* compared with sensitive strain RW1053.

Strain	Nalidixic acid	Norfloxacin	Ofloxacin	Pefloxacin	Enoxacin	Ciprofloxacin	Ceftazidime	Gentamycin
RW1053	4	0.03	0.015	0.03	0.03	0.004	0.13	1
227	500	1	1	1	2	0.25	0.25	2
58	64	2	1	1	2	0.5	0.13	0.5
158	64	1	0.5	1	2	0.25	0.13	0.5
202	31	0.5	0.25	0.5	1	0.06	0.5	1
218	>1000	4	2	4	8	1	0.25	2
231	31	1	1	1	2	0.25	0.06	0.5
233	125	1	1	1	2	0.25	0.13	1
235	62	2	1	1	4	0.25	0.5	1

Properties of Gyrase A Protein Purified from Clinical Strains

Strains 227, 202 and 58 were chosen for further study. Isolate 227 was derived from a patient treated with enoxacin for an *Escherichia coli* urinary tract infection and was initially quinolone-sensitive. After the course of treatment (2 × 200 mg daily for five days), the strain was resistant to enoxacin. In fact, strain 227 is ~ 100-fold more resistant to enoxacin than sensitive *Escherichia coli*. Unlike strain 218 which grew very poorly, 227 was almost as highly resistant and showed good growth characteristics. The other strains, 202 and 58, were included as they display intermediate levels of resistance.

Gyrase A protein was purified from sensitive and resistant bacteria by the same procedure involving Polymin P and ammonium sulphate precipitation followed by chromatography on DEAE-Sepharose. Peak fractions from the column were free of the gyrase B protein and of nuclease activity and could be complemented with purified gyrase B subunit to reconstitute DNA gyrase activity. A DNA supercoiling assay (Figure 2) was used to examine the quinolone sensitivity of gyrase reconstituted using gyrase A subunit purified from strain 227 (lanes j–r) or from the sensitive K12 strain N4186 (lanes a–i). By including twofold increments in enoxacin concentration, it can be seen that supercoiling by drug-sensitive gyrase was 50 % inhibited (ID50) at ~ 0.5 µg/ml of enoxacin (compare lanes f and i). However, supercoiling activity reconstituted with 227 gyrase A subunit was inhibited only at very high enoxacin concentrations, around 64 µg/ml (compare lanes k and r). These results establish that 227 produces a highly enoxacin-resistant gyrase A protein. The response of strain 227 gyrase A protein to other quinolones was also compared to the drug-sensitive A subunit using the DNA supercoiling assay. The results are summarized in Table 2. Clearly, the DNA supercoiling activity generated using 227 gyrase A protein was resistant to each quinolone examined.

To determine whether changes in the gyrase A protein were a feature of other quinolone-resistant strains, we carried out a more limited study of strains

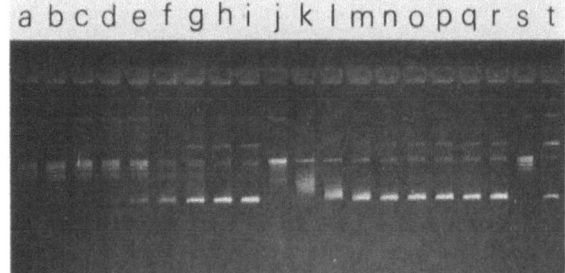

Figure 2: DNA supercoiling activity, reconstituted using gyrase A protein from clinical strain 227, showing high resistance to inhibition by enoxacin. Purified gyrase A protein (2 units) from quinolone-sensitive strain N4186 (a–i) or strain 227 (j–r) was complemented with excess gyrase B protein and DNA supercoiling activity was assayed in the absence and presence of enoxacin. Reactions contained relaxed pBR322 DNA (0.4 µg) and enoxacin at the following concentrations: 16, 8, 4, 2, 1, 0.5, 0.25, 0.12 µg/ml (lanes a–h), and at 125, 64, 32, 16, 8, 4, 2, 1 µg/ml (lanes j–q). No drug was included in lanes i and r. Relaxed and supercoiled pBR322 DNA markers are shown in lanes s and t, respectively.

202 and 58. Figure 3 compares nalidixic acid and norfloxacin inhibition of DNA supercoiling utilizing sensitive gyrase A protein (top wells) and strain 202 gyrase A subunit (bottom wells), reconstituted with wild-type gyrase B protein. For nalidixic acid (lanes a–g), the ID50 for the sensitive and 202 subunits are 32 µg/ml (compare top lanes f and g) and ~ 125 µg/ml (compare bottom lanes d and g), respectively. A similar analysis for norfloxacin (lanes i–o) gave ID50s of ~ 0.5 µg/ml and 4 µg/ml for sensitive and 202 subunit supercoiling assays, respectively. Results for gyrase A protein from strain 58 were similar and are given in Table 2. Thus, three independent clinical isolates appear to contain an altered gyrase A subunit responsible for conferring cross-resistance to quinolones.

Further Characterization of Strain 227 Quinolone-Resistant Gyrase A Protein

Affinity chromatography of 227 gyrase A protein on novobiocin-Sepharose was used to obtain a highly

Table 2: Quinolone concentrations causing 50 % inhibition (ID50) of DNA supercoiling by gyrase A proteins from clinical strains when assayed using excess gyrase B protein under standard conditions.

Strain		ID50 (µg/ml)				
		Norfloxacin	Ofloxacin	Pefloxacin	Ciprofloxacin	Enoxacin
N4186 (*gyr* A w.t.)	32	0.5	< 4	< 8	2	0.5
227	250	64	32	64	16	64
202	125	4	ND	ND	ND	ND
58	125	> 8	ND	ND	ND	ND

ND = not determined.

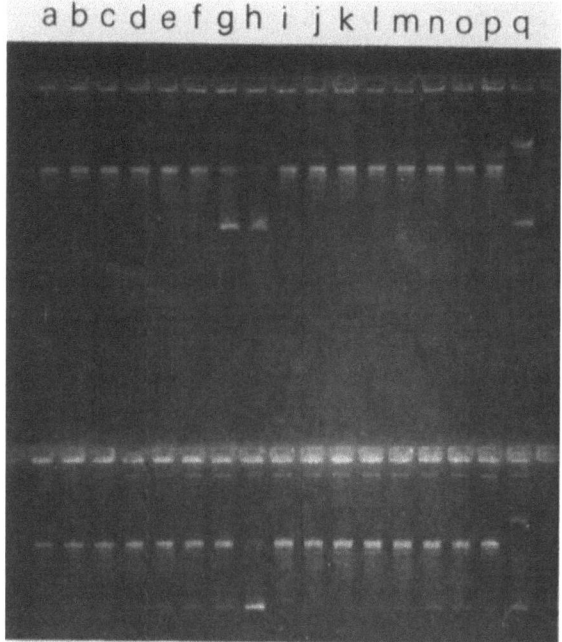
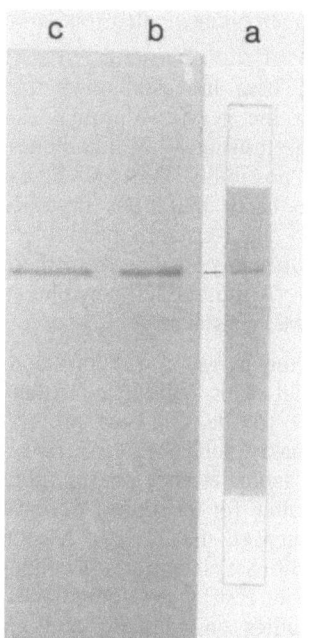

Figure 3: Gyrase A protein from clinical strain 202 is resistant to inhibition by both nalidixic acid and norfloxacin. DNA supercoiling activity was assayed in the presence of excess gyrase B protein as described in Figure 2. Reactions in top wells contained quinolone-sensitive gyrase A subunit (strain N4186); bottom wells, strain 202 gyrase A protein. In each case, lanes a–f contained nalidixic acid at 1000, 500, 250, 125, 64, 32 µg/ml; lane g contained no drug addition; lanes i–o contained norfloxacin at 64, 32, 16, 8, 4, 2, 1 µg/ml. Relaxed and supercoiled pBR322 DNA markers are included in lanes p and h, q, respectively.

Figure 4: Gel electrophoresis (a) and Western blot analysis (b) of gyrase A protein purified from strain 227. Ten percent polyacrylamide-SDS gels were run and either stained with Coomassie Blue (a) or Western blotted (b, c) using a rabbit anti-gyrase A antiserum. Lane c contained purified wild-type gyrase A protein.

purified preparation. Electrophoresis in polyacrylamide/SDS gels showed that the preparation contained essentially a single major band of relative molecular weight 97,000 that comigrated with authentic purified gyrase A protein from N4186 (Figure 4a). Western blot analysis using an anti-gyrase A protein rabbit polyclonal antiserum showed that the 97 kDa band was indeed gyrase A protein (Figure 4b, c). These observations establish that the gyrase A protein in strain 227 did not apparently undergo major structural alteration. The availability of highly purified 227 gyrase A protein enabled us to test whether it promoted quinolone-mediated DNA cleavage when incubated with gyrase B subunit and plasmid DNA, as would be expected with drug-sensitive gyrase (4, 23). Using 5 µg/ml of enoxacin, no DNA breakage could be demonstrated (data not shown). Thus both DNA supercoiling and DNA breakage activities of the 227 gyrase A protein are refractory to quinolones.

Discussion

Previous studies of quinolone resistance in bacteria have been restricted almost entirely to laboratory strains. Thus, genetic studies of spontaneous nalidixic acid- and norfloxacin-resistant mutants of *Escherichia coli* have implicated several chromosomal genes (30, 31, 34, 35). Low level resistance has been mapped to a number of loci including *omp* F (permeability) (35) and *gyr* B (44). High level resistance has been linked to the *gyr* A locus (4, 35). However, these studies are not necessarily informative about the mechanism of clinical resistance.

We have now shown conclusively that the gyrase A subunit is often implicated in high level clinical resistance to quinolones in uropathogenic strains. Eight nalidixic acid resistant strains (Table 1) were all found to exhibit high level cross-resistance to a collection of different quinolones. When the gyrase A protein was purified from several of these strains, it reconstituted a quinolone-resistant DNA supercoiling activity when gyrase B subunit was added (Table 2). Moreover, the supercoiling activity was also cross-resistant to other quinolones. As expected, the newer quinolones were more potent than nalidixic acid in inhibiting bacterial growth. This difference was also mirrored by the susceptibility of gyrase to inhibition in vitro (Table 2). However, in general much higher levels of quinolones were required to inhibit DNA supercoiling in vitro compared to the bacterial MICs.

The approach followed here has established that mutational alteration of the gyrase A protein can be important in clinical resistance to quinolones. We cannot exclude the possibility that the clinical isolates we studied also carry mutations in other genes that contribute to the resistance phenotype. However, for strain 227 it seems possible from these and other results that gyr A mutation(s) contributes the majority of the observed resistance.

We have characterized the gyrase A subunit from strain 227 in some detail. This quinolone-resistant protein is similar in size to the wild-type protein. This suggests that no major polypeptide rearrangement has occurred and indicates that one or more point changes are responsible for resistance. We have recently cloned and sequenced the 227 gyr A gene and shown that residue 83 (Ser) is important in conferring clinical sensitivity or resistance to quinolones. Interestingly, genetic studies on nalidixic acid resistant laboratory strains of *Escherichia coli* have also implicated residue 83 in high level resistance (45). Thus, the nature of mutations in gyr A responsible for drug resistance is now being uncovered. Mutations in the gyrase B subunit conferring low level resistance have also been described (46).

The molecular mechanism by which quinolones inhibit DNA gyrase is at present unknown. The drugs could bind directly to the enzyme. Alternatively, gyrase could recognize quinolone molecules bound to DNA as suggested by Shen and Pernet (47) and others (48). In either case, mutations in gyrase giving rise to quinolone resistance could conceivably exert an effect by reducing binding of the drug to the enzyme. Clearly, investigation of the enzymatic properties of quinolone-resistant gyrase subunits promises to play an important role in revealing the mode of action of antibacterial quinolone agents.

Acknowledgements

We thank Drs. Laura Piddock and Marty Gellert for strains and Dr. Mike Hayes for helpful discussion. This work was supported by SERC-CASE and Cooperative awards (jointly with Glaxo), by a postdoctoral fellowship under the SERC Molecular Recognition Initiative, by an SERC postgraduate studentship and by a Douglas Hems Memorial award.

References

1. **Smith, J. T.:** The 4-quinolone antibacterials. Pharmaceutical Journal 1984, 233: 299–305.
2. **Fisher, L. M.:** DNA gyrase and the mode of action of 4-quinolone antibacterial agents. Fortschritte der Antimikrobiellen und Antineoplastischen Chemotherapie 1987, Band 6–10, 1585–1589.
3. **Gellert, M., Mizuuchi, K., O'Dea, M. H., Nash, H. A.:** DNA gyrase: an enzyme that introduces superhelical turns into DNA. Proceedings of the National Academy of Sciences USA 1976, 73: 3872–3876.
4. **Gellert, M., Mizuuchi, K., O'Dea, M. H., Itoh, T., Tomizawa, J.-I.:** Nalidixic acid resistance: a second genetic character involved in DNA gyrase activity. Proceedings of the National Academy of Sciences USA 1977, 74: 4772–4776.
5. **Bourgignon, G. J., Levitt, M., Sternglanz, R.:** Studies on the mechanism of action of nalidixic acid. Antimicrobial Agents and Chemotherapy 1973, 4: 479–486.
6. **Goss, W. A., Deitz, W. H., Cook, T. M.:** Mechanism of action of nalidixic acid. Journal of Bacteriology 1965, 89: 1068–1074.
7. **Menzel, R., Gellert, M.:** Regulation of the genes for *Escherichia coli* DNA gyrase: homeostatic control of DNA supercoiling. Cell 1983, 34: 105–113.
8. **Gellert, M.:** DNA topoisomerases. Annual Reviews of Biochemistry 1981, 50: 879–910.
9. **Wang, J. C.:** DNA topoisomerases. Annual Reviews of Biochemistry 1985, 54: 665–697.
10. **Brown, P. O., Cozzarelli, N. R.:** A sign inversion mechanism for enzymatic supercoiling of DNA. Science 1979, 206: 1081–1083.
11. **Mizuuchi, K., Fisher, L. M., O'Dea, M. H., Gellert, M.:** DNA gyrase action involves the introduction of transient double-strand breaks into the DNA. Proceedings of the National Academy of Sciences USA 1980, 77: 1847–1851.
12. **Fisher, L. M., Mizuuchi, K., O'Dea, M. H., Ohmori, H., Gellert, M.:** Site-specific interaction of DNA gyrase with DNA. Proceedings of the National Academy of Sciences USA 1981, 78: 4165–4169.
13. **Liu, L. F., Wang, J. C.:** *Micrococcus luteus* gyrase: active components and a model for its supercoiling of DNA. Proceedings of the National Academy of Sciences USA 1978, 75: 2098–2102.
14. **Morrison, A., Cozzarelli, N. R.:** Contacts between DNA gyrase and its binding site on DNA. Proceedings of the National Academy of Sciences USA 1981, 78: 1416–1420.
15. **Kirkegaard, K., Wang, J. C.:** Mapping the topography of DNA wrapped around gyrase by nucleolytic and chemical probing of complexes of unique DNA sequences. Cell 1981, 23: 721–729.
16. **Higgins, N. P., Peebles, C. L., Sugino, A., Cozzarelli, N. R.:** Purification of subunits of *Escherichia coli* DNA gyrase and reconstitution of enzymic activity. Proceedings of the National Academy of Sciences USA 1978, 75: 1773–1777.
17. **Mizuuchi, K., O'Dea, M. H., Gellert, M.:** DNA gyrase: subunit structure and ATPase activity of the purified enzyme. Proceedings of the National Academy of Sciences USA 1978, 75: 5960–5963.
18. **Gellert, M., O'Dea, M. H., Itoh, T., Tomizawa, J. C.:** Novobiocin and coumermycin inhibit DNA supercoiling catalyzed by DNA gyrase. Proceedings of the National Academy of Sciences USA 1976, 73: 4474–4478.
19. **Sugino, A., Higgins, N. P., Brown, P. O., Peebles, C. L., Cozzarelli, N. R.:** Energy coupling in DNA gyrase and the mechanism of action of novobiocin. Proceedings of the National Academy of Sciences USA 1978, 75: 4838–4842.
20. **Morrison, A., Cozzarelli, N. R.:** Site specific cleavage of DNA by *Escherichia coli* DNA gyrase. Cell 1979, 17: 175–184.

21. Horowitz, D. S., Wang, J. C.: Mapping the active site tyrosine of *Escherichia coli* DNA gyrase. Journal of Biological Chemistry 1987, 262: 5339–5344.
22. Lockshon, D., Morris, D. R.: Sites of reaction of *Escherichia coli* DNA gyrase on pBR322 in vivo as revealed by oxolinic acid-induced plasmid linearisation. Journal of Molecular Biology 1985, 181: 63–74.
23. Fisher, L. M., Barot, H. A., Cullen, M. E.: DNA gyrase complex with DNA: determinants for site-specific DNA breakage. EMBO Journal 1986, 5: 1411–1418.
24. Crumplin, G. C., Smith, J. T.: Nalidixic acid and bacterial chromosome replication. Nature 1976, 260: 643–645.
25. Snyder, M., Drlica, K.: DNA gyrase on the bacterial chromosome: DNA cleavage induced by oxolinic acid. Journal of Molecular Biology 1979, 131: 287–302.
26. Ryan, M. J.: Coumermycin A_1; a preferential inhibitor of DNA synthesis in *Escherichia coli*. I. In vivo characterisation. Biochemistry 1976, 15: 3769–3777.
27. Drlica, K., Snyder, M.: Superhelical *Escherichia coli* DNA: relaxation by coumermycin. Journal of Molecular Biology 1978, 120: 145–154.
28. Drlica, K., Engle, E. C., Manes, S. H.: DNA gyrase on the bacterial chromosome: possibility of two levels of action. Proceedings of the National Academy of Sciences USA 1980, 77: 6879–6883.
29. Drlica, K.: Biology of deoxyribonucleic acid topoisomerases. Microbiological Reviews 1984, 48: 273–289.
30. Hane, M. W., Wood, T. H.: *Escherichia coli* K12 mutants resistant to nalidixic acid: genetic mapping and dominance studies. Journal of Bacteriology 1969, 99: 238–241.
31. Yamagishi, J., Furutani, Y., Ohue, T., Inoue, S., Nakamura, S., Shimizu, M.: New nalidixic acid resistance mutations related to deoxyribonucleic acid gyrase activity. Journal of Bacteriology 1981, 148: 450–458.
32. Tenney, J. H., Maack, R. W., Chippendale, G. R.: Rapid selection of organisms with increasing resistance on subinhibitory concentrations of norfloxacin in agar. Antimicrobial Agents and Chemotherapy 1983, 23: 188–189.
33. Sato, K., Inoue, Y., Fujii, T., Aoyama, H., Inoue, M., Mitsuhashi, S.: Purification and properties of DNA gyrase from a fluoroquinolone-resistant strain of *Escherichia coli*. Antimicrobial Agents and Chemotherapy 1986, 30: 777–780.
34. Hirai, K., Aoyama, H., Suzue, S., Irikura, T., Iyobe, S., Mitsuhashi, S.: Isolation and characterisation of norfloxacin-resistant mutants of *Escherichia coli* K12. Antimicrobial Agents and Chemotherapy 1986, 30: 248–253.
35. Hooper, D. C., Wolfson, J. S., Souza, K. S., Tung, C., McHugh, G. L., Swartz, M. N.: Genetic and biochemical characterisation of norfloxacin resistance in *Escherichia coli*. Antimicrobial Agents and Chemotherapy 1986, 29: 639–644.
36. Zweerink, M. M., Edison, A.: Inhibition of *Micrococcus luteus* DNA gyrase by norfloxacin and 10 other quinolone carboxylic acids. Antimicrobial Agents and Chemotherapy 1986, 29: 598–601.
37. Inoue, Y., Sato, K., Fujii, T., Hirai, K., Inoue, M., Iyobe, S., Mitsuhashi, S.: Some properties of subunits of DNA gyrase from *Pseudomonas aeruginosa* PAO1 and its nalidixic acid-resistant mutant. Journal of Bacteriology 1987, 169: 2322–2325.
38. Robillard, N. J., Scarpa, A. L.: Genetic and physiological characterisation of ciprofloxacin resistance in *Pseudomonas aeruginosa* PAO. Antimicrobial Agents and Chemotherapy 1988, 32: 535–539.
39. Aoyama, H., Sato, K., Fujii, T., Fujimaki, K., Inoue, M., Mitsuhashi, S.: Purification of *Citrobacter freundii* DNA gyrase and inhibition by quinolones. Antimicrobial Agents and Chemotherapy 1988, 32: 104–109.
40. Aoyama, H., Sato, K., Kato, T., Hirai, K., Mitsuhashi, S.: Norfloxacin resistance in a clinical isolate of *Escherichia coli*. Antimicrobial Agents and Chemotherapy 1987, 31: 1640–1641.
41. Piddock, L. J. V., Diver, J. M., Wise, R.: Cross-resistance of nalidixic acid resistant *Enterobacteriaceae* to new quinolones and other antimicrobials. European Journal of Clinical Microbiology and Infectious Diseases 1986, 5: 411–415.
42. Mizuuchi, K., Mizuuchi, M., O'Dea, M. H., Gellert, M.: Cloning and simplified purification of *Escherichia coli* gyrase A and B proteins. Journal of Biological Chemistry 1984, 259: 9199–9201.
43. Staudenbauer, W. C., Orr, E.: DNA gyrase: affinity chromatography on novobiocin-Sepharose and catalytic properties. Nucleic Acids Research 1981, 9: 3589–3603.
44. Inoue, S., Ohue, T., Yamagishi, J., Nakamura, S., Shimizu, M.: Mode of incomplete cross resistance among pipemidic, piromidic and nalidixic acids. Antimicrobial Agents and Chemotherapy 1978, 14: 240–245.
45. Yoshida, H., Kojima, T., Yamagishi, J., Nakamura, S.: Quinolone-resistant mutations of the *gyr* A gene of *Escherichia coli*. Molecular and General Genetics 1988, 211: 1–7.
46. Yamagashi, J., Yoshida, H., Yamayoshi, M., Nakamura, S.: Nalidixic acid-resistant mutations of the *gyr* B gene of *Escherichia coli*. Molecular and General Genetics 1986, 204: 367–373.
47. Shen, L. L., Pernet, A. G.: Mechanism of inhibition of DNA gyrase by analogues of nalidixic acid: the target of the drugs is DNA. Proceedings of the National Academy of Sciences USA 1985, 82: 307–311.
48. Tornaletti, S., Pedrini, A. M.: Studies on the interaction of 4-quinolones with DNA by DNA unwinding experiments. Biochemica et Biophysica Acta 1988, 949: 279–287.

Mechanisms of Nonbacterial
Anti-Infective Drugs

Mechanisms of Antoretroviral Compounds in Inhibition of Viral and Cellular DNA Polymerases

K. Ono[*]

> Many antiretroviral agents have been designed to target the reverse transcriptase molecule. Most if not all of these compounds have, however, some degree of in vitro cytotoxicity and/or in vivo side effects. Selectivity of an antiviral compound depends, at least in part, on its enzyme specificity for inhibition (i.e., different effectiveness for reverse transcriptase and host cell DNA polymerases). The inhibitory effects of various compounds, thus far proven to suppress reverse transcriptase, on the cellular DNA polymerases α, β and γ were examined. Many of these reverse transcriptase inhibitors were found to be more or less inhibitory to the host cell DNA polymerases as well. The results obtained by parallel testing of antiretroviral agents for the inhibition of eukaryotic DNA polymerases provide useful information about the selectivity of the compounds. Such findings also foster the modification of drug structures for improvement of the efficacies of antiviral potentials.

There are at least two kinds of retroviruses regarded as the causative agents of the current human infectious diseases adult T-cell leukemia (ATL) and acquired immune deficiency syndrome (AIDS). The causative viruses of ATL and AIDS have been designated as Human T-Lymphotropic Virus Type I (HTLV-I) and Human Immunodeficiency Virus (HIV), respectively. HTLV-I belongs to a group of oncoretroviruses that give rise to T-cell proliferation, whereas HIV is a member of the lentiretrovirus subfamily which destroys the host T-cells. Both ATL and AIDS have, however, a common feature in that after the virus infection there is a long latent period before clinical manifestations. In the case of HIV infection, various kinds of exogenous stimuli to the immune system, including viral and bacterial infections, seem to be necessary for the infection in seropositive persons to progress to a clinically evident state of immune deficiency. These stimuli may lead to viral gene activation with subsequent production of progeny viruses, creating cytopathic effects on the host $CD4^+$ cells. It is therefore especially important to suppress in vivo propagation of HIV in virus carriers with few or no clinical symptoms to prevent the development to AIDS.

Other than allopathic treatments toward intercurrent neoplasia (Kaposi's sarcoma) and/or opportunistic infections, there are at least two possible strategies on which chemotherapeutic approaches toward AIDS could be considered. These include (i) chemotherapy against the etiologic virus (HIV) with a drug(s) which has antiretroviral activity to block the replicative cycle of the virus, and (ii) reconstruction of the cellular immune system or activation of the immune functions by the use of biological response modifiers. In particular, interruption of the viral life cycle by treatment with an appropriate drug is a pre-requisite for the latter immunotherapy, because HIV is the primary cause of AIDS and reconstruction of the cellular immune system without prior antiviral treatment sometimes causes adverse effects. For these reasons, antiretroviral compounds have recently attracted special attention in the area of chemotherapeutic approaches to this serious viral disease.

It is thus obvious that the virus should be considered to be the primary target in the strategy of an adequate chemotherapy for AIDS (and probably for ATL, too), and one can easily imagine that there are several possible targets at various steps in the replicative cycle of the retroviruses. The main stages in the entire life cycle of the human pathogenic retroviruses and some of the potential targets for therapeutic intervention are summarized in Table 1.

Among the possible targets for antiretroviral agents, reverse transcriptase has long been considered to be the most attractive one, because the prominent difference between the replication cycle of the retrovirus and that of the host cell resides in the step of "reverse transcription" of the viral RNA to proviral DNA and the subsequent integration of the proviral DNA into host cell chromosomal DNA. A number of reverse transcriptase inhibitors have been described since discovery of RNA-directed DNA polymerase associated with retrovirus particles. Some of the representative inhibitors are classified by their in-

---

Laboratory of Viral Oncology, Aichi Cancer Center Research Institute, Chikusa-ku, Nagoya 464, Japan.

Table 1: Main stages in the replication cycle of human retroviruses and possible targets for chemotherapeutic intervention.

Stage	Example of potential target	Example of chemotherapeutic approach
Virus adsorption	gp120 of *env* protein	antibody to gp120
	virus receptor of the cell ($CD4^+$)	recombinant CD4
Reverse transcription	reverse transcriptase	enzyme inhibitors
Viral gene expression	viral mRNA	antisense oligodeoxynucleotide
	tat-III or art/trs protein	inhibitors
Viral component production	protease or glycosylase	inhibitors
Virus budding	assembly and budding process	interferon

Table 2: Inhibitors of reverse transcriptase.

Example of inhibitor	Inhibition mechanism
(I) Substrate or product analogues	
Arabinofuranosylnucleoside 5'-triphosphate (araNTP) (1, 2)	competition vs. corresponding dNTP[a]
2',3'-Dideoxynucleoside 5'-triphosphate (ddNTP) (3)	(i) competition vs. corresponding dNTP (ii) chain termination
Phosphonoformate (PFA) (4)	non-competition vs. dNTP & template·primer
(II) Template analogues	
2 and 2'-Substituted polynucleotide derivatives (5–8)	competition vs. template·primer
(III) Others	
Heteropolyanion	
5-tungsto-2-antimoniate (9)	competition vs. template·primer
21-tungsto-9-antimoniate (HPA23) (10)	competition vs. template·primer
Suramin[a] (11, 12)	competition vs. template·primer
Dye (Evans Blue, etc.)	competition vs. template·primer
Aurintricarboxylic acid	non-competition vs. dNTP & template·primer
Pyridoxal 5'-phosphate (13)	Schiff base formation with basic amino-acid(s) in active center of the enzyme (?)

[a]dNTP, 2'-deoxynucleoside 5'-triphosphate; suramin, hexasodium sym-bis(m-aminobenzoyl-m-amino-p-methylbenzoyl-l-naphthylamino-4,6,8-trisulfonate)carbamide.

hibition mechanisms and molecular targets in the reaction components of in vitro reverse transcription (Table 2). The inhibition mechanisms of these inhibitors will be presented and discussed later.

Reverse transcriptase is a DNA polymerase which catalyzes DNA snythesis on the RNA template by incorporating into the elongating DNA deoxynucleoside triphosphates, the bases of which are complementary to those of the template. In many points, however, the catalytic properties of reverse transcriptase are similar to those of host cell DNA polymerases. For this reason, almost all the inhibitors thus far proven to be effective to reverse transcriptase have also been found to be more or less inhibitory to cellular DNA polymerases; this may indicate one of the underlying mechanisms of these inhibitors which bring about in vitro cytotoxic effects as well as undesirable side effects in vivo. The purpose of this paper is to describe some of our findings on the enzyme selectivities of various antiretroviral compounds listed in Table 2, and to stress that parallel tests with both reverse transcriptase and cellular DNA polymerases are necessary for an exact evaluation of the inhibitory potential and selectivity of these antiretroviral compounds.

Materials and Methods

Chemicals. Various 2′, 3′-dideoxynucleoside 5′-triphosphates (ddNTP's; ddATP, ddCTP, ddGTP, ddTTP), $(rA)_n$, $(dT)_{12-18}$ and other poly- and oligo-nucleotides were obtained from P-L Biochemicals, USA. 3′-azido-2′,3′-dideoxythymidine 5′-triphosphate (AZTTP) was kind gift from Dr. M. Saneyoshi of Hokkaido University, Japan. Trisodium phosphonoformate was from Sigma Chemical, USA. Suramin and ammonium 21-tungsto-9-antimoniate (HPA23) were donated by Dr. H. Ohtomo of Gifu University, Japan, and by Dr. J.-C. Chermann of the Pasteur Institute, Paris, respectively. All tritium-labeled 2′-deoxynucleoside 5′-triphosphates were from the Radiochemical Centre, Amersham, England. Activated calf thymus DNA was the product of Worthington Biochemical, USA. DEAE-cellulose paper disc (DE81, ϕ 23 mm) was obtained from Whatman, UK.

Reverse Transcriptase and Eukaryotic DNA Polymerases. For most of the experiments in this study, reverse transcriptase purified from Rauscher murine leukemia virus (RLV) was used, and in some cases, HIV-reverse transcriptase was also tested. RLV was obtained from the culture medium of an established virus-producing cell line, R-17, and reverse transcriptase was purified as described previously (14). HIV was obtained from the culture medium of a continuously infected CEM cell-line (15), and HIV particles were purified as described earlier (16, 17). The detergent-treated virus particles were used as the HIV-reverse transcriptase.

DNA polymerases α and γ were purified from mouse myeloma MOPC 104E as previously described (18, 19). DNA polymerase β was purified from rat ascites hepatoma AH130 cells as previously described (20). DNA polymerases α, β and γ were also purified from cultured human KBIII cells (12) and used for some experiments.

Assay for DNA Polymerases. DNA polymerase activities were measured under the optimized reaction conditions specified for each of the DNA polymerases. Some details of these assay conditions are summarized in Table 3. The assay conditions described in Table 3, however, are representative of the conventional assay methods which may be applicable for the first screening test of inhibitors, and when necessary, one can change the assay conditions by substituting the template·primers with an assay system more sensitive to inhibitors. These more detailed conditions have been summarized previously (21).

The polymerase reaction (50 μl total volume) was started by the addition of 5 μl enzyme. The reaction mixture was incubated at 37 °C for 30–60 min and stopped by adding 20 μl of 0.2 M EDTA and immersing in ice. Then a 50 μl aliquot of the mixture was transferred to a DE81 filter paper disc and processed for radioactivity counting as described by Lindell et al. (22).

Treatment of Data. All data obtained by kinetic experiments were treated by double reciprocal and Dixon plottings for the determination of inhibition mode and the K_i (inhibition constant) values of the inhibitors.

Results

2′, 3′-Dideoxynucleoside 5′-Triphosphates (ddNTP's). It had been reported that ddTTP inhibited the activities of reverse transcriptase and DNA polymerases β and γ but not DNA polymerase α under the conventional reaction conditions employed by many workers in

Table 3: Recommended assay conditions for reverse transcriptase and various DNA and RNA polymerases[a].

DNA and RNA polymerase	Template·primer	Reaction components and their concentrations						
		Template·primer concentration[b] (μg/ml)	Buffer[c]	pH	[^{3}H]labeled nucleotide and concentration (μM)	Unlabeled nucleotide and concentration (μM)	Divalent cation and concentration (mM)	K$^+$ concentration (mM)
α	activated DNA	80	Tris	8.5	one of the dNTP's, 10	other three dNTP's, 10 each	Mg^{2+}, 4	0
β	activated DNA	200	Tris	9	one of the dNTP, 10	other three dNTP's, 10 each	Mg^{2+}, 10	30
γ	$(rA)_n \cdot (dT)_{12-18}$	10 (10:1)[d]	Tris	7.5	dTTP, 1		Mn^{2+}, 0.1	70
Primase & RNA polymerase[f]	$(dC)_n$	40	Tris	8	GTP, 1000		Mg^{2+}, 8	0
TdT[f]	$(dA)_{12-18}$	6	KPi[e]	6.5	dGTP, 10		Mn^{2+}, 5	50
RT[f]	$(rA)_n \cdot (dT)_{12-18}$	10 (1:1)[d]	Tris	8.5	dTTP, 10		Mn^{2+}, 0.2 (MLV)[f] Mg^{2+}, 5 (HIV)[f]	130
Polymerase I[f]	activated DNA	100	Tris	7.5	dTTP, 10	other three dNTP's, 10 each	Mn^{2+}, 0.2	100

[a]All reaction mixtures contained 15 % (v/v) glycerol and 1 mM dithiothreitol. [b]Concentration with respect to the template in the case of synthetic homopolymers. [c]All buffer concentrations are 50–100 mM. [d]Numbers in parentheses are base ratios of template to primer. [e]KPi, potassium phosphate. [f]MLV, murine leukemia virus; HIV, human immunodeficiency virus; TdT, terminal deoxynucleotidyltransferase; RT, reverse transcriptase, RNA polymerase and DNA polymerase I from *Escherichia coli*.

the field of DNA polymerase research. Our previous report, however, revealed that DNA polymerase α also could be inhibited by ddTTP when Mg^{2+} was replaced by Mn^{2+} in the reaction mixture (23). A more detailed study showed that all four ddNTP's inhibited DNA polymerase α activity (24), and some of these data are summarized in Table 4 together with those of DNA polymerases β and γ and RLV-reverse transcriptase.

As shown in Table 4, RLV-reverse transcriptase was inhibited by all four ddNTPs in competitive fashion with respect to the corresponding dNTP. Ki values, however, varied depending on the template·primer used. For example, when $(rA)_n \cdot (dT)_{12-18}$ was used, Ki for ddTTP was determined to be 9.3 μM, which is smaller than Km for dTTP (20 μM), and the ratio of Ki to Km (Ki/Km) was 0.47. With $(rC)_n \cdot (dG)_{12-18}$, both Km for dGTP (130 μM) and Ki for ddGTP

Table 4: Kinetic constants of RLV-reverse transcriptase and various murine DNA polymerases for dNTP's & ddNTP's.

DNA polymerase	Template·primer	Substrate			Inhibitor		
		[³H] dNTP	Unlabeled dNTP	Km for [³H]dNTP (μM)	ddNTP	Ki for ddNTP (μM)	Ki/Km
RLV-reverse transcriptase	$(rA)_n \cdot (dT)_{12-18}$	dTTP	–	20	ddTTP	9.3	0.47
	$(rC)_n \cdot (dG)_{12-18}$	dGTP	–	130	ddGTP	55	0.42
	endogenous viral RNA	dATP	dCTP, dGTP dTTP	0.5	ddATP	3.68	7.4
		dCTP	dATP, dGTP dTTP	1.1	ddCTP	0.47	0.43
		dGTP	dATP, dCTP dTTP	0.3	ddGTP	0.99	3.3
		dTTP	dATP, dCTP dGTP	0.2	ddTTP	0.04	0.2
α[a]	activated calf thymus DNA	dATP	dCTP, dGTP dTTP	1.7	ddATP	0.115	0.068
		dCTP	dATP, dGTP dTTP	2.0	ddCTP	0.095	0.048
		dGTP	dATP, dCTP dTTP	1.8	ddGTP	0.035	0.019
		dTTP	dATP, dCTP dTTP	1.8	ddTTP	0.035	0.019
	$(dA)_n \cdot (dT)_{12-18}$	dTTP	–	27.0	ddTTP	1.1	0.041
β	activated calf thymus	dATP	dCTP, dGTP dTTP	4.9	ddATP	0.56	0.11
		dCTP	dATP, dGTP dTTP	10.8	ddCTP	1.25	0.12
		dGTP	dATP, dCTP dTTP	5.3	ddGTP	0.48	0.09
		dTTP	dATP, dCTP dGTP	15.4	ddTTP	1.6	0.10
γ	activated calf thymus DNA	dATP	dCTP, dGTP dTTP	0.29	ddATP	0.23	0.79
		dCTP	dATP, dGTP dTTP	0.22	ddCTP	0.02	0.09
		dGTP	dATP, dCTP dTTP	0.13	ddGTP	0.06	0.46
		dTTP	dATP, dCTP dGTP	0.16	ddTTP	0.15	0.94
	$(rA)_n \cdot (dT)_{12-18}$	dTTP	–	0.56	ddTTP	0.003	0.005

[a] Ki's were determined under the assay conditions with Mn^{2+} (Reference No. 24).

(55 μM) were much higher than those for dTTP and ddTTP with $(rA)_n \cdot (dT)_{12-18}$. However, Ki/Km with $(rC)_n \cdot (dG)_{12-18}$ (0.42) is similar to that with $(rA)_n \cdot (dT)_{12-18}$ (0.47), indicating the similar degree of competition potential of ddTTP and ddGTP against the respective natural substrates, dTTP and dGTP.

When the inhibitions by ddNTPs were examined under "endogenous" reaction conditions with detergent-treated RLV virions (i.e., intrinsic viral RNA as the template·primer), Ki values for ddTTP (0.04 μM) and ddCTP (0.47 μM) were lower than those for ddATP (3.68 μM) and ddGTP (0.99 μM), and the ratios (Ki/Km) are again much lower with the pyrimidine dideoxy compounds (0.2–0.43) than with the purine dideoxy compounds (7.4 and 3.3) (Table 4).

DNA polymerase α was inhibited by all ddNTPs, and the Ki values obtained under the assay conditions with activated DNA (in the presence of Mn^{2+}) range from relatively narrow concentrations of 0.035 μM for ddTTP and ddGTP to 0.115 μM for ddATP; Ki/Km values (0.019–0.068) were much lower than those of the reverse transcriptase. When the template·primer was replaced by $(dA)_n \cdot (dT)_{12-18}$ with Mn^{2+}, both Km for dTTP and Ki for ddTTP increased to 27 μM and 1.1 μM, respectively. However, the Ki/Km value (0.041) was similar to those determined with activated DNA.

In the case of DNA polymerase β, all four ddNTPs showed relatively similar Ki's (0.48–1.6 μM) and Ki/Km values (0.09–0.12). On the other hand, ddCTP was the strongest inhibitor of DNA polymerase γ with activated DNA as the template·primer (Ki, 0.02 μM; Ki/Km, 0.09). ddTTP was a particularly strong inhibitor for γ-polymerase with $(rA)_n \cdot (dT)_{12-18}$ as the template·primer as shown by the smallest Ki (3 nM) and Ki/Km (0.005).

3'-Azido-2', 3'-Dideoxythymidine 5'-Triphosphate (AZTTP). Among the several 3'-modified ddTTP's tested thus far, AZTTP has been shown to be the most potent inhibitor of RLV-reverse transcriptase (25). Its Ki value was 42 nM (Table 5), which is much smaller than that of the mother compound ddTTP (9.3 μM; Table 4). When the effect of AZTTP was examined with other DNA polymerases, only DNA polymerase γ was found to be equally sensitive to inhibition by AZTTP. The Ki of γ-polymerase for AZTTP was 50 nM, but Ki/Km was much higher (0.28) than that of the reverse transcriptase (0.002), indicating stronger inhibition potential to reverse transcriptase than to γ-polymerase (Table 5). DNA polymerases α and β were almost insensitive to inhibition by this compound under the assay conditions with activated DNA. With $(dA)_n \cdot (dT)_{12-18}$ and Mn^{2+}, however, α-polymerase was sensitive to this drug as shown by the small Ki (0.72 μM) and Ki/Km (0.027) values.

Phosphonoformate (PFA). PFA was highly specific for reverse transcriptase as shown by a small Ki value (0.23 μM) (Table 6). Other than reverse transcriptase, only DNA polymerase α was slightly inhibited by PFA with a large Ki value (7.7 μM), which is much higher than Km for dTTP (1.1 μM).

Suramin and HPA23. Suramin and HPA23 have been shown to be competitive inhibitors for template·primer binding to reverse transcriptase (10, 11). We confirmed this and determined the Ki values to be 0.54 μM for suramin and 0.40 μM for HPA23 (Table 7). Besides reverse transcriptase, DNA polymerase α was strongly inhibited by both of these compounds. The Ki value for HPA23 (0.024 μM) was, however, much smaller than that for suramin (0.35 μM). Furthermore, HPA23 was also inhibitory to DNA polymerase

Table 5: Characterization of inhibition of various murine DNA polymerases by 3'-azido-2',3'-ddTTP (AZTTP).

DNA polymerase	Template·primer	[³H]dNTP	Substrate Unlabeled substrate	Km for [³H]dTTP (μM)	Ki of AZTTP (μM)	Ki/Km
α	activated calf thymus DNA	dTTP	dATP, dCTP dGTP	3.4	NI[a]	–
	$(dA)_n \cdot (dT)_{12-18}$	dTTP	–	27.0	0.72	0.027
β	activated calf thymus DNA	dTTP	dATP, dCTP dGTP	23.8	SI[a]	–
γ	$(rA)_n \cdot (dT)_{12-18}$	dTTP	–	0.18	0.05	0.28
Rauscher leukemia viral	$(rA)_n \cdot (dT)_{12-18}$	dTTP	–	20	0.042	0.002

[a]NI, no inhibition; SI, slight inhibition.

Table 6: Characterization of inhibition of various human DNA polymerases by phosphonoformate (PFA).

DNA polymerase	Template · primer	Variable substrate	Km for dNTP (μM)	Inhibition Mode	Ki (μM)	Ki/Km
α	activated calf thymus DNA	activated calf thymus DNA	–	NC[a]	–	–
		dTTP	1.1	NC	7.7	7.0
β	activated calf thymus DNA	–	–	NI[a]	–	–
γ	$(rA)_n \cdot (dT)_{12-18}$	–	–	NI	–	–
Rauscher leukemia viral	$(rA)_n \cdot (dT)_{12-18}$	$(rA)_n \cdot (dT)_{12-18}$	–	NC	–	–
		dTTP	20	NC	0.23	0.01

[a]NC, noncompetitive; NI, no inhibition.

Table 7: Characterization of inhibition of reverse transcriptase and various eukaryotic DNA polymerases by suramin and HPA23.

DNA polymerase	Template · primer	Variable substrate	Inhibition by suramin[a] Mode	Ki (μM)	Inhibition by HPA23[b] Mode	Ki (μM)
α	activated calf thymus DNA	activated DNA	competitive	0.35	noncompetitive	0.024
		dTTP	noncompetitive	–	noncompetitive	–
β	activated calf thymus DNA	–	slightly inhibited	–	slightly inhibited	–
γ	$(rA)_n \cdot (dT)_{12-18}$	$(rA)_n \cdot (dT)_{12-18}$	slightly inhibited	–	competitive	0.020
		dTTP			noncompetitive	–
Murine leukemia viral	$(rA)_n \cdot (dT)_{12-18}$	$(rA)_n \cdot (dT)_{12-18}$	competitive	0.54	competitive	0.40
		dTTP	noncompetitive	–	noncompetitive	–

[a] DNA polymerases α, β and γ purified from human KBIII cells were used (Reference No. 12).
[b] DNA polymerases α, β and γ purified from mouse myeloma cells were used (Reference No. 36).

γ with a small Ki value (0.020 μM). All these results indicate that both suramin and HPA23 are equally inhibitory to the purified DNA polymerases.

Discussion

It is now evident that many of the antiretroviral compounds which effectively inhibit reverse transcriptase activity are also inhibitory to various cellular DNA polymerases. These reverse transcriptase inhibitors can be classified by their inhibition mechanisms into two groups: (a) compounds which compete with the nucleotide substrate for binding to the enzyme, and (b) agents which disturb the template · primer binding to the polymerases. Among the nucleotide analogue inhibitors, ddNTPs show unique inhibitory action in the DNA synthesizing reaction. All of the ddNTPs have low efficiency as substrate (their incorporation rate is very low when compared to that of the normal substrate, dNTP) but high inhibition potential not only for reverse transcriptase but also for cellular DNA polymerases when adequate reaction conditions are provided (Table 4). Once incorporated into the growing DNA, ddNTP acts as a chain terminator because it lacks the 3'-OH group necessary for further DNA chain elongation. Thus ddNTP has dual functions in the inhibition of DNA synthesis: (a) as an enzyme inhibitor (25), and (b) as a chain terminator (26).

AZTTP, a modified ddTTP, has relatively high selectivity of inhibition toward reverse transcriptase. It was not inhibitory to DNA polymerase α and was slightly inhibitory to DNA polymerase β when activated DNA was used as the template · primer (Table 5). The Ki value of AZTTP for reverse transcriptase was as low as 42 nM, which is much smaller than the Ki value of the mother compound ddTTP (9.3 μM) and the Km value of dTTP (20 μM). AZTTP is also inhibitory to DNA polymerase γ with a similar Ki value (50 nM). Interestingly, α-polymerase was sensitive to inhibition by AZTTP when the assay system with $(dA)_n \cdot (dT)_{12-18}$ was employed. This fact implies that AZTTP has inhibitory potential toward DNA polymerase α, which is responsible for cellular DNA replication. Both 3'-azido-2',3'-dideoxythymidine (AZT) and 2',3'-dideoxycytidine (ddC) have been reported to be the most potent antiretroviral nucleosides which block the in vitro infectivities of both HIV and HTLV-I against the host T-cells (27). These nucleosides are phosphorylated by the host cell kinase system and become an active triphosphate form which strongly inhibits reverse transcriptase and also inhibits, although to a lesser extent, the activities of the host cell DNA polymerases as deduced from the data in Tables 4 and 5. It seems thus reasonable that these nucleosides bring about secondary effects such as hematologic disorders when long-term treatment of patients with these drugs is attempted.

Phosphonoformate is an anionic compound which is though to interact with DNA polymerase at the site where pyrophosphate is split off during the DNA polymerization process. As far as we have examined, this compound is highly specific for reverse transcriptase (Ki = 0.23 μM) (Table 6). Other than reverse transcriptase, only DNA polymerase α was inhibited by this compound (Ki value 7.7 μM), although to a much lesser extent (Table 6). The results of this study seem to be inconsistent with the previous report that a much higher PFA concentration (1000 μM) was required to reduce cell proliferation and cellular DNA synthesis to 50% in HeLa cells and human lung cells (28). Again in contradiction to our results, relatively higher PFA concentrations (> 100 μM) were required to achieve an inhibition of HIV replication, and much higher concentration of PFA (350 μM) protected the host ATH8 cells against the cytopathic effect of HIV (29). These discrepancies will be discussed later.

Various polyoxotungstate have been shown to exhibit both in vitro and in vivo antiviral activity to Friend leukemia virus (30), rabies virus (31), etc. Ammonium 5-tungsto-2-antimoniate, a member of polyoxotungstate family, and suramin were already shown to be inhibitors of reverse transcriptase in vitro (9, 10). Recently, another polyoxotungstate HPA23 has been shown to inhibit in vivo HIV production in AIDS patients (32), and a target of HPA23 seems to be HIV-associated reverse transcriptase, since the enzyme activity was strongly inhibited by this compound (10). During the course of the treatment with this drug, however, some side effects such as thrombocytopenia appeared (32). This prompted us to examine the inhibition potential of HPA23 against cellular DNA polymerases (33). Both DNA polymerases α and γ were, as expected, strongly inhibited, and some of the kinetic constants are shown in Table 7. In all cases of inhibition of the polymerase reaction by HPA23, the mode of inhibition was a competitive type with respect to the template · primer, indicating that the drug interferes with the binding of the DNA or RNA template to the polymerases. It should be noted that DNA polymerase α was particularly sensitive to inhibition by HPA23.

Suramin was first synthesized during World War I and since then it has long been used as an antitrypanosomal agent for the chemotherapy and prophylaxis of African trypanosomiasis (sleeping sickness). This compound has been shown to inhibit a large variety of enzymes in vitro, including glycolytic enzymes such as hexokinase and succinic dehydrogenase, ATPase and bacterial RNA polymerase, etc. (12). A recent finding that suramin is a potent inhibitor of reverse transcriptase from a number of retroviruses (11) led to in vitro and clinical tests which investigated its ability to inhibit HIV production as well as its potential suitability as an anti-AIDS drug. Although suramin suppressed the virus production in vitro (34) and in vivo (35), the long-term treatment regimen yielded various secondary effects such as renal insufficiency, etc; such side effects were likewise observed with trypanosomiasis patients treated with suramin. It is now clear, from Table 7, that suramin inhibits DNA polymerase α activity with a Ki value similar to that of reverse transcriptase, which may explain at least a part of the undesirable side effects observed. We have tested two other anionic compounds (Evans Blue, which is structurally related to suramin, and aurintricarboxylic acid) for the inhibition of cellular DNA polymerases and obtained results similar to those of the tests with suramin. Namely, they inhibit both reverse transcriptase and DNA polymerases by competing with the template · primers for binding to the enzyme (unpublished observation).

Finally, a comment should be added as to the enzymatic evaluation of an antiretroviral compound. There are always some discrepancies between the results of the cell culture test and those of the enzymatic test when evaluating the potential and selectivity of an antiretroviral compound as described previously, for example, for phosphonoformate. Strong potential and/or high selectivity of an antiviral compound observed in the inhibition of DNA polymerase and/or reverse transcriptase does not necessarily reflect the situation in vivo, because in intact cells, cellular DNA polymerases may exist in an organized state with associated cofactor(s) or enzyme(s) and therefore the sensitivities to exogenously added drugs may be different from those exhibited by the purified enzymes (12). In conclusion, the potential and the selectivity of an antiretroviral compound may depend on any one or more of the following factors: (a) easier permeability through the membrane of the target cell; (b) greater affinity to the reverse transcriptase than to the DNA polymerases α, β and γ; and (c) easier accessibility to reverse transcriptase in the cytoplasm than to the host cell DNA polymerases (α and β in the nucleus, and γ in the mitochondria) (11, 12). In fact, it has been shown that suramin, for example, does not show any inhibitory effect on the growth of host cells at concentrations which could probably block the infectivity and the cytopathic effect of HIV by inhibiting the reverse transcriptase activity (34). It is thus concluded that the cell culture test performed in parallel with the enzymatic test is desirable for the prediction of the inhibitory potential of an antiretroviral drug. Nevertheless, the findings of enzymatic studies, such as those described in this paper, will foster the modification of drug structures for improvement of the efficacies of antiviral potentials.

Acknowledgements

The author is grateful to M. Ogasawara, Y. Kojima, Y. Iwata, H. Nakane, T. Matsumoto, and N. Kojima for their assistance in various experiments. This work was supported in part by a Grant-in-Aid for Cancer Research from the Ministry of Education, Science and Culture of Japan. Skillful technical assistance of Mrs. S. Shinmura for preparing the manuscript is greatly appreciated.

References

1. Matsukage, A., Ono, K., Ohashi, A., Takahashi, T., Saneyoshi, M.: Inhibitory effect of 1-β-D-arabinofuranosylthymine 5'-triphosphate and 1-β-D-arabinofuranosylcytosine 5'-triphosphate on DNA polymerases from murine cells and oncornavirus. Cancer Research 1978, 38: 3076–3079.
2. Ono, K., Ohashi, A., Yamamoto, A., Matsukage, A., Takahashi, T., Saneyoshi, M., Ueda, T.: Inhibitory effects of 9-β-D-arabinofuranosylguanine 5'-triphosphate and 9-β-D-arabinofuranosyladenine 5'-triphosphate on DNA polymerases from murine cells and oncornavirus. Cancer Research 1979, 39: 4673–4680.
3. Smoler, D., Molineux, I., Baltimore, D.: Direction of polymerization by the avian myeloblastosis virus deoxyribonucleic acid polymerase. Journal of Biological Chemistry 1971, 246: 7697–7900.
4. Sundquist, B., Öberg, B.: Phosphonoformate inhibits reverse transcriptase. Journal of General Virology 1979, 45: 273–281.
5. De Clercq, E., Billiau, A., Hobbs, J., Torrence, P. F., Witkop, B.: Inhibition of oncornavirus functions by 2'-azido polynucleotides. Proceedings of the National Academy of Sciences USA 1975, 72: 284–288.
6. De Clercq, E., Fukui, T., Kakiuchi, N., Ikehara, M., Hattori, M., Pfleiderer, W.: Influence of various 2- and 2'-substituted polyadenylic acids on murine leukemia virus reverse transcriptase. Cancer Letters 1979, 7: 23–37.
7. De Clercq, E., Billiau, A., Hattori, M., Ikehara, M.: Inhibition of oncornavirus functions by poly(2-methylthioinosinic acid). Nucleic Acids Research 1975, 2: 2305–2313.
8. Fukui, T., De Clercq, E.: Inhibition of murine leukemia virus reverse transcriptase by 2-halogenated polyadenylic acids. Biochemical Journal 1982, 203: 755–760.
9. Chermann, J.-C., Sinoussi, F., Jasmin, C.: Inhibition of RNA-dependent DNA polymerase of murine oncornavirus by ammonium-5-tungsto-2-antimoniate. Biochemical and Biophysical Research Communications 1975, 65: 1229–1236.
10. Dormont, D., Spire, B., Barré-Sinoussi, F., Montagnier, L., Chermann, J.-C.: Inhibition of RNA-dependent DNA polymerases of AIDS and SAIDS retroviruses by HPA-23 (ammonium-21-tungsto-9-antimoniate). Annales de l'Institut Pasteur/Virology 1985, 136: 75–84.
11. De Clercq, E.: Suramin: a potent inhibitor of reverse transcriptase of RNA tumor viruses. Cancer Letters 1979, 8: 9–22.
12. Ono, K., Nakane, H., Fukushima, M.: Differential inhibition of various deoxyribonucleic and ribonucleic acid polymerases by suramin. European Journal of Biochemistry 1988, 172: 349–353.
13. Modak, M. J.: Pyridoxal 5' phosphate: a selective inhibitor of oncornaviral DNA polymerases. Biochemical and Biophysical Research Communications 1976, 71: 180–187.
14. Nakajima, K., Ono, K., Ito, Y.: Interconversion of molecular size of the DNA polymerase from Rauscher leukemia virus. Intervirology 1974, 3: 332–341.
15. Foley, G. E., Lazarus, H., Farber, S., Uzman, B. G., Boone, B. A., McCarthy, R. E.: Continuous culture of human lymphoblasts from peripheral blood of a child with acute leukemia. Cancer 1965, 18: 522–529.
16. Barré-Sinoussi, F., Chermann, J.-C., Rey, F., Nugeyre, M. T., Chamaret, S., Gruest, J., Dauguet, C., Axler-Blin, C., Vézinet-Brun, F., Rouzioux, C., Rozenbaum, W., Montagnier, L.: Isolation of a T-lymphotropic retrovirus from a patient at a risk for acquired immune deficiency syndrome (AIDS). Science 1983, 220: 868–871.
17. Rey, M. A., Spire, B., Dormont, D., Barré-Sinoussi, F., Montagnier, L., Chermann, J.-C.: Characterization of the RNA-dependent DNA polymerase of a new human T-lymphotropic retrovirus (lymphadenopathy-associated virus). Biochemical and Biophysical Research Communications 1984, 121: 126–133.
18. Matsukage, A., Sivarajan, M., Wilson, S. H.: Studies on DNA α-polymerase of mouse myeloma: partial purification and comparison of three molecular forms of enzyme. Biochemistry 1976, 15: 5305–5314.
19. Matsukage, A., Bohn, E. W., Wilson, S. H.: On the DNA polymerase III of mouse myeloma: partial purification and characterization. Biochemistry 1975, 14: 1006–1020.
20. Ono, K., Ohashi, A., Tanabe, K., Matsukage, A., Nishizawa, M., Takahashi, T.: Unique requirements for template-primers of DNA polymerase β from rat ascites hepatoma AH130 cells. Nucleic Acids Research 1979, 7: 715–726.
21. Ono, K.: Discrimination of cellular and viral DNA polymerases in retrovirus-infected cells: principle and applications. Bulletin de l'Institut Pasteur 1987, 85: 3–35.
22. Lindell, T. J., Weinberg, F., Morris, P. W., Roeder, R. G., Rutter, W. J.: Specific inhibition of nuclear RNA polymerase II by α-amanitin. Science 1967, 170: 447–449.
23. Ono, K., Ogasawara, M., Matsukage, A.: Inhibition of the activity of DNA polymerase α by 2',3'-dideoxythymidine 5'-triphosphate. Biochemical and Biophysical Research Communications 1979, 88: 1255–1262.
24. Ono, K., Ogasawara, M., Iwata, Y., Nakane, H.: Inhibition of DNA polymerase α by 2',3'-dideoxyribonucleoside 5'-triphosphates: effect of manganese ion. Biomedicine & Pharmacotherapy 1984, 38: 382–389.

25. Ono, K., Ogasawara, M., Iwata, Y., Nakane, H., Fujii, T., Sawai, K., Saneyoshi, M.: Inhibition of reverse transcriptase activity by 2′,3′-dideoxythymidine 5′-triphosphate and its derivatives modified on the 3′ position. Biochemical and Biophysical Research Communications 1986, 140: 498–507.
26. Atkinson, M. R., Deutcher, M. P., Kornberg, A., Russel, A. F., Moffat, J. G.: Enzymatic synthesis of deoxyribonucleic acid. XXXIV. Termination of chain growth by 2′,3′-dideoxyribonucleotide. Biochemistry 1969, 8: 4897–4904.
27. Mitsuya, H., Broder, S.: Strategies for antiviral therapy in AIDS. Nature 1987, 325: 773–778.
28. Stenberg, K., Larsson, A.: Reversible effects on cellular metabolism and proliferation by trisodium phosphonoformate. Antimicrobial Agents and Chemotherapy 1978, 14: 727–730.
29. Balzarini, J., Mitsuya, H., De Clercq, E., Broder, S.: Comparative inhibitory effects of suramin and other selected compounds on the infectivity and replication of human T-cell lymphotropic virus (HTLV-III)/lymphadenopathy-associated virus. International Journal of Cancer 1986, 37: 451–457.
30. Jasmin, C., Chermann, J.-C., Herve, G., Teze, A., Souchay, P., Boy-Loustau, C., Raybaud, N., Sinoussi, F., Raynaud, M.: In vivo inhibition of murine leukemia and sarcoma viruses by the heteropolyanion 5-tungsto-2-antimoniate. Journal of National Cancer Institute 1974, 53: 469–474.
31. Tsiang, H., Atanasiu, P., Chermann, J.-C., Jasmin, C.: Inhibition of rabies virus in vitro by the ammonium-5-tungsto-2-antimoniate. Journal of General Virology 1978, 40: 665–668.
32. Rozenbaum, W., Dormont, D., Spire, B., Vilmer, E., Gentilini, M., Griscelli, C., Montagnier, L., Barré-Sinoussi, F., Chermann, J.-C.: Antimoniotungstate (HPA23) treatment of three patients with AIDS and one with prodrome. Lancet 1985, i: 450–451.
33. Ono, K., Nakane, H., Matsumoto, T., Barré-Sinoussi, F., Chermann, J.-C.: Inhibition of DNA polymerase α activity by ammonium 21-tungsto-9-antimoniate (HPA23). Nucleic Acids Research Symposium Series 1984, Number 15: 169–172.
34. Mitsuya, H., Popovic, M., Yarchoan, R., Matsushita, S., Gallo, R. C., Broder, S.: Suramin protection of T cells in vitro against infectivity and cytopathic effect of HTLV-III. Science 1984, 226: 172–174.
35. Broder, S., Yarchoan, R., Collins, J. M., Lane, H. C., Markham, P. D., Klecker, R. W., Redfield, R. R., Mitsuya, H., Hoth, D. F., Gelmann, E., Groopman, J. E., Resnick, L., Gallo, R. C., Myers, C. E., Fauci, A. S.: Effects of suramin on HTLV-III/LAV infection presenting as Kaposi's sarcoma or AIDS-related complex: clinical pharmacology and suppression of virus replication in vivo. Lancet 1985, ii: 627–630.
36. Ono, K., Nakane, H., Barré-Sinoussi, F., Chermann, J.-C.: Differential inhibition of various mammalian DNA polymerase activities by ammonium 21-tungsto-9-antimoniate (HPA23). European Journal of Biochemistry 1988, in press.

Effects of Drugs on Lipids and Membrane Integrity of Fungi

N. H. Georgopapadakou

The frequency of fungal infections is increasing as a result of the successful use of antibacterials and the proliferation of immunocompromised patients. With the exception of 5-fluorocytosine, all clinically useful antifungals act upon the membrane lipids, inhibiting either their biosynthesis (azoles, allylamines, morpholines) or their function (polyenes). The fungal, in particular the candidal, membrane is reviewed as a target for antifungals. The effects of selected antifungals on lipid biosynthesis and membrane integrity and the implications of these effects on activity and toxicity are also discussed.

The frequency of fungal infections in humans has steadily increased in recent years as a result of advances in other therapeutic areas (organ transplantation, cancer chemotherapy, broad-spectrum antibacterial therapy), the use of invasive medical procedures (catheters, intravenous devices) and the emergence of the human immunodeficiency virus (1–3). Thus, opportunistic fungal infections are treated empirically in immunocompromised patients, especially when there is fever of unknown origin and the patient has not responded to broad-spectrum antibacterials (4).

Important fungal pathogens are listed in Table 1. The most common opportunistic pathogen is *Candida albicans*, an organism normally found as a commensal in the oral cavity and gastrointestinal tract of humans (5). *Candida albicans* is a dimorphic fungus, growing in the yeast form when part of the normal flora and in the hyphal form during tissue invasion (6). In the yeast form, *Candida albicans* resembles *Saccharomyces cerevisiae*, and this extensively studied organism, though haploid, has often been used as a model for the diploid *Candida albicans*.

Compounds currently in clinical use against *Candida albicans* are the polyene antibiotics, the azole derivatives, and 5-fluorocytosine (5-FC) (7) (Figure 1). With the exception of the last compound, all are targeted to act against the membrane. The fungal cell wall, a structure essential to the fungus but lacking in the mammalian cell, would seem to be an ideal target for antifungal agents. To date, however, agents active against the cell wall have not found clinical use in human mycoses.

This review focuses on the envelope (cell wall plus membrane) of *Candida albicans* and the effects of clinically important antifungal agents. The envelope, in particular the plasma membrane, is reviewed in terms of its composition, function, and biosynthesis of individual components. Antifungal targets are highlighted and the effects of antifungal agents on lipid biosynthesis and membrane function are discussed. Effects on cell-wall biosynthesis and cell morphology are also noted, as these processes are functionally connected with the plasma membrane and may be part of the microbial response to antifungal agents.

The Fungal Envelope: Composition, Biosynthesis, and Function

Cell Wall

The cell wall of fungi is a multilayer structure composed mostly of carbohydrate. Like its bacterial counterpart, it determines cell shape, confers rigidity and strength, and prevents lysis from osmotic shock. It also functions, by virtue of its limited porosity, as a permeability barrier for large molecules (8). In *Candida albicans*, the cell wall consists primarily of glucan and mannoproteins (9). Glucan is a mixture of branched β-1,3- and β-1,6-linked glucose polymers (10), while mannoproteins are branched mannose polymers attached to a protein through a GlcNAc-GlcNAc group and an arginine residue. Chitin, a linear β-1,4-linked GlcNAc homopolymer, is a minor but essential cell wall component associated with the septum (yeast form) and the apical region (hyphal form) (11).

Both glucan and chitin are synthesized on the cytoplasmic surface of the plasma membrane (12). They are then extruded and deposited on the outer surface as microfibrils which subsequently aggregate to form crystalline structures (13). As is discussed later in

Department of Chemotherapy (58/2), Hoffmann-La Roche Inc., Nutley, New Jersey 07110, USA.

Table 1: Fungal infections in man (Data from Reference No. 64).

Disease	Host site	Etiologic agent
Dermatophytoses	skin and hair	*Epidermophyton floccosum*
		Microsporum spp.
		Trichophyton spp.
Candidosis	skin, mucous membranes, systemic	*Candida albicans*
Aspergillosis	external ear and lungs	*Aspergillus fumigatus*
Blastomycosis	skin, lungs, systemic	*Blastomyces dermatidis*
Coccidioidomycosis	skin, lungs, systemic	*Coccidioides immitis*
Cryptococcosis	skin, meninges, lungs, systemic	*Cryptococcus neoformans*
Histoplasmosis	lungs, spleen, liver	*Histoplasma capsulatum*

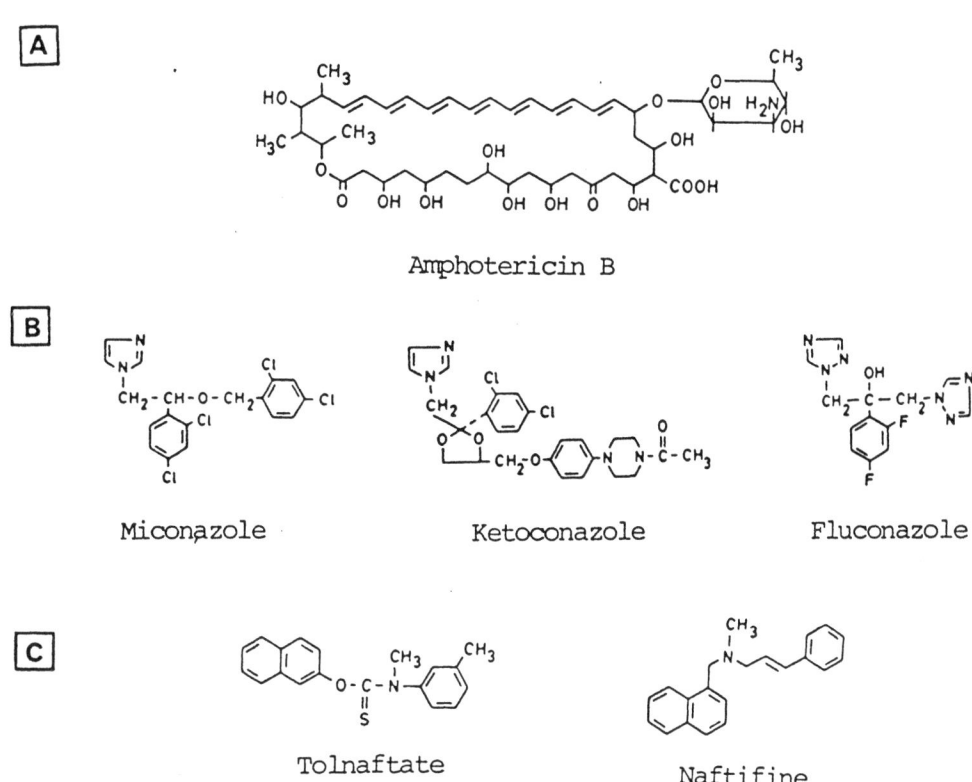

Figure 1: Structures of representative polyenes (A), azoles (B), and allylamines/thiocarbamates (C).

this review, the process of synthesis, secretion, and assembly of cell-wall polymers is influenced by the nature of the membrane, which in turn is determined by its lipid composition.

Glucan synthesis is assayed in spheroplasts of *Candida albicans* (14), as glucan synthase in isolated membranes is insensitive to the standard inhibitors papulacandin, echinocandin, and aculeacin (Georgopapadakou and Smith, unpublished results). Chitin synthesis is assayed in permeabilized cells or isolated membranes (11, 15). In either system, chitin synthase activity is sensitive to standard inhibitors. For example, the IC50 for polyoxin D is 1 μM (15). As in *Saccharomyces cerevisiae* (16, 17), there may be more than one chitin synthase in *Candida albicans*, each making a topologically distinct form of chitin (septal, glucan-associated). Most if not all chitin synthase is produced in the zymogen form and is subsequently activated by proteolysis (11, 18).

Plasma Membrane

The plasma membrane of fungi has the typical lipid bilayer structure with phosphatidylcholine, phosphatidylethanolamine, and ergosterol (or zymosterol) as major lipids (19, 20). It functions as a barrier between the cytoplasm and the environment, regulating

Table 2: Effects of antifungal agents on membrane integrity of *Candida albicans*.

Antifungal agent	Concentration (μm)	Total release of Potassium (%)	Total release of Aminoisobutyric (%)	Percent of cells stained with methylene blue
None		<5	<5	0
Polyenes				
Amphotericin B	10	100	97	100
Nystatin	10	100	97	100
Azoles				
Clotrimazole	100	<5	20	0
Econazole	100	47	98	0
Miconazole	100	66	94	60
Ketoconazole	100	<5	20	0
Allylamines, thiocarbamates				
Naftifine	100	<5	30	0
Tolnaftate	100	<5	<5	0

the transport of molecules in and out of the cells. It is also the matrix for the various membrane-bound enzymes, including those involved in cell-wall biosynthesis. The composition of the plasma membrane of *Candida albicans* has been discussed previously (21, 22). The effects of antifungal agents on the membrane integrity of *Candida albicans* are given in Table 2.

Ergosterol is the major fungal sterol and is an essential component of the fungal membrane, being analogous to cholesterol in mammalian cells. Inhibition of its biosynthesis leads to inhibition of fungal growth, though not to cell lysis (23). An important difference between fungi and mammalian cells is the absence of a sterol uptake system in the former. Thus, exogeneous sterols are not normally incorporated into the yeast membrane (24). It has been suggested that ergosterol has at least two types of function in membranes: (a) a nonspecific, "bulk" function in the regulation of membrane fluidity and integrity; and (b) a specific, "sparking" function in the regulation of cell growth and proliferation (25–28). The former is the traditional function for ergosterol; it requires large amounts of sterol (hence the name "bulk") and is not specific for ergosterol. The latter apparently involves control of some membrane-associated processes, requires minute amounts of sterol (hence the name "sparking") and is specific for ergosterol. Compounds which inhibit ergosterol biosynthesis substantially but not completely are likely to affect "bulk" ergosterol only and thus the extent of growth inhibition may depend on the nature of the intermediates that accumulate.

Ergosterol Biosynthesis

Ergosterol biosynthesis can be divided into four stages: (a) formation of mevalonate; (b) successive polymerizations leading to squalene; (c) cyclization to lanosterol; and (d) modifications leading to ergosterol. The enzymes involved in the first stage are mitochondrial, in the second mostly cytosolic, and in the third and fourth microsomal (29). There are several steps in ergosterol biosynthesis which can be blocked (Figure 2).

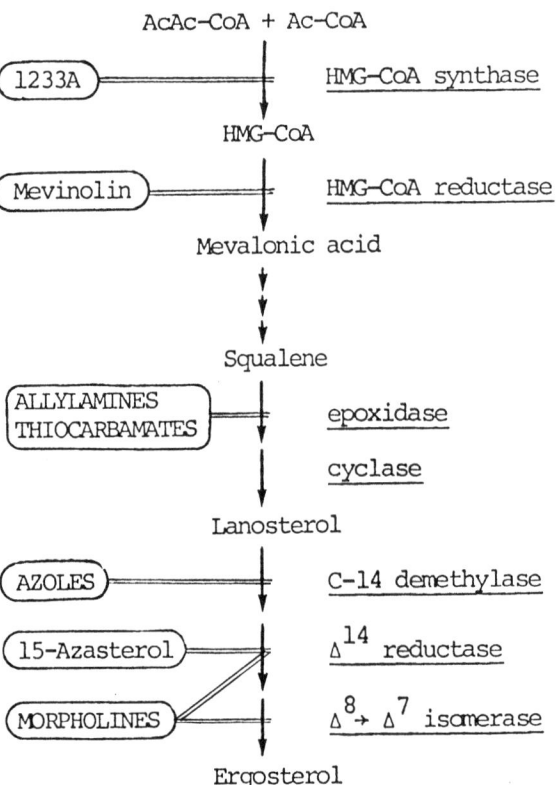

Figure 2: Biosynthesis of ergosterol showing the sites of inhibition by some antifungals. Clinically useful antifungals are in capital letters.

As in cholesterol biosynthesis, the rate-limiting enzyme of ergosterol biosynthesis is 3-hydroxy-3-methylglutaryl CoA reductase (HMG-CoA reductase) (30). Inhibitors of this enzyme, such as the sesquiterpenes mevinolin and compactin (31), have been of little value as antifungals because of their poor permeability. HMG-CoA synthase is another key enzyme in cholesterol biosynthesis and is a target for hypocholesteremic agents such as the β-lactone 1233A (32). However, 1233A apparently has no antifungal activity, probably due to permeability limitations.

Squalene epoxidase and squalene cyclase, targets for hypocholesteremic agents before HMG-CoA reductase emerged as the preferred target, are also targets for antifungal agents. Squalene epoxidase is the more attractive of the two, as accumulation of squalene may be less damaging to the host than accumulation of 2,3-oxidosqualene (33).

The biosynthetic steps following cyclization to lanosterol are complex because of pathway multiplicity (34). Nevertheless, two steps of particular interest are the cytochrome P-450-dependent C-14 demethylase reaction and the $\Delta^8 - \Delta^7$ isomerase reaction. These are targets, respectively, of the azole and morpholine antifungals.

Membrane Assays

The biosynthesis of ergosterol and other fungal lipids is determined by examining the relative incorporation of radiolabeled precursors into the different lipids. Membrane integrity, on the other hand, is determined by examining the barrier function of the membrane. The assays are also used to study the mode of action of antifungal agents.

In Vivo Lipid Biosynthesis

Candida albicans is grown in the presence of [^{14}C] acetate and the antifungal agent. Lipids are extracted from the cells, spearated by thin-layer chromatography (TLC), and radioactivity in the different bands is determined. Individual fatty acids are further separated by gas chromatography/mass spectrometry and quantified (22).

In Vitro Lipid Biosynthesis

Candida albicans cells are ruptured with glass beads, then incubated with a radiolabeled lipid precursor, usually [^{14}C] acetate, and the antifungal agent. Lipids are extracted, separated as above, and incorporation of radioactivity is measured by liquid scintillation counting (LSC). Densitometry is not used to determine incorporation of radioactivity in lipids, as non-radioactive ergosterol causes darkening of the X-ray film during autoradiography. Individual fatty acids are further separated by gas chromatography and quantified by liquid scintillation counting (22).

Membrane Integrity

Assays for membrane integrity are based on the release of intracellular substances (potassium, aminoisobutyric acid) or the entry of substances that are normally excluded (methylene blue) (22). In the potassium efflux assay, cells are incubated with the antifungal agent,, removed by centrifugation, and the amount of potassium released in the supernatant is determined with a flame photometer. In the radiolabel release assay, cells are first loaded with [^{14}C] aminoisobutyric acid, a nonmetabolizable amino acid, then incubated with the antifungal agent. Cell-associated radioactivity is determined by liquid scintillation counting after washing the cells. In the methylene blue exclusion assay, cells are incubated with the antifungal and then treated with methylene blue. The number of stained cells is determined by counting them in a hemocytometer.

Effects of Antifungal Agents

Polyenes

The polyene macrolide antibiotics, introduced in the late 1950s, are produced by *Streptomyces* species (35, 36). They are characterized by a very large lactone ring with a sugar (usually mycosamine) attached to it through a glycosidic bond (Figure 1). The lactone ring is amphipathic, consisting of a rigid lipophilic chain of four to seven conjugated double bonds and a flexible hydrophilic region with a number of hydroxyl groups. Polyenes are broad-spectrum, fungicidal antibiotics with a low incidence of resistance. Their mode of action involves binding to sterols in the cell membrane, resulting in membrane disruption and formation of transmembrane pores (37). This leads to increased permeability, leakage of cytoplasmic contents (especially potassium ions), and eventual cell death (38). Although polyenes interact both with ergosterol and cholesterol, clinically useful polyenes such as amphotericin B have higher affinity for ergosterol than cholesterol (39). The membrane effects of polyenes have been exploited in combination therapy, especially with 5-FC (40).

Amphotericin B and nystatin, at concentrations of 10 μM, completely abolish the barrier function of the plasma membrane in all three assays (Table 2). Neither compound affects lipid biosynthesis in vivo at concentrations up to 0.1 µM.

Azoles

Azole derivatives, introduced in the late 1960s, represent the single largest class of antifungals. They are synthetic compounds characterized by a free imidazole or triazole ring linked through a C-N bond to an aromatic ring (Figure 1). They remain the subject of intense research interest and have been covered in several recent reviews (41–44). They are generally fungistatic, with broad-spectrum antifungal activity. Their primary mode of action involves inhibition of ergosterol biosynthesis at the C-14 demethylation step, a cytochrome P-450-dependent reaction ubiquitous in fungi. This leads to accumulation of methylated sterols, including lanosterol, and a decrease in the ergosterol-to-methylated sterol ratio (Table 3). IC50s, defined as the concentration where the ergosterol-to-methylated sterol ratio is decreased to 50 % of control, range from ~ 1 nM for ketoconazole to ~ 100 nM for fluconazole (UK 49,858). For some azoles, these values are lower than the IC50s for the C-14 demethylase reaction (45), possibly due to azole accumulation in the cytoplasm (46). Consistent with inhibition of ergosterol, azoles antagonize the effects of amphotericin B (47).

Azoles also decrease the unsaturated-to-saturated fatty acid ratio, and cause a shift from C_{18} to C_{16} fatty acids (Table 4). The effects on fatty acids occur in vivo only, suggesting that they are probably secondary to ergosterol inhibition (22). Chitin synthase is stimulated by azoles in vivo, probably as a result of ergosterol depletion in the plasma membrane (Figure 3) (48, 49). Paradoxically, azoles seem to inhibit *Candida albicans* conversion to the hyphal form, which is normally associated with high levels of chitin synthase activity (11, 50). A possible explanation is that the increase in chitin synthase is secondary

Table 3: Effect of antifungal agents in vivo on *Candida albicans* sterols.

Antifungal agent	Concentration (µM)	Erg/DMS + TMS[a]	Sterols/Squalene
None		10.9	18.6
Azoles			
Econazole	0.01	3.4	ND
Tioconazole	0.003	4.1	ND
Ketoconazole	0.003	4.0	ND
Bifonazole	0.1	4.0	ND
Fluconazole	0.3	4.2	ND
Allylamines, Thiocarbamates			
Naftifine	10	ND	5.5
Terbinafine	0.01	ND	5.4
Tolnaftate	100	ND	10.2
Tolciclate	0.3	ND	8.2

[a] Erg/DMS + TMS, ergosterol: (dimethylsterol + trimethylsterol) ratio. In untreated cells, ergosterol is 12 %, DMD + TMS < 1 %, and squalene < 1 % of total lipids.
ND = not determined.

Table 4: Effect of antifungal agents in vivo on *Candida albicans* fatty acids.

Antifungal agent	Concentration (µM)	Fatty acid (% of total)					
		16:0	16:1	18:0	18:1	18:2	18:3
None		26	20	4	30	15	5
Azoles							
Clotrimazole	1	39	16	9	14	16	6
Econazole	1	40	15	10	14	16	6
Miconazole	1	38	16	10	12	19	6
Ketoconazole	1	42	13	8	14	18	6
Allylamines, thiocarbamates							
Naftifine	10	37	18	5	22	14	4
Tolnaftate	100	36	20	6	20	15	3

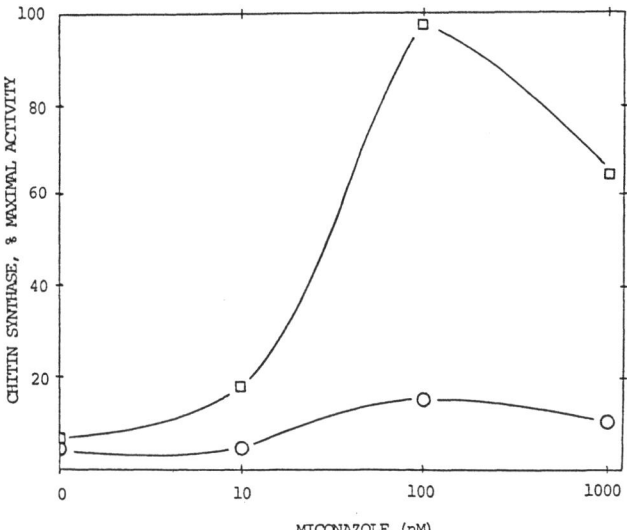

Figure 3: Chitin synthase activity of *Candida albicans* grown in the presence of miconazole. Activity was measured in spheroplast membranes before (o—o) and after (□—□) activation with trypsin (15).

to defective chitin or impaired cell division, produced under conditions of ergosterol depletion (51). In addition, clotrimazole, econazole and miconazole damage the plasma membrane directly, though at much higher concentrations (Table 2) (23).

Allylamines

Allylamines, introduced in the mid-1970s, and the structurally related thiocarbamates, introduced in the early 1960s, are also synthetic compounds (Figure 1) (52–54). They are active primarily against dermatophytes, their activity against *Candida albicans* being limited possibly by permeability (55). Their mode of action involves inhibition of lanosterol epoxidase leading to accumulation of squalene (56–59). IC50s, defined as the concentration where the sterol-to-squalene ratio is decreased to 50 % of control, range from $< 1 \mu M$ for terbinafine (SF 86-327) to 100 μM for tolnaftate (Table 3). Like azoles, allylamines decrease the unsaturated-to-saturated fatty acid ratio and cause a shift from C_{18} to C_{16} fatty acids in vivo (Table 4).

Morpholines

Tridermoph and several morpholine derivatives developed in the early 1970s are synthetic compounds used primarily as agricultural fungicides (60). Amorolfine (Ro 14-4767), a compound structurally related to fenpropimorph, has activity against several human pathogens (61) and shows promise as a topical antifungal. The mode of action of morpholines involves inhibition of $\Delta^8 - \Delta^7$ isomerase and Δ^{14} reductase reactions in ergosterol biosynthesis (62). The dual action may lead to lower incidence of resistance.

Conclusion

The fungal envelope remains the most attractive target for antifungal agents. Polyenes are still the most effective compounds for systemic mycoses, and liposomal formulations may reduce their toxicity (61). Azoles are becoming increasingly popular in the treatment of systemic infections, even in immunocompromised patients. Nevertheless, the nature of the molecular targets poses some inherent limitations. With polyenes, the close structural similarity of ergosterol to cholesterol leads to damage of mammalian cells. With azoles, the similarity of the cytochrome P-450-dependent C-14 demethylase reaction to the mammalian cytochrome P-450-dependent reactions of steroid hormone synthesis is the basis for their endocrine side effects. In addition, azoles which lack direct membrane effects are only fungistatic.

Such concerns should not distract from the progress made in all classes of ergosterol synthesis inhibitors, particularly the azoles, following elucidation of their mechanism of action. Thus, triazoles have higher specificity for the fungal enzyme, few side effects and more favorable pharmacokinetics than imidazoles. Significantly, some azoles may accumulate in *Candida albicans*, leading to increased antifungal activity (46). Progress has also been made with the allylamines. Terbinafine is a more potent and specific inhibitor of the fungal squalene epoxidase than naftifine.

Fungal cell-wall biosynthesis has been studied less extensively, and inhibitors of the various processes have been exclusively natural products. Lack of penetration has prevented the emergence of a chitin synthase inhibitor with anticandidal activity while toxicity problems may have slowed the development of glucan synthase inhibitors as antifungals. Yet, cell-wall targets are potentially fungicidal and more selective than ergosterol biosynthesis. This, together with the spectacular success of cell-wall targeted antibacterials, is a cause for optimism.

References

1. Meunier-Carpentier, F., Kiehn, T. E., Armstrong, D.: Fungemia in the immunocompromised host. Changing patterns, antigemia, high mortality. American Journal of Medicine 1981, 71: 363–370.

2. Horn, R., Wong, B., Kiehn, T. E., Armstrong, D.: Fungemia in a cancer hospital: changing frequency, earlier onset, and results of therapy. Reviews of Infectious Diseases 1985, 7: 646–655.
3. Clumeck, N., Hermans, P., De Wit, S.: Current problems in the management of AIDS patients. European Journal of Clinical Microbiology 1988, 7: 2–10.
4. DeGregorio, M. W., Lee, W. M., Linker, C. A., Jacobs, R. A., Ries, C. A.: Fungal infections in patients with acute leukemia. American Journal of Medicine 1982, 73: 543–548.
5. Odds, F. A.: *Candida* and candidosis. Leicester University Press, Leicester, UK, 1979.
6. Shepherd, M. G., Poulter, R. T. M., Sullivan, P. A.: *Candida albicans:* biology, genetics, and pathogenicity. Annual Review of Microbiology 1985, 39: 579–614.
7. Medoff, G., Brajtburg, J., Kobayashi, G. S.: Antifungal agents useful in therapy of systemic fungal infections. Annual Reviews of Pharmacology and Toxicology 1983, 23: 303–330.
8. Zlotnik, H., Fernandez, M. P., Bowers, B., Cabib, E.: *Saccharomyces cerevisiae* mannoproteins form an external cell wall polymer that determines wall porosity. Journal of Bacteriology 1984, 159: 1018–1026.
9. Sullivan, P. A., Chiew, Y. Y., Molloy, C., Templeton, M. D., Shepherd, M. G.: An analysis of the metabolism and cell wall composition of *Candida albicans* during germ-tube formation. Canadian Journal of Microbiology 1983, 29: 1514–1525.
10. Gopal, P. K., Shepherd, M. G., Sullivan, P. A.: Analysis of wall glucans from yeast, hyphal and germ-tube forming cells of *Candida albicans*. Journal of General Microbiology 1984, 130: 3295–3301.
11. Braun, P. C., Calderone, R. A.: Chitin synthesis in *Candida albicans*: Comparison of yeast and hyphal forms. Journal of Bacteriology 1978, 135: 1472–1477.
12. Cabib, E., Roberts, R.: Synthesis of the yeast cell wall and its regulation. Annual Reviews of Biochemistry 1982, 51: 763–793.
13. Kreger, D. R., Kopecka, M.: On the nature and formation of the fibrilar nets produced by protoplasts of *Saccharomyces cerevisiae* in liquid media: an electron microscopic, X-ray diffraction and chemical study. Journal of General Microbiology 1975, 92: 207–220.
14. Baguley, B. C., Rommele, G., Gruner, J., Wehrli, W.: Papulacandin B: an inhibitor of glucan synthesis in yeast spheroplasts. European Journal of Biochemistry 1979, 97: 345–351.
15. Georgopapadakou, N. H., Smith, S. A.: Chitin synthase in *Candida albicans*: comparison of digitonin-permeabilized cells and spheroplast membranes. Journal of Bacteriology 1985, 162: 826–829.
16. Sburlati, A., Cabib, E.: Chitin synthase 2, a presumptive participant in septum formation in *Saccharomyces cerevisiae*. The Journal of Biological Chemistry 1986, 261: 15147–15152.
17. Orlean, P.: Two chitin synthases in *Saccharomyces cerevisiae*. The Journal of Biological Chemistry 1987, 262: 5732–5739.
18. Hardy, J. C., Gooday, G. W.: Stability and zymogenic nature of chitin synthase from *Candida albicans*. Current Microbiology 1983, 9: 51–54.
19. Wassef, M. K.: Fungal Lipids. Advances in Lipid Research 1977, 15: 159–232.
20. Kaneko, H., Hoschara, M., Tanaka, M., Itch, T.: Lipid composition of 30 species of yeast. Lipids 1976, 11: 837–844.
21. Marriott, M. S.: Isolation and chemical characterization of plasma membranes from the yeast and mycelial forms of *Candida albicans*. Journal of General Microbiology 1975, 86: 115–132.
22. Georgopapadakou, N. H., Dix, B. A., Smith, S. A., Freudenberger, J., Funke, P. T.: Effect of antifungal agents on lipid biosynthesis and membrane integrity in *Candida albicans*. Antimicrobial Agents and Chemotherapy 1987, 31: 46–51.
23. Sud, I. J., Feingold, D. S.: Heterogeneity of action mechanisms among antimycotic imidazoles. Antimicrobial Agents and Chemotherapy 1981, 20: 71–74.
24. Lewis, T. A., Taylor, F. R., Parks, L. W.: Involvement of heme biosynthesis in control of sterol uptake by *Saccharomyces cerevisiae*. Journal of Bacteriology 1985, 163: 199–207.
25. Rodriguez, R. J., Taylor, F. R., Parks, L. W.: A requirement for ergosterol to permit growth of yeast sterol auxotrophs on cholestanol. Biochemical and Biophysical Research Communications 1982, 106: 435–441.
26. Ramgopal, M., Bloch, K.: Multiple functions for sterols in *Saccharomyces cerevisiae*. Proceedings of the National Academy of Sciences USA 1983, 80: 712–715.
27. Pinto, W. J., Lozano, R., Sekula, B. C., Nes, W. R.: Stereochemically distinct roles for sterol in *Saccharomyces cerevisiae*. Biochemical and Biophysical Research Communications 1983, 112: 47–54.
28. Rodriguez, R. J., Low, C., Bottema, C. D. K., Parks, L. W.: Multiple functions for sterols in *Saccharomyces cerevisiae*. Biochimica et Biophysica Acta 1985, 837: 336–343.
29. Nishino, T., Hata, S., Taketani, S., Yabusaki, Y., Katsuki, H.: Subcellular localization of the enzymes involved in the late stage of ergosterol biosynthesis in yeast. Journal of Biochemistry 1981, 89: 1391–1396.
30. Boll, M., Lowel, M., Still, J., Berndt, J.: Sterol biosynthesis in yeast. 3-Hydroxy-3-methylglutaryl-coenzyme A reductase as a regulatory enzyme. European Journal of Biochemistry 1975, 54: 435–444.
31. Endo, A.: Compactin (ML-236B) and related compounds as potential cholesterol-lowering agents that inhibit HMG-CoA reductase. Journal of Medicinal Chemistry 1985, 28: 401–405.
32. Omura, S., Tomoda, H., Kumagai, H., Greenspan, M., Yodkovitz, J. B., Chen, J. S., Alberts, A. W., Martin, I., Mochales, S., Monaghan, R. L., Chabala, J. C., Schwartz, R. E., Patchett, A. A.: Potent inhibitory effect of antibiotic 1233A on cholesterol biosynthesis which specifically blocks 3-hydroxy-3-methylglutaryl coenzyme A synthase. The Journal of Antibiotics 1987, 40: 1356–1357.
33. Baldwin, B. C.: Fungicidal inhibitors of ergosterol biosynthesis. Biochemical Society Transactions 1983, 11: 659–663.
34. Pierce, A. M., Pierce, H. D. Jr., Unrau, A. A., Oehlschlager, A. C.: Lipid composition and polyene antibiotic resistance of *Candida albicans* mutants. Canadian Journal of Biochemistry 1979, 56: 135–142.
35. Hamilton-Miller, J. M. T.: Fungal sterols and the mode of action of the polyene antibiotics. Advances in Applied Microbiology 1977, 17: 109–135.
36. Hammond, S. M.: Biological activity of polyene antibiotics. Progress in Medicinal Chemistry 1977, 14: 105–283.
37. Andreoli, T. E.: On the anatomy of amphotericin B-cholesterol pores in lipid membranes. Kidney International 1973, 4: 337–345.
38. Hammond, S. M., Lambert, P. A., Klinger, B. N.: The mode of action of polyene antibiotics: induced potassium leakage in *Candida albicans*. Journal of General Microbiology 1974, 81: 325–330.
39. Teerlink, T., De Kruijff, B., Demel, R. A.: The action of pimaricin, etruscomycin, and amphotericin B on liposomes with varying sterol content. Biochimica et Biophysica Acta 1980, 599: 484–492.

40. Medoff, G., Kobayashi, G. S., Kwan, C. N., Schlessinger, D., Venkov, P.: Potentiation of rifampin and 5-fluorocytosine as antifungal antibiotics by amphotericin B. Proceedings of the National Academy of Sciences USA 1972, 69: 196–199.
41. Gravestock, M. B., Ryley, J. F.: Antifungal chemotherapy. Annual Reports in Medicinal Chemistry 1984, 19: 127–136.
42. Berg, D., Buchel, K.-H., Plempel, M., Regel, E.: Antimycotic sterol biosynthesis inhibitors. Trends in Pharmacological Sciences 1986, 7: 233–238.
43. Richardson, K., Marriott, M. S.: Antifungal agents. Annual Reports in Medicinal Chemistry 1987, 22: 159–167.
44. Fromtling, R. A.: Overview of medically important antifungal azole derivatives. Clinical Microbiology Reviews 1988, 1: 187–217.
45. van den Bossche, H., Willemsens, G., Marichal, P.: Anti-*Candida* Drugs – the biochemical basis for their specificity. In: O'Leary, W. M. (ed.): Critical Reviews in Microbiology. Volume 15. CRC Press, Boca Raton, Fla., 1987, p. 57–72.
46. Boiron, P., Drouhet, E., Dupont, B., Improvisi, L.: Entry of ketoconazole into *Candida albicans*. Antimicrobial Agents and Chemotherapy 1987, 31: 244–248.
47. Brajtburg, J., Kobayashi, D., Medoff, A., Kobayashi, G. S.: Antifungal action of amphotericin B in combination with other polyene or imidazole antibiotics. The Journal of Infectious Diseases 1982, 146: 138–146.
48. Pesti, M., Campbell, J. M., Peberdy, J. F.: Alteration of ergosterol content and chitin synthase activity in *Candida albicans*. Current Microbiology 1981, 5: 187–190.
49. Takeo, K., Nishimura, K., Miyaji, M.: Resistance of the neck plasma membrane between the mother and the bud of *Saccharomyces cerevisiae* and *Candida albicans* to amphotericin B-induced deformation. FEMS Microbiology Letters 1987, 48: 321–324.
50. Borgers, M., De Brabander, M., van den Bossche, H., Van Cutsem, J.: Promotion of pseudomycelium formation of *Candida albicans* in culture: a morphologic study of the effects of miconazole and ketoconazole. Postgraduate Medicine 1979, 55: 687–691.
51. Roncero, C., Valdivieso, M. H., Ribas, J. C., Duran, A.: Effect of calcofluor white on chitin synthases from *Saccharomyces cerevisiae*. Journal of Bacteriology 1988, 170: 1945–1949.
52. Georgopoulos, A., Petranyi, G., Mieth, H., Drews, J.: In vitro activity of naftifine, a new antifungal agent. Antimicrobial Agents and Chemotherapy 1981, 19: 386–389.
53. Petranyi, G., Ryder, N. S., Stutz, A.: Allylamine derivatives: new class of synthetic antifungal agents inhibiting fungal squalene epoxidase. Science 1984, 224: 1239–1241.
54. Bianchi, A., Monti, G., de Carneri, I.: Tolciclate: further antimycotic studies. Antimicrobial Agents and Chemotherapy 1977, 12: 429–430.
55. Barrett-Bee, K. J., Lane, A. C., Turner, R. W.: The mode of antifungal action of tolnaftate. Journal of Medical Veterinary Mycology 1986, 24: 155–160.
56. Paltauf, F., Daum, G., Zuder, G., Hogenauer, G., Schulz, G., Seidl, G.: Squalene and ergosterol biosynthesis in fungi treated with naftifine, a new antimycotic agent. Biochimica et Biophysica Acta 1982, 712: 268–273.
57. Ryder, N. S., Dupont, M.-C.: Inhibition of squalene epoxidase by allylamine antimycotic compounds. Biochemical Journal 1985, 230: 765–770.
58. Morita, T., Nozawa, Y.: Effects of antifungal agents on ergosterol biosynthesis in *Candida albicans* and *Trichophyton mentagrophytes:* differential inhibitory sites of naphthiomate and miconazole. Journal of Investigative Dermatology 1985, 85: 434–437.
59. Ryder, N. S., Frank, I., Dupont, M.-C.: Ergosterol biosynthesis inhibition by the thiocarbamate antifungal agents tolnaftate and tolciclate. Antimicrobial Agents and Chemotherapy 1986, 29: 858–860.
60. Himmele, W., Pommer, E.-H.: 3-Phenylpropylamines, a new class of systemic fungicides. Angewandte Chemie, International Edition (English) 1980, 19: 184–189.
61. Polak, A.: Antifungal activity in vitro of Ro 14-4767/002, a phenylpropyl-morpholine. Sabouraudia 1983, 21: 205–213.
62. Baloch, R. I., Mercer, E. I., Wiggins, T. E., Baldwin, B. C.: Inhibition of ergosterol biosynthesis in *Saccharomyces cerevisiae* and *Ustilago maydis* by tridemorph, fenpropimorph, and fenpropidin. Phytochemistry 1984, 23: 2219–2226.
63. Mehta, R., Lopez-Berestein, G., Hopfer, R., Mills, K., Juliano, R. L.: Liposomal amphotericin A is toxic to fungal cells but not to mammalian cells. Biochimica et Biophysica Acta 1984, 770: 230–234.
64. Weinberg, E. D.: Antifungal agents. In: Foye, W. O. (ed.): Principles of Medicinal Chemistry. Lea and Febinger, Philadelphia, 1981, p. 809–816.

Membrane Changes Induced by Praziquantel

P. Andrews*, A. Harder

The mechanism of action of praziquantel, an anthelmintic effective against all trematodes and cestodes, is reviewed. Comparative studies of the effects of praziquantel and cationic amphiphilic drugs on the carbohydrate metabolism of *Schistosoma mansoni* have resulted in investigations into the interaction of praziquantel with phospholipids. The primary event is an interaction of praziquantel with membrane acidic phospholipids and Ca^{2+} ions, causing a transition in phospholipid organisation from the bilayer to the hexagonal phase. The resulting influx of calcium into the parasite induces muscular contractions. Hexagonal phases are associated with membrane fusion, a process which could lead to tegumental vacuolation. The stereospecific action of praziquantel could be explained by a hypothetical receptor mediating the primary interaction. Muscular contraction and tegumental damage are obvious effects of praziquantel, occurring within seconds after exposure. All other effects are indirect, resulting from perturbations of the environment of membrane-associated enzymes and the disruption of regulatory processes in the parasite.

Praziquantel is a broad-spectrum anthelmintic drug effective against two related groups of helminth parasites: the tapeworms, or cestodes, and the flukes, or trematodes (Figure 1). It has been available for the control of cestode and trematode infections in humans, companion animals and lifestock since about 1980. Today, praziquantel is one of the anthelmintics on the World Health Organization's List of Essential Drugs. It is considered the drug of choice for the treatment of human trematode infections, including those caused by schistosomes, liver- and lung flukes. It is the only drug effective against cysticercosis, an infection caused by larval tapeworms. Further, it is the only drug reliably effective against the dog tapeworm *Echinococcus*, thus making possible the prevention of hydatidosis, another form of larval tapeworm disease in humans.

Research aimed at elucidating the mode of action of praziquantel was initiated soon after the discovery of the anthelminitic potential of the then novel class of pyrazinoisoquinoline compounds in 1972. The purpose was to provide a rational basis for the intelligent and successful use of praziquantel in humans and animals. As a result of the concerted effort of researchers in many countries and laboratories, praziquantel is now a well studied drug with a mechanism of action that has been revealed to the molecular level. Most of the experiments conducted have been done using mice infected with either *Schistosoma mansoni* or isolated schistosomes.

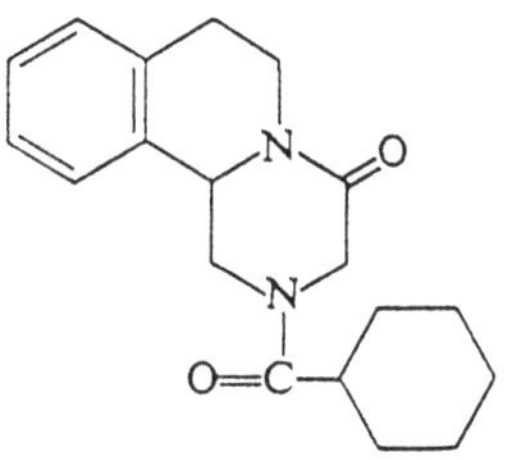

$C_{19}H_{24}N_2O_2$
mol.wt.: 312.42

Figure 1: Structural formula of praziquantel: 2-cyclohexyl-carbonyl [1, 2, 3, 6, 7, 11b] hexahydro-4H-pyrazino [2, 1-a] isoquinolin-4-one.

A detailed description of many aspects of praziquantel, including chemistry, metabolism, pharmacokinetics, toxicology and especially therapeutic efficacy in animals, has been compiled (1). A useful summary of the clinical use of praziquantel for the treatment of schistosomiasis and of other human trematode infections is found in the proceedings of two symposia (2, 3). The use of praziquantel as a cestocide has been summarized (4) and knowledge on the mechanism of antischistosomal action of praziquantel has also been reviewed (5).

Description of Schistosomes

Schistosomes are digenetic trematodes or flukes. Their life cycle involves an aquatic snail which releases larvae (cercariae) that actively infect man

Institut für Parasitologie, 5090 Leverkusen-Bayerwerk, FRG.

when he has contact with water. Once in the human body, the flukes migrate from the skin via the lungs to their appropriate location in the circulatory system, where they mature and begin to lay large numbers of eggs. A small fraction of the eggs passes through the capillary walls and adjoining tissues into the intestine or the bladder. When the excreta are released into water, larvae (miracidia) hatch from the eggs and infect the snail intermediate host. The larger fraction of the eggs is retained in the vasculature and tissues where the decaying eggs give rise to micro-embolisms and granulomatous reactions. The multitudinous eggs that accumulate in the tissues of the infected host are the pathogens of schistosomiasis or bilharzia, a disease which presently afflicts some 200 million people. A further 500–600 million are exposed to the threat of infection. The geographical distribution is wide, ranging from Iran to most of Africa, to parts of Latin America, and from China to Indonesia.

Schistosomes live in the portal or mesenteric veins of their host, and their body surface, the tegument, has developed some remarkable features. The primary functions of the tegument are the protection of the parasite against the host's immune attack and the maintenance of survival. In terms of protection the parasite incorporates host antigens on its tegumental surface and so camouflages itself effectively. In terms of survival the tegument serves as an important site of nutrient uptake and ion and water regulation. It further contains various enzymes; for example, it is a site of ATP generation both by oxidative pathways and from reduced glutathione, and it maintains a membrane potential of -35 to -41 mV. The ionic composition of the tegument is different from that of the serum bathing the parasite and also from that of erythrocytes. All these phenomena suggest the existence of a proton pump operating in the tegument of schistosomes which maintains ionic gradients and a pH value of the tegument of 7.8 (6). The tegument of schistosomes is much more than a mere envelope – it is an organ in its own right.

The surface of the tegument is studded with pits and spines. The pits lead to branched and sometimes interconnected channels which contain serum. The enormous increase in surface area of the parasite imparted by pits and channels is undoubtedly of value for an absorptive organ. Histologically, the tegument is a syncytium with a thickness of about 4 μm. Its cell nuclei are sunk below the circular muscle layer. The apical surface of the tegument is a specialized version of the normal phospholipid bilayer membrane, a so-called heptalaminate membrane, which is formed by the stacking of two trilaminate membranes on top of each other. The significance of this special adaptation is not understood, but it is known to occur in other blood-dwelling flukes and may be related to the intravascular habitat. The tegument is not a static structure. On the contrary, its components are subject to rapid rates of turnover. The heptalaminate surface membrane, with a half-life of about two to three hours, appears to be replaced continually by material provided through multilaminate vesicles produced in the cell bodies of the tegument (7).

Threshold Concentration of Praziquantel

A prerequisite for an analysis of the mechanism of action of a drug is information on the concentrations to which the parasites are exposed when the host is given a therapeutic dose. Schistosomes live in the vasculature and thus drug levels determined in samples of peripheral venous blood give a good approximation of the levels actually encountered by the parasite. One slight complication is that some schistosome species live in the portal vein, in which the concentration of praziquantel is known to be elevated during the phase of enteric absorption of praziquantel. Favourable to the calculation of concentrations encountered is the lack of antischistosomal effect of the praziquantel metabolites formed by the mammalian host. Thus, only the unchanged drug has to be considered. Further, while schistosomes take up praziquantel readily, they only bind it loosely and drug is readily lost in drug-free media. As far as is revealed by ^{14}C-autoradiography, praziquantel is evenly distributed through all organ systems of the parasite. Finally, it has been shown that schistosomes lack the ability to degrade praziquantel (8).

The simultaneous study of the pharmacokinetics and therapeutic efficacy of praziquantel in animal models allows the estimation of a threshold concentration to which the parasite must be exposed in order to be eliminated, as well as the time period involved. The threshold concentration is somewhat less than 10^{-6} M, and the period of exposure required is about six hours. These conditions are met in patients receiving antischistosomal therapy (5). Only those effects of praziquantel that are induced by concentrations of about 10^{-6} M are likely to be relevant for the understanding of the mechanism of action of praziquantel against schistosomes and other susceptible parasites.

Morphological Effects of Praziquantel

When schistosomes encounter 10^{-6} M praziquantel, either in vitro or in a treated animal, there are two very striking reactions. Firstly, an almost instantaneous spastic paralysis of the parasite's musculature occurs, and secondly, rapid structural damage to the surface of the tegument ensues. Within 30 seconds of exposure to 0.5×10^{-6} M praziquantel, schistosomes develop many bleb-like structures which can be seen from the outside and which are protrusions of the surface membrane (Figure 2). The outer surface of the tegumental membrane appears unchanged, at least as measured by intensity staining using Thièry's periodic acid Schiff silver proteinate reaction for carbohydrate, which shows that the surface coat remains intact (9). This tegumental blebbing is followed within minutes by increasing vacuolation which develops from the basal region of the tegument, and by the formation of larger balloon-like surface exudates, which are still contained by the tegumental membrane. Immunologically the parasite surface begins to change. Previously unexposed parasite antigens are exposed within 30 minutes of treating the mouse host (10). These additional epitopes evidently appear in the absence of any effects on surface-located host erythrocyte antigens (11). The process of vacuolation and ballooning of the tegument continues and eventually parts of the tegument are sloughed off. Within four hours after treating the mouse host, phagocytic cells are found associated with the parasite. Invasion of the parasite's body by phagocytes is in full progress after 17 hours of treatment and results in the lysis of the parasitic tissues within a few days.

How tegumental damage is brought about cannot be answered by morphological and ultrastructural studies. Similar tegumental alterations have also been observed in schistosomes exposed to many different conditions or compounds such as, hypo- or hypertonic media, in vitro culture, hyperimmune serum, complement, major basic protein, lectins and several antischistosomal substances. It thus appears that the morphologically visible damage is not directly related to the nature of the noxious agent encountered by the schistosome, but rather a general reaction to adverse conditions. One point, however, is noteworthy. Praziquantel induces surface blebbing within seconds, while many minutes or hours are required by the other agents. Praziquantel causes tegumental alterations qualitatively similar to those found in schistosomes in a large number of other digenetic trematodes living in the lungs, livers or intestines of their hosts and also in all of the several cestode species studied so far (1). The extent of tegumental damage caused varies between species.

Muscular Contraction

Contraction of the schistosome musculature can be monitored more exactly than the development of surface damage. Half maximal contraction is obtained just 11 seconds after the addition of 10^{-6} M praziquantel (12). The praziquantel-induced contraction depends on the presence of Ca^{2+} ions. Depletion of external calcium or addition of an excess of magnesium abolishes drug-induced concentration. Most inhibitors of known neurotransmitters of *Schistosoma mansoni*, as well as other pharmacologically active agents, do not antagonize the contraction-inducing effect of praziquantel. This lack of interaction of praziquantel with neuroreceptive sites together with the requirement for calcium ions has led to the idea that praziquantel directly or indirectly activates a calcium-dependent contraction of the parasite's musculature. It has been shown that 10^{-6} M praziquantel induces a rapid increase in the rate of uptake of external calcium into schistosomes, which is already measurable after one minute. However, it has not yet been shown that the concentration of Ca^{2+} ions actually increases within schistosome muscle cells when they contract under the influence of praziquantel.

The possibility that praziquantel acts like an ionophore has also been investigated. Although some ionophores (X537 and A23187) were shown to induce contraction in schistosomes, praziquantel

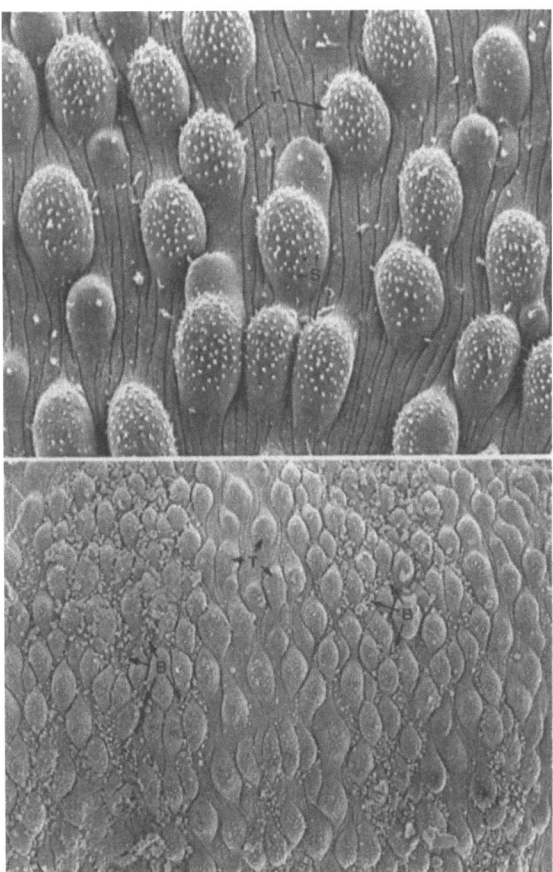

Figure 2: Scanning electron micrograph of the dorsal tegument of male *Schistosoma mansoni* provided with tubercles (T) and spines (S). (above) Untreated control, × 950. (below) After 60 min exposure to 30 μM praziquantel. The tegumental surface shows numerous bleb-like lesions (B), × 300.

does not behave like an ionophore in that it does not transfer Na^+ or Ca^{2+} ions from an aqueous medium into an organic phase (12). Another possibility that might have explained the action of praziquantel on calcium flux was ruled out when it was found that the calcium channel blocker D-600 did not prevent praziquantel-induced muscular contractions in schistosomes (13). Further, La^{3+} and Co^{2+} ions, known to interfere with Ca^{2+} binding and flux across biological membranes in experiments with other tissues, were also without effect on praziquantel-induced contraction (12). Fluoxetine was the only pharmacological agent that interfered with both the influx of calcium and the induction of muscular contraction. All these experiments suggest that praziquantel affects calcium flux across biological membranes by interaction with sites not classically associated with the regulation of Ca^{2+} transport.

Carbohydrate Metabolism

Besides the very rapid effects of praziquantel on schistosomes there are numerous other effects which only become apparent after several minutes or hours of exposure to praziquantel. These effects include changes in the ionic composition of the parasite, inhibition of various enzyme activities, and changes in carbohydrate, protein and nucleotide metabolism (5). It was from a study of these secondary effects that the next step toward unraveling the mechanism of action of praziquantel developed

The finding that fluoxetine interferes with the ability of praziquantel to induce contractions led to an investigation of the effect of fluoxetine and other cationic amphiphilic drugs and praziquantel on the carbohydrate metabolism of *Schistosoma mansoni* (14). Five amphiphilic cationic drugs-chlorpromazine, imipramine, amitryptiline, propranolol and fluoxetine- and the electrically neutral praziquantel all stimulate glucose uptake and lactate excretion in a qualitatively similar way. Quantitatively, however, there are differences. The five amphiphilic drugs are almost identical, with a maximal stimulatory effect at concentrations from 10^{-5} to 10^{-4} M and inhibition at 10^{-3} M. Praziquantel is more effective, being maximally stimulatory at 10^{-7} M and inhibitory above 10^{-6} M. Combination experiments during which schistosomes were first incubated with 5×10^{-5} M chlorpromazine or fluoxetine followed by the addition of 10^{-7} M praziquantel did not result in a reduced stimulation of glucose uptake and lactate excretion. Addition of higher concentrations of praziquantel, however, abolished the chlorpromazine-induced stimulatory effects. This can be explained by a higher affinity of praziquantel than that of chlorpromazine for the same binding site.

The combined effects of serotonin and praziquantel on the carbohydrate metabolism were also studied, because serotonin receptors had been implicated as possibly mediating the effects of praziquantel (15). The stimulatory effect of serotonin on glucose uptake and lactate release was not observed in parasites that had already been stimulated by the addition of 10^{-3} M fluoxetine or 10^{-5} M praziquantel. At lower concentrations of both drugs serotonin can exert its stimulatory effect. One of the amphiphilic drugs studied, fluoxetine, is a specific inhibitor of serotonin uptake in mouse brain and in schistosomes. It has been found that praziquantel inhibits serotonin uptake of *Schistosoma mansoni* as effectively as fluoxetine. Both drugs inhibit the sodium dependent and the sodium independent serotonin uptake by approximately 40% at a concentration of 10^{-5} M. At the same concentration praziquantel also inhibits glucose uptake and lactate excretion, while fluoxetine is not inhibitory but enhances glucose uptake as well as lactate excretion. This indicates that praziquantel is not a specific inhibitor of serotonin uptake. Its inhibitory effect is presumably caused by a perturbation of the tegumental environment of receptor proteins. A similar explanation has been suggested for the inhibitory effect of praziquantel on two other tegumental enzyme systems: the ATPase of *Schistosoma mansoni* (16) and different phosphatases of the cestode *Cotugnia digonopora* (17).

Amphiphilic cationic drugs such as chlorpromazine are known to affect different membrane-associated processes. They stabilize membranes, as seen by the decrease of relative hemolysis and the replacement of Ca^{2+} ions from membranes, and they release serotonin from rat mast cells indicating a change in the permeability to uncharged solutes through membranes. A certain range of concentrations ($0.3-1 \times 10^{-4}$ M chlorpromazine) is known as the range of prelysis, and it is just in this range of concentrations that chlorpromazine induces maximal glucose uptake, lactate excretion and also maximal motility of *Schistosoma mansoni*. Praziquantel and the amphiphilic cationic drugs have qualitatively similiar effects on the carbohydrate metabolism. Therefore, it is not unreasonable to assume that praziquantel is also a membrane-affecting drug.

Praziquantel − Phospholipid Interactions

Calcium ions are generally known to be involved in motility, muscle contraction, and the regulation of carbohydrate metabolism. Further, maintenance of membrane structure and function are governed by Ca^{2+} ions. Therefore, regarding schistosomes, it appears reasonable to assume that those effects of praziquantel which can be observed or recorded rapidly (contraction, permeability changes, tegumental damage), and those processes that can only be measured after minutes or hours (changes in the carbohydrate metabolism, serotonin uptake or enzyme activities), are sequelae of the same primary effect: changes in the distribution of calcium within the parasite that result from altered membrane properties. This conclusion is supported by the observation that four events — therapeutic efficacy against schistosomes in animal studies, induction of tegumental surface damage, muscular contraction and paralysis, and calcium influx — are all maximal in the presence of the levorotatory stereo-isomer, while the dextrorotatory stereo-isomer of praziquantel is virtually devoid of activity. This line of reasoning led to the next step toward understanding the mechanism of action of praziquantel, a step that was achieved by studying the interactions of synthetic phospholipids with praziquantel, fluoxetine and other amphiphilic drugs.

The investigations required the use of a model membrane, because tegumental phospholipids of Schistosoma mansoni can only be prepared in very small amounts. Further, the exact composition of these lipids and their distribution across the schistosomal tegument are not known. The best approximation is derived from the composition of the multilaminate vesicles, which are contained in the tegument and which are thought to be incorporated into the surface of schistosomes; the main components of their phospholipids are acidic phosphatidylserine (15 % of total phospholipids), neutral phosphatidylethanolamine (25 %) and phosphatidylcholine (28 %) (18). The initial studies were conducted using differential thermal analysis, a method which allows the measurement of stability of phospholipid membranes (phosphatidylglycerol) in the presence of different drugs and ions. A second method used was electron microscopy, which reveals possible structural alterations of the model membranes.

Imipramine and fluoxetine, which belong to the cationic drugs, increase the fluidity of acidic phospholipid membranes (phosphatidylglycerol), while praziquantel has only a small effect. The Ca^{2+} ion-induced stabilization is much lower in the presence of the positively charged drugs than in the presence of praziquantel, which has no net charge. Electron microscopy reveals that the amphiphilic drugs do not alter the structure of acidic phospholipid vesicles, while praziquantel induces a drastic alteration in the organization of acidic phospholipid vesicles, which then appear to be clumped together (19).

With respect to the alteration of membrane properties, it is quite obvious that there are important differences between praziquantel, which is electrically neutral, and the amphiphilic drugs, which carry positive charges. The latter are able to displace Ca^{2+} ions from membranes and thus reduce the amount of Ca^{2+} ions bound to membranes, while praziquantel enhances the permeability of Ca^{2+} ions through membranes. This difference of effect on membrane-associated Ca^{2+} ions could explain why the paralysis induced by these drugs in schistosomes is spastic in the case of praziquantel and flaccid in the case of the amphiphilic drugs. Spastic paralysis is provoked by the influx of Ca^{2+} ions, while the inability to contract, which results from reduced binding of Ca^{2+} ions to the membranes, leads to flaccidly paralyzed schistosomes. Under the electron microscope praziquantel appears to induce fusion processes between acidic phospholipid vesicles. Such phenomena are usually associated with, and can only be explained by, changes in the organization of the phospholipid molecules.

To study possible structural alterations of phospholipids that could explain how membranes change their permeability to ions, ^{31}P-nuclear magnetic resonance spectroscopy has been used. This technique allows the study of the effect of drugs, ions and temperature on the transition between the three different phases that a phospholipid can adopt: the bilayer phase, in which biological membranes are normally organised; the isotropic phase (vesicles, inverted vesicles, micellar, cubic or rhombic structures); and the hexagonal phase. The latter consists of hexagonally packed lipidic cylinders in which the polar headgroups are oriented toward an internal aqueous channel of nearly 20 Å diameter. This hexagonal organization of lipid molecules cannot maintain a permeability barrier which is otherwise well maintained by a membrane in the bilayer phase (20, 21). The formation of hexagonal structures is known to facilitate the fusion of membranes, a process which is involved in secretion and is thought to be the basis of the rapid vesiculation and vacuolation occurring in the schistosomal tegument in the presence of praziquantel.

A phospholipid dispersion consisting of phosphatidylethanolamine and phosphatidylserine with a molar ratio of 2:1, which corresponds to the assumed composition of tegumental lipids, gives a mixture of isotropic and bilayer signals, i.e. the isotropic and the bilayer phases coexist (Figure 3). When Ca^{2+} ions are present, a mixture of hexagonal and bilayer phases exists. The addition of praziquantel to the phospholipid mixture (molar ratio 1:1) results in the formation of a pure isotropic phase. The simultaneous presence of praziquantel and Ca^{2+} ions gives rise to a complete transition to the hexagonal phase when the experiment is performed at 35 °C. The ratio of lipid to calcium is not critical — it can range from 4:1 to 1:1. The degree of transition to the hexagonal phase is less marked when the lipid mixture contains an increased amount of phosphatidylethanolamine. At a molar ratio of phosphatidyl-

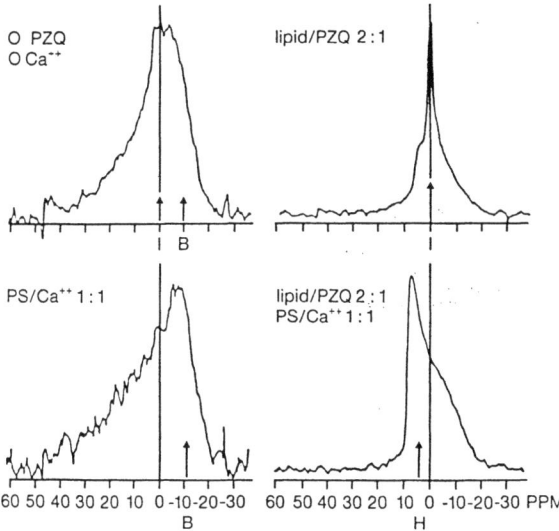

Figure 3: ^{31}P-NMR-spectra of mixtures off egg-yolk phosphatidylethanolamine and bovine brain phosphatidylserine (PS) (molar ratio 2:1) without any addition; after addition of praziquantel (PZQ) (lipid/drug molar ratio 2:1); after the addition of Ca^{2+} (PS/Ca^{2+} molar ratio 1:1); and after the simultaneous addition of praziquantel and Ca^{2+} (lipid/drug molar ratio 2:1, PS/Ca^{2+} molar ratio 1:1) at 25 °C. The arrows indicate the position of the signals obtainable from the three phases: B = bilayer, H = hexagonal, I = isotropic.

ethanolamine to phosphatidylserine of 4:1, there is only a partial transition to the hexagonal phase at 25 °C, while there is a pronounced but not exclusive transition to the hexagonal phase at 35 °C.

These experiments show that praziquantel is capable of inducing conformational transitions in artificial phospholipid membranes known to be associated with an increase in permeability to ions under conditions that attempt to simulate the natural situation: a molar ratio of phosphatidylethanolamine to phosphatidylserine of 2:1 (as is presumed to exist in the tegumental lipids of schistosomes), the presence of Ca^{2+} ions, and physiological temperatures of 25° and 35 °C. There is no proof yet that similar transitions occur in natural schistosomal membranes. Electron microscopy after freeze fracture preparation of schistosomal membranes may reveal such changes. However, concentrations of praziquantel as low as 3×10^{-6} M (equivalent to a lipid to drug ratio of 50:1) have still resulted in the formation of hexagonal phases. This is in good agreement with the threshold concentration in serum of 10^{-6} M which has been derived from therapeutic experiments.

In the absence of calcium, the amphiphilic drugs fluoxetine and imipramine behave like praziquantel. All three drugs induce an isotropic phase when added to the phospholipid mixture. The further addition of Ca^{2+} ions, however, reveals important differences. Fluoxetine also induces hexagonal structures, but fails to increase membrane permeability. This apparent discrepancy, induction of hexagonal structures without concomitant permeability increase, can be resolved, however. Fluoxetine is positively charged and imparts this charge to the internal aqueous channel of the hexagonal structures. Thus, cations are repelled and this effectively prevents the permeation of Ca^{2+} ions through the internal channel (22). Imipramine, another positively charged amphiphilic drug, induces lamellar structures in the presence of Ca^{2+} ions. Again, positive charges are imparted to the lamellae with the result that Ca^{2+} ions are displaced from the membrane. In order to cause an increase in the ion permeability of the phospholipid membrane it is not sufficient for a drug to induce hexagonal structures alone. The charge which the drug imparts is important, too. An increase in permeability to positively charged ions is only achieved if the hexagonal phase is induced by an electrically neutral drug like praziquantel.

A crucial question is whether praziquantel has the same stereospecificity of effect in the artificial phospholipid system employed as it is know to have against schistosomes in host organisms. It has been found that the levorotatory stereo-isomer is slightly more effective than the dextrarotatory stereo-isomer in inducing the transition of hexagonal phases. This lack of a profound difference in the effects of the two steric forms of praziquantel is the reason for postulating the existence of a stereospecific link between membrane and drug. This link is likely to be a receptor protein. Such a receptor has been described for an antischistosomally active benzodiazepine, a compound which induces influx of calcium and muscular contraction in a way similar to praziquantel (12, 23). The postulated praziquantel receptor of schistosomes remains to be characterized. Such a stereospecific praziquantel receptor should also occur in other trematodes and cestodes and should not be found in nematodes and mammals. The occurrence of a receptor could then explain why the effects of praziquantel are essentially restricted to those parasitic helminths possessing a syncytial tegument.

Conclusion

The present knowledge of how praziquantel affects schistosomes can be summarized in a model (Figure 4). The primary effect of praziquantel is the alteration of the permeability of the tegumental membrane by perturbations which result from an interaction between negatively charged phospholipids, Ca^{2+} ions and the electrically neutral drug molecule. The effect on the phospholipid membrane is presumably me-

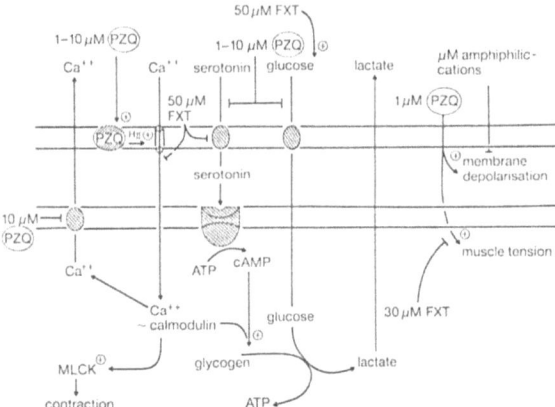

Figure 4: Functional model of the effects of praziquantel showing a cross section through the schistosoma tegument containing protein receptors (hatched) in the outer (upper) and in the inner (lower) membrane of the tegument; ⟶ ⊕ denotes a stimulatory effect, ⟶ an inhibitory effect; H_{II} = hexagonal phospholipid phase, FXT = fluoxetine; MLCK = myosin light chain kinase; PZQ = praziquantel.

diated by a protein receptor which can distinguish between the two stereo-isomers of the drug, thus causing the observed stereospecificity of the effects of praziquantel. Once inside the parasite, Ca^{2+} ions act as second messengers and trigger contraction and glycogen breakdown. Some membrane-associated transport proteins, e.g. those specific for the uptake of serotonin or glucose or Ca^{2+}-ATPase, are inhibited indirectly by perturbances in their tegumental environment. Thus, the Ca^{2+}-ATPase, which normally pumps calcium from the parasite into the medium, is unable to control the rise of Ca^{2+} ion concentration within the parasite. This leads to a break-down of metabolic processes. One of the dire consequences is that the parasite loses its ability to repair tegumental surface lesions, which then exposes it to the attack of the immune system of the host. Phagocytic cells begin to invade the parasite within 17 hours after treatment of the host, a process terminating in the lysis of the tissues of the parasite within a few days.

One unexpected finding resulting from the analysis of the mechanism of action of praziquantel is that the effects induced in schistostomes are of a reversible nature. Repair of drug-induced lesions is prevented by the interaction of the immune system with the parasite, which is rendered susceptible to immune attack through tegumental damage and paralysis. The importance of this interaction can be seen in experiments with immunocompromised animals. Treatment has been shown to be less effective in immunocompromised than in immune competent animals (5). Pursuit of the search for synergistic effects between mechanisms involved in host-parasite interactions and agents that impair parasite-specific functions will result in the further progress in anthelmintic therapy.

References

1. **Andrews, P., Thomas, H., Pohlke, R., Seubert, J.:** Praziquantel. Medicinal Research Reviews 1983, 3: 147–200.
2. Proceedings of the Biltricide Symposium on African Schistosomiasis. Nairobi, February 24–26, 1980. Arzneimittelforschung 1981, 31: 535–618.
3. Proceedings of the International Symposium on Human Trematode Infections in Southeast and East Asia. Kyongju, Republic of Korea, October 19–21, 1983. Arzneimittelforschung 1984, 34: 1115–1242.
4. **Groll, E.:** Praziquantel. Advances in Pharmacology and Chemotherapy 1984, 20: 219–238.
5. **Andrews, P.:** Praziquantel: mechanisms of anti-schistosomal activity. Pharmacology and Therapeutics 1985, 29: 129–156.
6. **Huang, T.-Y.:** Biochemical characteristics of the tegument of *Schistosoma japonicum*. Archiv for Pharmaci og Chemi Scientific Edition 1987, 15: 65–75.
7. **Wilson, R. A., Barnes, P. E.:** The formation and turnover of the membranocalyx on the tegument of *Schistosoma mansoni*. Parasitology 1977, 74: 61–71.
8. **Andrews, P., Thomas, H., Weber, H.:** The in vitro uptake of ^{14}C-praziquantel by cestodes, trematodes and a nematode. Journal of Parasitology 1980, 60: 920–925.
9. **Becker, B., Mehlhorn, H., Andrews, P., Thomas, H., Eckert, J.:** Light and electron microscopic studies on the effect of praziquantel on *Schistosoma mansoni*, *Dicrocoelium dendriticum* and *Fasciola hepatica* (Trematoda) in vitro. Zeitschrift für Parasitenkunde 1980, 63: 113–128.
10. **Xiao, S. H., et al.:** The appearance of surface antigen of *Schistosoma japonicum* recovered from infected mice after treatment with pyquiton. Shanghai Journal of Immunology 1981, 1: 9–15.
11. **Harnett, W., Kusel, J. R.:** Increased exposure of parasite antigens at the surface of adult male *Schistosoma mansoni* exposed to praziquantel in vitro. Parasitology 1986, 93: 401–405.
12. **Pax, R., Bennett, J. L., Fetterer, R.:** A benzodiazepine derivative and praziquantel: effects on musculature of *Schistosoma mansoni* and *Schistosoma japonicum*. Naunyn-Schmiedeberg's Archives of Pharmacology 1978, 304: 309–315.
13. **Fetterer, R. H., Pax, R. A., Bennett, J. L.:** Praziquantel, potassium and 2,4-dinitrophenol: analysis of their action on the musculature of *Schistosoma mansoni*. European Journal of Pharmacology 1980, 64: 31–38.
14. **Harder, A., Andrews, P., Thomas, H.:** Chlorpromazine, other amphiphilic cationic drugs and praziquantel: effects on carbohydrate metabolism of *Schistosoma mansoni*. Parasitology Research 1987, 73: 245–249.
15. **Harder, A., Abbink, J., Andrews, P., Thomas, H.:** Praziquantel impairs the ability of exogenous serotonin to stimulate carbohydrate metabolism in intact *Schistosoma mansoni*. Parasitology Research 1987, 73: 442–445.
16. **Nechay, B. R., Hillman, G. G., Dotson, M. J.:** Properties and drug sensitivity of adenosine triphosphatases from *Schistosoma mansoni*. Journal of Parasitology 1980, 66: 596–600.

17. **Pampori, N. A.:** Enzymes of isolated brush border membrane of *Cotugnia digonopora* and their insensitivity to anthelmintics in vitro. Veterinary Parasitology 1985, 18: 13–19.
18. **McDiarmid, S. S., Podesta, R. B., Rahman, S. M.:** Preparation and partial characterization of a multilamellar body fraction from *Schistosoma mansoni*. Molecular Biochemical Parasitology 1982, 5: 93–105.
19. **Harder, A., Andrews, P., Thomas, H.:** Praziquantel: mode of action. Biochemical Society Transactions 1986, 15: 68–70.
20. **Cullis, P. R., Hope, M. J., Nayar, R., Tilcock, C. P. S.:** Roles of phospholipids in exocytosis. In Horrocks, L. A., Kanfer, J. N., Procellati, G. (ed.): Phospholipids in the nervous system. Raven Press, New York, 1985, p. 71–86.
21. **Cullis, P. R., Hope, M. J., De Kruijff, B., Verkleij, A. J., Tilcock, C. P. S.:** Structural properties and functional roles of phospholipids in bioligical membranes. In: Kuo, F. (ed.): Phospholipids and cellular regulation. CRC Press, Boca Raton, Fla., 1985, p. 1–59.
22. **Harder, A., Goossens, J., Andrews, P.:** Influence of praziquantel and Ca^{2+} on the bilayer-isotropic-hexagonal transition of model membranes. Molecular and Biochemical Parasitology 1988, 29: 55–60.
23. **Bennett, J. L.:** Characteristics of antischistosomal benzodiazepine binding sites in *Schistostoma mansoni*. Journal of Parasitology 1981, 66: 742–747.

Mechanisms of Action of Antimalarial Drugs

W. Peters*

Multiple-drug resistance in the malignant tertian parasite, *Plasmodium falciparum*, has become a major global public health problem during the past three decades. Few drugs are available to prevent or treat infections with such parasites and relatively little is known about the modes of action of even such widely used compounds as chloroquine or primaquine. However, much has been learned from investigations of the methods by which the parasites develop resistance to various antimalarials. This paper reviews new data concerning the uptake of drugs, their attachment to such parasite substrates as malaria pigment and calmodulin, and possible effects on various enzymes. Recent research on new antimalarials such as artemisinin is evaluated. Caution is recommended on the use of new compounds for monotherapy because of the high risk of the development of further drug-resistant parasite strains.

Antimalarial drugs differ from most other antimicrobial agents in that more has been learned about their mechanisms of action because of the ability of the target organisms to become resistant to them than through a straightforward study of their activity against sensitive *Plasmodium*. Indeed it is only in recent years that even the most basic knowledge of, for example, the pharmacokinetics and metabolism of such long established compounds as primaquine and amodiaquine, has been revealed. It is something of a paradox, also, that the increasing problem of drug resistance has led to a revival of interest in the longest established antimalarial, quinine, and its congeners, as well as the discovery of a previously unknown class of blood schizontocides of plant origin, the sesquiterpene lactones typified by artemisinin, that have been used as febrifuges in China for the past 2,000 years or more. Although the field of malaria chemotherapy has been reviewed extensively since 1970 (1, 2), the problem of resistance has increased at such a pace that it has become essential to assess anew all the previous publications. Even since the latest tome on the subject appeared in 1987 (3), many new data have accumulated on the possible modes of action of antimalarials, on the geographical spread of drug resistance, and on the manner in which parasites appear to develop ways of evading drug action. Yet few new antimalarial drugs are on the horizon in spite of the rapidly increasing threat posed, in particular, by multiple drug-resistant strains of the malignant tertian parasite, *Plasmodium falciparum*.

Since malaria parasites are unfamiliar to many classical microbiologists, this review will commence with a brief account of these protozoa and their life cycles, physiology, biochemistry and interactions with their vertebrate hosts. This will be followed by a mention of the newer models available for the study of antimalarial drug action, the spectrum (albeit limited) of currently available compounds and the recent history of drug resistance. No attempt will be made to summarize the vast volume of data that has only recently been reviewed (3). Instead, attention will be focused on those observations and hypotheses that have been published since the author's 1987 work went to press, i.e. late in 1986.

The Malaria Parasites

The life cycles of the malaria parasites that infect man are summarised in Figure 1. *Plasmodium vivax* and *Plasmodium ovale* share the ability to produce true relapses by virtue of the existence of a dormant, intrahepatocytic stage, the hypnozoite. Although long suspected to exist on the basis of circumstantial evidence, the nature of this unicellular parasite which develops from sporozoites was first demonstrated only as recently as 1980 by Krotoski and his associates. Further investigation by these workers has now confirmed by direct observation of liver biopsies in the *Plasmodium cynomolgi*-rhesus model (which runs a close parallel to *Plasmodium vivax* and *Plasmodium ovale*) that primaquine is able to eliminate the hypnozoites, whereas the dihydrofolate reductase inhibitors proguanil and pyrimethamine cannot (4), thus explaining the long recognised failure of the latter compounds either to serve as causal prophylactics or radical curative agents against the relapsing plasmodia of man.

Department of Medical Protozoology, London School of Hygiene and Tropical Medicine, London WC1E 7HT, UK.

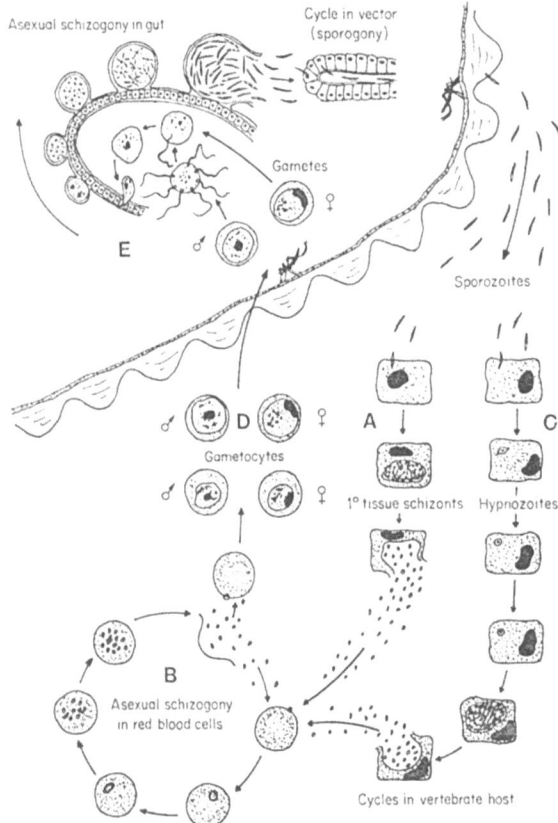

Figure 1: Diagram of the life cycle of a relapsing malaria species, *Plasmodium vivax*, showing sites of action of antimalarial drugs. A. causal prophylactics; B. blood schizontocides; C. hypnozoitocides (anti-relapse drugs); D. gametocytocides; E. sporontocides. (Original by L. Williams, reproduced by permission of Academic Press from Reference No. 3 with modifications).

Physiology and Biochemistry

Few new facts have emerged since the subject was last reviewed (3). However, recent observations on the influence of calmodulin antagonists and calcium channel blockers on the reversal of drug resistance which are reviewed below have focused attention on the vital importance of calcium metabolism in the intraerythrocytic stages of the parasites. Studies on inhibitors of polyamine metabolism such as difluoromethylornithine (DFMO) similarly have drawn attention to the metabolic pathways associated with transmethylation and nucleic acid synthesis, pathways in which S-adenosylmethionine holds a key position. DFMO has been shown to inhibit significantly the maturation of intrahepatic schizonts, as well as the asexual, intraerythrocytic stages of *Plasmodium falciparum* in vitro (5). Of several antagonists of ornithine decarboxylase tested, only DFMO was active in vivo (against *Plasmodium berghei* in the mouse model) (6). Recently attention has been recalled to the phenomenon of the "leakiness" which the malaria parasite induces in its host erythrocyte. This permits an increased traffic of substrates to and from the parasite.

However, this alone appears to be insufficient without the production by the parasite of new transmembrane pump proteins especially for the entry of anions. The unique biophysical properties of these new proteins may, it has been suggested, open "a cornucopia of new potential avenues for the chemotherapy of malaria" (7). One example of a compound based on this hypothesis is the zinc chelator, dipicolinic acid, which inhibits the growth of *Plasmodium falciparum* in vitro by depriving the parasites of the zinc ions essential to their metabolism.

The Host-Parasite Interface

The failure of chemotherapy to cure a number of parasitic infections in patients whose immune defences are compromised by drug treatment or AIDS brings into prominence the maxim that no drug, in the absence of an adequate host immune response, is truly parasiticidal. In rodents infected with *Plasmodium chabaudi* and pretreated with hydrocortisone, for example, chloroquine and quinine fail to inhibit parasitaemia (8). A further problem could arise if the agent in question, in addition to being antiparasitic, also reduces the host's humoral or cellular responses. This charge has been leveled by several investigators against such antimalarials as chloroquine, mefloquine (9), quinine, primaquine, pyrimethamine and artemisinin. It is generally accepted, however, that any such immunosuppressive action is either absent or insignificant at the blood levels associated with malaria prophylaxis or therapy.

In Vitro Experimental Models

A major advance was made when, in 1976, methods for the continuous culture of *Plasmodium falciparum* in red cells were described. However, a method to culture in vitro the exoerythrocytic intrahepatic stages evaded the medical community until 1980 when French investigators described a simple technique using *Plasmodium yoelii* in monolayers of rat hepatocytes. From the original rodent model has evolved a technique that lends itself to the relatively easy evaluation of the direct action of drugs on the intrahepatic parasites. In this model the parasites were shown to be highly sensitive to pyrimethamine. Chloroquine and mefloquine were inactive (10). The hepatic stages of all the other human *Plasmodium* species have now been cultured in vitro and forms probably representing hypnozoites have been demonstrated in cultures of *Plasmodium vivax*. No data have been published to date on the effect of pyrimethamine on these stages in vitro but it would be surprising if this compound (inactive as a hypnozoitocide in vivo) should prove to be effective in vitro. Primaquine, the only hypnozoitocide in clinical use, has a significant activity against the hepatic stages of *Plasmodium yoelii* in vitro and is known to have a true causal prophylactic action against *Plasmodium falciparum* in vivo (being, however, too toxic to be employed in the latter capacity). Evidence so far, therefore, indicates that the rodent model will probably be invaluable in identifying agents that are true causal prophylactics against non-relapsing parasites such as *Plasmodium falciparum*, but of little value as a model for relapsing species such as *Plasmodium vivax*.

Currently Available Blood Schizontocides

In contrast to the flood of antibacterial agents that have been introduced, only one new antimalarial has been marketed in the past 35 years in the Western world, although two or three others have been introduced on a limited commercial basis by the Chinese pharmaceutical industry. This state of affairs exists not because a surfeit of effective antimalarials is already available, but because of the reluctance of the pharmaceutical industry worldwide to invest in the development of antiparasitic agents destined largely for countries of the Third World, and this in the face of a rapidly growing problem of multiple drug resistance. Two organisations have been responsible for most of the antimalarial research and development since the 1950s: The U.S. Army Research and Development Command, and the UNDP/World Bank/WHO Special Programme for Research and Training in Tropical Diseases (the TDR programme). Antimalarials currently on the open market or available in limited quantities through national health agencies are listed in Table 1.

From over 300,000 compounds screened in the U.S. Army programme, one drug, mefloquine, is being progressively made available commercially and a second, halofantrine, is currently in early field trials. Both are aminoalcohol analogues of quinine (Figure 2) and it seems that the mode of action (essentially as blood schizontocides) of all three is similar. Their main differences lie in their pharmacokinetics, metabolism and toxicity. Only in the past few years has it been demonstrated that the quinine congener, quinidine, is marginally more active against multiple drug-resistant *Plasmodium falciparum* than quinine and it now appears that cinchonine is still more active. For reasons that are not yet entirely clear, a mixture of all three compounds appears to be marginally more

Table 1: Antimalarials currently available for clinical use.

Generic name	Availability		Indications
	Open market	Through government agencies	
Chloroquine	+	+	blood schizontocide against drug-sensitive *Plasmodium falciparum* and other species
Amodiaquine	+	+	as chloroquine
Quinine	+	+	blood schizontocide against drug-resistant *Plasmodium falciparum* or any serious infection with this parasite
Mefloquine	limited	limited	blood schizontocide against drug-resistant *Plasmodium falciparum*
Halofantrine	–	in advanced trials	as mefloquine
Pyrimethamine	+	+	limited prophylactic use against drug-sensitive parasites
Proguanil	+	limited	limited prophylactic use against drug-sensitive parasites
Fansidar[R]	+	+	prophylaxis or therapy of drug-resistant *Plasmodium falciparum*
Maloprim[R]	+	+	prophylaxis of drug-resistant *Plasmodium falciparum*
Fansimef[R]	limited	limited	prophylaxis or therapy of drug-resistant *Plasmodium falciparum*
Artemisinin	limited	limited	therapy of drug-resistant *Plasmodium falciparum*
Artemether	–	limited	therapy of drug-resistant *Plasmodium falciparum*
Primaquine	+	+	radical cure of *Plasmodium vivax*; gametocytocidal action against *Plasmodium falciparum*

active than any of the individual components in vivo (11).

Of the potent 4-aminoquinoline antimalarials, chloroquine has retained pride of place as the safest and cheapest. Even though amodiaquine (which can also be looked on as a Mannich base) is dose for dose more active than chloroquine and was beginning to suggest itself as a replacement for chloroquine against

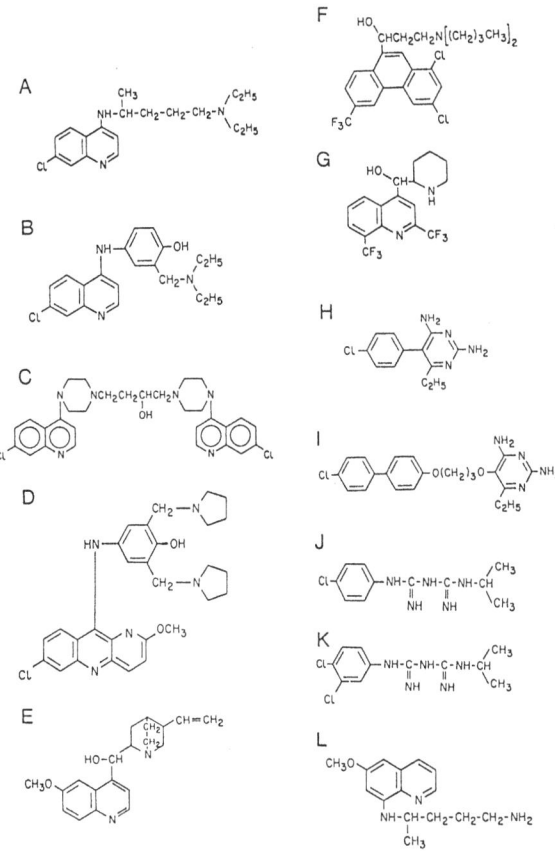

Figure 2: Chemical structures of antimalarial drugs. A. chloroquine; B. amodiaquine; C. hydroxypiperaquine; D. pyronaridine; E. quinine; F. halofantrine; G. mefloquine; H. pyrimethamine; I. M & B 35,769; J. proguanil; K. chlorproguanil; L. primaquine.

strains of *Plasmodium falciparum* that are resistant to chloroquine, recent evidence of its toxicity has detracted largely from its use. A remarkably high incidence of hepatotoxicity and agranulocytosis in individuals who received repeated, prophylactic dosage is surprising in the light of its apparent safety in the past. Whether this toxicity is associated with the parent compound or its desethyl metabolite (amodiaquine has recently been shown to act as a rapidly metabolised prodrug in man), awaits clarification. Furthermore, in some areas, e.g. Brazil, amodiaquine is now no more effective than chloroquine (12).

Compounds Currently Under Investigation

The bis-quinazoline, hydroxypiperaquine (Figure 2), introduced on a limited basis in a few countries of the Far East and Southwest Pacific, was derived by Chinese investigators from a compound code named 12,278 RP (dichlorquinazine) which was described over 30 years ago by researchers at Rhône Poulenc, but discarded as having no significant advantage over chloroquine against chloroquine-resistant infections in experimental animals (3). Following up the Mannich bases, the Chinese have synthesised pyronaridine, a compound that combines some of the structural features of the amodiaquine analogue, amopyroquine, and of mepacrine. This compound, which has been shown to be active in vitro and in vivo against multiple drug-resistant *Plasmodium falciparum*, is currently being evaluated more widely under TDR auspices.

Little progress has been made in the field of dihydrofolate reductase inhibitors. Unlike pyrimethamine, proguanil has retained its reputation as a prophylactic agent against *Plasmodium falciparum* even in areas where multiple drug-resistant *Plasmodium falciparum* is prevalent, although the extent to which this superiority will be borne out by hard data is an open question. Attention is currently being directed toward the evaluation of chlorproguanil, a dichlor analogue of proguanil which was reputed, seemingly without adequate justification, to have so much longer a half-life than proguanil that it could afford prophylactic cover after single weekly doses of 20 mg rather than proguanil at 100 to 200 mg per day. Current pharmacokinetic studies as well as reports of its partial failure as a prophylactic, especially in East Africa, have cast doubt as to whether chlorproguanil will really find a place in clinical use (13). What is beyond doubt is that certain combinations of dihydrofolate reductase inhibitors with sulphonamides or dapsone have a highly synergistic action, sufficient in many instances to control parasites that are resistant to the components used individually. Pyrimethamine-sulfadoxine (Fansidar) proved to be very effective both as a prophylactic and a radical curative agent against chloroquine-resistant *Plasmodium falciparum* for some 15 years before strains additionally resistant to this compound began to emerge. (3). Pyrimethamine-dapsone (Maloprim) has not been used for therapy and may be marginally more useful in the prophylaxis of such strains than Fansidar, although not everywhere. In Papua New Guinea breakthroughs have recently been reported of chloroquine plus Maloprim (14). Unfortunately, both antifol combinations are under a shadow, the long-acting sulfadoxine component being associated with severe cutaneous reactions in a small proportion of individuals who have received it (usually in repeated or overdosage), and the dapsone component leading to agranulocytosis in sensitive subjects (3). The principle of combining such potent antifol antimalarials with sulphonamides or dapsone is, nevertheless, too valuable to discard lightly. Proguanil has been shown to potentiate with dapsone (3) or with short-acting sulphonamides such as sulfisoxazole or sulfamethoxazole (15) and a study is currently underway on the combination of chlorproguanil with dapsone (16), a logical combination based on the similar half-lives of the triazine metabolite of chlorproguanil and of the sulphone. Preliminary clinical trials have also been reported on a new pyrimidine antifol, M & B 35,769, which is analogous to pyrimethamine. Although this was more active than pyrimethamine against some strains of Plasmodium which were resistant to pyrimethamine, inconsistent results have been obtained so far in man. The most recent series of antimalarials to have been introduced, albeit so far on a limited scale, is that based on the sequiterpene lactone, artemisin, the main active principle of the common plant *Artemisia annua* Linnaeus (Compositae) (17). This is discussed further below.

The Recent History of Drug Resistance

For a detailed account of the emergence of resistance to currently available antimalarials in parasites affecting man, reference should be made to the author's recent review (3). The problem of drug resistance is restricted essentially to *Plasmodium falciparum* but, since this is the most dangerous parasite of all, the problem has taken on unprecedented dimensions. On the African continent, for example, this parasite is responsible for over 90% of all infections and nearly all of the million or more deaths that are estimated to be due primarily to malaria each year. Firstly chloroquine- and now multiple drug-resistant strains of this parasite, which first made their appearance in East Africa ten years ago, have been identified during the past year in more and more countries of West Africa, so that at the time of writing, they are without doubt established in most of the endemic countries of this continent. Although chloroquine retains its value for the time being in most of West Africa, at least for treatment of acute falciparum malaria in semi-immune indigenous patients, this is by no means true in East and Central Africa where some infections are now showing a significant loss of response even to quinine, which has, up to now, been a major line of defence against such strains. Fansidar, which has probably been overemployed in areas where it was not needed, is also losing its efficacy, both over an increasing geographical area and in degree. It is ominous that strains of *Plasmodium falciparum* with a poor response to mefloquine have been identified both in East Africa and, most serious of all, in West Africa (18), where this compound had never been available. That such strains readily become resistant to halofantrine has been demonstrated both in rodent malaria (19) and in falciparum infection in man.

Although there are, to date, no clinical data to suggest that any strains of *Plasmodium falciparum* with resistance to artemisinin or its analogues have appeared, it must be only a matter of time before such strains are observed. It is very easy, under experimental conditions, to develop resistance to artemisinin or its analogues (3, 20) in *Plasmodium falciparum* in vitro or in the rodent parasite, *Plasmodium berghei* in vivo. Moreover, strains resistant to mefloquine have been seen to have a reduced sensitivity to artemisinin (W. K. Milhous, personal communication).

Several observations have accumulated to indicate that, in contrast to most drug-resistant microorganisms, chloroquine- and poly-resistant *Plasmodium falciparum* are dominant over sensitive parasites. Only recently has the opportunity arisen to observe whether the resistance can diminish in the absence of drug selection pressure. Both in Vietnam and in Thailand (Table 2) chloroquine has been practically abandoned for the past decade or more because of the very high level of chloroquine resistance, and replaced by pyrimethamine-sulfadoxine and quinine. In each country there are indications that *Plasmodium falciparum* infections are now beginning to show a more normal response to chloroquine both in vivo and in vitro (21, 22). If further monitoring bears out this trend there may yet be a possibility of deploying chloroquine once again at some future date. Should that situation arise, however, it will be vital to plan with great care a new strategy for the use of antimalarials, and to incorporate a strict control over drug distribution.

Modes of Drug Action

Drug Uptake Mechanisms

One of the interesting phenomena associated with a number of blood schizontocides, even in such chemically diverse classes as the 4-aminoquinolones and sesquiterpene lactones, is their high level of concentration in parasitised erythrocytes. Chloroquine, a lysosomotropic compound, is taken up, probably by both passive and active transport mechanisms (23), into the trophozoite food vacuoles (Figure 3), whereas in contrast to this, artemisinin is associated with other membranes within the parasites (24). While the

Table 2: Changes in in vitro chloroquine responses of *Plasmodium falciparum* isolates in Thailand, 1981–1986. Adapted from Reference No. 22.

Year	No. of isolates examined	EC_{50}[a]	EC_{90}	EC_{95}
		(chloroquine 10^{-6} moles litre^{-1} blood)		
1981	15	3.3	7.4	9.3
1983	24	1.3	5.6	8.4
1984	22	1.4	5.0	7.2
1985	37	0.9	5.79	9.7
1986	32	0.47	3.19	5.47

[a] EC_{50} = 50% effective concentration.

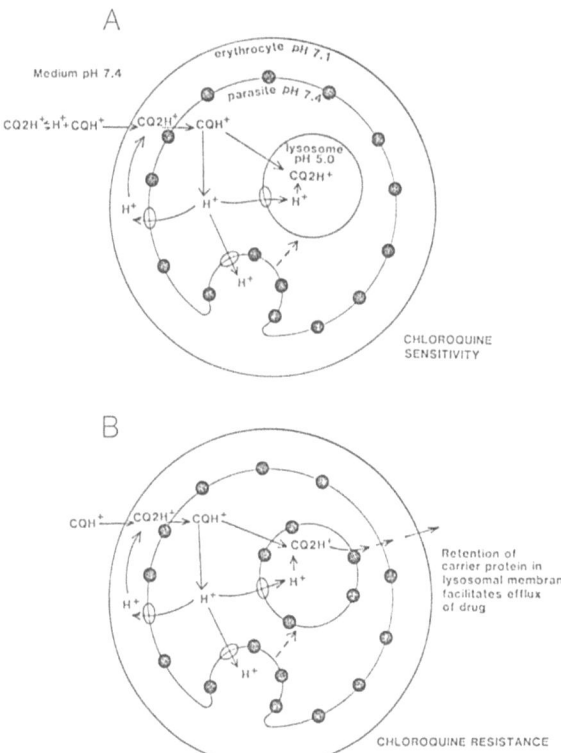

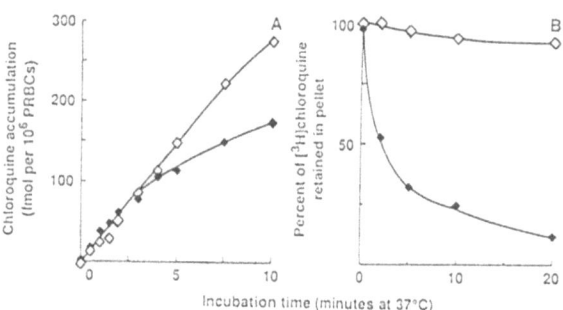

Figure 3: Model of the mechanisms of concentration of chloroquine in (A) a drug-sensitive and (B) drug-resistant *Plasmodium* trophozoite within an erythrocyte. • = parasite membrane carrier (permease) which binds diprotonated drug; ⊖→ = ATP-driven proton pump; CQ2H$^+$ = diprotonated chloroquine (membrane-impermeant); CQH$^+$ = monoprotonated chloroquine (membrane-permeant). (Original by courtesy of Dr. D. C. Warhurst).

Figure 4: Chloroquine accumulation and efflux in vitro from erythrocytes containing a chloroquine-sensitive strain of *Plasmodium falciparum* (Haiti 135 – open diamond) or a chloroquine-resistant strain (Indochina I – closed diamond). While the initial rates of accumulation were the same in both strains, the rate of efflux was markedly increased from the erythrocytes containing resistant parasites. (From Reference No. 25, reproduced by kind permission of the authors and Science, copyright 1987 by the American Association for the Advancement of Science).

rate and method of uptake of chloroquine have been extensively studied, what was not formerly appreciated was that the parasites also possess a mechanism for eliminating the drug. Thus the level of concentration is a fine balance between drug influx and efflux. It has been known for a long time that the concentration of chloroquine in erythrocytes that contain chloroquine-resistant parasites is less than that in red cells containing drug-sensitive parasites. The initial rate of accumulation has now been shown to be similar in both strains. What does differ is the rate of efflux which is significantly higher from drug-resistant than drug-susceptible parasites (Figure 4) (25).

The mechanism of chloroquine concentration has been the subject of several hypotheses, ranging from simple passage across a pH gradient from plasma to host cell cytoplasm, to binding with ferriprotoporphyrin IX (FP IX), with active transport from erythrocyte cytoplasm to parasite cytoplasm to parasite food vacuole achieved by means of a carrier protein. In a recent review of all the available data (26) the role of binding with ferriprotoporphyrin IX has been dismissed and the importance of movement along a pH gradient has received renewed attention. Chloroquine accumulates in the parasites as a weak base and is able to inhibit the activity of parasite proteases within the food vacuoles by increasing the pH (27), thus depriving the parasites of essential aminoacids that they would otherwise obtain from the digestion of ingested haemoglobin. An earlier suggestion that chloroquine, mepacrine and quinine kill malaria parasites through their ability to intercalate with DNA has long been dismissed. The quinine analogue, mefloquine, does not intercalate. Moreover, recent studies have shown that chloroquine, primaquine, mefloquine and halofantrine do not significantly stimulate the double-strand cleavage of *Plasmodium berghei* DNA and are poor in vitro inhibitors of topoisomerase-catalysed reactions (28).

In addition to the above mechanisms of drug concentration, infected red cells develop new permeability pathways, becoming "leaky". These pathways are permeable to small non-electrolytes and to anions but not to cations. It has been proposed that parasite polypeptides produce structural defects in the red cell membrane, the phospholipids of which form a "selectivity filter", and that drugs could be targeted into infected erythrocytes by designing them with the properties they would require to permeate across the filter (7).

Chloroquine and Malaria Pigment

When the malaria trophozoite digests haemoglobin of its host cell, the residual iron-containing porphyrin is deposited in it as an insoluble pigment, haemozoin. It has been suggested that this is formed by the removal of aminoacids from haemoglobin with the transitory formation of the highly lytic substance, FP IX, which is rapidly sequestered by complexing with one or more polypeptides of parasite origin.

These have been isolated but not yet completely characterized. (The chloroquine-FP IX complex, unlike FP IX itself, promotes the peroxidative cleavage of unsaturated phospholipids in liposomes of rat liver in vitro (29)). As chloroquine binds avidly with FP IX to form an even more highly lytic complex, is was suggested that this was the basis for the plasmodical activity of the drug. However, no ultrastructural evidence has ever been obtained to indicate that lysis of parasite membranes occurs in parasitised red cells exposed to therapeutic concentrations of chloroquine.

Antimalarials and Calcium Metabolism

Calcium ions (Ca^{2+}) are essential for many vital metabolic functions in eukaryotes and it has been shown recently that calmodulin is present in the cytoplasm and at the apices of merozoites of *Plasmodium falciparum* intraerythrocytic trophozoites, its content being proportional to the age of the parasites (30). The immunomodulating antibiotic, cyclosporin A, has been known for some years to inhibit the growth of *Plasmodium berghei* in mice, and this, as well as a number of analogues that lack any significant action on the immune system, inhibits *Plasmodium falciparum* in vitro, but no obvious explanation has been found for this activity. Cyclosporin A has since been shown to bind to calmodulin, as well as to reverse resistance of tumour cells to vincristine. It has now been shown by radioimmunoassay and immunoelectron microscopy that cyclosporin A is concentrated in the food vacuoles of *Plasmodium falciparum*

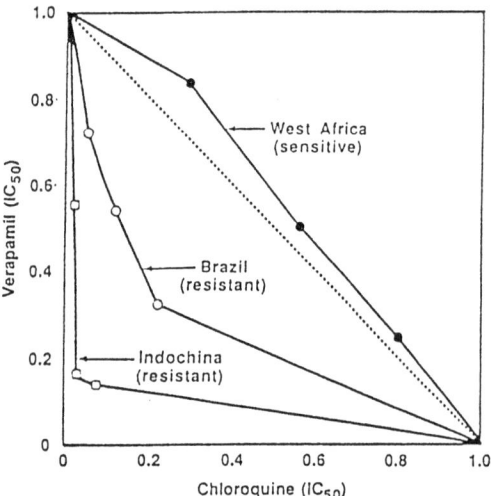

Figure 5: The synergistic effect of chloroquine and verapamil against chloroquine-sensitive and drug-resistant *Plasmodium falciparum* in vitro. The control IC 50s normalised to one unit refer to the individual compounds used alone. The IC 50s of the combinations are plotted as fractions of the control IC 50s. (From Reference No. 32 by kind permission of the authors and Science, copyright 1987 by the American Association for the Advancement of Science).

and dispersed within the parasite cytoplasm. The binding of this compound was competitive with another calmodulin inhibitor, W-7, and with chloroquine. From a study of the structural requirements for calmodulin antagonism it was found that the level of activity of several blood schizontocidal antimalarials "reflected their reported anti-calmodulin effect." (30) In this context the localisation of mepacrine in the region of the apical complexes of the merozoites, noted some years ago (31), may take on a new significance. Mepacrine was the most active antimalarial tested in vitro in the recent study. These workers also noted that a number of Ca^{2+} channel blockers had some inhibitory action on the growth of *Plasmodium falciparum*, one of the most effective being verapamil, which also has a direct effect on calmodulin. Moreover, a significant antagonism was detected between several antimalarials (mepacrine, chloroquine, quinine) and cyclosporin A, especially when tested against a multiple drug-resistant strain of *Plasmodium falciparum*.

Reversal of Chloroquine Resistance

It is particularly pertinent, therefore, that verapamil has now been shown to restore the inhibitory action of chloroquine against such drug-resistant parasites in vitro, but not against drug-sensitive parasites (Figure 5) (32).

Multiple drug resistance in *Plasmodium falciparum* and chloroquine resistance in the NS strain of *Plasmodium yoelii* are associated with a decrease in the concentration of the drug in infected red cells (3). Various types of multiple drug resistance in tumour cells have been attributed to the existence of a membrane-associated protein, P-170 glycoprotein, which is believed to protect cells against noxious substances in a non-specific manner by pumping them out, a process that almost certainly requires energy (33). Its action is apparently blocked by the calcium channel blocker verapamil, which is an inhibitor of Ca^{2+}-activated ATPase, so that higher concentrations of the antitumour agents remain in the cytoplasm of the tumour cells. Amplification of the gene coding for P-170 may underlie the phenomenon of multiple drug resistance. To date, however, there is no evidence that a similar protein exists on the surface of malaria parasites. A wide range of other calcium channel blockers besides verapamil, e.g. diltiazem, vinblastine, daunomycin (32) and flunarizine (34), reverse the excess efflux of chloroquine that has been found in multiple drug resistant *Plasmodium falciparum* in vitro. Verapamil also restores the activity of chloroquine in vivo against the chloroquine-resistant *Plasmodium yoelii* NS strain (unpublished data), which we consider to be a valuable model for chloroquine-resistant *Plasmodium falciparum*.

Against the hypothesis that verapamil reverses chloroquine resistance through its action as a channel blocker is the possibility that the uptake of this compound, unlike for example, anti-tumour agents such as colchicine and vincristine, is an energy-dependent mechanism. It has been postulated that chloroquine uptake requires the participation of a glucose-dependent permease to drive diprotonated drug from the erythrocyte cytoplasm into the parasite cytoplasm (which is of a higher pH) (23). However, it is probable that the initial process of uptake is essentially that of the passage of the weakly monoprotonated drug from the plasma into the erythrocyte and then, at a later phase of uptake, from the parasite cytoplasm into the parasite food vacuoles (which can be regarded as lysosomal equivalents). Since increased chloroquine efflux has now been demonstrated in resistant malaria parasites, the parallel with tumour cells appears to be close. The permease hypothesis could, however, account also for the increased efflux if chloroquine is permitted to return from the food vacuoles into the parasite cytoplasm from which it could again pass back to the erythrocyte cytoplasm, then the plasma (Figure 5). In highly chloroquine-resistant *Plasmodium berghei* RC trophozoites, chloroquine is generally dispersed in the parasite cytoplasm in contrast to drug-sensitive parasites in which it is concentrated in food vacuoles (35).

Action of Drugs on Parasite Proteases and Monooxygenases

In highly resistant, RC-type strains of *Plasmodium berghei* (in contrast to the *Plasmodium yoelii* NS strain which is, as mentioned above, probably a better model for chloroquine-resistant *Plasmodium falciparum*), there is clearly a marked increase in the quantitiy of the food vacuoles and of endoprotease activity. No significant differences, however, were detected between the proteases of drug-sensitive and chloroquine-resistant *Plasmodium falciparum* (36). It has been suggested that chloroquine, in the form of a complex with FP IX, exerts its action by inhibiting these proteases, but the concentrations at which this occurs are far higher than those believed to be reached even in the food vacuoles after exposure to therapeutic doses.

As the concentrations of several microsomal monooxygenases and cytochrome P-450 have been reported to be considerably raised in RC-type *Plasmodium berghei*, it has been suggested that chloroquine resistance in such parasites is due to their enhanced ability to detoxify this compound (37). A number of compounds inhibit monooxygenase activity in liver microsomes, among them chloramphenicol, phenylhydrazine and a copper-lysine complex, copper(lysine)$_2$, and also, interestingly, verapamil (38). The copper derivative is claimed to reverse resistance in RC-type *Plasmodium berghei* when administered in vivo to infected mice together with an otherwise ineffective dose of chloroquine. The complex alone is inactive (39). If confirmed, this observation could offer another interesting new avenue to the search for compounds that will reverse chloroquine resistance. It is pertinent to observe in this context that both chloroquine itself and verapamil are also inhibitors of hepatic drug metabolising enzymes.

Antimalarial Action of Endoperoxidases

The discovery of the active constituent of the traditional Chinese anti-pyretic plant Qinghao (*Artemisia annua*, Linnaeus, Compositae) has opened a novel avenue for the synthesis of antimalarial endo-peroxidases (17). Artemisinin, a sesquiterpene lactone, is a rapidly acting blood schizontocide which is effective against all species of human malaria parasites, including multiple drug-resistant *Plasmodium falciparum*. Its action is limited to the asexual intraerythrocytic stages and it has no causal nor hypnozoitocidal action (40). In view of the poor solubility of artemisinin itself a number of semi-synthetic analogues have been produced by substitution of the lactone on position 12 (Figure 6). Clinical trials in China and Burma have demonstrated that two derivatives, sodium artesunate and artemether, are more active than the parent compound and both have been given parenterally in place of quinine with great success in the treatment of severe falciparum malaria (3). Because of indications that sodium artesunate solutions are not chemically stable, a new, soluble analogue, arteether, is currently being developed for clinical trial (41). An esteric

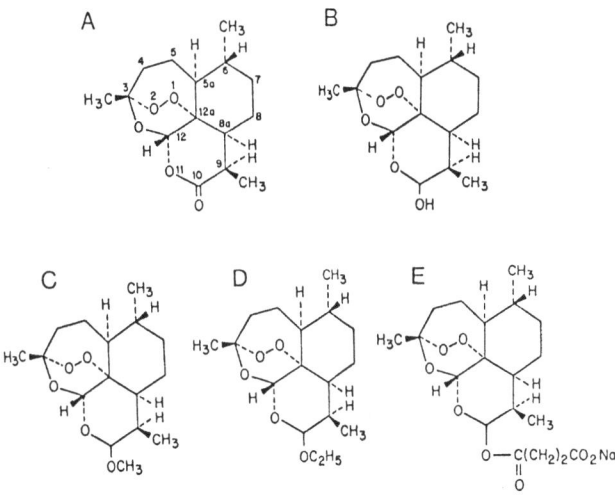

Figure 6: Chemical structures of antimalarial sesquiterpene lactones. A. artemisinin; B. dihydroartemisinin; C. artemether; D. arteether; E. sodium artesunate.

analogue, artelinic acid, which is also soluble and stable in a weakly alkaline solution, has also been found to be more active than artemisinin, with the same spectrum of action against multiple drug-resistant *Plasmodium falciparum* (42).

It is likely that all these compounds are converted rapidly in vivo to the dihydro form which is the active metabolite. The earliest antiparasitic effect of the sesquiterpene lactones, which are highly concentrated in the region of the membranes of intraerythrocytic trophozoites (24), is an interference with energy production. This is followed by a reduction of DNA synthesis, probably resulting from inhibition of mRNA polymerase activity. Purine synthesis has been shown to be blocked in *Plasmodium berghei* at the level of inosine monophosphate dehydrogenase (43). In *Plasmodium falciparum* in vitro, hypoxanthine incorporation into DNA is inhibited, as is the incorporation of isoleucine into protein, the first of these being very rapid in onset. Metabolic degradation by reduction of the peroxide bridge renders the compounds inactive. At the ultrastructural level, dihydroartemisinin has been shown to produce early changes in the parasite membranes, disorganisation of the ribosomes, and later, the formation of a nucleus-like structure in the nucleus. The compound does not produce malaria pigment or changes in the food vacuoles (24). It has been suggested that the artemisinin molecule binds to parasite membranes by virtue of its sterol-like structure. It seems possible that the selective attachment to parasite as distinct from erythrocyte membranes is related to their different lipid compositions.

One of the features of the treatment of human malaria with artemisinin and its analogues is the high recrudescence rate (up to about 10%), which is not necessarily related to the selection of drug-resistant parasites, although at least *Plasmodium berghei* does readily become resistant to the compounds. It has been shown that parasites in younger erythrocytes are less sensitive to these drugs than those in more mature host cells and there is some evidence suggesting that their action is not mediated by the release of oxygen radicals, even though their structures would suggest this (44). In this context it is interesting to note that two methoxylated flavones enhanced the action of artemisinin against *Plasmodium falciparum* in vitro, and it seems possible that flavones which exist in *Artemisia annua* together with artemisinin may actually have a synergistic effect when the crude plant is used (45).

Synergism has been demonstrated against both *Plasmodium falciparum* in vitro (46) and *Plasmodium berghei* in vivo (47) between artemisinin and aminoalcohols such as mefloquine and halofantrine, the effect being particularly marked in strains resistant to such compounds. On the contrary, combinations of artemisinin with dihydrofolate reductase inhibitors or the potentiating pyrimethamine-sulfadoxine mixture (Fansidar) showed an antagonistic effect. Tetracycline was also synergistic with artemisinin against both drug-sensitive and chloroquine-resistant *Plasmodium falciparum*, while primaquine was synergistic with artemisinin only against the resistant parasite strain. In *Plasmodium berghei* infected mice, the potentiation with primaquine was also observed in a primaquine-resistant strain. The potentiation with mefloquine, primaquine, tetracycline and clindamycin was found also in a rodent infection with artemisinin-resistant *Plasmodium berghei*. These observations have obvious implications for the deployment of the sesquiterpene lactone derivatives in the chemotherapy of multiple drug-resistant *Plasmodium falciparum* and in the prevention of the emergence of resistance to the sesquiterpenes themselves.

Recent Studies on the Mode of Action of Primaquine

It is remarkable that the 8-aminoquinoline compound primaquine was widely used for the radical cure of infections with *Plasmodium vivax* (by virtue of its hypnozoitocidal action) for three decades before any serious studies were carried out on its pharmacokinetics. It is now recognised that the parent compound has a short half-life in man, probably between four and six hours. Moreover, it now appears very likely that its hypnozoitocidal activity is due not to the parent compound but to one or more metabolites (48). Recent studies with in vitro models of intrahepatic schizonts of rodent malaria parasites, as well as in vivo studies with putative metabolites, have indicated that several 8-aminoquinolines which, unlike primaquine itself, are virutally inactive against the intraerythrocytic stages, have a marked effect on tissue stages. The 6-hydroxy, 5-hydroxy, 5,6-hydroxy and 6-methoxy 8-aminoquinolines are about three times as active against tissue stages as primaquine in vivo (49), although primaquine is relatively more active in the in vitro model (10). These observations may lead to the synthesis and evaluation of further analogues of these putative metabolites as substitutes for primaquine, which has the disadvantage of causing haemolysis of host red cells in subjects deficient in glucose 6-phosphate dehydrogenase. The mechanism of that action is probably related to the ability of the parent compound to accelerate the flux through the hexose monophosphate shunts of parasitised erythrocytes (50).

Conclusion

The advent of multiple drug resistance in *Plasmodium falciparum* has necessitated both a closer look at the way existing antimalarials work, and the ways in which parasites overcome the drugs. New chemical classes of antimalarials are required urgently, but finding new compounds is a lengthy and expensive process. It is therefore even more essential to seek ways of impeding the selection of drug-resistant parasites. Experimental data as well as hard clinical experience have long made it clear that *Plasmodium falciparum* has an exceptional ability to develop resistance to almost any type of antimalarial when selective pressure has been exerted with a single compound. The deployment of appropriately selected drug combinations (such as the potentiating combination of pyrimethamine with sulfadoxine) can undoubtedly delay that process, but not overcome it. The author has long crusaded for the strict limitation of the deployment of newly developed, "last ditch", reserve drugs such as mefloquine (or now halofantrine or artemisinin) for monotherapy, and especially for prophylaxis, except where the existence of multiple drug-resistant *Plasmodium falciparum* makes their use essential. There are good experimental data as well as philosophical reasons to support the use of drug combinations to impede the emergence of resistance to new compounds, rather than risking the loss of the individual components. It may also prove possible to reverse drug resistance once it occurs. The process of developing new compounds or making better use of old ones will be a painful one, but the task must be faced. Even if the much vaunted antimalarial vaccines reach fruition over the next decade, it will still be vital to have available potent, safe, antimalarial drugs to prevent infection and to treat any cases that do occur, especially with the malignant tertian parasite, *Plasmodium falciparum*.

Acknowledgements

Original studies carried out in the author's laboratory received partial support under various grants from the CHEMAL component of the UNDP/World Bank/WHO Special Programme for Research and Training in Tropical Diseases and from the U.S. Army Medical Research and Development Command, Department of the Army. I wish to acknowledge with thanks especially the skilled technical assistance of Mr. B. L. Robinson and invaluable advice from Dr. D. C. Warhurst.

References

1. Peters, W.: Chemotherapy and drug resistance in malaria. Academic Press, London, 1970.
2. Thompson, P. E., Werbel, L. M.: Antimalarial agents: chemistry and pharmacology. Academic Press, New York, 1972.
3. Peters, W.: Chemotherapy and drug resistance in malaria. Academic Press, London, 1987.
4. Jiang, J.-B., Bray, R. S., Krotowski, W. A., Canning, E. U., Liang, D. S., Huang, J.-C., Liao, J.-Y., Li, D.-S., Lun, Z.-R., Landau, I.: Observations on early and late post-sporozoite tissue stages in primate malaria. V. The effect of pyrimethamine and proguanil upon tissue hypnozoites and schizonts of *Plasmodium cynomolgi bastianellii*. Transactions of the Royal Society of Tropical Medicine and Hygiene 1988, 82: 56–58.
5. Assaraf, Y. G., Golenser, J., Spira, D. T., Messer, G., Bachrach, U.: Cytostatic effect of DL-*a*-difluoromethylornithine against *Plasmodium falciparum* and its reversal by diamines and spermidine. Parasitology Research 1987, 73: 313–318.
6. Bitonti, A. J., McCann, P. P., Sjoerdsma, A.: *Plasmodium falciparum* and *Plasmodium berghei*: effects of ornithine decarboxylase inhibitors on erythrocytic schizogony. Experimental Parasitology 1987, 64: 237–243.
7. Ginsburg, H., Stein, W. D.: New permeability pathways induced by the malarial parasite in the membrane of its host erythrocyte: potential routes for targeting of drugs into infected cells. Bioscience Reports 1987, 7: 455–463.
8. Targett, G. A. T.: Chemotherapy and the immune response in parasitic infections. Parasitology 1985, 90: 661–673.
9. Bygbjerg, I. C., Theander, T. G., Andersen, B. J., Flachs, H., Jepsen, S., Larsen, P. B.: In vitro effect of chloroquine, mefloquine and quinine on human lymphocyte proliferative responses to malaria antigens and other antigens/mitogens. Tropical Medicine and Parasitology 1986, 37: 245–247.
10. Millet, P., Landau, I., Peters, W.: In vitro testing of antimalarial exo-erythrocytic schizontocides in primary cultures of hepatocytes. Memorias do Instituto Oswaldo Cruz 1986, 81, Supplement II: 135–141.
11. Bunnag, D., Harinasuta, T., Vanijanonta, S., Looareesuwan, S., Chittamas, S., Punnavut, W., Berthe, J., Druilhe, P.: Treatment of chloroquine-resistant falciparum malaria with a combination of quinine, quinidine and cinchonine (LA 40221) in adults by oral and intravenous administration. Acta Leidensia 1987, 55: 139–149.
12. Kremsner, P. G., Zotter, G. M., Grainger, W., Feldmeier, H.: Amodiaquine-resistant malaria in Brazil. Lancet 1987, i: 684.
13. Watkins, W. M., Chulay, J. D., Sixsmith, D. G., Spencer, H. C., Howells, R. E.: A preliminary pharmacokinetic study of the antimalarial drugs proguanil and chlorproguanil. Journal of Pharmacy and Pharmacology 1987, 39: 261–265.
14. Edstein, M. D., Veenendal, J. R., Rieckmann, K. H., O'Donoghue, M.: Failure of dapsone/pyrimethamine plus chloroquine against falciparum malaria in Papua New Guinea. Lancet 1988, i: 237.
15. Pang, L., Limsomwong, N., Shanks, D., Karwacki, J., Singharaj, P., Schuster, B. G.: Malaria prophylaxis with proguanil plus sulfa regimens. Proceedings of the 27th International Congress of Military Medicine and Pharmacy, Interlaken, 4–11 May 1988, Military Department, Bern, p. 11.904: 1–6.
16. Watkins, W. M., Brandling-Bennett, A. D., Nevill, C. G., Carter, J. Y., Boriga, D. A., Howells, R. E., Koech, D. K.: Chlorproguanil/dapsone for the treatment of non-severe *Plasmodium falciparum* malaria in Kenya: a pilot sutdy. Transactions of the Royal Society of Tropical Medicine and Hygiene 1988, 82: (in press).
17. Klayman, D. L.: Qinghaosu (artemisinin): an antimalarial drug from China. Science 1985, 228: 1049–1055.
18. Oduola, A. M. J., Milhous, W. K., Salako, L. A., Walker, O., Desjardins, R. E.: Reduced in vitro susceptibility to mefloquine in West African isolates of *Plasmodium falciparum*. Lancet 1987, ii: 1304–1305.
19. Peters, W., Robinson, B. L., Ellis, D. S.: The chemotherapy of rodent malaria. XLII. Halofantrine and halofantrine resistance. Annals of Tropical Medicine and Parasitology 1987, 81: 639–646.

20. Li, C. S., Du, Y. L., Jiang, Q.: Development of Qinghaosu-resistant line of *Plasmodium berghei* ANKA and N strains. Acta Pharmaceutica Sinica 1986, 21: 811–815.
21. Jacquier, P., Druilhe, P., Felix, H., Diquet, B., Djibo, L.: Is *Plasmodium falciparum* resistance to chloroquine reversible in absence of drug pressure? Lancet 1985, ii: 270–271.
22. Thaithong, S., Suebsaeng, L., Rooney, W., Beale, G. H.: Evidence of increased chloroquine sensitivity in Thai isolates of *Plasmodium falciparum*. Transactions of the Royal Society of Tropical Medicine and Hygiene 1988, 82: 37–38.
23. Warhurst, D. C.: Antimalarial schizontocides: why a permease is necessary. Parasitology Today 1986, 2: 331–334.
24. Ellis, D. S., Li, Z. L., Gu, H. M., Peters, W., Robinson, B. L., Tovey, G., Warhurst, D. C.: The chemotherapy of rodent malaria. XXXIX. Ultrastructural changes following treatment with artemisinine of *Plasmodium berghei* infection in mice, with observations of the localization of [^{3}H]-dihydroartemisinine in *Plasmodium falciparum* in vitro. Annals of Tropical Medicine and Hygiene 1985, 79: 367–374.
25. Krogstad, D. J., Gluzman, I. Y., Kyle, D. E., Oduola, A. M. J., Martin, S. K., Milhous, K., Schlesinger, P. H.: Efflux of chloroquine from *Plasmodium falciparum*: mechanism of chloroquine resistance. Science 1987, 238: 1283–1285.
26. Ginsburg, H., Geary, T. G.: Current concepts and new ideas on the mechanism of action of quinoline-containing antimalarials. Biochemical Pharmacology 1987, 36: 1567–1576.
27. Krogstad, D. J., Schlesinger, P. H.: A perspective on antimalarial action: effects of weak bases on *Plasmodium falciparum*. Biochemical Pharmacology 1986, 35: 547–552.
28. Riou, J.-F., Gabillot, M., Philippe, M., Schrevel, J., Riou, G.: Purification and characterization of *Plasmodium berghei* DNA topoisomerases I and II: drug action, inhibition of decatenation and relaxation, and stimulation of DNA cleavage. Biochemistry 1986, 25: 1471–1479.
29. Sugioka, Y., Suzuki, M., Sugioka, K., Nakano, M.: A ferriprotoporphyrin IX-chloroquine complex promotes membrane phospholipid peroxidation. FEBS Letters 1987, 223: 251–254.
30. Scheibel, L. W., Colombani, P. M., Hess, A. D., Aikawa, M., Atkinson, C. T., Milhous, W. K.: Calcium and calmodulin antagonists inhibit human malaria parasites (*Plasmodium falciparum*): implications for drug design. Proceedings of the National Academy of Science USA 1987, 84: 7310–7314.
31. Warhurst, D. C., Thomas, S. C.: Localisation of mepacrine in *Plasmodium berghei* and *Plasmodium falciparum* by fluorescence microscopy. Annals of Tropical Medicine and Parasitology 1975, 69: 417–420.
32. Martin, S. K., Oduola, A. M. J., Milhous, W. K.: Reversal of chloroquine resistance in *Plasmodium falciparum* by verapamil. Science 1987, 235: 899–902.
33. Stark, G. R.: Progress in understanding multidrug resistance. Nature 1986, 324: 407–408.
34. Satayavivad, J., Wongsawatkul, O., Bunnag, D., Tan-Ariya, P., Brockelman, C. R.: Flunarizine and verapamil inhibit chloroquine-resistant *Plasmodium falciparum* growth in vitro. Southeast Asian Journal of Tropical Medicine and Public Health 1987, 18: 253–258.
35. Moreau, S., Prensier, G., Maalla, J., Fortier, B.: Identification of distinct accumulation sites of 4-aminoquinoline in chloroquine sensitive and resistant *Plasmodium berghei* strains. European Journal of Cell Biology 1986, 42: 207–210.
36. Vander Jagt, D. L., Hunsaker, L. A., Campos, N. M.: Comparison of proteases from chloroquine-sensitive and chloroquine-resistant strains of *Plasmodium falciparum*. Biochemical Pharmacology 1987, 36: 3285–3291.
37. Salganik, R. I., Pankova, T. G., Chekhonadskikh, T. V., Igonina, T. M.: Chloroquine resistance of *Plasmodium berghei*: biochemical basis and countermeasures. Bulletin of the World Health Organization 1987, 65: 381–386.
38. Edwards, D. J., Lavoie, R., Beckman, H., Blevins, R., Rubenfire, M.: The effect of coadministration of verapamil on the pharmacokinetics and metabolism of quinidine. Clinical Pharmacology and Therapeutics 1987, 41: 68–73.
39. Rabinovich, S. A., Kulikovskaya, I. M., Maksakovskaya, E. V., Chekhonadskikh, T. V., Pankova, T. G., Salganik, R. I.: Suppression of the chloroquine resistance of *Plasmodium berghei* by treatment of infected mice with a microsomal monooxygenase inhibitor. Bulletin of the World Health Organization 1987, 65: 387–389.
40. Peters, W., Li, Z.-L., Robinson, B. L., Warhurst, D. C.: The chemotherapy of rodent malaria. XL. The action of artemisinin and related sesquiterpenes. Annals of Tropical Medicine and Parasitology 1986, 80: 483–489.
41. Brossi, A., Venugopalan, B., Gerpe, L. D., Yeh, H. J. C., Flippen-Anderson, J. L., Buchs, P., Luo, X. D., Milhous, W., Peters, W.: Arteether, a new antimalarial drug: synthesis and antimalarial properties. Journal of Medicinal Chemistry 1988, 31: 645–649.
42. Lin, A. J., Klayman, D. L., Milhous, W. K.: Antimalarial activity of new water-soluble dihydroartemisinin derivatives. Journal of Medicinal Chemistry 1987, 30: 2147–2150.
43. Zhao, Y., Hall, I. H., Oswald, C. B., Yokio, T., Lee, K.-H.: Antimalarial agents. III. Mechanism of action of artesunate against *Plasmodium berghei* infection. Chemical and Pharmaceutical Bulletin (Tokyo) 1987, 35: 2052–2061.
44. Waki, S. Gu, H. M., Zhu, M. Y.: Sensitivity of malaria parasites to artemether (qinghaosu derivative) depends on host cell age. Transactions of the Royal Society of Tropical Medicine and Hygiene 1987, 81: 913–914.
45. Elford, B. C., Roberts, M. F., Phillipson, J. D., Wilson, J. M.: Potentiation of the antimalarial activity of qinghaosu by methoxylated flavones. Transactions of the Royal Society of Tropical Medicine and Hygiene 1987, 81: 434–436.
46. Chawira, A. N., Warhurst, D. C.: The effect of artemisinin combined with standard antimalarials against chloroquine-sensitive and chloroquine-resistant strains of *Plasmodium falciparum* in vitro. Journal of Tropical Medicine and Hygiene 1987, 90: 1–8.
47. Chawira, A. N., Warhurst, D. C., Robinson, B. L., Peters, W.: The effect of combinations of qinghaosu (artemisinin) with standard antimalarial drugs in the suppressive treatment of malaria in mice. Transactions of the Royal Society of Tropical Medicine and Hygiene 1987, 81: 554–558.
48. Wernsdorfer, W. H., Trigg, P. I. (ed.): Primaquine; pharmacokinetics, metabolism, toxicity and activity. John Wiley, Chichester, 1987.
49. Peters, W., Robinson, B. L.: The activity of primaquine and its possible metabolites against rodent malaria. In: Wernsdorfer, W. H., Trigg, P. I. (ed.): Primaquine; pharmacokinetics, metabolism, toxicity and activity. John Wiley, Chichester, 1987, p. 93–101.
50. Deslauriers, R., Butler, K., Smith, I. C. P.: Oxidant stress in malaria as probed by stable nitroxide radicals in erythrocytes infected with *Plasmodium berghei*. The effects of primaquine and chloroquine. Biochimica et Biophysica Acta 1987, 931: 267–275.

Pathogenic Microbial Mechanisms Susceptible to Drug Application

Bacterial Adherence in Pathogenicity

S. Normark*, S. Hultgren, B.-I. Marklund, G. Nyberg, A. Olsén, N. Strömberg, J. Tennent

Escherichia coli adhesins associated with extraintestinal infections such as acute pyelonephritis and neonatal meningitis are carbohydrate-binding proteins preferentially located at the tips of pili (fimbriae). Strategies to purify the adhesins prior to their polymerization into the pilus are discussed as a means to obtain structural and functional information concerning adhesin-receptor interactions. Such information is important for the future design of improved receptor analogues. The manner in which structural variation in an adhesin gene may yield antigenic and epitopic binding variants is also discussed. It is suggested that minor differences in the binding pocket of the adhesin may have major consequences on the tropism of the adhering organism. Finally, it is emphasized that bacterial adhesins may also recognize host proteins, and binding to matrix proteins as a means for bacterial attachment is briefly discussed.

Both primary pathogens and opportunistic bacteria that colonize mucosal surfaces must express adhesive properties in order to attach to the epithelium. Bacterial attachment is a means of colonizing the appropriate ecological niche to avoid being swept away by mucosal secretions, and may also be a first step in an invasive process. Furthermore, bacterial attachment may increase the efficiency by which toxins produced by the organism are targeted to their site of action. This may be particularly relevant in the intestinal tract, where proteolytic enzymes may inhibit the long-term effect of toxins.

Mucosal membranes are characterized by an extensive carbohydrate coat, contributed by the membrane glycoproteins and glycolipids as well as by the more loosely associated mucin glycoproteins. It is therefore not surprising that most bacterial adhesins have evolved to act as lectins, using carbohydrates as receptor sites. Some of these sites are present on glycoproteins such as mannose, which is recognized by Type 1 pili, while other carbohydrate receptors occur on glycolipids like the Galα1 → 4Gal moiety, which is present on the globoseries of glycolipids recognized by the majority of pyelonephritic *Escherichia coli* (1, 2). Many bacterial adhesins, such as those of *Mycoplasma pneumoniae,* recognize carbohydrate structures present on both glycoproteins and glycolipids. *Mycoplasma pneumoniae* may bind via the P1 adhesin (3) to NeuAcα2 → 3 (Galβ1 → 4GlcNAcβ1 → 3)$_n$, present in glycoconjugates (4, 5).

Department of Microbiology, University of Umeå, S-901 87 Umeå, Sweden.

There is a broad range of receptor affinities exhibited by the different adhesins. The lactose-binding adhesins present in many primary pathogens and opportunistic bacteria are defined as low-affinity binders by the criterion that soluble univalent lactose cannot inhibit the multivalent interaction between the microbe and a lactose-containing glycolipid (6, 7). It is not known why many bacteria have evolved adhesins that bind with a low affinity. One possible advantage of such adhesins could be that they are able to mediate bacterial attachment even in the presence of soluble receptor analogues that cannot inhibit their low-affinity adherence. In contrast, the Galα1 → 4Gal-specific attachment of pyelonephritic *Escherichia coli* is inhibited by soluble synthetic Galα1 → 4Gal (galabiose) and may therefore be referred to as a high-affinity binding (8). The Galα1 → 4Gal receptor is distributed throughout the urinary tract epithelium, and the ability of bacteria to bind to this receptor is an important virulence factor in urinary tract infections. Human urine does not normally contain soluble Galα1 → 4Gal analogues, which could explain the evolution in *Escherichia coli* of high-affinity binding to this receptor. Human urine contains high amounts of sialosylgalactosides, possibly explaining why the high-affinity S-fimbriae with specificity for these structures do not seem to be involved in urinary tract infections (T. Korhonen, personal communication).

Recent work has demonstrated that carbohydrate-specific bacterial adhesins may recognize the receptor in both an internal and terminal position (6, 7, 9). This work also showed that chemical groups distal as well as proximal to the oligosaccharide receptor site in the glycolipid may in some instances enhance binding and in others sterically interfere with receptor binding. Membranes from different tissues and species differ in their chemical composition and distribution of glycolipids, so that two adhesins recognizing different epitopes on the same oligosaccharide may have a markedly different tissue-binding distribution in vivo due to different responses to neighboring groups.

In recent years it has become evident that bacteria interact with components of the intracellular matrix as well as with membrane receptors. Binding to fibronectin, fibrinogen, laminin, vitronectin and collagen are common properties of both gram-positive and gram-negative bacteria. For wound pathogens such as *Staphylococcus aureus*, it is easy to imagine that binding to matrix proteins may be a virulence-associated property (10, 11, 12). Many epithelial cells contain receptors for matrix proteins which are important in cell differentiation and cell migration. These receptors belong to a common group of heterodimeric proteins termed integrins (13). Thus, bacterial adhesins that bind to cell-associated matrix proteins may resemble eukaryotic receptors that interact with these same proteins, marking a unique mechanism for bacterial attachment to cell surfaces.

A given microbe may express a multitude of different receptor-binding specificities. Most *Escherichia coli* isolates, for example, are able to express mannose-binding Type 1 pili. In addition, *Escherichia coli* associated with extraintestinal infections such as neonatal meningitis and urinary tract infections express other adhesins encoded in chromosomally located gene clusters. Finally, *Escherichia coli* strains associated with gastroenteritis express another set of adhesins that are usually plasmid-encoded (14). In each given situation it is difficult, if not impossible, to determine the relative importance of each binding specificity in the pathogenicity of the organisms. For an organism that is strictly a human pathogen, such as *Neisseria gonorrhoeae,* one would assume that each known adhesin has some role in the host-parasite interaction. Other organisms may have several hosts or may live as free-living saphrophytes. Different receptor-binding specificities in such organisms may reflect their ability to use several different ecological niches. To assess the individual role of one type of receptor-binding specificity, the corresponding adhesin must be cloned, the gene inactivated, and the mutated allele introduced into the original isolate, replacing the wildtype allele. Mutant and wildtype strains can then be compared in relevant infectious model systems. There are only a few situations documented where it has been possible to construct clean "knockout" mutations in adhesin genes (15). One reason for this is the unexpected complexity of the genetics of bacterial adhesins. Only recently have genes encoding distinct adhesins been characterized (16–19).

Escherichia coli is an excellent organism for studies aimed at a molecular understanding of bacterial attachment. *Escherichia coli* adhesins can be broadly divided into two major groups: those that are associated with filamentous surface polymers (pili adhesins), and those that are not associated with any particular surface structure (non-pili adhesins). *Escherichia coli* may express one or more pili adhesins either plasmid- or chromosomally-encoded in a single cell from distinct gene clusters (14). To date, only one non-pili adhesin, the chromosomally-encoded AFA-1, has been studied genetically (20).

Biogenesis of Galα1 → 4Gal-Binding P-pili in Uropathogenic *Escherichia coli*

Almost all *Escherichia coli* isolates associated with acute pyelonephritis in uncompromised children express mannose-resistant adhesins that bind to the P-blood group antigens on human uroepithelial cells (21, 22). The important portion of these glycolipid antigens necessary for binding was found to be a Galα1 → 4Gal moiety (1, 2, 9). Such digalactoside-specific binding is mediated by P-pili (22, 23). The chromosomal *pap* gene cluster specifying P-pili has been cloned from the uropathogenic *Escherichia coli* strain J96. This clone conferred mannose-resistant haemagglutination (MRHA) and the expression of P-pili on the *Escherichia coli* K12 strain HB101 (24). By way of subcloning, the *pap* gene cluster was localized within a 9.8 kb *Eco*RI-*Bam*HI fragment cloned in pPAP5 (25).

The genetic organization of the *pap* gene cluster (Figure 1) as well as the gene clusters encoding Type 1, S, K88 and K99 pili has been examined using molecular techniques (14). These systems were found to resemble each other in several important aspects. Each cluster contains two genes involved in regulation that map at the promoter proximal end. With the exception of the K88 cluster, the gene encoding the major pilin subunit is located immediately distal to the regulatory region. Each cluster also contains several accessory genes that specify proteins involved in the transport, export and assembly of the pili. The adhesin is the product of a gene distinct from that which encodes pilin, at least for the P, S and Type 1 pilus systems (16–19, 26, 27). Furthermore, it is interesting that the gene organization of the AFA-1 non-pili adhesin cluster (20) is similar to that of the pili gene clusters.

The bulk of the P-pilus consists of repeating subunits of PapA. Antiserum raised against purified P-pili was shown to inhibit MRHA and to block the binding of P-piliated bacteria to uroepithelial cells (28). Later, immunogold electron microscopy showed that the antiserum against the pili contained antibodies against

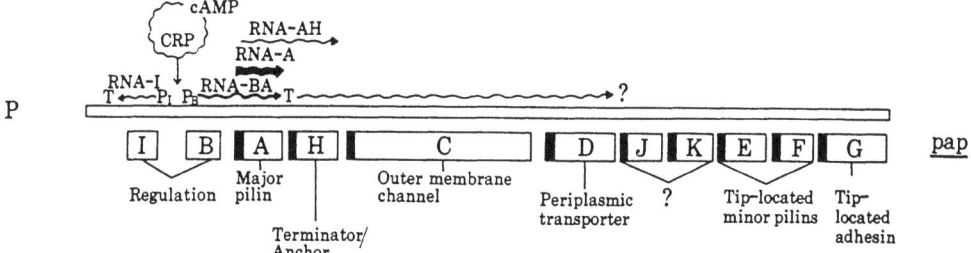

Figure 1: Structural and regulatory features of the *pap* gene cluster encoding P or Pap pili of serotype F13. The *pap* gene cluster from *Escherichia coli* strain J96 maps within the 9.8 kb *Eco*RI-*Bam*HI fragment of plasmid pPAP5 (25). The positions of the various Pap proteins are indicated. The *papI* and *papB* promoters, designated P_I and P_B, respectively, are shown together with the proposed regulatory targets of the PapI, PapB and CRP proteins. Messenger RNA transcripts emanating from P_I and P_B are depicted as wavy lines, while postulated transcriptional terminators are shown as stem and loop structures. Below, the proposed function for each of the pap gene products is given.

three pilus tip located proteins: PapE, PapF and PapG (29, 30). Linker insertion mutations and *trans*-complementation experiments revealed that the Galα1 → 4Gal-binding properties of the pilus resided in the PapG molecule (16). PapF was found to be required for bacterial binding and played an important role in initiating pilus assembly. The function of PapE was to firmly link the adhesin to the pilus (29). In addition to the PapG adhesin and the minor pilin, PapF, two other accessory *pap* gene products, PapC and PapD, are necessary for bacterial binding (25, 26). PapC is thought to be an outer membrane channel, and perhaps a polymerization center, for the surface localization of the P-pilus components (31), while PapD is essential for the stability of the various pilus components and also plays a role in the transport of the subunits to the polymerization center.

Type 1 pili, unlike flagella, are polymerized from the base, meaning that the pilus tip is formed initially in the biogenesis of pili (32). It is most likely that the related P-pili are also polymerized from the base. We have identified one *pap* gene product, PapH, that is important both for length determination and for the anchoring of the pilus to the bacterial cell envelope (30). The components in the P-pilus heteropolymer are structurally related, especially in their amino and carboxy termini (29, 33). We found that both the major and the minor pilus subunits, including the Galα1 → 4Gal-specific adhesin, occur as soluble complexes with the PapD transport protein in the periplasmic space prior to their polymerization into the growing pilus. It is likely that the conserved regions in the subunits are of importance both for interaction with PapD and for subunit interactions.

It has been possible by genetic analysis to obtain an understanding of regions of the polypeptides required for subunit interactions and to define a region on the adhesin that is important in recognizing the receptor. However, structural information based on crystallography data are badly needed. So far, it has not been possible to obtain crystals from purified pili. Likewise, adhesins purified from pili readily aggregate, making structural studies difficult (17). Our observation that the pilus subunits, including the adhesin, occur as individual soluble complexes in the periplasmic space with the transport protein, PapD, has opened new avenues to the crystallization of the pilus components. It has recently been possible to purify the PapD transport protein, and crystals have already been obtained (C. I. Brändén, personal communication). It has also been possible to isolate the dimeric complex between PapD and the pilus tip associated PapE protein. Also, the PapD-PapG adhesin complex has been isolated by utilizing the receptor-binding specificity of PapG (S. Hultgren, unpublished results). Briefly, periplasmic extracts overproducing PapD and PapG were run through a galabiose-sepharose column, after which the bound PapD-PapG adhesin complex was eluted with a synthetic receptor analogue. The preassembled adhesin in complex with PapD could thereby be eluted from the column.

Receptor Analogues and Drug Design

It has been suggested for some time that receptor analogues may be a novel strategy to combat bacterial infections at the level of the mucosal membranes. It has been demonstrated, using a mouse model for urinary tract infections, that receptor analogues prevented colonization of the kidney by the challenging *Escherichia coli* organism (34). It is likely that the interaction between the adhesin and its natural receptor is not optimal; by rational drug design, it should be possible to obtain receptor analogues with a higher affinity for the adhesin than the natural one. It is hoped that a detailed analysis of a PapG adhesin-receptor complex will yield data that enable the design of such high-affinity analogues to be delivered as polymeric structures to overcome the cooperativity of a multivalent bacterial interaction. Despite the lack of crystallographic data, it has already been possible to generate synthetic analogues that show a considerably higher inhibitory potency of hemagglutination than the galabiose receptor (J. Kihlberg, unpublished results).

The original method for binding of the cholera toxin to thin-layer chromatograms of glycolipids was recently extended to a solid-phase receptor-binding assay in which it was possible to identify the binding of bacteria, viruses or purified adhesins to specific glycolipids (35). The use of a large number of glycolipid derivatives has shown that bacterial adhesins frequently recognize a carbohydrate moiety, both in a terminal and an internal position in the carbohydrate chain. It has also been demonstrated that neighboring groups may both enhance or sterically interfere with bacterial binding (6, 7). When combined with molecular modelling, such analyses may provide information as to the region of the receptor saccharide that is recognized by the adhesin. Such analyses, currently performed by K.-A. Karlsson in Göteborg, will be an important complement to X-ray crystallography in rational drug design.

Epitopic Variation of Galα1 → 4Gal Adhesins and Bacterial Tropism

The primary observation by Karlsson and his associates that different lactose-binding bacteria seem to recognize different epitopes on the lactose molecules prompted us to see if epitopic variation also occurs for Galα1 → 4Gal-binding *Escherichia coli*. Four different cloned *Escherichia coli pap* operons were transformed into *Escherichia coli* HB101, and the receptor-binding properties were analyzed using the solid-phase receptor-binding assay. It was demonstrated that three of the clones bound strongly to almost all of the Galα1 → 4Gal-containing glycolipids tested and that one of these three clones differed in detailed specificity by binding only weakly to the P_1-antigen. Even more interesting, the fourth clone (*prs*) preferentially bound to the Forssman antigen (15), a Galα1 → 4Gal-containing glycolipid prevalent in sheep erythrocytes but not in human erythrocytes (36). Unlike the other three clones the *prs* clone failed to recognize the P^k- and P_1-blood group antigens and reacted only slightly with P antigen (globoside), the major human erythrocyte glycolipid. Hence, *Escherichia coli* expressing the PrsG adhesin agglutinated sheep but not human erythrocytes. The Forssman antigen is also present in the dog kidney. It is interesting to note that urinary tract infection *Escherichia coli* isolates from dogs frequently express P-like pili based on serology and Southern blot hybridization using *pap*-specific DNA as a probe. These strains, however, agglutinate dog and sheep erythrocytes rather than human erythrocytes and bind to dog kidney derived MDCK cells rather than to human T24 cells (37 and unpublished data). Many of these dog strains show binding specificities virtually identical to that mediated by *prs* (unpublished data). Since bacteria expressing the PrsG adhesin bind also to Galα1 → 4Gal-containing glycolipids carrying terminal saccharides other than the Forssman antigen (unpublished data), we are now convinced that there exist epitopic variants of Galα1 → 4Gal-binding adhesins that are restricted to subsets of the globoseries of Galα1 → 4Gal-containing glycolipids. It is possible that subtle differences in the receptor-binding pocket of the adhesin cause these differences in binding. In vitro mutagenesis in conjunction with X-ray crystallography will provide excellent tools for the molecular resolution of this situation. Possibly, epitopic variation may be a means for *Escherichia coli* to colonize the urinary tract of different species.

Adhesins and Immunoprophylaxis

Another approach to prevent bacterial attachment is through immunoprophylaxis. Bacterial pili are in general good antigens; however, protection is primarily obtained only against the homologous strain. This is due in part to the large variability in sequence and antigenicity of the major pilin subunit. It is not known today if the pilus-associated adhesin varies to the same extent as the major subunit. For P-pili, it is known that variants of PapG exist, some of which do not crossreact serologically (38). The mannose-specific adhesin on Type 1 pili might be antigenically more conserved (S. Abraham, personal communication). Vaccination trials with purified adhesins have not yet been tried in any system.

Escherichia coli Pili and Binding to Matrix Proteins

Since a pilus may be composed of several subunit proteins, it may be that a single pilus binds to more than one receptor. It has recently been demonstrated that *Escherichia coli* P and Type 1 pili mediate binding to fibronectin and other matrix proteins coated onto glass slides (J. Emödy, unpublished data). This binding seems to be mediated by the major pilin subunit. The interaction between P-pili and Type 1 pili with fibronectin is likely to be quite weak, since *Escherichia coli* expressing these two classes of pili do not bind soluble fibronectin. Nevertheless, there exist many *Escherichia coli* isolates that do bind soluble fibronectin. We have recently cloned the fibronectin-binding property of one such *Escherichia coli* isolate and shown that expression of the cloned gene in *Escherichia coli* HB101, enables this organism to bind soluble fibronectin (A. Olsén and S. Normark, unpublished data). The fibronectin-binding property was associated with the production of unusually curly pili. These results suggest that *Escherichia coli* can express pili organelles that specifically bind to matrix proteins. Since only one gene product is required for the production of curly pili, we suppose that it encodes the major subunit of these pili, which is most likely the fibronectin-binding adhesin.

Pili Adhesins in Other Gram-Negative Organisms

It is not yet known if adhesive pili in organisms other than *Escherichia coli* bind through their major subunit, or if specific adhesins are associated with these pili. *Neisseria gonorrhoeae, Neisseria meningitidis, Pseudomonas aeruginosa, Bacteroides nodosus* and *Moraxella bovis* express pili in which the major subunits are highly similar (39). Residues 1 to 20 are identical in all of these pilins except for a few highly conserved substitutions. It has not yet been shown whether this class of pili are heteropolymers. Even though a purified pili preparation from *Neisseria gonorrhoeae* contains small amounts of other proteins, it is not known if these proteins are associated with the pilus or not (40). In *Neisseria gonorrhoeae*, genes involved in pilus biogenesis other than the major subunit gene have not yet been reported. It is likely that genes required for secretion and assembly of the gonococcal pilus will soon be identified. The lactose-specific binding property recently found in strains of *Neisseria gonorrhoeae* is also expressed in variants that do not express pili (6). These results demonstrate that *Neisseria gonorrhoeae* expresses at least one carbohydrate-binding specificity that is not mediated by the pilin subunit itself.

Concluding Remarks

Bacterial attachment is a far more complex process than previously anticipated. Many carbohydrate-specific adhesins are only minor components of pili heteropolymers and are therefore produced in very low quantities by the cell. The development of receptor analogues as a novel strategy to prevent or treat infections requires a detailed understanding of the interactions between the adhesin and its receptor. Understanding the biogenesis pathway for pili makes it possible to purify the adhesin prior to its assembly into the pilus. In its pre-assembled stage the adhesin is a soluble complex with a transport protein that should enable crystallization of the adhesin in the presence of its receptor. It is hoped that this strategy, applied to the Galα1 → 4Gal-specific adhesin of uropathogenic *Escherichia coli*, will give specific as well as general information needed to design receptor analogues in a rational fashion.

References

1. Leffler, H., Svanborg-Edén, C.: Chemical identification of a glycosphingolipid receptor for *Escherichia coli* attaching to human urinary tract epithelial cells and agglutinating human erythrocytes. FEMS Microbiology Letters 1980, 8: 127–134.
2. Källenius, G., Möllby, R., Svensson, S. B., Winberg, J., Lundblad, A., Cedergren, B.: The P^k antigen as receptor for the hemagglutinin of pyelonephritic *Escherichia coli*. FEMS Microbiology Letters 1980, 297–302.
3. Hu, P. C., Cole, R. M., Huang, Y. S., Graham, J. A., Gardner, D. E., Collier, A. M., Clyde, W. A.: *Mycoplasma pneumoniae* infection: role of a surface protein in the attachment organelle. Science 1982, 216: 313–315.
4. Loomes, L. M., Clemura, K.-I., Feizi, T.: Interaction of *Mycoplasma pneumoniae* with erythrocyte glycolipids of I and i antigen types. Infection and Immunity 1985, 47: 15–20.
5. Loomes, L. M., Clemura, K.-I., Childs, R. A., Paulson, J. C., Rogers, G. N., Scudder, P. R., Michalski, J.-C., Hounsell, E. F., Taylor-Robinson, D., Feizi, T.: Erythrocyte receptors for *Mycoplasma pneumoniae* are sialylated oligosaccharides of Ii antigen type. Nature 1984, 307: 560–563.
6. Strömberg, N., Deal, C., Nyberg, G., Normark, S., So, M., Karlsson, K.-A.: Identification of carbohydrate structures which are possible receptors for *Neisseria gonorrhoeae*. Proceedings of the National Academy of Sciences of the USA 1988, 85: 4902–4906.
7. Strömberg, N., Ryd, M., Lindberg, A. A., Karlsson, K.-A.: Studies on the binding of bacteria to glycolipids. Two species of *Propionibacterium* apparently recognize separate epitopes on lactose of lactosylceramide. FEBS Letters 1988, 232: 193–198.
8. Leffler, H., Svanborg-Edén, C.: Glycolipids as receptors for *Escherichia coli* lectins or adhesins. In: Mirelman, D. (ed.): Microbial lectins and agglutinins. Wiley, New York, 1986, p. 83–111.
9. Bock, K., Breimer, E. M., Brignole, A., Hansson, G. C., Karlsson, K.-A., Larson, G., Leffler, H., Samuelsson, B. E., Strömberg, N., Svanborg-Edén, C., Thurin, J.: Specificity of binding of a strain of uropathogenic *Escherichia coli* to Galα1 → 4Gal containing glycosphingolipids. Journal of Biological Chemistry 1985, 260: 8545–8551.
10. Kuusela, P.: Fibronectin binds to *Staphylococcus aureus*. Nature 1978, 276: 718–720.
11. Wadström, T., Switalski, L., Speziale, P., Rubin, K., Rydén, C., Fröman, G., Faris, A., Lindberg, M., Höök, M.: In: Jackson, G. J. (ed.): Pathogenesis of infection. Springer, Berlin, 1985, p. 193–207.
12. Flock, J.-I., Fröman, G., Jönsson, K., Guss, B., Signäs, C., Nilsson, B., Raucci, G., Höök, M., Wadström, T., Lindberg, M.: Cloning and expression of the gene for a fibronectin-binding protein from *Staphylococcus aureus*. EMBO Journal 1987, 6: 2351–2357.
13. Hynes, R.: Integrins: a family of cell surface receptors. Cell 1987, 48: 549–554.
14. Normark, S., Båga, M., Göransson, M., Lindberg, F. P., Lund, B., Norgren, M., Uhlin, B.-E.: Genetics and bio-

genesis of *Escherichia coli* adhesins. In: Mirelman, D. (ed.): Microbial lectins and agglutinins. Wiley, New York, 1986, p. 113–143.
15. Lund, B., Marklund, B.-I., Strömberg, N., Lindberg, F., Karlsson, K.-A., Normark, S.: Uropathogenic *Escherichia coli* can express serologically identical pili of different receptor binding specificity. Molecular Microbiology 1988, 2: 255–263.
16. Lund, B., Lindberg, F., Marklund, B.-I., Normark, S.: PapG is the α-D-galactopyranosyl-(1→4)-β-D-galactopyranose-binding adhesin of uropathogenic *Escherichia coli*. Proceedings of the National Academy of Sciences of the USA 1987, 84: 5898–5902.
17. Moch, T., Hoschlützky, H., Hacker, T., Kröncke, K.-P., Jann, K.: Isolation and characterization of the α-sialyl-β-2,3-galactosyl specific adhesin from fimbriated *Escherichia coli*. Proceedings of the National Academy of Sciences of the USA 1987, 84: 3462–3466.
18. Maurer, L., Orndorff, P. E.: Identification and characterization of genes determining binding and pilus length of *Escherichia coli* Type 1 pili. Journal of Bacteriology 1987, 169: 640–645.
19. Mimion, F. C., Abraham, S. N., Beachy, E. H., Gougen, J. D.: The genetic determinant of adhesive function in Type 1 fimbriae of *Escherichia coli* is distinct from the gene encoding the fimbrial subunit. Journal of Bacteriology 1986, 165: 1033–1036.
20. Labigne-Roussel, A., Falkow, S.: Distribution and degree of heterogeneity of the afimbrial-adhesin-encoding operon (*afa*) among uropathogenic *Escherichia coli* isolates. Infection and Immunity 1988, 56: 640–648.
21. Källenius, G., Möllby, R., Svensson, S. B., Helin, I., Hultberg, H., Cedergren, B., Winberg, J.: Occurrence of P-fimbriated *Escherichia coli* in urinary tract infections. Lancet 1981, ii: 1369–1372.
22. Väisänen, V., Elo, J., Tallgren, L. G., Siitonen, A., Mäkelä, P. H., Svanborg-Edén, C., Källenius, G., Svensson, S. B., Hultberg, H., Korhonen, T.: Mannose-resistant haemagglutination and P antigen recognition are characteristic of *Escherichia coli* causing primary pyelonephritis. Lancet 1981, ii: 1366–1369.
23. O'Hanley, P., Lark, D., Normark, S., Falkow, S., Schoolnik, G. K.: Mannose-sensitive and Gal-Gal binding *Escherichia coli* pili from recombinant strains. Journal of Experimental Medicine 1983, 158: 1713–1719.
24. Hull, R. A., Gill, R. E., Hsu, P., Minshew, B. H., Falkow, S.: Construction and expression of recombinant plasmids encoding Type 1 or D-mannose-resistant pili from a urinary tract infection *Escherichia coli* isolate. Infection and Immunity 1981, 33: 933–938.
25. Lindberg, F. P., Lund B., Normark, S.: Genes of pyelonephritic *Escherichia coli* required for digalactoside specific agglutination of human cells. EMBO Journal 1984, 3: 1167–1173.
26. Norgren, M., Normark, S., Lark, D., O'Hanley, P., nik, G., Falkow, S., Svanborg-Edén, C., Båga, M., Uhlin, B.-E.: Mutations in *Escherichia coli* cistrons affecting adhesion to human cells do not abolish Pap pili fiber formation. EMBO Journal 1984, 3: 1159–1165.

27. Hacker, J., Schmidt, G., Hughes, C., Knapp, S., Marget, M., Goebel, W.: Cloning and characterization of genes involved in production of mannose-resistant neuraminidase-susceptible (X) fimbriae from a uropathogenic 06:K15:H31 *Escherichia coli* strain. Infection and Immunity 1985, 47: 434–440.
28. Korhonen, T. K., Leffler, H., Svanborg-Edén, C.: Binding specificity of piliated strains of *Escherichia coli* and *Salmonella typhimurium* to epithelial cells, *Saccharomyces cerevisiae* cells, and erythrocytes. Infection and Immunity 1981, 32: 796–804.
29. Lindberg, F., Lund, B., Normark, S.: Gene products specifying adhesion of uropathogenic *Escherichia coli* are minor components of pili. Proceedings of the National Academy of Sciences of the USA 1986, 83: 1891–1895.
30. Lindberg, F., Lund, B., Johansson, L., Normark, S.: Localization of the receptor-binding protein at the tip of the bacterial pilus. Nature 1987, 328: 84–87.
31. Norgren, M., Båga, M., Tennent, J. M., Normark, S.: Nucleotide sequence, regulation and functional analysis of the *papC* gene required for cell surface localization of Pap pili of uropathogenic *Escherichia coli*. Molecular Microbiology 1987, 1: 169–178.
32. Lowe, M. A., Holt, S. C., Eisenstein, B. I.: Immunoelectron microscopic analysis of elongation of type 1 fimbriae of *Escherichia coli*. Journal of Bacteriology 1987, 169: 157–163.
33. Båga, M., Norgren, M., Normark, S.: Biogenesis of *Escherichia coli* Pap-pili: PapH, a minor pilin subunit involved in cell anchoring and length modulation. Cell 1987, 49: 241–251.
34. Svanborg-Edén, C., Freter, T., Hagberg, L., Hull, R., Hull, S., Leffler, H., Schoolnik, G.: Inhibition of experimental ascending urinary tract infection by an epithelial cell surface receptor analogue. Nature 1982, 298: 560–562.
35. Hansson, G. C., Karlsson, K.-A., Larson, G., Strömberg, N., Thurin, J.: Carbohydrate-specific adhesion of bacteria to thin-layer chromatograms: a rationalized approach to the study of host cell glycolipid receptors. Analytical Biochemistry 1985, 146: 158–163.
36. Momoi, M., Yamakawa, T.: Glucosamine-containing sphingolipids from sheep erythrocytes. Journal of Biological Chemistry 1978, 84: 317–325.
37. Garcia, E., Hamers, A., Bergmans, H., Bernard, A., van der Zeijst, B., Gaastra, W.: Adhesion of canine and human uropathogenic *Escherichia coli* and *Proteus mirabilis* strains to canine and human epithelial cells. Current Microbiology 1988, (in press).
38. Lund, B., Lindberg, F., Normark, S.: Structure and antigenic properties of the tip-located P-pilus proteins of uropathogenic *Escherichia coli*. Journal of Bacteriology 1988, 170: 1887–1894.
39. Elleman, T. C.: Pilins of *Bacteroides nodosus*: molecular basis of serotypic variation and relationships to other bacterial pilins. Microbiological Reviews 1988, 52: 233–247.
40. Muir, L., Strugnell, R. A., Davies, J. K.: Proteins that appear to be associated with pili in *Neisseria gonorrhoeae*. Infection and Immunity 1988, 56: 1743–1747.

Haemophilus Influenzae Gene Expression and Bacterial Invasion

E. R. Moxon*, J. S. Kroll, J. N. Weiser

The pathogenesis of bacterial meningitis involves several sequential events: acquisition of the causative organism by a susceptible individual, nasopharyngeal colonisation, invasion of the respiratory epithelium resulting in bacteraemia, haematogenous dissemination, invasion of the blood-brain barrier, and the occurrence of inflammatory changes in the sub-arachnoid space followed by bacterial replication within the central nervous system. The molecular basis of the bacterial invasiveness of *Haemophilus influenzae*, a major cause of meningitis in infants and young children, has been investigated through the application of genetic techniques and the use of a biologically relevant experimental rat model of meningitis. Genes for capsular polysaccharide and lipopolysaccharide are important determinants of *Haemophilus influenzae* virulence and contribute to the invasive potential of the organism by enhancing intravascular survival. The genes for the type b capsule confer greater efficiency in evading host clearance mechanisms than do the genes for the other capsular polysaccharides. This enhanced survival has at least two important potential pathophysiological consequences, since there is a direct relationship between the magnitude of bacteraemia and the probability of meningitis, and since increased blood-brain barrier permeability is directly related to the number of bacteria in the cerebrospinal fluid.

More than 50 years ago, Margaret Pittman recognised that virtually all cases of invasive *Haemophilus influenzae* disease were caused by capsulate strains, and that of the six antigenically distinct serotypes designated a through f, those expressing the type b (polyribosyl-ribitol phosphate) polysaccharide capsule accounted for more than 90% of infections, including meningitis (1).

The pathogenesis of bacterial meningitis involves several sequential events: acquisition of the bacterium following transmission from another individual, respiratory tract (nasopharyngeal) colonisation, invasion of the respiratory tract resulting in bacteraemia, haematogenous dissemination, invasion of the blood-brain barrier, and, finally, the occurrence of inflammatory changes within the sub-arachnoid space and meninges followed by bacterial multiplication within the central nervous system (CNS) (Figure 1). Although strains of *Haemophilus influenzae* capable of causing meningitis are described as invasive, the term fails to capture the specific nature of the biological events or the complex molecular interactions between host and microbe which determine the subsequent pathogenic events. Furthermore, it does not impart any sense of the temporal or quantitative contribution of the cumulative co-evolutionary changes in the genes of both host and microbe.

Several determinants have been implicated as contributors to the pathogenic potential of *Haemophilus influenzae* (Table 1), and the genes controlling their expression can be studied through the application of the techniques of molecular biology. In this report *Haemophilus influenzae* meningitis will serve as a model to illustrate how the molecular determinants of microbial invasiveness in the pathogenesis of meningitis have been studied.

Gene Expression and Bacterial Invasion

The availablity of an experimental model of *Haemophilus influenzae* meningitis in infant rats provides a useful tool for studying the determinants of microbial invasiveness, since virulence can be studied

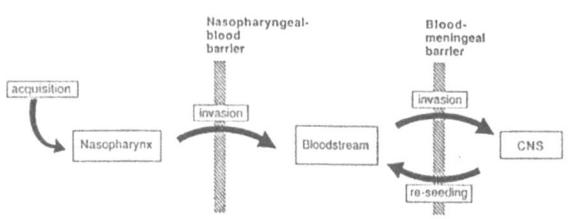

Figure 1: Pathogenetic sequence for bacterial meningitis caused by *Haemophilus influenzae* type b.

---

* Infectious Diseases Unit, Department of Paediatrics, John Radcliffe Hospital, Headington, Oxford OX3 9DU, UK.

Table 1: Putative virulence determinants of *Haemophilus influenzae*.

1. Capsular polysaccharide
2. Lipopolysaccharide
3. Outer membrane proteins
4. Pilus proteins
5. IgA$_1$ proteases
6. Factors affecting ciliated epithelium

only in a biologically relevant system. In the infant rat model of *Haemophilus influenzae* bacteraemia and meningitis (2), the bacteria must cross both epithelial and endothelial cell barriers (Figure 1) to result in meningitis. To investigate the genetic basis of *Haemophilus influenzae* invasiveness, the avirulent strain Rd was transformed using RNA obtained from a virulent type b strain (Eagan) (3). In contrast to the non-invasive behaviour of Rd, type b transformants of Rd were found to be highly virulent for rats: following intranasal inoculation, meningitis resulted. This experiment indicates that molecules of DNA from Eagan can be taken up by strain Rd and, when integrated into the chromosome by homologous recombination, can render the transformants invasive. Subsequent studies have sought to identify the genes involved and the mechanisms through which their expression mediates the invasive phenotype.

In further studies the transformation of Rd by whole cell genomic DNA from Eagan resulted in two distinct genotypes. These transformants differed in the amount of type b capsule elaborated, in their lipopolysaccharide (LPS) phenotype and in their virulence potential (4). The recipient in the transformation, strain Rd, was originally obtained from Dr. G. Leidy and has been used as a prototype strain in many laboratories. It is a spontaneous, capsule-deficient variant of a capsulate type d clinical isolate obtained from the nasopharynx of an asymptomatic New Yorker in about 1940. (personal communication, G. Leidy). The donor type b strain, Eagan, was originally isolated from the cerebrospinal fluid (CSF) of a child with meningitis (5). Of the several iridescent colonies produced by transformation, Rd:b$^+$:01 and Rd:b$^+$:02 were two that differed in their LPS phenotype, as reveabled by examination with SDS-PAGE and silver staining (4). Using an ELISA, Rd:b$^+$:01 was found to elaborate about twice as much b capsule as did Rd:b$^+$:02. Nonetheless, Rd:b$^+$:02 was found to be more virulent than Rd:b$^+$:01 following intranasal, intraperitoneal or intracisternal challenge (4, 6). The relative virulence of Rd, Rb$^+$:01 and Rb$^+$:02 (and related variants of these strains) has established the independent contribution of capsule and of LPS genes in virulence, providing insights into their role in the pathogenesis of meningitis.

Genetic Basis of Capsule Expression and its Role in Virulence

Cloning of the chromosomal locus for type b capsule expression (*cap* b) from Eagan has made it possible to investigate the contribution of capsule genes to virulence and to understand why the transformation of Rd resulted in the different transformants. The chromosomal locus for type b capsule (*cap* b) contains a duplication of approximately 17 kilobases (kb) organised in a directly repeated configuration (7), loci within each copy being involved in capsule production (8). This duplication has been found to be a feature of almost all type b strains based on an analysis of type b isolates obtained from all over the world (9). Using DNA cloned from *cap* b as probes in Southern hybridisation analyses, the chromosomal DNA of Rd was found to possess a residual *cap* locus which contained a small stretch of DNA with homology to *cap* b. This small region of the chromosome – a kilobase or less in size – is duplicated in Eagan but not in Rd. Thus, when Rd is transformed with chromosomal DNA from Eagan, the integration of either the entire duplication, as found in Rd:b$^+$:01, or, alternatively, only one complete copy, as found in Rd:b$^+$:02, can occur (Figure 2).

An important conclusion from these observations is that duplication of genes in *cap* b is not necessary for type b capsule expression, nor does it enhance virulence (6, 10). Rd:b$^+$:02 defines a reduced locus

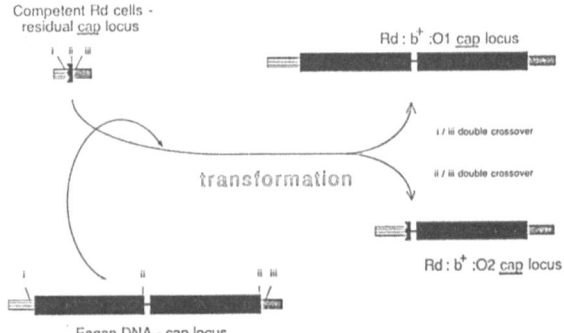

Figure 2: Schematic representation of the transformation of competent, capsule-deficient strain Rd-cells using DNA obtained from serotype b strain Eagan as the donor. The residual *cap* locus found in Rd has three segments of DNA (i, ii and iii) which have sequence homology to DNA in the *cap* locus of the serotype b donor, strain Eagan, as shown. As segment ii is present in duplicate in Eagan, homologous recombination (double-crossover) can result in two outcomes in which *cap* DNA from the donor (Eagan) is integrated into the target locus in Rd to give capsulate transformats. Recombination involving segments i and iii yields the duplicated *cap* locus of Rd:b$^+$:01, while crossover between ii and iii yields the single-copy locus of Rd:b$^+$:02.

comprising a single copy of the 17 kb repeat together with about 1.3 kb of DNA (designated the 'bridge' region) found between the 17 kb repeats in the Eagan (wild-type) *cap* b locus (10, 11). Thus, the greater virulence of Rd:b^+:02 is most likely attributable to the altered LPS, although the molecular basis for the change in LPS found in Rd:b^+:02 remains uncertain. Apparently, there are genes within or linked to *cap* b that are involved in LPS expression (4, 12). Neither of the capsule-deficient strains, Rd or Rd:b^-:02, causes invasive disease in infant rats, although each is able to colonise the nasopharynx. (Obtained from Rd:b^+:02, Rd:b^-:02 is a spontaneous, capsule-deficient variant that has sustained a defined mutation in a region essential for type b capsule expression (8)). Therefore, capsule is essential for the occurrence of one or more of the events following colonisation which determine the potential of *Haemophilus influenzae* to penetrate respiratory epithelium, enter the bloodstream and cause sustained bacteraemia.

Following intravenous inoculation, Rd is rapidly cleared from the blood, whereas the type b transformants are not. This shows that capsule mediates intravascular survival once the organism has reached the bloodstream. A crucial unanswered question concerns the influence of type b capsule on the events that precede the entry of *Haemophilus influenzae* into the blood, i.e. penetration of the organism through or between respiratory epithelium and its subsequent translocation into the lumen of the endothelium of blood vessels. Similarly, the determinants of penetration through the blood-meningeal-CSF barrier are unknown. However, a critical magnitude of bacteraemia ($>10^3$ organisms/ml) appears necessary (but not sufficient) for the occurrence of meningitis (13) and suggests that dose-related bacterial-induced injury to one or more components of the blood-brain barrier may be important. In the absence of specific data on this issue, suffice it to emphasise that there is no requirement for type b capsule to be a determinant of cellular invasion.

If capsule-deficient organisms were capable of successful translocation from the nasopharynx into the bloodstream, or from the bloodstream into the CNS, the results of the experimental infection in the infant rat would be adequately explained on the basis of the rapid clearance of bacteria from the blood. Since sustained, high density bacteraemia is a critical factor in the pathogenesis of meningitis, and type b strains are by far the most common cause, the question remains as to what extent type b capsule mediates the greater virulence potential of such strains. To investigate this question further, transformants of Rd:b^-:02 to each of the six different capsular types were obtained. The capsule-deficient variant Rd:b^-:02 was chosen as the recipient because it could be transformed at relatively high frequency (as compared to Rd) to each of the six capsular serotypes. Physical mapping of the transformants has shown that they differ solely in that region of the chromosome which contains the DNA conferring type-specificity. These transformants shared identical phenotypic characteristics such as outer membrane proteins, LPS, and biotype, but differed in capsular phenotype. Following intranasal challenge of infant rats, only the serotype a and b transformants consistently caused bacteraemia, but the type b transformant was significantly more virulent. It is of particular interest that both type a and type b polysaccharide polymers include ribitol phosphate, which is not found in the other four capsules.

These results provide strong evidence that type b capsule genes are critical for maximal virulence. Furthermore, recent studies (6) have identified an important role for type b capsule in the pathogenesis of meningeal inflammation and altered blood-brain barrier permeability (BBBP) as a consequence of the role of capsule in enhancing survival within the subarachnoid space. Altered BBBP is related primarily to the number of bacteria and the number of inflammatory cells in the meninges and CSF; interestingly, clearance of bacteria from the CSF did not correlate with the magnitude of the CSF pleocytosis.

Genetic Basis of LPS Expression and its Role in Virulence

The most reasonable explanation for the greater virulence of Rd:b^+:02, when compared to Rd:b^+:01, is that it reflects structural differences in the respective LPS molecules of the two strains. Several lines of evidence support a role for *Haemophilus influenzae* LPS as a virulence factor, and the structural basis for the pathogenic potential of these molecules is currently under investigation. LPS molecules of *Haemophilus influenzae* lack the repetitive terminal sugars characteristic of the smooth LPS molecules ('O' antigenic determinants) of *Enterobacteriaceae* (4, 12, 14).

The core oligosaccharides comprise the neutral sugars glucose, galactose and heptose, and may also contain N-acetyl glucosamine (14). Preliminary compositional analysis indicate that Rd:b^+:01 possesses terminal glucose and galactose, whereas Rd:b^+:02 lacks terminal galactose (personal communication, S. Zamze). This finding is consistent with the differences observed in the reactivity of the strains with monoclonal antibodies specific for terminal *Haemophilus influenzae* lipo-oligosaccharide epitopes (4). Variations in lipo-oligosaccharide epitopes associated with altered virulence have also been reported by Kimura et al (15). A deep rough mutant of Rd:b^+:02 (Rd:b^+:I69), lacking all oligosaccharide sugars except KDO, was found to be avirulent for rats (16). Taken together, these findings indicate that the structure of the core oligosaccharides, in concert with capsule, determines the efficiency with which *Haemophilus influenzae* evade host mechanisms. These mechanisms in turn are mediated through the serum bactericidal and opsonic activity of complement, antibodies and phagocytic cells.

Using monoclonal antibodies, Kimura and Hansen (15, 17) have shown that the lipo-oligosaccharides of *Haemophilus influenzae* exhibit phase-variation. This variation appears to be regulated by complex transcriptional mechanisms involving the glycosyl transferase genes, which are responsible for the assembly of the core oligosaccharides. Each LPS molecule may exhibit phase variation of several epitopes (defined by reactivity with monoclonal antibodies), and therefore each bacterial cell can express an extensive repertoire of LPS molecules. It is tempting to speculate that this variation in LPS expression provides an effective and elegant mechanism through which individual organisms can adapt to and avoid host immune responses in the pathogenesis of invasive disease. Furthermore, since asymptomatic carriage is far more common than disease, particular surface-exposed oligosaccharides may be selected by colonising strains, and this would provide a mechanism by which *Haemophilus influenzae* could adapt to different hosts. The variant oligosaccharides could mimic the glycosidic residues of host cell receptors against which host immune responses presumably would be constrained.

Acknowledgements

This work is supported in part by The Medical Research Council, The Meningitis Trust and The Lister Institute. Dr. J. Simon Kroll is a Lister Institute Research Fellow and Dr. Jeffrey N. Weiser is a Research Fellow of the Pediatric Service of Johnson & Johnson. The authors wish to thank Mrs. Sheila Hayes for her expert and invaluable help in preparing the manuscript.

References

1. **Pittman, M.:** Variation and type specificity in the bacterial species *Haemophilus influenzae*. Journal of Experimental Medicine 1931, 53: 471–493.
2. **Moxon, E. R., Smith, A. L., Averill, D. R., Smith, D. H.:** *Haemophilus influenzae* meningitis in infant rats after intranasal inoculation. Journal of Infectious Diseases 1974, 129: 154–162.
3. **Moxon, E. R., Vaughn, K. A.:** The type b capsular polysaccharide as a virulence dterminant of *Haemophilus influenzae*: studies using clinical isolates and laboratory transformants. Journal of Infectious Diseases 1981, 153: 517–534.
4. **Zwahlen, A., Rubin, L. G., Moxon, E. R.:** Contribution of lipopolysaccharide to pathogenicity of *Haemophilus influenzae*: comparative virulence of genetically-related strains in rats. Microbial Pathogenesis 1986, 1: 465–473.
5. **Anderson, P., Johnston, R. B., Smith, D. H.:** Human serum activities against *Haemophilus influenzae* type b. Journal of Clinical Investigation 1972, 51: 31–38.
6. **Lesse, A., Scheld, W. M., Zwahlen, A., Moxon, E. R.:** Role of cerebrospinal fluid pleocytosis and *Haemophilus influenzae* type b capsule on blood-brain barrier permeability during experimental meningitis in the rat. Journal of Clinical Investigation 1988, 82: 102–109.
7. **Hoiseth, S. K., Moxon, E. R., Silver, R. P.:** Genes involved in *Haemophilus influenzae* type b capsule expression are part of an 18-kilobase tandem duplication. Proceedings of the National Academy of Science, USA 1986, 83: 1106–1110.
8. **Ely, S., Tippett, J., Kroll, J. S., Moxon, E. R.:** Mutations affecting expression and maintenance of genes encoding the type b capsule of *Haemophilus influenzae*. Journal of Bacteriology 1986, 167: 44–48.
9. **Allan, I., Loeb, M. R., Moxon, E. R.:** Limited genetic diversity of *Haemophilus influenzae* (type b). Microbial Pathogenesis 1987, 2: 139–145.
10. **Kroll, J. S., Moxon, E. R.:** Capsulation and gene copynumber at the *cap* locus of *Haemophilus influenzae* type b. Journal of Bacteriology 1988, 170: 859–864.
11. **Kroll, J. S., Hopkins, I., Moxon, E. R.:** Capsule loss in *Haemophilus influenzae* type b occurs by recombination-mediated disruption of a gene essential for polysaccharide export. Cell 1988, 53: 347–356.
12. **Zwahlen, A., Winkelstein, J. A., Moxon, E. R.:** Surface determinants of *Haemophilus influenzae* pathogenicity: comparative virulence of capsular transformants in normal and complement-depleted rats. Journal of Infectious Diseases 1983, 148: 385–394.
13. **Moxon, E. R., Ostrow, P. T.:** *Haemophilus influenzae* meningitis in infant rats: the role of bacteremia in the pathogenesis of the age-dependent inflammatory responses in cerebrospinal fluid. Journal of Infectious Diseases 1977, 135: 303–307.
14. **Zamze, S. E., Moxon, E. R.:** Composition of the lipopolysaccharide from different capsular serotype strains of *Haemophilus influenzae*. Journal of General Microbiology 1987, 133: 1443–1451.
15. **Kimura, A., Patrick, C. C., Miller, E. E., Cope, L. D., McCracken, G. H., Hansen, E. J.:** *Haemophilus influenzae* type b lipo-oligosaccharide: stability of expression and association with virulence. Infection and Immunity 1987, 55: 1979–1986.
16. **Zwahlen, A., Rubin, L. G., Connelly, C. J., Inzana, T. J., Moxon, E. R.:** Alteration of the cell wall of *Haemophilus influenzae* type b by transformation with cloned DNA: association with attenuated virulence. Journal of Infectious Diseases 1985, 152: 485–492.
17. **Kimura, A., Hansen, E. J.:** Antigenic and phenotypic variations of *Haemophilus influenzae* type b lipopolysaccharide and their relationship to virulence. Infection and Immunity 1986, 51: 69–79.

Coordinate Regulation of Bacterial Virulence Genes

W. Goebel, J. Hacker

Bacterial virulence is a multifactorial process often governed by a complex set of properties termed virulence factors. The degree of virulence is essentially influenced by the expression of the genes determining these factors. There is growing evidence that virulence genes are frequently regulated by *trans*-acting proteins which lead to the coordinate expression of several or even all of these genes. In addition, virulence is often controlled by physical (pH, temperature, osmolarity) and/or nutrient (e. g. amino acids, metal ions) parameters, which seem to directly influence the expression of the coordinate regulatory proteins. The best studied examples of coordinate regulatory elements are the genes *tox*R of *Vibrio cholerae*, *vir* of *Bordetella pertussis* and *fur* of *Escherichia coli*. Others, like *vir*F of *Yersinia enterocolitica*, *agr* of *Staphylococcus aureus* and *mry* of *Streptococcus pyogenes*, may exhibit similar functions. Experimental evidence is presented which suggests that genes involved in virulence of *Listeria monocytogenes* and of uropathogenic *Escherichia coli* strains may also be coordinately regulated.

Recent genetic studies of bacterial pathogens indicate that virulence is multifactorial and governed by multiple genes (1, 2). This appears to be obvious, considering that extracellular bacteria normally adhere to specific host cells, escape the host's defense system, and damage host cells by synthesizing a variety of exotoxins. Intracellular bacteria, on the other hand, have to possess properties which render them invasive not only for phagocytes, but (often) also for non-professional phagocytic cells, and which allow them to evade the intracellular milieu of the host cells. These virulence factors are governed by genetic determinants which often consist of several genes (e. g. determinants for fimbriated and non-fimbriated adhesins of *Escherichia coli*, of the hemolysin determinant of *Escherichia coli*) which must be coordinately regulated in order to guarantee the efficient expression of the phenotype (e. g. formation of an adhesion pilus, hemolysin secretion, etc.).

The genetic determinants encoding virulence are located on plasmids, on the chromosome, or more rarely, on phage genomes, and are sometimes physically linked. For example, the genes for heat-labile enterotoxin can be located on the same plasmid as the colonization factors (3), and the close proximity of the genes encoding P-pilus adhesion (*pap*) to those determining hemolysin has been demonstrated in uropathogenic *Escherichia coli* strains (4). In most cases, however, examined virulence determinants are dispersed over the chromosome or are even located on different genomes (e. g. plasmid and chromosome). Nevertheless, even in the latter cases the coordinate loss of several virulence determinants has been observed (5). Mutants were isolated in *Bordetella pertussis* that had lost hemolysin, filamentous hemagglutinin, adenylate cyclase, pertussis toxin, and dermonecrotic toxin, all substances which have been attributed to virulence (6). Likewise, spontaneous loss of several extracullular proteins, including hemolysin and toxic shock syndrome toxin (TSST), was reported in *Staphylococcus aureus* (7). Cholera Toxin (CT) and CT-coregulated pilus (TCP) (essential for *Vibrio cholerae* colonization) are jointly lost, together with other proteins of yet unidentified properties in *Vibrio cholerae* (8). Moreover, these factors are all controlled in a coordinate manner by physiological parameters such as osmolarity, pH, temperature, and the presence of certain amino acids (e. g. Asn) (8). Coordinate regulation of several genes, including virulence determinants, by iron has been observed (9). Plasmid-encoded virulence genes in *Yersinia enterocolitica* and *Yersinia pseudotuberculosis* are influenced by Ca^{2+} and temperature (10). The coordinate loss of hemolysin, of several adhesion pili, and of serum resistance in certain uropathogenic *Escherichia coli* strains as a consequence of the deletion of a large chromosomal insert carrying the *hly* genes has recently been described (5).

These observations suggest coordinate genetic regulation of virulence determinants by *trans*-acting factor(s) which are able to recognize crucial, common regulatory

---

Institut für Genetik und Mikrobiologie, Röntgenring 11, 8700 Würzburg, FRG.

sites on the individual virulence determinants. Some of these *trans*-acting regulators have been recently characterized genetically and in part biochemically. In this paper we will summarize some of the recent developments which have contributed to the molecular understanding of the rather complex regulation of bacterial virulence. Factors involved in coordinate regulation of virulence may also prove to be interesting targets for the development of new chemotherapeutical concepts in controlling bacterial diseases. Several examples of coordinate regulation of virulence genes will be discussed: a) *Tox*R-mediated regulation in *Vibrio cholerae*; b) Vir-mediated regulation in *Bordetella pertussis*; c) *Fur* iron regulation in *Escherichia coli* and *Shigella* spp.; d) *Agr*-controlled gene expression of *Staphylococcus aureus*; and e) *Mry*-mediated gene regulation in *Streptococcus pyogenes*. In addition, new data will be presented which suggest a similar type of regulation in uropathogenic *Escherichia coli* strains and, possibly, also in *Listeria monocytogenes*.

Regulation of Virulence in *Vibrio cholerae* by *Tox*R

The *tox*R gene encodes a 32.5-kDa transmembrane DNA binding protein (8, 11, 12) that activates transcription of the cholera toxin operon (*ctx*AB). Null mutations in *tox*R eliminated not only the expression of cholera toxin (*ctx*) but also the production of proteins that were previously known to be physiologically regulated, similar to *ctx*, by osmolarity, pH, temperature and the presence of certain amino acids (e.g. Asn). Using transposon Tn*pho*A insertions into the chromosome of *Vibrio cholerae*, Calderwood and co-workers (13) have identified 10–12 genes that are apparently *tox*R regulated. Among these are the major subunit of a pilus colonization factor (toxin co-regulated pilus, *tcp*) of *Vibrio cholerae* and an outer membrane protein. Thus it appears that *Vibrio cholerae* possesses at least 12 different *tox*R-activated genes, some (maybe even most) of which are involved in virulence. *Tox*R represents a transmembrane protein (8, 11–13) with the N-terminal end located in the cytoplasm and the C-terminal end in the periplasm, which appears to be unusual for a transcriptional activator. However, toxR seems to recognize physical and nutrient parameters (pH, osmolarity, temperature, amino acid composition); therefore it is reasonable to assume that this "sensing" is achieved via the periplasmic C-terminal part of the ToxR protein. DNA binding by ToxR is accomplished by the cytoplasmic N-terminal part of this protein, which exhibits remarkable homology with other transcriptional activator proteins such as PhoB, VirG, OmpR and SfrA (12). While most DNA binding proteins recognize dyad symetrical sequences, the DNA sequence recognized by ToxR is a tandemly (eightfold) repeated sequence, TTTTGAT, located 56 bp upstream of the transcriptional start site for *ctx*. A model for the possible function of ToxR has been recently proposed by Miller et al. (12).

Vir in *Bordetella pertussis*

The involvement of a *trans*-acting regulation factor, termed Vir in the gene expression for pertussis toxin (*ptx*), filamentous hemagglutinin (*fha*), hemolysin (*hly*), dermonecrotic toxin (*dnt*) and extracellular adenylate cyclase (*cya*) of *Bordetella pertussis*, was first demonstrated by Weiss and Falkow (6). These virulence factors are also regulated by Mg^{2+} and nicotinic acid in the growth medium. Moreover, in the case of *Bordetella pertussis*, two phases (I and III) exist during which these virulence factors are expressed (phase I) or not expressed (phase III). Thus the vir^+ state is similar to phase I or low $Mg^{2+}/$nicotinate. Using Tn*pho*A transposon mutagenesis, Calderwood et al. (12) identified 17 phosphatase-active fusions that were *vir*-regulated. Interestingly, two types of *vir*-regulated genes were identified. In addition to *pho*A fusions that were activated by vir^+ growth conditions, they also found genes that were repressed by vir^+ conditions and activated by vir^- conditions (high Mg^+/nicotinate). It was further shown that the latter genes (termed "vir-repressed genes", *vrg*) are indeed directly repressed by the Vir protein, suggesting that Vir may exhibit a dual regulatory function. Sequence analysis of several *vir*-activated and-repressed genes have been performed. Rappuoli and Gross (14, 15) identified a 170 bp DNA sequence upstream of the starting site for the *ptx* gene (*vir*-activated), with structures typical of binding site for regulatory proteins: a palindromic sequence in position -182 to -170, and a 21 bp sequence in position -157 to -137 repeated after two turns of the DNA helix. Deletions in one of these repeat elements in the presence of Vir led to a significant reduction of gene expression, suggesting that the repeated sequence may represent the binding site for Vir. Removal of the sequence between -180 to -171 resulted in a significant increase in gene expression, suggesting that this palindromic sequence may also be involved in the regulation of *ptx* transcription. It is interesting to note that *Bordetella parapertussis* and *Bordetalla bronciseptica*, both of which contain the *ptx* gene but are incapable of expressing it, carry a large number of mutations in the region between -170 and $+1$. Analysis of a larger number of *vir*-activated *pho*A fusions indicated a repeated sequence near the starting site of transcription (13). Interestingly, a highly homologous repeat sequence (a near perfect 20 bp dyad repeat) was identified within the coding region of a gene that is *vir*-repressed (15). This homology in the repeats in *vir*-activated and *vir*-repressed promoters suggests that this common region may be the binding site for the Vir protein. Although the molecular nature of the Vir gene product is presently unknown, preliminary data (R. Rappuoli, personal communication) indicate that the active Vir component may be composed of more than one polypeptide. Thus, the *vir* locus may be a master switch, and its expression or non-expression would determine the pathogenic character of the bacterium. It has been suggested (15) that the level of expression of *vir* may be modulated by the environmental influences known to affect the pathogenic character of this organism (see above).

Gene Expression by *Fur*

Once bacteria have entered a mammalian host, iron is an important environmental signal and may therefore lead to coordinate expression of a number of virulence determinants. Iron regulation is mediated by the *fur* locus, which was first identified in *Escherichia coli* as a gene whose product represses a variety of iron-scavenging systems when sufficient iron is present in the environment (9, 16). Several important bacterial toxins, including the Shiga toxin from *Shigella dysenteriae* (17), the Shiga-like toxin (Slt) of certain *Escherichia coli* strains (17, 18), and the diphtheria toxin of *Corynebacterium diphtheriae* (9), have been shown to be regulated by iron. It was suggested that in *Escherichia coli*, iron functions as a co-repressor which, in combination with the *fur* gene product, may repress transcription of the iron regulated genes. It has been shown (18) that fur$^-$ mutations produce an iron-constitutive expression for the *slt* genes (*slt*A, B, with only 12 bp separating the two genes). Furthermore, a 21 bp element of dyad symmetric was identified immediately upstream of the promoter transcribing *slt*A, B. This sequence proved to be homologous to similar sequences located in front of several other iron-regulated genes in *Escherichia coli*. Recently, Calderwood and Mekalanos (18) have directly demonstrated, by inserting a synthetic oligonucleotide representing the *fur* consensus sequence between the *omp*F promoter and the *lac*Z structural gene, that this sequence indeed is the operator site to which the Fur-iron complex binds, thereby repressing transcription of the adjacent genes.

*Vir*F as a Regulatory Element of the Exported Virulence Proteins of *Yersinia*

Virulence in *Yersinia enterocolitica* is mainly determined by genes located on a plasmid (pYV, 70 kb). These virulence genes are expressed best at 37 °C in a medium containing no calcium (19). A 20 kb region of pYV containing at least four genes, *vir*A, B, C and F, appears to be responsible for this calcium/temperature dependence of virulence (10, 20). Under "virulent conditions" these bacteria secrete several proteins (Yop-proteins). The *yop* genes are scattered over pVY, but are located outside of the "calcium region". While mutations in *vir*A, B and C reduced transcription of a cloned *yop* gene (yop51) (21), mutation in *vir*F abolished transcription entirely. It was further shown that *vir*F acts as positive regulator of transcription not only for *yop* genes of *Yersinia enterocolitica* but also for those of *Yersinia pseudotuberculosis*. The transcription of *vir*F appears to be thermo-dependent, which explains the temperature-dependence of virulence of *Yersinia enterocolitica*. Furthermore, a mutation in *vir*F suppresses the calcium requirement for growth at 37 °C. Preliminary data suggest that virF gene product is a protein of about 21 kDa. The functions of *vir*A, B and C remain unclear. Thus it appears that *vir*F may function as a *trans*-acting transcription activator for a coordinate regulation of the *yop* genes, the products of which are important for the expression of virulence.

Evidence for Coordinate Regulation of Virlence Determinants in Uropathogenic *Escherichia coli*

Most uropathogenic *Escherichia coli* strains possess properties which appear to contribute to virulence (22). The most frequently occurring virulence factors are hemolysin, specific iron transport systems, serum resistance, 0- and K- antigens, and adhesive fimbriae of different receptor specificities (P, S, M, and others). The *Escherichia coli* hemolysin, which acts as cytotoxin, may be located on the chromosome or on transmissible plasmids (23). The plasmid-encoded *hly*-genes of *Escherichia coli* appear to be transcribed from two initation sites, one located in front of *hly*C, reading the genes *hly*C, A and B, and another one located within *hly*B, transcribing *hly*D. Both initiations sites may consist of more than one promoter sequence which do not correspond to the normal consensus sequence of *Escherichia coli* promoters (W. Goebel and I. Then, unpublished results). These promoters are activated by an enhancer-like element, which is located about 1.5 kb upstream of the first promoter in front of *hly*C. The sequence of this element, termed *hly*R, has been determined and its function was analysed by introduction of deletions into *hly*R (24). These studies indicated that *hly*R acts in *cis*, but is orientation dependent and contains several sites which may act as binding sites for host regulatory proteins. *Hly*R enhances synthesis and secretion of *Hly*A 50- to 100-fold. Whether the expression of the other hly gene products is stimulated to a similar extent has not yet been determined. The

DNA sequence of the 5' upstream regulatory region in front of *hly*C is quite different between the plasmid- and the chromosome-encoded *hly* determinants. It is still unknown whether the *hly*R-like sequence also enhances expression of chromosomal *hly* genes and whether *hly*R plays a role in coordinate regulation of hemolysin with other virulence factors. A recent report (25) suggests that all four chromosomal genes (*hly*C, A, B and D) may be transcribed as a polycistronic m-RNA.

In contrast to the plasmid-encoded hemolysin-determinant which is activated by a *cis*-acting DNA sequence, fimbrial adhesins are regulated by trans-acting factors. For the determinant coding for S-fimbrial adhesins (*sfa*), two strong promoters arranged in inverse orientation are located next to the 5' end of the gene cluster and a weak promoter is located in front of the fimbrillin structural gene *sfa*A (Figure 1). Two proteins, SfaB (12 kDa) and SfaC (8 kDa) are encoded by the *sfa*A-upstream region of the *sfa* determinant. Protein- and operon fusions of *sfa*-specific sequences to the genes *pho*A and *lac*Z, coding for the enzymes alkaline phosphatase and β-galactosidase, respectively, and subsequent complementation tests have been used to demonstrate that both proteins, SfaB and SfaC, act as positive regulatory factors and are necessary for the full transcriptional activity of the *sfa* determinant (T. Schmoll, W. Goebel and J. Hacker, unpublished results). An arrangement of regulatory factors similar to *sfa* was detected for the P-fimbrial determinant *pap* (pili associated with pyelonephritis), whereas type I fimbrial determinants, which code for mannose-sensitive adherence factors, seem to be regulated in a different fashion (26). It was further demonstrated in complementation tests that the SfaB and SfaC proteins (and also the corresponding gene products of the *pap* gene cluster) are able to *trans*-complement other intact but non-expressed adhesin determinants which may be located either on plasmids or on the chromosome (T. Schmoll, and J. Hacker, unpublished results).

The two virulence determinants described here, coding for hemolysin and fimbrial adhesins, are very often physically linked on the *Escherichia coli* chromosome (4, 5). These gene clusters can be located on large chromosomal inserts. These inserts, up to 100 kb in size and flanked by short direct repeats, are deleted at relatively high frequencies, probably by recombination between the two direct repeated sequences at the termini of the inserts (Figure 2). The localization of hemolysin- and fimbrial determinants on such inserts and their elimination from the chromosome by deletions have been demonstrated for several uropathogenic *Escherichia coli* strains belonging to serogroups 06 and 018 (5, 27). Specific deletion events which resemble those demonstrated first for hemolysin and fimbrial genes in *Escherichia coli* have also been recently observed in *Haemophilus influenzae* strains. In *Haemophilus* spp. these chromosomal deletions led to a non-capsulated phenotype of encapsulated isolates (28). The deletion of inserts carrying hemolysin gene clusters and a determinant which codes for P-related fimbriae (*prf*) in the uropathogenic *Escherichia coli* 06 strain 536 results in a coordinate elimination of the expression of S-fimbriae, type I fimbriae and serum resistance (5). As indicated in Table 1, it was shown that the structural genes for S- and type I-fimbriae (*sfa* and *fim*) are still present in the chromosome of the deletion mutants but are not transcribed. The functional integrity of the *sfa* genes was demonstrated by cloning the genes in *Escherichia coli* K-12, where they express high levels of fimbriae. These data argue for the presence of a *trans*-acting factor, presumably located in the vicinity of the *hly* and *prf* determinants, which may influence the expression of the *sfa* and the type I gene clusters.

To characterize more precisely additional regulatory factors which are not physically linked to S adhesin determinants, Tn5 mutants were isolated from the Sfa-positive *Escherichia coli* strain 536. As indicated in Table 2 and Figure 3, three types of mutants which affected the expression of Sfa were identified.

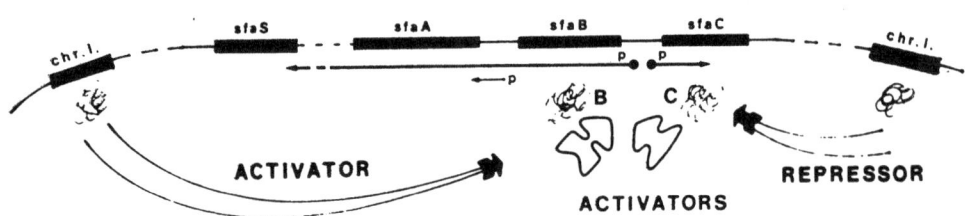

Figure 1: Arrangement of genes which influence the expression of the S-fimbrial adhesin determinant (*sfa*). The genes *sfa*B and *sfa*C code for two activator proteins. The abbreviation chr.1. marks chromosomal loci which negatively or positively influence the expression of *sfa*. The gene *sfa*A codes for the S fimbrillin, *sfa*S is responsible for the S adhesin. The location of promoter regions are indicated by arrows and "p".

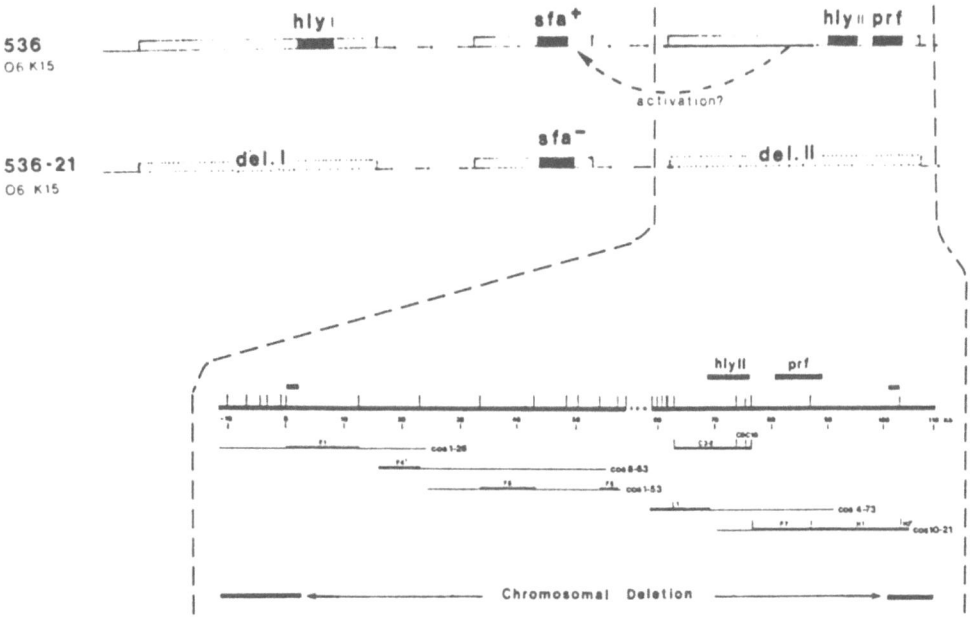

Figure 2: Arrangement of virulence determinants of the uropathogenic strain 536 and the nonpathogenic mutant 536-21. In the lower part of the figure a precise physical map of the *hly/prf* specific insert is given.

Table 1: Virulence properties of *Escherichia coli* strain 536 and its mutants.

Virulence genes determining	Strains			
	536	536-21	536-114	536-25
Hemolysin I	active	deleted	deleted	active
Hemolysin II	active	deleted	active	deleted
P-related fimbriae	active	deleted	active	deleted
S-fimbrial adhesin	active	reduced expression	active	reduced expression
Type I fimbriae	active	reduced expression	active	reduced expression
Serum resistance	active	reduced or no expression	active	reduced or no expression

Table 2: Analysis of S-fimbrial adhesin (Sfa) production of Tn5 mutants inserted into the chromosome of *Escherichia coli* 536.

Strain	Locus of Tn5-insertion	HA-Titer[a]
536 WT	–	1:8
536-21	–	1:2
536/17B1	*sfa* determinant	–
536/17A5	negative- acting locus	1:32
536/5F2	positive- acting locus	1:2
536/5A7	positive- acting locus	1:2
536/16B5	random	1:8

[a]S-specific hemagglutination with bovine RBCs.

Mutants with Tn5 insertions in the *sfa* structural genes were completely non-fimbriated. In addition, mutants which led to an increase or a decrease in Sfa-expression indicated by S-specific hemagglutination were isolated. These mutants had the Tn5 element inserted into chromosomal loci different from the *sfa* gene cluster, as demonstrated by DNA-DNA hybridizations (see Figure 3). The isolation of these mutant argues for the existence of chromosomal sites which code for *trans*-acting factors influencing the regulation of this adhesion determinant. Studies are underway to elucidate the identity of these sites and their similarity to the loci, which are located next

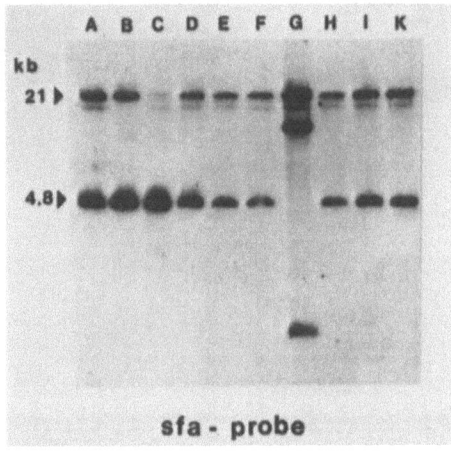

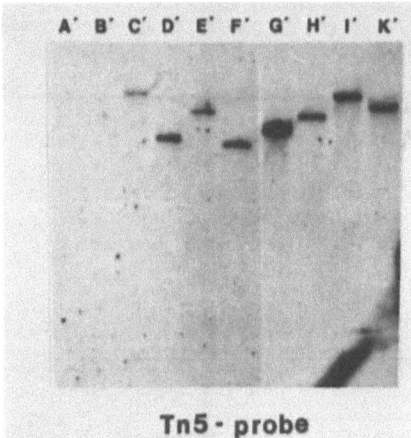

Figure 3: Southern hybridization of EcoRI-cleaved chromosomal DNAs of strain 536 (Sfa+, lanes A, A'), mutant 536-21 (Sfa−, lanes A, A') and various Tn5 mutants of strain 536 (lanes C, C' to K, K'), including mutant 536/17B1 (lane G, G'), which carries the Tn5-transposon inserted into the *sfa* structural genes. The DNAs were hybridized with nick-translated 32-P labeled probes. The 9,5 kb EcoRV fragment of plasmid pANN801-13 (*sfa*-probe; Reference No. 27) and the 4,5 kb HindIII fragment of Tn5 (Tn5 probe; Reference No. 27) were used as probes.

to the *hly* and *prf* genes and which also influence the expression of fimbriae.

The integration host factor (IHF) protein of *Escherichia coli*, which is encoded by the *him* genes, was also identified as a co-factor for the expression of type I fimbriae (29, 30). In addition, the expression of two of three fimbriae which are encoded by the CFAII plasmid of enterotoxigenic *Escherichia coli* strains (CS1, CS2, CS3) is strongly dependent on an as yet unidentified *trans*-acting host factor (31). It seems therefore that the influence of *trans*-acting factors on the expression of virulence genes is a general feature of pathogenic *Escherichia coli* strains and is not restricted to particular isolates. Circumstantial evidence also exists for coordinate regulation of virulence genes in *Shigella dysenteriae* (2).

Coordinate Regulation in Pathogenic Gram-Positive Bacteria

Coordinate regulation of virulence, although more thoroughly studied in the described gram-negative bacteria, seems to also occur in gram-positive bacteria. Recsei et al. (7) described the coordinate regulation of exoprotein gene expression in *Staphylococcus aureus* by a *trans*-activator element termed *agr* (accessory gene regulator). At least some of the genes affected by *agr* are known virulence factors, e.g. toxin (hemolysin) and toxic shock syndrome toxin (TSST). A common regulatory element has also been postulated for the apparent coordinate expression of the M protein and colony opacity in group A Streptococci (32). Whereas virtually nothing is known about the significance of opacity, the M protein, which is anti-phagocytic, is the major virulence factor in these bacteria. Whether the recently identified *mry* locus, a gene required for high-level expression of the M protein, serves as a coordinate regulatory element is unknown (33).

Using Tn916 transposon mutagenesis, hemolysin (listeriolysin)-negative mutants in *Listeria monocytogenes* were recently obtained. It was further shown that listeriolysin represents a major virulence factor essential for the intracellular survival of these facultative intracellular bacteria. One class (class I) of listeriolysin-negative mutants carries the transposon in the structural gene, *lis*A, and synthesizes a truncated lisA gene product (34). The other class (class II) of hly− mutants carries the transposon outside of the structural *lis*A gene (M. Leimeister-Wächter and T. Chakraborty, personal communication), about 1 kb upstream of the *lis*A structural gene. Class II mutants do not synthesize a protein cross-reacting with listeriolysin antibodies (34). In addition, comparison of the protein patterns from class II hly− mutants with those of class I mutants and the wild-type hly+ strain indicates the loss of several other proteins (in addition to listeriolysin) in class II but not in class I mutants. Among the missing proteins is at least one other protein which appears to be a major immunodominant antigen of *Listeria monocytogenes* (like listeriolysin). This protein reacts with several antisera obtained from patients infected with *Listeria monocytogenes*, and with antibodies raised against the "soluble antigen" of *Listeria monocytogenes*. Soluble antigen induces protective T-cell immunity and may therefore contain the major protective T-cell stimulating antigens of *Listeria monocytogenes*. The mutation of class II mutants may affect a coordinate regulatory element which activates the expression of listeriolysin and other extracellular proteins possibly involved in virulence of *Listeria monocytogenes*.

Conclusion

Regulation of virulence genes in bacterial pathogens may occur on two levels. Genes determining a simple virulence factor, e.g. an adhesion pilus, a capsule, etc., are often arranged in operon-like structures controlled by *cis* and *trans*-acting positive and/or negative regulatory elements (DNA sequences and protein factors) which allow the coordinate expression of the components necessary for the individual virulence phenotype (e.g. formation of an adhesion pilus, synthesis and secretion of hemolysin in *Escherichia coli*, capsule synthesis, etc.). This regulation occurs mainly on the transcriptional level but post-transcriptional events (stability of m-RNA, direct translational and post-translational controls) may also be involved. In addition there is growing evidence that the multifactorial virulence property is coordinately regulated by environmental parameters (temperature, pH, metal ions, nutrients), the action of which appears to be mediated by *trans*-acting regulatory elements. These elements recognize specific DNA sequences located in front of several (or even all) virulence operons and guarantee their coordinate expression. Furthermore, there is evidence that this second-level coordinate regulation of virulence is widespread among bacterial pathogens. Thus far, more precise biochemical characterization exists only for the *tox*R element, the putative structure of which suggests a bifunctional property of this protein: one part of the transmembrane polypeptide, located in the periplasmic space, may sense environmental parameters, whereas the other (cytoplasmic) part seems to interact directly with the DNA. It remains to be investigated whether this feature is a more common structure of elements involved in the coordinate regulation of bacterial virulence. Whether drugs will be found which specifically interact with such virulence-controlling elements is an extremely interesting question.

Acknowledgements

The authors thank J. Hess, A. Ludwig, I. Then, M. Ott and T. Schmoll for allowing us to cite unpublished data. Our own research included in this report was supported by grants from the Deutsche Forschungsgemeinschaft (SFB 165-B4 and Ha 1434/1-5).

References

1. Goebel, W.: Genetic approaches to study virulence in bacteria. Current Topics in Microbiology Immunology 1985, 118: 1–283.
2. Goebel, W.: Intracellular bacteria. Current Topics in Microbiology Immunology 1988, 138: (in press).
3. Sack, B. R.: Human diarrhoeal disease caused by enterotoxigenic *Escherichia coli*. Annual Reviews in Microbiology 1975, 29: 333–353.
4. Low, D., Lark, V., Lark, D., Schoolnik, G., Falkow, S.: The operons governing the production of hemolysin and mannose-resistant hemagglutination are closely linked in *Escherichia coli* serotype 04 and 06 isolates from urinary tract infections. Infection and Immunity 1984, 43: 353–358.
5. Knapp, S., Hacker, J., Jarchau, T., Goebel, W.: Large, unstable inserts in the chromosome affect virulence properties of uropathogenic *Escherichia coli* 06 strain 536. Journal of Bacteriology 1986, 168: 22–30.
6. Weiss, A. A., Falkow, S.: Genetic analysis of phase change of *Bordetella pertussis*. Infection and Immunity 1984, 43: 263–269.
7. Recsei, P., Kreiswirth, B., Schlievert, P., Gruss, A., Novick, R. P.: Regulation of exotoxin gene expression in *Staphylococcus aureus* by *agr*. Molecular and General Genetics 1986, 202: 58–61.
8. Taylor, R. K., Miller, V. L., Furlong, D. B., Mekalanos, J. J.: Use of phoA gene fusions to identify a pilus colonization factor coordinately regulated with cholera toxin. Proceedings of the National Academy of Sciences USA 1987, 84: 2833–2837.
9. Neilands, J. B.: Microbial envelope proteins related to iron. Annual Reviews of Microbiology 1982, 36: 285–309.
10. Cornelis, G., Sory, M.-P., Laroche, Y., Derclaye, I.: Genetic analysis of the plasmid region controlling virulence in *Yersinia enterocolitica* 0:9 by mini-mu insertions and lac gene fusions. Microbial Pathogenesis 1986, 1: 349–359.
11. Betley, M. J., Miller, V. L., Mekalanos, J. J.: Genetics of bacterial enterotoxins. Annual Reviews of Microbiology 1986, 40: 577–605.
12. Miller, V. L., Taylor, R. K., Mekalanos, J. J.: Cholera toxin transcriptional activator ToxR is a transmembrane DNA binding protein. Cell 1987, 48: 271–279.
13. Calderwood, S., Knapp, S., Peterson, K., Taylor, R., Mekalanos, J.: Coordinate regulation of virulence determinants. Zentralblatt für Bakteriologie 1988, (Supplement) 17: 169–175.
14. Rappuoli, R., Arico, B., Bartolini, A., Gross, R., Perugini, M., Pizza, M. G.: Pertussis toxin. Zentralblatt für Bakteriologie 1988, (Supplement) 17: 19–28.
15. Gross, R., Rappuoli, R.: Positive regulation of pertussis toxin expression. Proceedings of the National Academy of Sciences USA 1988, 85: 3913–3917.
16. Braun, V.: Regulation of iron uptake in *Escherichia coli*. in: Schlesinger, D. (ed.): Microbiology. American Society for Microbiology, Washington, DC, 1983, p. 301–305.
17. O'Brien, A. D., Newland, J. W., Miller, S. F., Holmes, R. J., Smith, H. W., Formal, S. F.: Shiga-like toxin-converting phages from *Escherichia coli* strains that cause hemorrhagie colitis or infantile diarrhoea. Science 1984, 226: 694–696.
18. Calderwood, S. B., Mekalanos, J. J.: Iron regulation of shiga-like toxin expression in *Escherichia coli* is mediated by the fur locus. Journal of Bacteriology 1987, 169: 4759–4764.
19. Gemski, P., Lazere, J. R., Casey, T.: Plasmid associated with pathogenicity and calcium dependency of *Yersinia enterocolitica*. Infection and Immunity 1980, 27: 682–685.
20. Bölin, J., Forsberg, A., Norlander, L., Skurnik, M., Wolf-Watz, H.: Identification and mapping of the temperature-inducible, plasmid-encoded proteins of *Yersinia* spp. Infection and Immunity 1988, 56: 343–348.

21. Cornelis, G., Vanootheghem, J.-C., Sory, M.-P., Michiels, T., Biot, T., Sluiters, C.: Genetic regulation of the exported virulence protein (YOPs) of *Yersinia*. Zentralblatt für Bakteriologie 1988, (Supplement) 17: 231–232.
22. Hacker, J., Hof, H. Emödy, L., Goebel, W.: Influence of cloned *Escherichia coli* hemolysin genes, S-fimbriae and serum resistance on pathogenicity in different animal models. Microbial Pathogenesis 1987, 1: 533–547.
23. Hacker, J., Hughes, C.: Genetics of *Escherichia coli* hemolysin. Current Topics in Microbiology Immunology 1985, 118: 139–162.
24. Vogel, M., Hess, J., Then, I., Juarez, A., Goebel, W.: Characterization of a sequence (hlyR) which enhances synthesis and secretion of hemolysin in *Escherichia coli*. Molecular and General Genetics 1988, 212: 76–84.
25. Welch, R. A., Pellet, S.: Transcriptional organization of the *Escherichia coli* hemolysin genes. Journal of Bacteriology 1988, 170: 1622–1630.
26. Baga, M., Göransson, M., Normark, S., Uhlin, B. E.: Transcriptional activation of a Pap pilus virulence operon from uropathogenic *Escherichia coli*. EMBO Journal 1985, 4: 3887–3893.
27. Hacker, J., Schmoll, T., Ott, M., Marre, R., Hof, H., Jarchau, T., Knapp, S., Then, I., Goebel, W.: Genetic structure and expression of virulence determinants from uropathogenic *Escherichia coli* strains. Reviews of Infectious Diseases 1988, 9: (in press).
28. Hoiseth, S. K., Moxon, E. R., Siver, R. P.: Genes involved in *Haemophilus influenzae* type b capsule expression are part of an 18-kilobase tandem duplication. Proceedings of the National Academy of Sciences USA 1986, 83: 1106–1110.
29. Eisenstein, B. I., Swet, D. S., Vaughn, V., Friedman, D. I.: Integration host factor is required for the DNA inversion that controls phase variation in *Escherichia coli*. Proceedings of the National Academy of Sciences USA 1987, 84: 6506–6510.
30. Dorman, C. J., Higgins, C. F.: Fimbrial phase variation in *Escherichia coli*: Dependence on integration host factor and homologies with other site-specific recombinases. Journal of Bacteriology 1987, 169: 3840–3843.
31. Baylan, M., Smyth, C. J.: Mobilization of CS fimbriae associated plasmids of enterotoxigenic *Escherichia coli* of serotype 06: K15: H16 or H− into various wild-type hosts. FEMS Microbiology Letters 1985, 29: 83–89.
32. Simpson, W. S., Cleary, P. P.: Expression of M-type 12 protein by a group A *Streptococcus* exhibits phaselike variation: evidence for coregulation of colony opacity determinants and M protein. Infection and Immunity 1987, 55: 2448–2455.
33. Caparon, M. G., Scott, J. R.: Identification of a gene that regulates expression of M protein, the major virulence determinant of group A streptococci. Proceedings of the National Academy of Sciences USA 1987, 84: 8677–8681.
34. Kathariou, S., Metz, P., Hof, H., Goebel, W.: Tn*916*-induced mutations in the hemolysin determinant affecting virulence of *Listeria monocytogenes*. Journal of Bacteriology 1987, 169: 1291–1297.

Microbial Drug Resistance

Transposon Transfer of Drug Resistance

F. H. Kayser*, B. Berger-Bächi

Bacterial DNA is a dynamic molecule, subject to extensive structural rearrangements. The main mechanism for restructuring of bacterial genomes is the illegitimate recombination between heterologous DNA sequences, a process made possible by transposable DNA elements. Bacterial transposons can be divided into three classes. Class I transposons comprise the insertion sequence (IS) elements as well as the composite transposons, class II transposons include the Tn3-elements, and class III transposons form a group of elements possessing properties not found in classes I and II. Integration of transposons into foreign DNA can occur as "conservative transposition", in which the element moves from a donor to a recipient site, or in a mode called "replicative transposition", in which the transposon is copied as part of its movement. Besides insertion, transposable DNA can promote deletion, inversion, excision, or the fusion of two complete replicons. The mechanisms of illegitimate recombination described have contributed significantly to the evolution of drug resistance in clinically important bacteria. Molecular data suggest that many drug resistance genes have evolved in antibiotic-producing microorganisms. Mobilization of these determinants was initially made possible by transposable DNA elements. The rapid spread of determinants through bacterial populations then occurred via plasmids and bacteriophages. Mutations in resistance genes of transposons resulted in the evolution of determinants coding for resistance to new antimicrobials.

Soon after the introduction of antibiotics into clinical practice, it became apparent that bacteria have a remarkable capacity to adapt to the presence of drugs in their natural environment by becoming resistant to them. During the 1940s and 1950s resistance was thought to arise solely by mutation and selection. The first suspicion that there was something unusual about the inheritance of resistance came with the observation of irreversible loss of resistance in some strains. Genetic investigations stimulated by these observations showed that resistance is often due to extrachromosomal DNA elements called R-(resistance) factors or R-plasmids, and that such R-plasmids can be transferred from cell to cell and throughout bacterial populations via conjugation or transduction (1). It was believed that such R-plasmids were the fundamental genetic units contributing to the clinical problem of drug resistance.

In the last 15 years, however, evidence has accumulated that many antimicrobial resistance genes are located on small genetic elements which can move around or "transpose" from one location to the other independently from the host recombination system (2–4, and Berg, D., Howe, M. (ed.): Mobile DNA. American Society for Microbiology, Washington, DC, 1988, in press). These elements encode all the genetic information necessary to bring about their own movement, and, in addition, contain the genetic information for resistance. Resistance (R)-transposons can be found integrated into the bacterial chromosome and as parts of plasmids or bacteriophages. It now appears that these R-transposons are the fundamental genetic units of bacterial drug resistance. This review focuses on the contribution of transposons in the evolution of drug resistance in bacteria.

General Structure of Bacterial Transposons

The DNA molecule, as carrier of the genetic information, is dynamic and subject to rearrangements. Two specialized forms of recombination for restructuring the chromosome can be distinguished. Both are responsible for reassorting, adding or deleting genetic information. The site specific recombination system is responsible for single reciprocal crossover between short homologous segments. An example of site specific recombination is integration and excision of bacteriophage lambda and Tn554. The transpositional recombination system comprises specific DNA vectors — transposable elements or transposons — which can move from one genetic location to an other.

Institute of Medical Microbiology, University of Zürich, Gloriastraße 30/32, CH-8028 Zürich, Switzerland.

Transpositional recombination is distinct and independent of the conventional homologous recombination.

The DNA sequences responsible for transposition are linear pieces of DNA that range in size from less than 1 to 23 kilobase pairs (kb). With rare exceptions, these segments contain nucleotide sequences repeated in inverse orientation at both ends (IRs). The inverted repeats (IRs) of different transposons vary both in size — 8 to 40 base pairs (bp) — and in the degree of conservation. They provide the recognition sites for the element's transposase(s), an enzyme necessary for the translocation process. The transposase also recognizes a short segment of the target DNA (3 to 13 bp). When a transposon integrates into this target, the recognition sequence is duplicated in direct orientation, i.e. direct repeats (DRs), as a consequence of the mechanism of insertion. Thus, after transposition, the transposed DNA is flanked by one copy each of the target sequence. Exceptions from this general structure do exist.

Classes of Bacterial Transposons

For convenience it has become customary to divide bacterial transposons into three classes (Figure 1, Table 1). Class I transposons comprise the Insertion Sequences (IS) and the composite transposons. Insertion sequence elements are normal constituents of bacterial chromosomes and plasmids. They represent the simplest class of transposable DNA, since their genetic functions are concerned only with the ability to translocate. Insertion sequence elements have a size range of 750–1600 bp. They have one or two open reading frames that code for the transposase, which acts only in *cis*, that is, on transposon ends on the same DNA-molecule as the transposase gene. The most frequent transpositional event seen with an IS element is a simple insertion. A DNA element flanked by two IS modules in inverted or in direct orientation forms a composite transposon. Often a divergence is observed between the right and the left IS elements, and only one element remains functional. This is sufficient for transposition of the entire composite element. The central region carries markers unconnected with transposition, for instance drug resistance markers. Because composite transposons usually have four IS ends that can be used in recombination, the interaction with a target sequence allows a wide possibility of genetic rearrangements.

Class II transposons form the family of Tn3-like elements and contain two genes necessary for transposition: *tnp*A encoding a transposase and *tnp*R encoding a resolvase, which is a site-specific recombinase. Both gene products are able to act in *trans*, in contrast to the IS transposase (see above). In addition, class II transposons contain an internal cointegrate resolution site called *res*, and often, antibiotic resistance determinants as well. Class III transposons are flanked by terminal inverted repeats of 35–40 bp and duplicate a target sequence in direct repeats upon integration. Tn3-like elements display a *cis* acting transposition immunity.

Class III transposons, finally, comprise an increasing number of genetic elements that fit neither into class I or II. Belonging to this class is Tn554, a site-specific transposable element of staphylococcal origin which carries resistance to the macrolide-lincosamide-streptogramin B antibiotics and to spectinomycin (5).

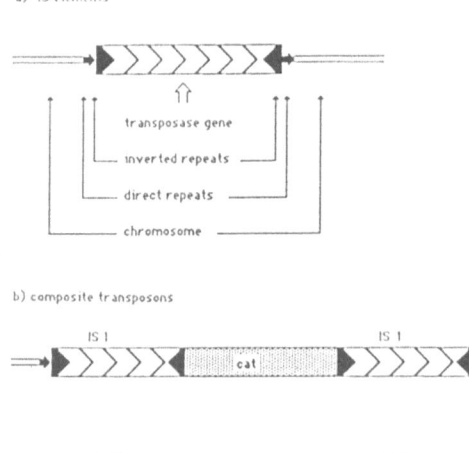

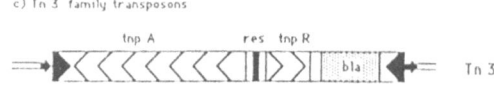

Figure 1: General structure of transposable DNA elements.
a. Insertion sequence (IS) elements. The simplest transposons known. Each codes only for the proteins (usually one) needed to sponsor its own transposition.
b. Composite transposons are flanked by IS modules in either direct (Tn9) or inverted (Tn10) orientation. The central region carries markers unconnected with transposition. The marker *cat* of Tn9 codes for chloramphenicol acetyltransferase, *tet*B for the tetracycline resistance protein of class B.
c. Tn3-like transposons consist of two genes whose products are needed for transposition: *tnp*A codes for a transposase. The gene *tnp*R codes for a protein which acts as a repressor for *tnp*A and *tnp*R and simultaneously provides the resolvase function. The *tnp*R gene product binds to an intercistronic control region called *res* (for resolution). *Res* is the site for resolution of the intermediate cointegrate formed in replicative transposition. The gene *bla* of Tn3 encodes production of TEM-type betalactamase.

Table 1: Examples of transposable elements[a].

Element	Size	Source	Resistance[b]	Remarks[c]
Insertion sequences				
IS*1*	768 bp	Enterobacteriaceae	–	23 bp TRs; 9 bp TDs
IS*10*-R	1329 bp	Enterobacteriaceae	–	22 bp TRs; 9 bp TDs
IS*50*-R	1531 bp	Enterobacteriaceae	–	9 bp TRs; 9 bp TDs
IS*903*	1057 bp	Enterobacteriaceae	–	18 bp TRs; 9 bp TDs
IS*431*-L	800 bp	Staphylococcus	–	22 bp TRs
Composite transposons				
Tn*5*	5700 bp	Enterobacteriaceae	Kan	IS*50*-R functional, IS*50*-L non-functional. Modules in inverted orientation.
Tn*9*	2638 bp	Enterobacteriaceae	Chl	IS*1* modules in direct orientation.
Tn*10*	9300 bp	Enterobacteriaceae	Tet	IS*10*-R functional, IS*10*-L reduced function. Inverted IS modules.
Tn*903*	3100 bp	Enterobacteriaceae	Kan	IS*903* modules in inverted orientation.
Tn*4001*	4700 bp	Staphylococcus	Kan/Gen/Tob	IS*256* (1350 bp) inverted modules.
Tn*3*-like elements				
Tn*3*	4957 bp	Enterobacteriaceae	Amp	38 bp TRs; 5 bp TDs
Tn*21*	19.6 kbp	Enterobacteriaceae	Mer-Sul-Str/Spe	38 bp TRs
Tn*551*	5300 bp	Staphylococcus	MLS	40 bp TRs; 5 bp TDs. Transposes preferentially to the chromosome.
Class III transposons				
Tn*916*	16.4 kbp	Enterococcus	Tet	Conjugative; chromosome
Tn*1545*	25.3 kbp	Streptococcus pneumoniae	Tet-MLS-Kan	Conjugative; chromosome
Tn*554*	6691 bp	Staphylococcus	MLS-Spe	Site-specific insertion into *att*554 of chromosome; asymmetric ends; no TRs and TDs.

[a] References 2, 3, 4 and Berg, D., Howe, M. (ed.): Mobile DNA. American Society for Microbiology, Washington, DC, 1988, in press.
[b] Amp = ampicillin; Chl = Chloramphenicol; Gen = gentamicin; Kan = kanamycin; MLS = macrolide/lincosamide/streptogramin B; Mer = mercury; Spe = spectinomycin; Str = streptomycin; Tet = tetracycline; Tob = tobramycin. Abbreviations separated by a slash (/) indicate resistance to drugs mediated by the same gene product.
[c] TRs = terminal repeats; TDs = target duplications.

Tn*554* has asymmetric ends, without inverted or direct terminal repeats; there is no target duplication upon transposition. Tn*554* is strictly site-specific, integrating into the staphylococcal chromosome exclusively at a site called *att*554; is shows a high frequency of transposition. Thus, Tn*554* resembles integrative bacteriophages.

A special group of class III transposons are the conjugative elements Tn*916* and derivatives (6), and Tn*1545* (7), both ubiquitous among streptococci. The self-transmissible, chromosomal Tn*916* (16.4 kb) of the enterococci carries the tetracycline resistance marker *tet*M, which promotes conjugative transfer independent of the plasmid-mediated conjugation system of *Enterococcus faecalis* to a broad range of hosts such as *Staphylococcus*, *Bacillus*, *Acholeplasma* and *Mycoplasma* species. Tn*916* found in a *Clostridium difficile* wild type strain has been shown to mediate *tet*M transfer from this organism to *Staphylococcus aureus* (8). The 25.3 kb element Tn*1545* is a self-transmissible transposon of *Streptococcus pneumoniae* that codes for resistance to tetracycline (*tet*M), kanamycin (*aph*A) and the macrolide-lincosamide-streptogramin B antibiotics (*erm*B) (7). It transposes to different sites within a cell. The element can be conjugally transferred among the streptococci including group N lactic streptococci. It can also be transferred by mixed cultivation to enterococci, *Staphylococcus aureus*, *Bacillus thuringiensis* and *Listeria monocytogenes*.

Transposition Models

The central property of transposons is their ability to integrate into foreign DNA sequences. This nonhomologous recombination is different from conventional recombination mediated by the *rec*A system of the host. Transposition is catalysed by the transposon-encoded transposase. The two general modes of transposition, conservative and replicative, are distinguished by the fate of the donor site. In conservative transposition, the transposing element moves as a physical entity from a donor site to a recipient site. The fate of the donor site is yet unclear. The donor replicon might be destroyed or the damage caused by loss of the transposon might be repaired. In replicative transposition, the transposon is copied as part of its movement. One copy remains at the original site whereas a new copy is inserted at the new site.

Several models have been proposed to describe the molecular events in conservative and replicative transposition (4). The first stage in both transposition modes is cleavage of the transposon at both ends and cleavage of the target molecule at sites staggered by 5–9 bp. Then, each end of the transposon is joined to one of the protruding single strands of the target to form an intermediate between the donor and the recipient replicon. In conservative transposition, the second stage comprises the filling of the staggered cuts of the recipient replicon. Thus, the product is a recipient replicon, in which the transposon has been inserted between direct repeats of the target sequence. Conservative replication is typical for class I transposons. In replicative transposition, the second stage involves duplication of the transposon and formation of an intermediate cointegrate. After recombination at the *res* site of the two copies of the transposable element, the cointegrate is resolved in a reaction called resolution, involving the enzyme resolvase. Thus, the original donor and a receptor replicon which has gained the transposed sequence flanked by direct repeats is obtained. Replicative transposition is typical for class II transposons. Transposable elements can insert into various loci of the receptor replicon at random; some show more or less preference for hot spots (for instance A—T rich regions), and few insert into specific sites.

Further Types of DNA Rearrangements

In addition to the intermolecular transposition described above, transposons can promote other types of DNA rearrangements that can influence the resistance phenotype of cells. Insertion of a copy of an IS element in the same direction at a second site near its original location can result in recombination between the two and deletion of the DNA, leaving one copy of the IS on the chromosome. Reciprocal recombination between two IS elements in inverted orientation results in the inversion of the DNA between the IS sequences. Excision of transposable elements is also observed. Excision can be precise, restoring the DNA sequence to its previous state before insertion, or imprecise, leaving a remnant of the transposon behind, possibly extending into the DNA flanking the transposon. Excision does not require transposon-coded functions, but probably occurs by some cellular mechanism that generates spontaneous deletions between closely spaced repeated sequences.

An important reaction for the evolution of multi-resistance plasmids mediated by transposons is replicon fusion (9). When IS elements are involved in this process, the resulting dual replicons are relatively stable. Class II transposons will not mediate stable cointegrates due to resolution by the resolvase of these elements. However, class II elements which lack one of the IRs, although no longer able to transpose, can mediate transposition-like recombination that generates fused replicons.

Evolution of Drug Resistance

Antibiotics were introduced into medicine less than 50 years ago. Despite this short period of time, today one can find examples of organisms resistant to most of the drugs marketed. Questions therefore arise regarding the origin of resistance genes and the mechanisms of the rapid spread of resistance through bacterial populations.

It seems that spontaneous mutation followed by environmental selective pressure acting on the mutant has contributed only slightly to the problem of drug resistance. An example of this process if resistance to nalidixic acid, which develops exclusively by chromosomal mutation. Classic or legitimate recombination between homologous DNA sequences also seems to have had only a minor influence on the development of drug resistance. Yet the rapid evolution of drug-resistant bacteria has resulted from processes allowing for the reassortment of genetic information and thus for the rapid evolution of chromosome structure (10). These processes comprise the various forms of illegitimate recombination brought about by transposable DNA elements, as well as mechanisms of the distribution of DNA through bacterial populations such as transfer via conjugative plasmids or transducing bacteriophages that have a broad host range. The following paragraphs outline some examples of the importance of transposable DNA for the evolution of drug resistance.

Many drug resistance genes code for drug inactivating or modifying enzymes. Resistance depending on such mechanisms cannot be created in the test tube. The question then arises of where these resistance genes originated. Comparison of the amino acid sequences of five types of 3'-aminoglycoside phosphotransferases [APH(3')] from gram-negative and gram-positive bacteria, from a butirosin-producing *Bacillus circulans* culture, and from a neomycin-producing *Streptomyces fradiae* strain indicates that these enzymes have diverged from a common ancestor (11). The structural data support the concept that antibiotic-producing bacteria were the source of the resistance determinants. In these organisms such determinants probably are necessary for the survival of the organism. Dissimination to other bacteria then was made possible through acquisition of the R-determinants by transposable DNA segments. The composite transposons Tn5 and Tn903 contain the genes for APH(3') types I and II, respectively, which are closely related. The IS elements flanking the transposons, IS50 and IS903, respectively, are unrelated. Thus, the APH(3') genes must have been acquired independently by the two elements (12).

One of the best examined examples for broad dissemination of resistance genes via transposons and plasmids is presented by the tetracycline resistance determinant (13). Five classes of determinants (tetA–E) often found on transposons were identified in gram-negative rod bacteria. The class B determinants is found in Enterobacteriaceae as well as in Haemophilus species. In the latter, the determinant is part of a transposon almost identical to Tn10, which was originally discovered in Enterobacteriaceae. Three different tetracycline resistance determinants have been described in streptococci: classes L, M and N. The marker tetM is part of the conjugative transposon Tn916. DNA : DNA hybridization studies have demonstrated homology between the tetM originally found in streptococci and determinants observed in Gardnerella, Ureaplasma, Neisseria, Mycoplasma and Staphylococcus species. Recently, it was shown that Clostridium difficile can bear a transposon very similar to the streptococcal transposon Tn916, and that it can be transferred to Staphylococcus aureus by mixed cultivation (8). Genetic experiments on beta-lactamase-producing Haemophilus influenzae suggest that the antibiotic resistance transposon Tn3 was introduced from Enterobacteriaceae into phenotypically cryptic plasmids naturally residing in a few strains of Haemophilus. This event resulted in the evolution of conjugative antibiotic resistance plasmids which consequently were able to spread through this genus (14).

Plasmids carrying multiple resistance markers might have developed by successive integration of various R-transposons into plasmid DNA (15) or by replicon fusion (9). R-plasmids such as R1, R6 and R 100 have structures consistent with their formation via IS1-mediated cointegrate formation. They also carry two sequences capable of functioning as replication origins. Besides the evolution of multi-resistance plasmids, another potentially important aspect of replicon fusion would be the addition of a non-transposable R-determinant from a non-conjugative to a conjugative plasmid, and, hence, rapid distribution of the respective R-marker.

Transposons are not subject to the constraints of plasmids for replication in various hosts. They can jump from an incompatible plasmid into endogenous plasmids of a host or even into the host's chromosome. Analysis of resistance to multiple antibiotics in an Acinetobacter strain causing epidemic infections in a hospital revealed that very probably the strain was infected with a conjugative resistance plasmid of the hospital flora. Since the plasmid could not be maintained stably in the Acinetobacter host, transposition of a 16 Md DNA sequence mediating resistance to gentamicin, streptomycin, chloramphenicol, sulfamethoxazole and tetracycline into the host chromosome occurred (16).

There are a number of observations that suggest transfer of genes from gram-positive to gram-negative organisms. A staphylococcal insertion sequence-like element, IS431, recently has been sequenced and shown to have similarity to IS26 of Proteus vulgaris (17). The kanamycin resistance gene aphA, coding for APH(3') type III, and thought to be specific to gram-positive cocci, has been detected in Campylobacter coli (18). High level resistance to the macrolide-lincosamide-streptogramin B antibiotics in Escherichia coli has been found to be due to a resistance determinant (ermBC) which is almost identical to erm genes described for streptococcal plasmids and for transposon Tn917 of Enterococcus faecalis (19). Since plasmids of gram-positive bacteria cannot be stably maintained in gram-negative organisms, it seems likely that the observed flux of resistance genes was made possible by illegitimate integration processes.

Discussion

Over the last decade basic science has provided important insights into the origin of drug resistance genes and the mechanism of their spread through bacterial populations. The explanations lie in the fact that DNA is a dynamic molecule and is subject to structural rearrangements. Besides mutation and legitimate recombination between homologous sequences, restructuring of DNA is mainly due to illegitimate recombination between heterologous sequences made possible by transposable DNA elements. Three classes of transposable DNA can be distinguished. Class I comprises the IS elements and composite transposons, class II includes the Tn3-like transposons, and class III forms a group of transposons neither fitting into class I or II. With rare exceptions, transposable elements have inverted repeats at their ends and trigger the duplication of a target sequence (direct repeats) upon integration. The central property of transposable DNA is its ability to integrate into foreign DNA. Two general modes of transposition exist. In conservative transposition, the transposing element moves from a donor site to a recipient site without duplication. In replicative transposition, the transposon is copied as part of the movement. In addition to simple insertion, transposable DNA can promote other types of DNA rearrangements which might influence the resistance phenotype of the host: deletion, inversion, excision or replicon fusion.

Although attempts to reconstruct evolutionary events are always circumstantial at best, there is strong evidence that transposons have greatly contributed to the problem of drug resistance in clinically important bacteria. These elements are the fundamental genetic units of drug resistance, possessing the ability to jump into bacterial chromosomes, plasmids and virus genomes of highly divergent sequences. Via transmissible plasmids and bacteriophages serving as vectors, these resistance units can be distributed through bacterial populations. In the presence of antibiotics providing the appropriate selective pressure, mutations in the resistance genes located on transposons can result in the evolution of markers encoding resistance to new drugs — as exemplified by the development of resistance to third generation cephalosporins. Point mutations in genes coding for beta-lactamases normally ineffective against these cephalosporins has resulted in determinants of enzymes with a substrate spectrum that also included third generation cephalosporins (20, and Abstracts No. 517–522, 27th Interscience Conference on Antimicrobial Agents and Chemotherapy, New York, 1987). Many important contributions to this subject not discussed here have been provided by distinguished colleagues. This brief review describes only some examples of the importance of transposable DNA for the evolution of antibiotic resistance.

References

1. Watanabe, T.: Infective heredity of multiple drug resistance in bacteria. Bacteriological Reviews 1963, 27: 87–115.
2. Kleckner, N.: Transposable elements in prokaryotes. Annual Review of Genetics 1981, 15: 341–404.
3. Shapiro, J. A. (ed.): Mobile genetic elements. Academic Press, Orlando, Fla., 1983, p. 1–688.
4. Grindley, N. D. F.: Transpositional recombination in prokaryotes. Annual Review of Biochemistry 1985, 54: 863–896.
5. Murphy, E., Huwyler, L., Bastos, M.: Transposon Tn554: complete nucleotide sequence and isolation of transposition-defective and antibiotic-sensitive mutants. EMBO Journal 1985, 4: 3357–3365.
6. Franke, A. E., Clewell, D. B.: Evidence for a chromosomeborne resistance transposon (Tn916) in Streptococcus faecalis that is capable of conjugal transfer in the absence of a conjugative plasmid. Journal of Bacteriology 1981, 145: 494–502.
7. Courvalin, P., Carlier, C.: Tn1545: a conjugative shuttle transposon. Molecular and General Genetics 1987, 206: 259–264.
8. Hächler, H., Kayser, F. H., Berger-Bächi, B.: Homology of a transferable tetracycline resistance determinant of Clostridium difficile with Streptococcus (Enterococcus) faecalis transposon Tn916. Antimicrobial Agents and Chemotherapy 1987, 31: 1033–1038.
9. Bennett, P. M., Heritage, J., Comanducci, A., Dodd, H. M.: Evolution of R plasmids by replicon fusion. Journal of Antimicrobial Chemotherapy 1987, 18, Supplement C: 103–111.
10. Syvanen, M.: The evolutionary implications of mobile genetic elements. Annual Review of Genetics 1984, 18: 271–293.
11. Trieu-Cuot, P., Courvalin, P.: Evolution and transfer of aminoglycoside resistance genes under natural conditions. Journal of Antimicrobial Chemotherapy 1987, 18, Supplement C: 93–102.
12. Grinsted, J.: Evolution of transposable elements. Journal of Antimicrobial Chemotherapy 1987, 18, Supplement C: 77–83.
13. Levy, S. B.: Resistance to the tetracyclines. In: Bryan, L. E. (ed.): Antimicrobial drug resistance. Academic Press, Orlando, Fla., 1984, p. 191–240.
14. Laufs, R., Riess, F. C., Jahn, G., Fock, R., Kaulfers, P. M.: Origin of Haemophilus influenzae R factors. Journal of Bacteriology 1981, 147: 563–568.
15. Wiedemann, B., Meyer, J. F., Zühlsdorf, M. T.: Insertions of resistance genes into Tn21-like transposons. Journal of Antimicrobial Chemotherapy 1987, 18, Supplement C: 85–92.
16. Devaud, M., Kayser, F. H., Bächi, B.: Transposon-mediated multiple antibiotic resistance in Acinetobacter strains. Antimicrobial Agents and Chemotherapy 1982, 22: 323–329.
17. Barberis-Maino, L., Berger-Bächi, B., Weber, H., Beck, W. D., Kayser, F. H.: IS431, a staphylococcal insertion sequence-like element related to IS26 from Proteus vulgaris. Gene 1987, 59: 107–113.
18. Trieu-Cuot, P., Gerbaud, G., Lambert, T., Courvalin, P.: In vivo transfer of genetic information between gram-positive and gram-negative bacteria. EMBO Journal 1985, 4: 3583–3587.
19. Brisson-Noël, A., Arthur, M., Courvalin, P.: Evidence for natural gene transfer from gram-positive cocci to Escherichia coli. Journal of Bacteriology 1988, 170: 1739–1745.
20. Kliebe, C., Nies, B. A., Meyer, J. F., Tolxdorff-Neutzling, R. M., Wiedemann, B.: Evolution of plasmid-coded resistance to broad spectrum cephalosporins. Antimicrobial Agents and Chemotherapy 1985, 28: 302–307.

Bacterial Proteins Involved in Antimicrobial Drug Resistance

C. C. Sanders

Antimicrobial drug resistance is a predictable response to the use of antibiotics. Among clinical isolates, this response most often involves the production of a drug-inactivating enzyme. Such enzymes have severely limited the clinical usefulness of many antimicrobial agents. Furthermore, their appearance and spread among microbial populations often reflect use and misuse of various antimicrobial agents. For example, the spread of chloramphenicol acetyltrans-ferase among strains of *Salmonella typhi* worldwide has caused many problems for the treatment of typhoid fever. Dissemination of this enzyme among *Haemophilus influenzae* and *Bacteroides fragilis* in the future could pose many new therapeutic problems. A variety of aminoglycoside inactivating enzymes affecting one or many members of this drug class have evolved. The prevalence of resistance to specific aminoglycosides varies widely from country to country and reflects not only aminoglycoside utilization patterns but also the prevalence of specific genes encoding the various inactivating enzymes. For β-lactam drugs, the β-lactamases are by far the most common mechanism of resistance encountered among clinical isolates. These enzymes comprise a diverse family of serine proteases and their dissemination maong both gram-positive and gram-negative bacteria has greatly influenced the efficacy of β-lactam drugs. All in all, an understanding and appreciation of these inactivating enzymes is essential for new drug design.

Antibiotic resistance is a worldwide problem associated with the use, misuse and overuse of antimicrobial agents (1–7). Over the last decade, various task forces have been formed to study the problems posed by drug resistance (8–10), and a multinational group, the Alliance for the Prudent Use of Antibiotics, has arisen to compile and disseminate information about resistance (3). Despite numerous problems associated with data collection and evaluation, several worldwide trends are amply clear. Drug resistance is a predictable response to antibiotic use; genes for resistance are continuing to spread to new species; and there is greater morbidity and mortality associated with infections due to resistant bacteria (1–8). Although a major thrust for combating these problems has always been the development of newer antimicrobial agents, it has become clear that an understanding of the mechanisms responsible for resistance at a molecular level is an essential component of new drug design.

There are three major mechanisms whereby bacteria may resist the effects of antimicrobial agents. These include (i) production of drug inactivating enzymes, (ii) alteration of the drug's target, and (iii) diminished permeability. Of these three, the production of drug inactivating enzymes is by far the most prevalent mechanism responsible for resistance in clinical isolates of both gram-positive and gram-negative bacteria. In naturally susceptible species, the genetic information responsible for the production of such enzymes may arise via acquisition of a plasmid or via mutation of a chromosomal or plasmid derived gene. Thus, the prevalence of genes encoding drug inactivating enzymes increases in any environment in which there is high volume use of antibiotics affected by such enzymes.

The antibiotic era has been ongoing sufficiently long to allow an historical analysis of drug inactivating enzymes as an indicator of drug use and microbial response to it. Thus, this overview will examine enzymes affecting three major groups of antibiotics: chloramphenicol, the aminoglycosides and the β-lactam antibiotics. It will examine not only the molecular actions of the enzymes but also the past, present and future impact of their dissemination worldwide upon therapeutic approaches for infectious diseases (Table 1).

Chloramphenicol

Resistance to chloramphenicol is usually mediated by chloramphenicol acetyltransferase, an enzyme that acetylates the 3- and 1-hydroxyl groups of chloramphenicol (11). This enzyme in both gram-positive and gram-negative bacteria is usually plasmid medi-

---

Department of Medical Microbiology, Creighton University School of Medicine, Omaha, Nebraska 68178, USA.

Table 1: Impact of drug inactivating enzymes on therapy for infectious diseases.

Antibiotic	Enzyme	Therapeutic Problems Past/Present	Present/Future
Chloramphenicol	Acetyltransferase	Typhoid fever	Meningitis due to *Haemophilus influenzae*
Aminoglycosides	ANT (2″), AAC(3)	Infections due to gentamicin-resistant bacteria	
	AAC (6′)		Infections due to amikacin-resistant bacteria
Penicillins/ cephalosporins	Penicillinase TEM β-lactamase	Staphylococcal infections PPNG infections	Enterococcal infections Infections due to bacteria resistant to newer cephalosporins
		Meningitis due to *Haemophilus influenzae*	Infections due to bacteria resistant to β-lactamase inhibitor/β-lactam combinations
	Chromosomal β-lactamases	*Enterobacter, Serratia, Pseudomonas* infections	Infections due to multiply resistant mutants of *Enterobacter, Serratia*, and *Pseudomonas* spp.

ated (12). Its dissemination among strains of *Salmonella typhi* has caused many therapeutic problems during outbreaks of typhoid fever in Mexico, India, Vietnam, Thailand, Korea, Formosa, Bangladesh, Chile and Peru (13, 14). Although rarely encountered in clinical isolates of *Haemophilus influenzae* (15, 16) and *Bacteroides fragilis* (17–19), subsequent dissemination of chloramphenicol acetyltransferase among strains of these species could pose significant therapeutic problems. Such problems have been encountered in Spain where *Haemophilus influenzae* resistant to both ampicillin and chloramphenicol have been recovered (20).

Aminoglycosides

A variety of aminoglycoside inactivating enzymes are produced by both gram-positive and gram-negative bacteria (21). These inactivate one or many aminoglycosides by N-acetylation (AAC), 0-phosphorylation (APH), or 0-nucleotidylyation (ANT). Depending upon the drug and the site modified, this produces partial or complete loss of bioactivity. Most aminoglycoside inactivating enzymes are plasmid-mediated and can be associated with multiresistant transposons (21). The prevalence of resistance to specific aminoglycosides varies widely and reflects not only aminoglycoside utilization patterns but also prevalence of specific genes encoding the various inactivating enzymes (8, 21). For example, in countries that utilize gentamicin or its derivatives to a greater extent than amikacin, the most prevalent enzymes are ANT(2″) and AAC(3) (8, 21–24). In the Far East, however, where amikacin and similar kanamycin-family aminoglycosides are widely used, AAC(6′) is most prevalent (8, 21, 23). This selective pressure favoring the appearance and dissemination of specific enzymes producing aminoglycoside resistance is best illustrated by epidemiological studies performed at individual hospitals. At the New York Veterans Administration Medical Center, an increase from 2 % to > 7 % in amikacin resistance mediated by AAC(6′) was observed over an 18-month period (25). This increase coincided with a three-fold increase in amikacin utilization within the institution. Similarly, during a nine-month period at the San Juan de Dios hospital in Santiago, Chile, when amikacin was the sole aminoglycoside used, AAC(6′) mediated resistance to amikacin was found in 42 strains of Enterobacteriaceae (26). Such resistance had not been encountered in this hospital previously. Although all institutions that have switched to amikacin as the primary aminoglycoside have not seen similar increases in resistance (27), this probably reflects the absence of genes encoding the appropriate enzyme(s) among the hospital flora. In such institutions, dissemination of amikacin resistance merely awaits introduction of the appropriate gene(s).

Beta-Lactam Antibiotics

β-lactamases are a diverse family of microbial enzymes that hydrolyze the cyclic amide bond of susceptible β-lactam antibiotics. Recent advances in protein chemistry and molecular biology techniques have shown that they belong to a super family of serine proteases which also includes the penicillin-binding proteins (PBPs), the targets of the β-lactam drugs

(28). Thus, it appears that the β-lactamases and PBPs share a common ancestry and the former probably evolved from the latter as a response by bacteria to β-lactams in their environment. Although β-lactamases can be encoded by either plasmid or chromosomal genes, the former have been particularly important in the rising prevalence of β-lactam resistance among clinical isolates as well as its dissemination to diverse species.

Plasmid-Mediated Enzymes

Perhaps the best example of spread of a plasmid almost completely throughout all strains of a species is the production of penicillinase by *Staphylococcus aureus*. Today over 80% of strains worldwide produce penicillinase (29). Fortunately, the introduction of penicillinase-resistant penicillins solved most of the therapeutic problems posed by this enzyme. Although this penicillinase has essentially been the only β-lactamase of gram-positive bacteria to cause therapeutic problems, recent reports of β-lactamase in clinical isolates of *Streptococcus faecalis* may be cause for future concern (30).

Among gram-negative bacteria, there are many diverse plasmid-mediated β-lactamases (31–33). Dissemination of one specific enzyme, TEM, and its close relatives within the Richmond and Sykes Class III enzymes has had a profound effect on therapeutic approaches to a variety of infections. Although the predominance of the TEM β-lactamase among Enterobacteriaceae was recognized in the mid-1960s, it did not spread to *Haemophilus influenzae* until the early 1970s. Epidemiologic studies performed during the mid 1970s in various parts of the world showed the prevalence of β-lactamase-producing *Haemophilus influenzae* to vary between 0 and 8% (8, 34, 35). Later surveys performed in the late 1970s and early 1980s showed the prevalence increasing to 6–15% (15, 34–36). Most recent surveys of isolates recovered during 1986 indicate that resistance is still increasing (15, 16, 37). Among nine European countries included in a recent survey, β-lactamase production was found in 17% (62 of 372) of all isolates of *Haemophilus influenzae* serotype b and 11% (214 of 1961) of non-serotype b isolates (37). A national collaborative study performed in the U.S. showed 32% (240 of 757) of serotype b and 16% (320 of 2,054) of non-serotype b *Haemophilus influenzae* produced β-lactamases (15). This introduction and dissemination of the TEM β-lactamase necessitated the use of chloramphenicol in initial treatment of *Haemophilus influenzae* meningitis. More recently, several of the newer β-lactamase resistant cephalosporins have become preferred therapy (38).

In June 1975, Stanley Falkow predicted the acquisition of plasmid-mediated penicillinase in *Neisseria gonorrhoeae* (39). One year later, the first clinical isolates of penicillinase-producing *Neisseria gonorrhoeae* (PPNG) appeared independently in the Far East and West Africa (8). This enzyme was also a TEM β-lactamase. PPNG now constitutes over 50% of clinical isolates recovered in many areas of Asia and Africa, while in the USA, UK, and parts of Europe, less than 20% of isolates are PPNG (8). However, even within these areas there are high prevalence regions. In 1985, within the state of Florida, approximately 40% of cases of gonorrhea in Miami (south Florida) were due to PPNG while in Jacksonville (north Forida), only 5% were due to PPNG (40). Florida, New York City and Los Angeles account for over 70% of PPNG cases in the U.S. (40). In areas of high PPNG prevalence, the drug of choice for therapy of gonorrhea has switched from penicillin to spectinomycin or one of the newer β-lactamase stable cephalosporins.

Early surveys of β-lactamases in Enterobacteriaceae and *Pseudomonas aeruginosa* showed a much greater prevalence of TEM and related Richmond and Sykes Class III β-lactamases over other plasmid-mediated enzymes (31–33). These enzymes are responsible for ampicillin resistance in *Escherichia coli* and *Proteus mirabilis*, cephalosporin resistance in *Klebsiella pneumoniae* and much of the carbenicillin resistance in *Pseudomonas aeruginosa*. Recent surveys reveal that the predominance of TEM β-lactamases over other plasmid-mediated enzymes persists to this day (41–44) in Enterobacteriaeceae despite the discovery of numerous additional enzymes (45, 46) and spread of plasmids between *Pseudomonas aeruginosa* and Enterobacteriaceae (47). For *Pseudomonas aeruginosa*, the widespread use of carbenicillin and congeners has led away from a dominance of TEM β-lactamases to a greater prevalence of PSE-1 and PSE-4 (two TEM related Class III enzymes) as well as OXA-1 and OXA-2 (two Richmond and Sykes Class V enzymes) (33, 48, 49). In an attempt to circumvent the therapeutic problems posed by these plasmid-mediated β-lactamases, two approaches have been taken. The first involves the development of β-lactamase inhibitors while the second centers on the design of enzyme-resistant antibiotics. Both approaches have been fairly successful in specific areas; however, both have also led to new problems with β-lactamases.

The introduction of combinations containing a suicide (irreversible) inhibitor of β-lactamase and a β-lactam antibiotic returned many bacteria that produced plasmid-mediated enzymes back into the inhibitory spectrum of enzyme labile drugs (50, 51). These combinations include for example clavulanic acid plus amoxicillin or ticarcillin, and sulbactam plus ampicillin or cefoperazone. The microbial response to this approach is just beginning to be seen. In a recent examination of 34 clavulanic acid/ticarcillin-resistant Enterobacteriaceae, two major mechanisms were found to be responsible for this resistance in strains of *Escherichia coli* and *Klebsiella pneumoniae* (52). The first mechanism involved production of high levels of TEM or SHV β-lactamases. These enzymes, although still susceptible to inhibition by calvulanic acid, were present at too great a level to allow sufficient inhibition to occur to bring the ticarcillin activity against the strains down to a clinically achievable range. The second mechanism involved the production of PSE-1, an enzyme heretofore found only rarely in Enterobacteriaceae (47). This enzyme, although susceptible to inhibition by clavulanic acid, hydrolyzes ticarcillin so rapidly that effective inhibition is once again not possible. It remains to be seen if Enterobacteriaceae with these resistance mechanisms become more prevalent as the use of combinations containing β-lactamase inhibitors becomes more widespread.

A second strategy to counteract resistance produced by plasmid-mediated β-lactamases in gram-negative bacteria has involved the design of enzyme-resistant drugs. These include numerous newer generation cephalosporins. Unfortunately, in various areas of Europe, Tunisia and elsewhere, the microbial response to this approach is already being seen (53–60). Enterobacteriaceae have now been recovered that are resistant to one or more of the newer cephalosporins by virtue of the production of plasmid-mediated β-lactamases. These enzymes are not unique, but appear to be derivatives of the older TEM and SHV β-lactamases (53, 60). A mutation in the structural gene which alters the substrate profile of the enzymes seems to have occurred. Fortunately, all such enzymes examined to date are still highly susceptible to inhibition by clavulanic acid. Thus, therapeutic problems posed by them may be solved by the use of inhibitor/cephalosporin combinations.

Chromosomal Beta-Lactamases

Although the plasmid-mediated β-lactamases of gram-negative bacteria continue to cause numerous therapeutic problems, those enzymes encoded by the bacterial chromosome are becoming increasingly important clinically. Once again, the reason for this is the recent development of various β-lactamase stable compounds. Two major groups of enzymes are involved. The first is an oxyiminocephalosporinase produced characteristically by indole-positive strains of *Klebsiella pneumoniae,* i.e. *Klebsiella oxytoca* (61). This enzyme belongs to Richmond and Sykes Class IV and is often referred to as the K1 enzyme (31). This broad spectrum β-lactamase hydrolyzes penicillins including cloxacillin, the oxyiminocephalosporins (e.g. cefuroxime and cefotaxime) and aztreonam. Thus, use of some of the newer β-lactams will select for a greater prevalence of *Klebsiella oxytoca* in the environment. Although susceptible to inhibition by clavulanic acid, this enzyme when produced at high levels confers resistance to clavulanic acid/ticarcillin combinations (52).

In 1976, Matthew and Harris (62) showed that virtually every gram-negative bacterium possesses a chromosomally encoded β-lactamase. Most of these enzymes are constitutively expressed at very low levels and do not contribute to β-lactam resistance. However, in certain species, the enzymes are inducible (31, 63). These inducible β-lactamases are primarily cephalosporinases of Richmond and Sykes Class I and are not susceptible to inhibition by clavulanic acid (31, 63). They are characteristically found in *Citrobacter freundii, Enterobacter* spp., *Serratia* spp. and *Pseudomonas aeruginosa* and are responsible for the resistance of most of these organisms to ampicillin, older cephalosporins and cephamycins. This resistance arises because these β-lactam antibiotics are good inducers of the enzyme and are hydrolyzed by it. Thus, these compounds have never been clinically useful against such organisms. However, over the last ten years newer cephalosporins and monobactams have been developed which are much less susceptible to hydrolysis by the chromosomal cephalosporinases and appear to be highly active in vitro against organisms possessing them. Nevertheless, when these new β-lactams have been used to treat infections caused by organisms with inducible β-lactamases, a rapid emergence of resistance has been observed in a number of instances (63). This resistance has been found to be due to the selection by the newer drugs of mutants expressing extremely high levels of chromosomal cephalosporinase. The expression of inducible β-lactamases is governed by an extremely complex array of regulatory genes which has not been completely elucidated to date (64). However, mutation in one regulatory gene, *amp*D, is responsible for conversion of the normally inducible expression of chromosomal cephalosporinase to high level and in many instances constitutive expression of the enzyme (65). This mutation occurs spontaneously in cells possessing an inducible β-lactamase at a frequency of 10^{-6} to 10^{-7} (63). Such mutants are resistant to multiple β-lactam antibiotics including all of the penicillins, cephalosporins and monobactams (63).

Many of the newer β-lactam antibiotics create a selective pressure favoring growth of such mutants over wild-type cells. This selective pressure arises because the drugs are generally poor inducers of chromosomal cephalosporinases in wild-type cells and are much more resistant to hydrolysis by these enzymes than are the older β-lactams (63). Thus, only those cells constitutively expressing high levels of enzyme, i.e. *amp*D mutants, are able to survive in the presence of the newer β-lactams. It is therefore not surprising that when the drugs are used in a given environment the prevalence of such mutants increases significantly.

The selection of *amp*D mutants from strains possessing inducible cephalosporinases has been responsible for a number of clinical problems associated with the use of many of the newer β-lactam antibiotics (66). These include the emergence of mutants with multiple β-lactam resistance in 14% to 56% of patients infected with organisms possessing inducible β-lactamases and in whom the newer drugs were used for therapy (66). In 25% to 75% of these patients, clinical failure was associated with resistance. The spread of such mutants within the hospital environment has posed additional problems as outbreaks of nosocomial infections ensued. Such outbreaks have been most common in burns units, intensive care units, cancer centers and cystic fibrosis units, where there is a clustering of patients at risk of infection with organisms possessing inducible β-lactamases (66). Although the new carbapenems are active against such mutants and have been used successfully to treat infections caused by them, the major clinical problems posed by organisms with inducible β-lactamases still await a more general solution. Until then, the newer β-lactams should be used judiciously to keep these problems to a minimum.

References

1. Kunin, C. M.: Antibiotic resistance – a world health problem we cannot ignore. Annals of Internal Medicine 1983, 99: 859–860.
2. Jackson, G. G.: Antibiotic policies, practices and pressures. Journal of Antimicrobial Chemotherapy 1979, 5: 1–4.
3. Levy, S. B.: Antibiotic resistance. Infection Control 1983, 4: 195–197.
4. Finland, M.: Emergence of antibiotic resistance in hospitals, 1935–1975. Reviews of Infectious Diseases 1979, 1: 4–21.
5. McGowan, J. E. Jr.: Antimicrobial resistance in hospital organisms and its relation to antibiotic use. Reviews of Infectious Diseases 1983, 5: 1033–1048.
6. Cooke, D., Salter, A. J., Phillips, I.: Antimicrobial misuse, antibiotic policies and information services. Journal of Antimicrobial Chemotherapy 1980, 6: 435–443.
7. Holmberg, S. D., Soloman, S. L., Blake, P. A.: Health and economic impacts of antimicrobial resistance. Reviews of Infectious Diseases 1987, 9: 1065–1078.
8. O'Brien, T. F. and the Members of Task Force 2: Resistance of bacteria to antibacterial agents: report of Task Force 2. Reviews of Infectious Diseases 1987, Supplement 3, 9: S244–S260.
9. Antimicrobial Agents Committee: Report from the Antimicrobial Agents Committee. Journal of Infectious Diseases 1987, 156: 700–705.
10. World Health Organization Scientific Working Group on Antibacterial Resistance: Control of antibiotic-resistant bacteria: memorandum from a WHO meeting. Bulletin of the World Health Organization 1983, 61: 423-433.
11. Shaw, W. V.: The enzymatic acetylation of chloramphenicol by extracts of R factor-resistant *Escherichia coli*. Journal of Biological Chemistry 1967, 242: 687–693.
12. Smith, A. L., Burns, J. L.: Resistance to chloramphenicol and fusidic acid. In: Bryan, L. E. (ed.): Antimicrobial Drug Resistance. Academic Press, New York, 1984, p. 293–315.
13. Bryan, J. P., Rocha, H., Scheld, W. M.: Problems in salmonellosis: rationale for clinical trials with newer β-lactam agents and quinolones. Reviews of Infectious Disease 1986, 8: 189–207.
14. Farrar, W. E.: Antibiotic resistance in developing countries. Journal of Infectious Diseases 1985, 152: 1103–1106.
15. Doern, G. V., Jorgensen, J. H., Thornsberry, C., Preston, D. A., Tubert, T., Redding, J. S., Maher, L. A.: National collaborative study of the prevalence of antimicrobial resistance among clinical isolates of *Haemophilus influenzae*. Antimicrobial Agents and Chemotherapy 1988, 32: 180–185.
16. Howard, A. J., Williams, H. M.: The prevalence of antibiotic resistance in *Haemophilus influenzae* in Wales. Journal of Antimicrobial Chemotherapy 1988, 21: 251–260.
17. DeAlmeida, A. E. C. C., DeUzeda, M.: Susceptibility to five antimicrobial agents of strains of the *Bacteroides fragilis* group isolated in Brasil. Antimicrobial Agents and Chemotherapy. 1987, 617–618.
18. Tally, F. P., Chuchural, G. J. Jr., Jacobus, N. V., Gorbach, S. L., Aldridge, K., Cleary, T., Finegold, S. M., Hill, G., Iannini, P., O'Keefe, P., Pierson, C.: Nationwide study of the susceptibility of the *Bacteroides fragilis* group in the United States. Antimicrobial Agents and Chemotherapy 1985, 28: 675–677.
19. Bourgault, A.-M., Harding, G. K., Smith, J. A., Horsman, G. B., Marrie, T. J., Lamothe, F.: Survey of anaerobic susceptiblity patterns in Canada. Antimicrobial Agents and Chemotherapy 1986, 30: 798–801.
20. Campos, J., Garcia-Tornel, S., Gairi, J. M., Fabregues, I.: Multiply resistant *Haemophilus influenzae* type b causing meningitis: comparative clinical and laboratory study. Journal of Pediatrics 1986, 108: 879–902.
21. Davies, J. E.: Resistance to aminoglycosides: mechanisms and frequency. Reviews of Infectious Diseases 1983, Supplement 2, 5: S261–S267.
22. Maes, P.: Evaluation of the resistance mechanisms of gentamicin-resistant gram-negative bacilli and their susceptibility to tobramycin, netilmicin and amikacin. Journal of Antimicrobial Chemotherapy 1985, 15: 283–289.
23. Shimizer, K., Kumada, T., Hsieh, W.-C., Chung, H.-Y., Chong, Y., Hare, R. S., Miller, G. H., Sabatelli, F. J., Howard, J.: Comparison of aminoglycoside resistance patterns in Japan, Formosa, and Korea, Chile, and the United States. Antimicrobial Agents and Chemotherapy 1985; 28: 282–288.
24. Kettner, M., Navarová, J., Langsádl, L.: Aminoglycoside resistance patterns in clinical isolates of Enterobacteriaceae from Czechoslovakia. Journal of Antimicrobial Chemotherapy 1987, 20: 383–387.
25. Levine, J. F., Maslow, M. J., Leibowitz, R. E., Pollock, A. A., Hanna, B. A., Schaefler, S., Simberkoff, M. S., Rahal, J. J. Jr.: Amikacin-resistant gram-negative bacilli: correlation of occurrence with amikacin use. Journal of Infectious Diseases 1985, 151: 295–300.
26. Nhieu, G. T. U., Goldstein, F. W., Pinto, M. E., Acar, J. F., Collatz, E.: Transfer of amikacin resistance by closely related plasmids in members of the family Enterobacteraceae isolated in Chile. Antimicrobial Agents and Chemotherapy 1986, 29: 833–837.

27. Price, K. E., Kresel, P. A., Farchione, L. A., Siskin, S. B., Karpow, S. A.: Epidemiological studies of aminoglycoside resistance in the U.S.A. Journal of Antimicrobial Chemotherapy 1981, Supplement A, 8: 89–105.
28. Ghuysen, J.-M.: Bacterial active-site serine, penicillin-interactive proteins and domains. Mechanism, structure and evolution. Reviews of Infectious Diseases 1988, 10: 726–732.
29. O'Brien, T. F. and the International Survey of Antibiotic Resistance Group: Resistance to antibiotics at medical centers in different parts of the world. Journal of Antimicrobial Chemotherapy 1986, Supplement C, 18: 243–253.
30. Murray, B. E., Mederski-Samoraj, B. D.: Transferable beta-lactamase: a new mechanism for in vitro penicillin resistance in *Streptococcus faecalis*. Journal of Clinical Investigation 1983, 72: 1168–1171.
31. Richmond, M. H., Sykes, R. B.: The β-lactamases of gram-negative bacteria and their possible physiologic role. Advances in Microbial Physiology 1973, 9: 31–88.
32. Matthew, M.: Plasmid mediated β-lactamases of gram-negative bacteria: properties and distribution. Journal of Antimicrobial Chemotherapy 1979; 5: 349–358.
33. Medieros, A. A.: β-lactamases. British Medical Bulletin 1984, 40: 18–27.
34. Williams, J. D., Moosdeen, F.: Antibiotic resistance in *Haemophilus influenzae:* epidemiology, mechanisms, and therapeutic possibilities. Reviews of Infectious Diseases 1986, Supplement 5, 8: S555–S560.
35. Jokipii, L., Jokipii, A. M. M.: Emergence and prevalence of β-lactamase producing *Haemophilus influenzae* in Finland and susceptibility of 102 respiratory isolates to eight antibiotics. Journal of Antimicrobial Chemotherapy 1980, 6: 623–631.
36. Scheifele, D. W.: Ampicillin-resistant *Haemophilus influenzae* in Canada: nationwide survey of hospital laboratories. Canadian Medical Association Journal 1979, 121: 198–202.
37. Machka, K., Braveny, I., Dabernat, H., Dornbush, K., VanDyck, E., Kayser, F. H., VanKlingeren, B., Mittermayer, H., Perea, E., Powell, M.: Distribution and resistance patterns of *Haemophilus influenzae:* a European cooperative study. European Journal of Clinical Microbiology 1988, 7: 14–24.
38. McCracken, G. H. Jr., Nelson, J. D., Kaplan, S. L., Overturf, G. D., Rodriguez, W. J., Steele, R. W.: Consensus report: antimicrobial therapy for bacterial meningitis in infants and children. Pediatric Infectious Disease Journal 1987, 6: 501–505.
39. Falkow, S., Elwell, L. P., deGraaff, J., Heffron, F., Mayer, L.: A possible model for the development of plasmid-mediated penicillin resistance in the gonococcus. In: Catterall, R. D., Nicol, C. S. (ed.): Sexually Transmitted Disease, Academic Press, London, 1976, p. 120–133.
40. Anonymous: Penicillinase-producing *Neisseria gonorrhoeae* migrating northward. Alliance for the Prudent Use of Antibiotics, 1986, 4: 1.
41. Stobberingh, E. E., Houben, A. W., vanBoven, C. P. A.: Cephalosporin resistance among gram-negative hospital strains and the prevalence of β-lactamase types. Antonie van Leeuwenhoek 1982, 48: 200–201.
42. Opferkuch, W., Cullmann, W.: Beta-lactamases in ampicillin-resistant Enterobacteriaceae. Infection 1983, Supplement 2, 11: S83–S84.
43. Roy, C., Segura, C., Tirado, M., Reig, R., Hermida, M., Teruel, D., Foz, A.: Frequency of plasmid-determined beta-lactamases in 680 consecutively isolated strains of Enterobacteriaceae. European Journal of Clinical Microbiology 1985, 4: 146–147.
44. Simpson, I. N., Knothe, H., Plested, S. J., Harper, P. B.: Qualitative and quantitative aspects of β-lactamase production as mechanisms of β-lactam resistance in a survey of clinical isolates from faecal samples. Journal of Antimicrobial Chemotherapy 1986, 17: 725–727.
45. Medeiros, A. A., Cohenford, M., Jacoby, G. A.: Five novel plasmid-determined β-lactamases. Antimicrobial Agents and Chemotherapy 1985, 27: 715–719.
46. Bush, K., Sykes, R. B.: Characterization and epidemiology of β-lactamases. In: Peterson, P. K., Verhoef, J. (ed.): Antimicrobial Agents Annual 2, Elsevier, Amsterdam, 1987, p. 371–382.
47. Medeiros, A. A., Hedges, R. W., Jacoby, G. A.: Spread of a *"Pseudomonas-*specific" β-lactamase to plasmids of enterobacteria. Journal of Bacteriology 1982, 149: 700–707.
48. Williams, R. J., Livermore, D. M., Lindridge, M. A., Said, A. A., Williams, J. D.: Mechanisms of beta-lactam resistance in British isolates of *Pseudomonas aeruginosa*. Journal of Medical Microbiology 1984, 17: 283–293.
49. Jouvenot, M., Bonin, P., Michel-Briand, Y.: Frequency of β-lactamases that are markedly active against carbenicillin in *Pseudomonas aeruginosa* strains isolated in a medical school hospital. Journal of Antimicrobial Chemotherapy 1983, 12: 451–458.
50. Bush, K., Sykes, R. B.: β-lactamase inhibitors in perspective. Journal of Antimicrobial Chemotherapy 1983, 11: 97–107.
51. Neu, H. C.: The role of β-lactamase inhibitors in chemotherapy. Pharmacology and Therapeutics 1985, 30: 1–18.
52. Sanders, C. C., Iaconis, J. P., Bodey, G. P., Šamonis, G.: Resistance to ticarcillin/potassium clavulanate among clinical isolates of Enterobacteriaceae: role of PSE-1 and high levels of TEM-1 and SHV-1 and problems with false susceptibility in disk diffusion tests. Antimicrobial Agents and Chemotherapy 1988, (in press).
53. Kliebe, C., Nies, B. A., Meyer, J. F., Tolxdorff-Neutzling, R. M., Wiedemann, B.: Evolution of plasmid-coded resistance to broad-spectrum cephalosporins. Antimicrobial Agents and Chemotherapy 1985, 28: 302–309.
54. Sirot, D., Sirot, J., Labia, R., Morand, A., Courvalin, P., Darfeuille-Michaud, A., Perroux, R., Cliezel, R.: Transferable resistance to third-generation cephalosporins in clinical isolates of *Klebsiella pneumoniae:* identification of CTX-1, a novel β-lactamase. Journal of Antimicrobial Chemotherapy 1987, 20: 323–334.
55. Sirot, J., Labia, R., Thabaut, A.: *Klebsiella pneumoniae* strains more resistant to ceftazidime than to other third-generation cephalosporins. Journal of Antimicrobial Chemotherapy 1987, 20: 611–612.
56. Spencer, R. C., Wheat, P. F., Winstanley, T. G., Cox, D. M., Plested, S. J.: Novel β-lactamase in a clinical isolate of *Klebsiella pneumoniae* conferring unusual resistance to β-lactam antibiotics. Journal of Antimicrobial Chemotherapy 1987, 20: 919–921.
57. Bauernfeind, A., Hörl, G.: Novel R-factor borne β-lactamase of *Escherichia coli* conferring resistance to cephalosporins. Infection 1987, 15: 257–259.
58. Redjeb, S. B., Yaghlane, H. B., Boujnah, A., Philippon, A., Labia, R.: Synergy between clavulanic acid and newer β-lactams on nine clinical isolates of *Klebsiella pneumoniae, Escherichia coli,* and *Salmonella typhimurium* resistant to third-generation cephalosporins. Journal of Antimicrobial Chemotherapy 1988, 21: 263–264.
59. Gutmann, L., Kitzis, M. D., Billot-Klein, D., Goldstein, F., TranVanNhieu, G., Lu, T., Carlet, J., Collatz, E., Williamson, R.: Plasmid mediated β-lactamase (TEM-7) involved in resistance to ceftazidime and aztreonam. Reviews of Infectious Disease 1988, 10: 860–866.

60. **Sougakoff, W., Goussard, S., Gerbaud, G., Courvalin, P.**: Plasmid-mediated resistance to third-generation cephalosporins due to point-mutations in TEM-type penicillinase genes. Reviews of Infectious Diseases 1988, 10: 879–884.
61. **Sanders, C. C.**: The chromosomal β-lactamases. In: Bryan, L. E. (ed.) Microbial drug resistance, Springer-Verlag, Berlin, (in press).
62. **Matthew, M., Harris, A. M.**: Identification of β-lactamases by analytical isoelectric focusing: correlation with bacterial taxonomy. Journal of General Microbiology 1976, 94: 55–67.
63. **Sanders, C. C.**: Chromosomal cephalosporinases responsible for multiple resistance to newer β-lactam antibiotics. Annual Review of Microbiology 1987, 41: 573–593.
64. **Lindberg, F., Lindquist, S., Normark, S.**: Genetic basis of induction and overproduction of chromosomal type I β-lactamase in non-fastidious gram-negative rods. Reviews of Infectious Diseases 1988, 10: 782–785.
65. **Lindberg, F., Lindquist, S., Normark, S.**: Inactivation of the *amp*D gene causes semiconstitutive overproduction of the inducible *Citrobacter freundii* β-lactamase. Journal of Bacteriology 1987, 169: 1923–1928.
66. **Sanders, W. E. Jr., Sanders, C. C.**: Inducible β-lactamases: clinical and epidemiological implications for use of newer cephalosporins. Reviews of Infectious Diseases 1988, 10: 830–838.

Persistent Herpes Simplex Virus Infection and Mechanisms of Virus Drug Resistance

H. J. Field

Herpes simplex virus (HSV) is susceptible to a variety of antiviral compounds, most of which are nucleoside analogues that interfere with DNA metabolism involving the virus enzymes DNA-polymerase and thymidine kinase. Single mutations in the virus genome give rise to resistant mutants following selection in vitro in the presence of a particular drug, and in this respect HSV is similar to several other viruses. Such mutants have been invaluable research tools. HSV is responsible for a variety of lesions which tend to be recurrent, owing to the special ability of the virus to remain latent in and reactivate from neural tissue. The consequences of this upon clinical resistance are discussed in the present review. In fact, clinical resistance in HSV infections has not yet become widespread but does appear to be especially important in immunocompromised patients, including those suffering from AIDS. HSV is proposed as an important model for the investigation of drug resistance in other, more complex organisms, and with respect to antiviral strategies against the human immunodeficiency virus.

Herpesviruses – Persistence and Latency

Herpesvirus Family. The Herpesviridae constitute a very large family of DNA-containing viruses associated with most if not all vertebrates. Several members of the family, for example, herpes simplex virus (HSV) of human origin were among the earliest virus infections to be recognised, and, being relatively easy to culture and study, the particles have been thoroughly characterised. However, although the entire nucleotide sequence has been determined for several herpes viruses, these viruses code for in excees of 70 separate polypeptides; this large coding potential means that many facets of the host-virus relationship of even the best known herpesviruses are still to be elucidated. As the various infections among animals and humans have become recognised, the single most notable feature of the family seems to be the unparalleled ability of these viruses to establish persistent, lifelong infections. Although infection of the natural host may lead to trivial or subclinical disease and the host immune responses may limit the pathology produced by the acute infection, typically the virus is not eradicated but remains in lifelong relationship with the host, maintaining the potential for future transmission, sometimes accompanied by recrudescent disease, for perhaps several decades after its original acquisition by that individual (1).

Herpesvirus and Neurological Latency. Six herpesvirus infections associated with man are currently recognised. Of these, HSV types 1 and 2 and varicella-zoster virus (VZV) have a particular predilection for neurological tissue. These viruses are able to establish latent infections within neurons, especially in the sensory ganglia, where the virus becomes quiescent. Recently is has become apparent that a small part of the virus genetic information is transcribed within the infected neurons and either this mRNA or its translation product probably has a role in maintaining the virus in the non-replicating state (2). Many herpes viruses among the animal kingdom show a relationship with neurons similar to that of the human "neurological" viruses, and together these types of viruses form a subgroup, the alpha herpes viruses (3). There are notable exceptions, for example the alpha herpesvirus of the horse – equine herpesvirus-1 – which does not appear to infect neurons. As will become apparent below, the nature of herpesvirus latency, at least as it occurs in neurons, poses particular problems with regard to antiviral chemotherapy, since the majority of compounds described to date interact with virus proteins which are expressed in the cells only during active virus replication. Furthermore, the prolonged presence of the virus in the host provides the possibility of extensive interaction with antiviral molecules and could consequently increase the likelihood of resistance development.

Queens' College, Cambridge, UK.

Herpes Simplex Virus and Acute Disease. Typically, HSV infects cells at a mucocutaneous junction where the primary infection established is often associated with vesicular lesions. These lesions heal in a few days but the virus has meanwhile translocated via axonal fibres to the neurons of sensory ganglia, where latent virus infection is established. From time to time the latent virus reactivates, giving rise to recurrent virus shedding at the mucosal surface, perhaps with recrudescent disease (1). Sometimes, either the initial infection or the recurrent virus multiplication is subclinical or associated with minimal disease. The intimate relationship between HSV (and VZV) and the nervous system during latency makes it remarkable that overt neurological damage is relatively rare. However, HSV encephalitis does occur spontaneously with a low incidence in the population (approximately $1/10^6$ per annum) (4). This is a devastating disease with a high mortality if untreated. Another situation in which permanent damage to the host may result is when the cornea of the eye is a focus of replication and recurrent ocular disease is established. Thirdly, HSV can be particularly severe in the neonate infected at or shortly after birth. Apart from these relatively rare, sporadic forms of disease, the other situation in which herpes viruses are a major cause of morbidity is when the immune status of the host is compromised. Typically, the pattern of HSV in these cases is one of chronic, gradually spreading lesions which, although not necessarily life-threatening, cause much suffering and may seriously complicate the management of the patient (5). Under these circumstances antiviral chemotherapy (e.g. acyclovir) has recorded its greatest success and in most cases the disease can be controlled by therapy or prevented by prophylaxis. However, it is also emerging that the immunocompromised host provides a situation in which viral drug resistance is particularly likely to become manifest.

Similarity between Herpes Simplex and AIDS. While herpes infections have been recognised for many centuries, human immunodeficiency virus (HIV) has only recently come to light. It is of course a member of the *Retroviridae*, a family which comprises viruses that are completely different from the herpesvirus at the biochemical level. In particular the retrovirus contains two copies of a relatively small, single-strand of RNA compared with the large double-stranded DNA genome of HSV, but there are points of similarity at both the molecular and pathological level which make a comparison useful. For example, both viruses encode the genetic information for a DNA polymerase and in both cases this enzyme has been a prime target for inhibition by or interaction with nucleoside analogues. Like HSV, HIV also appears to characteristically establish a persistent infection which is probably lifelong. DNA of the HIV becomes integrated into the chromosome of host cells and in this form it may become quiescent. This also suggests the possibility of functional latency with a potential for reactivation while providing the virus a haven in which to escape both the immune effector mechanisms and the effects of antiviral agents (6). HIV also interacts with the nervous system, and although it may have a completely different pathogenesis compared with herpes encephalitis (neural cells are not thought to be directly involved with HIV), a progressive neuropathy is encountered and this may require antiviral agents to penetrate the central nervous system to control this aspect of the infection. Finally, because it causes intense immunosuppression. HIV may be associated indirectly with recurrent and severe manifestations of herpesvirus infections in the compromised host.

Herpesviruses — Targets for Chemotherapy

Of all viruses, those which have been most sensitive to inhibitors are members of the *Herpesviridae*. There are a number of reasons for this. The diseases caused by these viruses are common and recurrent, and are therefore commercially attractive to the drug companies. The clinical signs are usually self-limiting, and this has at times encouraged premature judgement of efficacy. Most importantly, the virus codes for several enzymes, of which the thymidine kinase (TK) and DNA-polymerase are particularly useful targets for selective toxicity. Finally, there are numerous tissue cultures and animal models and even isolated enzyme systems in which potential inhibitors can readily be evaluated. Hundreds of compounds have shown some selective inhibition of HSV, at least in vitro. Of this large number several nucleoside analogues have shown clinical efficacy. Adenine arabinoside (Ara-A), iododeoxyuridine and trifluorothymidine have all been licensed for use in humans (7). More recently, acyclovir has been added to this list and is undoubtedly the most successful antiviral drug to date. Several other nucleoside analogues are likely to be used in humans in the future. The pyrophosphate analogues form a class of compounds that differ from the nucleoside analogues; however, they may also interact directly with HSV DNA-polymerase at the pyrophosphate binding site and thereby inhibit enzyme function (8). Phosphonoformate has shown promise in several animal models and has undergone trials in humans under the name "Foscarnet"; while this drug appears to have limited clinical potential for treating herpes infections, it has been very valuable in elucidating the mode of action of other compounds because of its interactions with herpesvirus and other virus-induced polymerases (see below).

Nucleoside and Related Inhibitors of Herpes Simplex Virus. The sensitivity of HSV to a wide range of chemical inhibitors is related to the fact that this virus encodes a group of enzymes (thought to number more than one dozen) mainly involved with nucleotide metabolism, (9) induced in infected cells during the active replication cycle. The successful drugs act by virtue of their formation of substrate analogues for one or more of these enzymes. Selective toxicity is possible because the substrate specificities of the virus-induced enzymes differ from their normal cellular counterparts. The enzyme of paramount importance in this respect is the HSV DNA-polymerase. The majority of drugs in use to date ultimately inhibit the DNA-polymerase or are incorporated by it into the virus DNA chain. Examples are the pyrophosphate analogue phosphonoformate, which interacts directly with the pyrophosphate binding site on the enzyme (8), and acyclovir which in the form of acyclovir-triphosphate competes effectively with the natural substrate dGTP and acts as a suicide inhibitor of the enzyme (10). The older drug iododeoxyuridine is thought to represent the case where the analogue triphosphate is actually incorporated into the virus DNA internally by the virus polymerase, creating abnormal virus genomes (11). A second enzyme of particular importance is the virus-encoded thymidine kinase, which in the case of HSV has a much wider substrate specificity than its cellular counterpart enzymes (12). HSV thymidine kinase phosphorylates acyclovir (and variety of other nucleoside analogues), thus producing active levels of the analogue triphosphate within infected cells while levels of acyclovir-triphosphate in uninfected cells remain low; this probably accounts for the very low toxicity of this drug.

Mechanisms of Drug Resistance

Microbial Resistance to Drugs. All microbes and even eukaryotic cells demonstrate an ability to subvert cytotoxic and cytostatic drugs by means of genetic change (13). Drug-resistant variants are strains which show a markedly decreased sensitivity to a given compound. The term is commonly applied to strains that fail to be inhibited by the drug at concentrations that are readily obtained in vivo. The sensitivity of the strain is usually determined by a convenient test performed in vitro. The mechanisms of drug resistance are numerous and vary widely in bacteria and eukaryotic cells. The mechanisms by which viruses can acquire resistance are probably restricted to the process by which mutations in the genome give rise to simple alteration in one or more virus proteins which in turn are relieved from the drug interaction.

Virus Resistance to Drugs. Mutants resistant to a variety of drugs have been isolated from several different viruses to date and some examples shown in Table 1 illustrate this diversity. Given the high mutation rate (14) and the enormous in vivo replication potential among viruses, it is clear that they could readily subvert therapy were it not true that severe constraints operate on the selection of mutant viruses during chemotherapy. This is suggested because development of resistance to drugs such as acyclovir appears to be relatively rare in humans compared with the ready selection of resistant mutants in tissue culture systems. The virus genome and the proteins it induces in the cell form a complex and highly interactive process. Many genetic loci and virus-induced products are likely to have multiple roles. It may be that the majority of resistant variants are less pathogenic than their progenitor strains.

Table 1: Examples of viruses in which drug resistance has been demonstrated. (Reference numbers in parentheses).

Virus family	Compounds[a]	Animals[b]	Man[c]
Pox			
vaccinia	thiosemicarbazones nucleoside analogues pyrophosphate analogues	yes	
Herpes			
HSV	numerous nucleoside	yes	yes
VZ	and pyrophosphate		yes(75)
CMV	analogues aphidicolin [ribavirin] [carbonoxalone]		yes(76)
Picorna			
polio	guanidine	yes	
foot&mouth			
rhinovirus	chalcones dichloroflavan rhodanine, arildone [flavone] [enviroxime]	yes	yes(77)
Toga			
sinbis	ribavirin		
Orthomyxo			
influenza A	amantadine	yes	yes(78)
fowl plague	rimantadine norakin [ribavirin]	yes	
Retro			
murine	phosphonofolmate		
retroviruses	coumermycin		
HIV	azidothymidine[d] (79)		

[a] Resistance obtained by passage in tissue culture in the presence of drug.
[b] Resistance obtained from experimentally infected, drug-treated animals.
[c] Resistance observed among clinical isolates.
[d] Shown by site specific mutagenesis using an isolated enzyme system.
[ ] = Resistance sought but not observed to date.

Occasionally, perhaps, a series of genetic changes gives rise to a virulent resistant clone. The immunocompromised host may provide a special environment which is less exacting for the infecting virus and in which less pathogenic variants have the opportunity to thrive. As discussed below, most examples of clinical resistance to acyclovir to date have been encountered in immunosuppressed patients.

Drug Resistant Variants as a Research Tool. Resistant variants have the potential to subvert effective clinical or prophylactic use of drugs, however, such mutants have enormous value in elucidating many aspects of virus-host-drug interactions. Some of these uses are summarised in Table 2. Perhaps of particular significance is that the demonstration of clinical resistance in vivo (when sensitive strains respond to therapy) is a clear indication of a direct effect upon virus replication by the drug in question. This proves that the drug is not working by some other effect such as the activation of macrophages or the inhibition of an intercurrent infection. Such an approach will be useful in the evaluation of certain novel compounds currently being used in AIDS chemotherapy. These principles have been established from experience with several drugs, especially the inhibitors of HSV. However, this experience gained with HSV forms an invaluable background when approaching newer problems such as the chemotherapy of HIV (6) or hepatitis B infections (15). This is particularly true when examining novel drugs with modes of action which are proposed to be completely different from compounds studied previously. One point which should be stressed is that the mutants which have been fully characterised in a number of different virus systems all suggest that a single point mutation leading to a single amino-acid substitution can be suffi-

Table 2: Some of the uses for which resistant mutants have been employed.

1. Elucidation of drug mode of action.
   a. Identification of virus products which interact with drug.
   b. Rational design of novel substrate analogues.
2. Proof of true selective toxicity.
   a. In tissue culture systems.
   b. In animal models and in man.
3. Genetic analysis.
   a. As phenotypic markers.
   b. Selection systems for marker rescue.
   c. Ready introduction of mutations into specific genes for functional analysis, e.g. effects on pathogenesis.
4. The study of clinical resistance.
   a. Defining the variety and nature of resistant mutants.
   b. The development of test systems for resistance detection.
   c. Defining circumstances for resistance development.
   d. Developing strategies to circumvent resistance.

cient to cause a 100-fold increase in resistance. It follows from the above account that drug resistance to many inhibitors of HSV is likely to involve changes in the genes encoding the thymidine kinase and DNA-polymerase. Mutant viruses obtained by selection in vitro and subsequently from infected patients have confirmed this hypothesis.

Mechanisms of Drug Resistance in Herpesviruses

Thymidine Kinase, I: TK-Defective Mutants. Foundation studies of Dubbs and Kit (16) in the early 1960s concerning the acquired resistance by strains of HSV to bromodeoxyuridine and iododeoxyuridine provided the first evidence that the elevation in thymidine kinase activity in HSV-infected cells resulted from the induction of a virus-coded protein with kinase function. It was apparent that loss of this function by a virus strain conferred resistance to drugs whose activity depended at least in part on phosphorylation within the infected cells by virus-coded enzymes. Characterization of individual resistant mutants suggested that such viruses induced truncated thymidine kinase polypeptides following premature termination at a stop codon (17). At this time drug resistance was already suspected to be a clinical problem, particularly in relation to the treatment of herpetic eye disease (18). With the advent of acyclovir interest once again focused on mechanisms of resistance, and one of the first papers to describe the novel compound (at that time known as acycloguanosine) recorded that temperature-sensitive mutants in the thymidine kinase locus were relatively insensitive to the drug (19). Two papers produced shortly after this showed unequivocally that the genetic lesions in a number of acyclovir-resistant mutants mapped to either the thymidine kinase or DNA-polymerase locus (20, 21). As expected, selection of thymidine kinase resistance to a particular analogue conferred resistance to other drugs which shared the requirement for virus thymidine kinase activation (22). It should also be noted that the degree of resistance depends on the type of cells in which the virus is replicating. In some cases the actual fold-increase in resistance is small, suggesting that cellular kinases may be bypassing the deficit in the virus itself (23). This is pertinent to the design of in vitro tests for screening clinical isolates for resistance. Although widely observed in tissue culture it is still unclear how these cellular effects are reflected in the variety of differentiated cells in which HSV replicates in the natural infection in humans.

Thymidine Kinase, II: Mutants Which Induce an Altered TK. While attempting to induce viruses with lesions confined to DNA-polymerase, Darby et al. inadvertently discovered a class of acyclovir-resistant mutants which induced a mutated thymidine kinase that retained phosphorylating function (24). The thymidine kinase unduced by such mutants was found to have a changed substrate specificity, resulting in resistance to one or more nucleoside analogues. The phenomenon was not confined to acyclovir, for example, analogous mutants were isolated following selection with bromovinyldeoxyuridine (25) and methoxymethyldeoxyuridine (26). The study of purified enzyme extracts of such mutants provided strong biochemical evidence that the change in sensitivity of the virus to inhibition was a direct result of changes in the biochemical properties of the enzyme as measured in vitro (27). Finally, a number of resistant mutants have now been analysed by means of DNA sequencing. The profound changes in the biochemical and biological properties of the mutant viruses result from single base changes leading to single amino acid substitutions in the thymidine kinase structural gene (28, 29). Clearly, the analysis of these mutants and others which are being characterised can provide valuable information about the conformation of the enzyme-active site and aid in the design of new analogues (30).

DNA-Polymerase. As stated above, the key enzyme involved in the inhibition of HSV by many nucleoside analogues is DNA-polymerase. Many mutants whose resistance maps to the DNA-polymerase locus have been isolated in tissue culture (31). Using a strategy similar to that described for the HSV thymidine kinase mutants, sequencing techniques revealed particular regions in the enzyme which are prone to vary (again as a result of single point mutations and consequent amino acid substitutions), leading to drug resistance to particular analogues (32, 33). Again, patterns of cross-resistance between compounds are complex but viruses selected for resistance to the pyrophosphate analogues, e.g. phosphonoformate, commonly have acquired co-resistance to nucleoside analogues (34).

Resistance in HSV Determined at Alternative Loci. To date, no other sites of drug resistance have been confirmed in HSV following selection of virus mutants resistant to nucleoside analogues. However, one of a series of putative DNA-polymerase mutants analysed by Larder et al. (33) revealed no nucleotide substitutions in the DNA-polymerase sequence. This led to speculation that other peptides involved in the polymerase complex could be likely candidates for resistance; one possibility is one of the DNA binding proteins. Mutants resistant to the drug aphidicolin (which is also an inhibitor of DNA-polymerase activity) have been isolated and the lesions were found to map to the major DNA binding protein (35). Given the complex interactions between the various virus-induced proteins, it will be surprising if other sites are not involved in resistance to nucleoside analogues such as acyclovir. Effective inhibitors of HSV which work independently of the thymidine kinase or DNA-polymerase pathway are very few in number. It has not proved possible to develop mutants resistant to ribavirin (36) or to the glycorhyzic acid derivative, carbonoxalone (D. J. Dargan, personal communication). For a drug to which no resistant mutants can be isolated, the possibility remains, until direct evidence proves otherwise, that the compound does not have a specific mode of antiviral action.

Resistant Mutants in Clinical Practice

Resistance in Ocular Herpes. From the outset, clinicians treating ocular HSV with nucleoside inhibitors gained the impression that drug resistance might account for clinical failure, although this was difficult to prove formally (37). In any case the efficacy of the early antiviral drugs was relatively poor and many other explanations may have accounted for failed therapy. However, clinicians continued to report that treatment failure could be overcome by switching to alternative drugs (38), and virus strains with biochemically proven resistance especially to iododeoxyuridine have been reported (39, 40). It appears that resistance following topical therapy in ocular herpes occurs more readily to iododeoxyuridine than to acyclovir both in animal models (see below) and in clinical practice, although there is no clear explanation yet as to why this should be so.

Resistance in Herpes Encephalitis. One of the most successful areas of deployment of antiherpetic drugs has been in the treatment of herpes encephalitis (41). Early studies with Ara-A proved it beyond doubt to be beneficial in improving survival and reducing sequelae. More recently, acyclovir was found to compare favourably with Ara-A (4). The total number of encephalitis cases treated to date is still very small compared with the more typical labial and genital forms of HSV infection, but it is worth mentioning that no evidence of clinical resistance has yet been observed and in no case has resistance been thought to have compromised the therapy. However, the examination of clinical isolates, including some obtained from encephalitis cases, revealed the presence of a small proportion of virions with lesions in the DNA-polymerase conferring drug resistance (42). But as stated, there is no evidence to suggest that these virions within the total population were significant in the viral response to the inhibitors used in the chemotherapy of herpes encephalitis.

Resistance in Labial and Genital Herpes. Since the introduction of acyclovir, the sensitivity of clinical isolates to the drug before, during, and after therapy has been closely monitored. In very large surveys the majority of clinical isolates show no decrease in sensitivity, although occasional isolates are encountered which appear to be resistant (43–45). Those resistant isolates which have been isolated and characterised fit very closely with laboratory mutants which have already been studied. The majority of resistant isolates are thymidine kinase-defective and this accounts for their loss of sensitivity. A very small number of strains possessing thymidine kinase with altered substrate specificity such that they are capable of phosphorylating thymidine but not acyclovir have been encountered (46), and at least one DNA-polymerase resistant mutant has been isolated from a human (47). It is of interest that a mutant strain of HSV type 2, whose thymidine kinase gene has been cloned and sequenced (12), contained a single base change as observed in the laboratory isolates examined previously. Furthermore one isolate of HSV type 1 with an altered DNA-polymerase was found to have a base substitution identical to one already encountered in a laboratory-selected mutant (G. K. Darby, personal communication).

Drug Resistance in Prophylactic HSV Therapy. Classically, herpes simplex infections follow a pattern of latency and recurrence. There are two situations where the frequency of virus shedding is such that the infection may be described as truly persistent. One situation, that of the immunocompromised host, will be considered separately below. In addition, certain individuals whose immune system is not measurably abnormal (although specific defects may exist) do suffer frequent if not continuous herpes lesions. Clearly there is a wide spectrum of a recurrent/persistent pattern of disease, but patients of this type have been candidates for long-term chronic prophylactic therapy with oral acyclovir. Such therapy is effective in suppressing virus replication and preventing recrudescent disease (48, 49). These clinical trials have been monitored particularly closely for the development of resistant strains. Breakthrough recurrences do occur and early observations suggested that these may be associated with reduced sensitivity to the drug (50). Although resistant isolates have been obtained there is no consistent pattern of resistance development, and contrary to the more pessimistic predictions, resistance has not emerged as the major cause of treatment failures; other explanations such as patient non-compliance with regular dosing regimens have been invoked (49). While accepting the evidence at face value — that drug resistance is not the major limiting factor — it would be foolish to discount completely a phenomenon which clearly exists and can result in treatment failure. We should continue to question the in vitro systems currently available for drug sensitivity testing in case they do not provide an accurate reflection of drug sensitivity in vivo (51–53). Methods for analysing drug sensitivity in vitro have been considered in detail elsewhere (54). Furthermore, the question of mixtures of virions with different phenotypes within a virus population has yet to be fully explored, a point which will be elaborated below.

Drug Resistance in the Immunocompromised Host. The majority of drug-resistant strains of HSV have been obtained from immunosuppressed patients (48, 55–58). There are two likely reasons for this. First, it is clear that virus replication may be prolonged, having a tendency toward true persistence. Second, and most important, the host-responses to infection are impaired and less pathogenic viruses that would not survive in the face of normal host responses may continue to replicate. However, even if some resistant viruses are less-pathogenic it is clear that they are capable of producing overt disease in this type of patient (59). A majority of mutant viruses isolated from immunocompromised patients have been found to be thymidine kinase-defective; such mutants are usually mixed together with normal virions (46, 60). When plaque-purified thymidine kinase-defective viruses have noticeably reduced pathogenicity when tested in a variety of animal models (61, 62). There is an extensive literature on the pathogenicity of thymidine kinase-defective HSV, the consensus being that such viruses have greatly reduced ability to establish latent infections and markedly less ability to damage the nervous system (of the non-human host) following potentially lethal inoculations, although these properties can be modified by the presence of wild-type (thymidine kinase-inducing) virus (63). Several examples exist of multiple disease episodes in patients in which acyclovir therapy has been employed and multiple isolates have been examined for evidence of resistance. An important observation in such patients is that following the development of resistance during a particular episode of disease, subsequent isolates may be of a sensitive virus phenotype (50). This is consistent with the view that the latent infection established with the pre-therapy sensitive virus was responsible for subsequent reactivations. It suggests that ganglionic neurons colonised during recurrent episodes of virus shedding do not necessarily contribute significantly to later reactivation events, although it is premature to conclude that this will not occur in some cases. It is becoming clear that drug resistance in the immunocompromised host is not confined to HSV. For example, cytomegalovirus strains resistant to dihydroxypropoxymethylguanosine have already been encountered in these patients (64) and it is likely that drug-resistant variants of a wide variety of other microbes will be found among such patients.

Models for Resistance Development in the Laboratory

Tissue Culture Models and Cell Free Systems. The development of resistant variants can be demonstrated readily in a variety of tissue culture systems. Resistance to thymidine kinase-mediated drugs such as acyclovir occurs with high frequency; the viruses multiply with kinetics similar to wild types and this poses a problem for the selection of mutants with more "subtle lesions". A variety of special selection systems have been devised to accomplish this; for example, thymidine kinase-transformed cells or serum-starved cells have been used to reduce the selective advantage of the thymidine kinase-deficient phenotype (24). More recently it has been possible to engineer recombinant viruses with deletions or mutations introduced into specific genes or base-specific loci (30). While these systems can give much insight into the mechanisms of resistance (63), the circumstances which may lead to clinical resistance can be approached more directly by the use of animal models.

Animal Models for Resistance Development. Three strategies exist for examining resistance development in animal models. Normal animals in which recurrences occur repeatedly, either naturally or following a reactivation stimulus, can be employed. The most suitable systems are guinea pig genital infections, rabbit eye infections in which epinephron iontophoresis is used to stimulate recurrences, or murine skin models in which local trauma is used to produce recurrences. The development of resistance to iododeoxyuridine has been observed in rabbits following repeated topical administration (65), but when effective chemotherapy with acyclovir has been employed in these models resistance has not readily been observed and this seems to reflect the observations in humans. The second approach is to repeatedly passage virus in animals receiving chemotherapy. This was first used to demonstrate poxvirus resistance in mice (66), and later, influenza virus resistance in mice, (67) and more recently, in chickens (68, 69). In these studies the viruses which were isolated appeared similar to tissue culture-selected mutants. The same strategy applied to HSV infection of mice also yielded a resistant virus population (70). Moreover, latent infections could be established in mice using such "resistant" inocula, and explantation of the ganglia yielded resistant, pathogenic populations of virions following reactivation from the cultured tissue (71). The third strategy for selection of resistant viruses has been to use immunocompromised animals, and in the case of HSV, this has proved to be the most efficient system. Nude (athymic) mice inoculated with HSV and treated with acyclovir develop chronic, indolent lesions from which resistant virus can be isolated (72). Similar results have been obtained with X-irradiated mice and mice treated with the immunosuppressive drug cyclosporin-A (unpublished observations). These experiments appear to provide situations which resemble closely the development of resistance in humans under the circumstances of immunosuppression, suggesting that they are good models for testing strategies such as drug combinations or the use of alternating drug regimens.

Role of Virus Mixtures. Both in humans and in the various animal models for resistance development it has been observed that virus isolates are often heterogeneous and contain virions with a resistant phenotype (46, 60). It is notable that a recently described (73) clinical isolate of HSV type 2, which induces thymidine kinase with altered substrate specificity, was also shown to contain a mixture of distinctly different viruses which could be separated by plaque purification. Animal experiments suggest that the properties of mixtures differ from the individual component strains studied in plaque-purified stock (70, 71). The existence of virus mixtures may be masked in some of the in vitro systems used to test for virus sensitivity (51, 52); however, it is likely that these mixtures play a very important role in HSV response to inhibitors and thus should be a focus of attention in future studies.

Transmission of Infection and Resistance. As the use of acyclovir becomes more widespread, secondary infections acquired from those already under chemotherapy will become more common. To date there is no evidence of a higher incidence of resistance in patients undergoing chemotherapy, but the results of experiments in animal models mentioned above and the observations of immunocompromised patients suggest that this is likely. Since resistance is possible and some resistant strains clearly have pathogenic potential, it is hard to believe that in time resistant strains will not become prevalent. However, whether the time scale be years or decades is hard to predict from our current knowledge of resistance mechanisms and infection models.

Future Prospects

Clinical Drug Resistant in Microbes. Despite our poor understanding of the role of resistance in clinical practice, resistance to nuceloside analogues is well understood at a biochemical level. Much work on how these changes in the virus may be reflected in the biological function of the virus has already been carried out in a variety of model systems. While resistance in bacteria and other microbes has been known and studied for much longer, these new observations in the relatively simple virus systems offer important models for phenomena which may have a much wider significance. For example, the effects of drug resistance mutations leading to changes in pathogenicity as well as the role of resistant components of mixtures can be researched more readily in virus systems and the observations can have relevance to larger and more complex microorganisms.

The use of nucleoside analogues to combat HIV is the beginning of a new era of antiviral therapy (74). The causative agent is completely different from that of HSV and the mechanisms of drug resistance, if encountered, will be different at the molecular level. However, the ways in which HSV resistance has been approached in the laboratory offer valuable experience and clear guidelines which should be helpful in approaching similar problems with new viral diseases.

References

1. Wildy, P., Field, H. J., Nash, A. A.: Classical herpes latency revisited. In: Mahy, B. W. J., Minson, A. C., Darby, G. K. (ed.): Virus persistence. Society for General Microbiology. Symposium 33, Cambridge University Press, Cambridge, 1982, p. 133–167.
2. Spivack, J. G., Fraser, N. W.: Expression of herpes simplex virus type 1 latency-associated transcripts in the trigeminal ganglia of mice during acute infection and reactivation of latent infection. Journal of Virolology 1988, 62: 1479–1485.
3. Roizman, B., Batterson, W.: Herpesviruses and their replication. In: Field, B. N., Knipe, D. M., Chanock, R. M., Melnick, J. L., Roizman, B., Shope, R. E. (ed.): Field's virology. Raven Press, New York, 1985, p. 497–526.
4. Whitley, R. J.: Treatment of human herpes virus infections with special reference to encephalitis. Journal of Antimicrobial Chemotherapy 1984, 14 (Supplement A): 57–74.
5. Whitley, R. J., Levin, M., Barton, N., Hershey, B. J., Davis, G., Keeney, R. E., Whelchel, J., Diethelm, A. G., Kartus, P., Soong, S.-J.: Infections due to herpes simplex virus in the immunocompromised host: natural history and acyclovir therapy. Journal of Infectious Diseases 1984, 150: 323–329.
6. Mitsuya, H., Broder, S.: Strategies for antiviral therapy in AIDS. Nature 1987, 325: 773–778.
7. Hovi, T.: Successful selective inhibitors of viruses. In: Field, H. J. (Ed.): Antiviral agents: development and assessment of antiviral chemotherapy. CRC Press, Fla., 1988, p. 1–21.
8. Oberg, B.: Antiviral effects of phosphonoformate (PFA, foscarnet sodium). Pharmacology and Therapeutics 1983, 19: 387–415.
9. Oberg, B.: Inhibitors of virus-specific enzymes. In: Stuart-Harris, C. H., Oxford, J. (ed.): Problems of antiviral therapy. Academic Press, London, 1983, p. 35–69.
10. Elion, G. B.: The biochemistry and mechanism of action of acyclovir. Journal of Antimicrobial Chemotherapy 1983, 12 (Supplement B): 9–17.
11. Prusoff, W. H., Fischer, P. H.: Basis for the selective antiviral and antitumour activity of pyrimidine nucleoside analogues. In: Walker, R. T., De Clercq, E., Eckstein, F. (ed.): Nucleoside analogues, chemistry, biology, and medical applications. Plenum Press, New York, 1979, p. 281–318.
12. Kit, S.: Thymidine kinase. Microbiological Science 1985, 2: 369–375.
13. Oxford, J. S., Field, H. J., Reeves, D. S. (ed.): Drug resistance in viruses, other microbes and eukaryotes. Academic Press, London, 1986, p. iii et seq.
14. Coen, D. M.: General aspects of virus drug resistance with special reference to herpes simplex virus. Journal of Antimicrobial Chemotherapy 1986, 18 (Supplement B): 1–10.
15. Thomas, H. C., Scully, L. J.: Antiviral therapy in hepatitis B infection. British Medical Bulletin 1985, 41: 374–380.
16. Dubbs, D. R., Kit, S.: Mutant strains of herpes simplex deficient in thymidine kinase-inducing activity. Virology 1964, 22: 493–502.
17. Summers, W. P., Wagner, M., Summers, W. C.: Possible peptide chain termination mutants in thymidine kinase gene of a mammalian virus, herpes simplex virus. Proceedings of the National Academy of Sciences USA 1975, 72: 4081–4084.
18. Coleman, V. R., Tsu, E., Jawetz, E.: "Treatment resistance" to idoxuridine in herpetic keratitis. Proceedings of the Society for Experimental Biology and Medicine 1968, 129: 761–765.
19. Elion, G. B., Furman, J. A., Fyfe, J. A., De Miranda, P., Beauchamp, L., Schaeffer, H. J.: Selectivity of action of an antiherpetic agent, 9-(2-(hydroxyethoxymethyl)guanine. Proceedings of the National Academy of Sciences USA 1978, 74: 5716–5720.
20. Coen, D. M., Schaffer, P. A.: Two distinct loci confer resistance to acycloguanosine in herpes simplex virus type 1. Proceedings of the National Academy of Sciences USA 1980, 77: 2265–2269.
21. Schnipper, L. E., Crumpacker, C. S.: Resistance of herpes simplex virus to acycloguanosine: role of viral thymidine kinase and DNA polymerase loci. Proceedings of the National Academy of Sciences USA 1980, 77: 2270–2273.
22. Field, H., MacMillan, A., Darby, G.: The sensitivity of acyclovir-resistant mutants of herpes simplex virus to other antiviral drugs. Journal of Infectious Diseases 1981, 143: 281–285.
23. Field, H. J., Darby, G., Wildy, P.: Isolation and characterization of acyclovir-resistant mutants of herpes simplex virus. Journal of General Virology 1980, 49: 115–124.
24. Darby, G., Field, H. J., Salisbury, S. A.: Altered substrate specificity of herpes simplex virus thymidine kinase confers acyclovir-resistance. Nature 1981, 289: 81–83.
25. Larder, B. A., Cheng, Y.-C., Darby, G.: Characterization of abnormal thymidine kinases induced by drug-resistant strains of herpes simplex virus type 1. Journal of General Virology 1983, 64: 523–532.
26. Veerisetty, V., Gentry, G. A.: Alterations in substrate specificity and physicochemical properties of deoxythymidine kinase of a drug-resistant herpes simplex virus type 1 mutant. Journal of Virology 1983, 46: 901–908.
27. Larder, B. A., Derse, D., Cheng, Y.-C., Darby, G.: Properties of purified enzymes induced by pathogenic drug-resistant mutants of herpes simplex virus. Evidence for virus variants expressing normal DNA polymerase and altered thymidine kinase. Journal of Biological Chemistry 1983, 285: 2027–2033.
28. Darby, G., Larder, B. A., Inglis, M. M.: Evidence that the "active centre" of the herpes simplex virus thymiine kinase involves an interaction between three distinct regions of the polypeptide. Journal of General Virology 1986, 67: 753–758.
29. Kit, S., Sheppard, M., Ichimura, H., Nusinoff-Lehrman, S., Ellis, N. M., Fyfe, J. A., Otsuka, H.: Nucleotide sequence changes in the thymidine kinase gene of herpes simplex virus type 2 clones from a patient treated with acyclovir. Antimicrobial Agents and Chemotherapy 1987, 31: 1483–1490.
30. Inglis, M. M., Darby, G.: Analyses of the role of the cystein 171 residue in the activity of herpes simplex virus

type 1 thymidine kinase by oligonucleotide-directed mutagenesis. Journal of General Virology 1987, 68: 39–46.
31. Coen, D. M., Chiou, H. C., Fleming, H. E., Jr., Leslie, L. K., Retondon, M. J.: Drug resistant and hypersensitive herpes simplex virus mutants: isolation and application to dissection of the pol locus. In: Rapp, F. (ed.): Herpesvirus. Allan R. Liss, New York, 1984, p. 373–385.
32. Honess, R. W., Purifoy, D. J. M., Young, D., Gopal, R., Cammack, N., O'Hare, P.: Single mutations at many sites within the DNA polymerase locus of herpes simplex viruses can confer hypersensitivity to aphidicolin and resistance to phosphonoacetic acid. Journal of General Virology 1984, 65: 1–17.
33. Larder, B. A., Kemp, S. D., Darby, G.: Related functional domains in virus DNA polymerase. EMBO Journal 1987, 6: 169–175.
34. Larder, B. A., Darby, G.: Virus drug-resistance: mechanisms and consequences. Antiviral Research 1984, 4: 1–42.
35. Chiou, H. C., Weller, S. K., Coen, D. M.: Mutations in the herpes simplex virus major DNA binding protein gene leading to altered sensitivity to DNA polymerase inhibitors. Virology 1985, 145: 213–226.
36. Allen, L. B., Fingal, C. M.: Failure of type 1 herpesvirus to develop resistance to Ribavirin. Antimicrobial Agents and Chemotherapy 1977, 12: 120–121.
37. Jawetz, E., Coleman, W. R., Dawson, C. R., Thygeson, P.: The dynamics of IUDR action in herpetic keratitis and the emergence of IUDR-resistance in vivo. Annals of the New York Academy of Science 1970, 173: 282–291.
38. McGill, J., Scott, G. M.: Viral keratitis. British Medical Bulletin 1985, 41: 351–356.
39. Hirano, A., Yumura, K., Kurimura, T., Katsumoto, T., Moriyama, H., Manabe, R.: Analysis of herpes simplex virus isolated from patients with recurrent herpes keratitis exhibiting "treatment resistance" to 5-iodo-2'-deoxyuridine. Acta Virologica 1979, 23: 226–230.
40. Funderburgh, M. L., Funderburgh, J. L., Chandler, J. W.: Thymidine kinase activity of ocular herpes simplex isolates resistant to IDUR therapy. Investigative Ophalmology and Visual Science 1986, 27: 1546–1548.
41. Anderson, J. R.: The chemotherapy of herpes simplex encephalitis in man. In Field, H. J. (ed.): Antiviral agents: the development and assessment of antiviral chemotherapy. CRC Press, Fla., 1988, p. 1–12.
42. Parris, D. S., Harrington, J. E.: Herpes simplex virus variants resistant to high concentrations of acyclovir exist in clinical isolates. Antimicrobial Agents and Chemotherapy 1982, 22: 71–77.
43. Barry, D. W., Lehrman, S. N., Ellis, M. N.: Clinical and laboratory experience with acyclovir-resistant herpes viruses. Journal of Antimicrobial Chemotherapy 1986, 18 (Supplement B): 75–84.
44. McLaren, C., Corey, L., Dekker, C., Barry, D. W.: In vitro sensitivity to acyclovir in genital herpes simplex virus from acyclovir-treated patients. Journal of Infectious Diseases 1983, 148: 868–875.
45. Collins, P., Oliver, N. M.: Sensitivity monitoring of herpes simplex virus isolates from patients receiving acyclovir. Journal of Antimicrobial Chemotherapy 1986, 18 (Supplement B): 103–112.
46. Martin, J. L., Ellis, M. N., Keller, P. M., Biron, K. K., Lehrman, S. N., Barry, D. W., Furmin, P. A.: Plaque autoradiographic assay for the detection and quantitation of thymidine kinase-deficient and thymidine kinase-altered mutants of herpes simplex in clinical isolates. Antimicrobial Agents and Chemotherapy 1985, 28: 181–187.
47. Parker, A. C., Craig, J. I. O., Collins, P., Oliver, N., Smith, I.: Acyclovir-resistant herpes simplex virus infection due to altered DNA polymerase. Lancet 1987, ii: 1461.
48. Anderson, H., Scarfe, J. H., Sutton, R. N. P., Hickmot, E., Brigden, D., Burke, C.: Oral acyclovir prophylaxis against herpes simplex virus in non-Hodgkin lymphoma and acute lymphoblastic leukaemia patients receiving remission induction chemotherapy. A randomised double blind, placebo controlled trial. British Journal of Cancer 1984, 50: 45–49.
49. Gold, D., Corey, L.: Acyclovir prophylaxis for herpes simplex virus infection. Antimicrobial Agents and Chemotherapy 1987, 31: 361–367.
50. Strauss, S. E., Takiff, H. E., Seidlin, M., Bachrach, S., Lininger, L., DiGiovanna, J. J., Western, K. A., Smith, H. A., Lehrman, S. N., Creagh-Kirk, T., Alling, D. W.: Suppression of frequently occurring genital herpes. A placebo-controlled double-blind trial with acyclovir. New England Journal of Medicine 1984, 310: 1545–1550.
51. Harmenberg, J., Sundqvist, V.-A., Gadler, H., Leven, B., Brannstrom, G., Wahren, B.: Comparative methods for detection of thymidine kinase-deficient herpes simplex virus type 1 strains. Antimicrobial Agents and Chemotherapy 1986, 30: 570–573.
52. Harmenberg, J., Wahren, B., Sundqvist, V.-A., Leven, B.: Multiplicity dependence of sensitivity of herpes simplex virus isolates to antiviral compounds. Journal of Antimicrobial Chemotherapy 1985, 15: 567–573.
53. Swierkosz, E. M., Scholl, D. R., Brown, J. L., Jollick, J. D., Gleaves, C. A.: Improved DNA hybridization method for detection of acyclovir-resistant herpes simplex virus. Antimicrobial Agents and Chemotherapy 1987, 31: 1465–1469.
54. Field, H. J.: Development of Antiviral Resistance. In: Field, H. J. (ed.): Antiviral agents, the development and assessment of antiviral chemotherapy. CRC Press, Fla., 1987, p. 127–149.
55. Burns, W. H., Saral, R., Santos, G. W., Laskin, O. L., Leithan, P. S., McLaren, C., Barry, D. W.: Isolation and characterisation of resistant herpes simplex virus after acyclovir therapy. Lancet 1982, i: 421–423.
56. Wade, J. C., Newton, B., McLaren, C., Flournoy, N., Keeney, R. E., Meyers, J. D.: Intravenous acyclovir to treat mucocutaneous herpes simplex virus infection after bone marrow transplantation. Annals of Internal Medicine 1982, 96: 265–269.
57. Crumpacker, C. S., Schnipper, L. E., Marlowe, S. I., Kowalsky, P. N., Hershey, B. J., Levin, M. J.: Resistance to antiviral drugs of herpes simplex virus isolated from a patient treated with acyclovir. New England Journal of Medicine 1982, 306: 343–346.
58. Field, H. J.: Resistance and latency. British Medical Bulletin 1985, 41: 345–350.
59. Bean, B., Fletcher, C., Englund, J., Lehrman, S. N., Ellis, M. N.: Progressive mucocutaneous herpes simplex infection due to acyclovir-resistant virus in an immunocompromised patient: correlation of viral susceptibilities and plasma levels with response to therapy. Diagnostic Microbiology and Infectious Disease 1987, 7: 199–204.
60. Christophers, J., Sutton, R. N. P.: Characterization of acyclovir-resistant and sensitive clinical isolates of herpes simplex virus from an immunocompromised patient. Journal of Antimicrobial Chemotherapy 1987, 20: 389–398.
61. Sibrack, C. D., Gutman, L. T., Wilfert, C. M., McClaren, C., St. Clair, M. H., Keller, P. M., Barry, D. W.: Pathogenicity of acyclovir-resistant herpes simplex virus type 1 from an immunodeficient child. Journal of Infectious Diseases 1982, 146: 673–682.

62. Field, H. J., Darby, G.: Pathogenicity in mice of strains of herpes simplex virus which are resistant to acyclovir in vitro and in vivo. Antimicrobial Agents and Chemotherapy 1980, 17: 209–216.
63. Field, H. J., Owen, L.: The problem of virus drug resistance in antiviral drug development. In: De Clercq, E., Walker, R. T. (ed.): Antiviral drug development: a multidisciplinary approach. Plenum Press, New York, 1988, p. 203–236.
64. Biron, K. K., Fyfe, J. A., Stanat, S. C., Leslie, L. K., Sorrell, J. B., Lambe, C. U., Coen, D. M.: A human cytomegalovirus mutant resistant to the nucleoside analog 9-([2-hydroxy-1(hydroxymethyl)ethoxy] methyl) guanine (BW B759U) induces reduced levels of BW B759U triphosphate. Proceedings of the National Academy of Science USA 1986, 83: 8769–8773.
65. Denis, J., Langois, M., Elkaim, M., Amiel, C., Aymard, M., Huraux, J. M.: HSV1 strain sensitivity in experimental rabbit keratitis: evolution under repeated topical IDU administrations. Current Eye Research 1987, 6: 39–45.
66. Appleyard, G., Way, H.: Thiosemicarbazone-resistant rabbitpox virus. British Journal of Experimental Pathology 1966, 47: 144–151.
67. Oxford, J. S., Logan, I. S., Potter, C. W.: In vivo selection of an influenza A2 strain resistant to amantadine. Nature 1970, 226: 82–83.
68. Webster, R. G., Kawaoka, Y., Bean, W. J.: Vaccination as a strategy to reduce the emergence of amantadine and rimantadine resistant strains of A/chick/Pennsylvania/83 (H5N2) influenza virus. Journal of Antimicrobial Chemotherapy 1986, 18 (Supplement B): 157–164.
69. Beard, C. W., Brugh, M., Webster, R. G.: Emergence of amantadine-resistant H5N2 avian influenza virus during a simulated layer flock treatment program. Avian Diseases 1987, 31: 533–537.
70. Field, H. J.: Development of clinical resistance to acyclovir in herpes simplex virus-infected mice receiving oral therapy. Antimicrobial Agents and Chemotherapy 1982, 21: 744–752.
71. Field, H. J., Lay, E.: Characterization of latent infections in mice after inoculation with herpes simplex virus which is clinically resistant to acyclovir. Antiviral Research 1984, 4: 43–52.
72. Ellis, M. N., Martin J. L., Lobe, D. C., Johnsrude, J. D., Barry, D. W.: Induction of acyclovir-resistant mutants of herpes simplex virus type 1 in athymic nude mice. Journal of Antimicrobial Chemotherapy 1986, 18 (Supplement B): 95–101.
73. Ellis, M. N., Keller, P. M., Fyfe, J. A., Martin, J. L., Rooney, J. F., Straus, S. E., Nusinoff Lehrman, S., Barry, D. W.: Clinical isolate of herpes simplex type 2 that induces thymidine kinase with altered substrate specificity. Antimicrobial Agents and Chemotherapy 1987, 31: 1117–1125.
74. De Clercq, E.: New selective antiviral agents active against AIDS viruses. Trends in Pharmacological Science 1987, 8: 339–345.
75. Shiraki, K., Ogino, T., Yamanishi, K., Takahashi, M.: Isolation of drug resistant mutants of varicella-zoster virus: cross resistance of acyclovir resistant mutant with phosphonoacetic acid and bromodeoxyuridine. Biken Journal 1983, 26: 17–23.
76. Biron, K. K., Fyfe, J. A., Stanat, S. C., Leslie, L. K., Sorrell, J. B., Lambe, C. U., Coen, D. M.: A human cytomegalovirus mutant resistant to the nucleoside analog 9-([2-hydroxy-1(hydroxymethyl)ethoxy]methyl) guanine (BW B759U) induces reduced levels of BW B759U triphosphate. Proceedings of the National Academy of Sciences USA 1986, 83: 8769–8773.
77. Al-Nakib, W., Yasin, S., Dearden, C. J.: In vitro and in vivo development of drug resistance by rhinoviruses. Antiviral Research 1988, 9: 128.
78. Pemberton, R. M., Jennings, R., Potter, C. W., Oxford, J. S.: Amantadine resistance in clinical influenza A (H3N2) and (H1N1) virus isolates. Journal of Antimicrobial Chemotherapy 1986, 18 (Supplement B): 135–140.
79. Larder, B. A., Purifoy, J. M., Powell, K. L., Darby, G.: Site-specific mutagenesis of AIDS virus reverse transcriptase. Nature 1987, 327: 716–717.

Pharmacology and Drug Delivery

Antiviral Therapy with Small Particle Aerosols

V. Knight*, B. Gilbert

The generation and use of small particle aqueous aerosols (1.23 μm aerodynamic mass median diameter, GSD = 2.0 μm) containing ribavirin is described. Administered via aerosol, ribavirin will be deposited rather uniformly on the surface of the nasopharynx, the tracheobronchial tree and in the pulmonary area. Examples of aerosol-delivered dosages found to be effective in the treatment of respiratory syncytial virus infection and influenza A and B virus infections are as follows: 12.8 mg of ribavirin/hour for a 6-month-old infant weighing 7.5 kg, and 56.2 kg of ribavirin/hour for a 25-year-old adult weighing 62.5 kg. Drugs which are relatively insoluble in aqueous solutions can also be administered in small particle aerosol by using liposomes as a vehicle. The preparation of enviroxime, a potent anti-rhinovirus drug, in liposomes for aerosol use is reported here. Its antiviral activity in liposomes was found to be undiminished, but its cellular toxicity was greatly reduced. It was well-tolerated by normal volunteers and studies are planned to determine its clinical efficacy.

In the past few years we have developed an aerosol method for the administration of antiviral drugs to the respiratory tract and have used this technique to successfully treat respiratory syncytial and influenza virus infections with ribavirin (1–4). We have also recently developed an aerosol method for the administration of the anti-rhinoviral drug, enviroxime, incorporated into liposomes (5–7). Methods of preparation and administration of drugs in small particle aerosol and for prediction of regional and total deposition in the respiratory tract are described for drugs administered in this way. Data on the clinical use of ribavirin aerosol is summarized, as are results of preclinical studies which suggest that enviroxime prepared in liposomes and administered in a small particle aerosol may be a suitable method of treating rhinovirus infections.

Principles of Small Particle Aerosol Treatment

Our greatest experience with small particle aerosol delivery of antiviral drugs has involved use of the Collison jet nebulizer. Recently, we have also done studies with the Puritan-Bennett jet nebulizer which delivers an aerosol similar to that of the Collison nebulizer. The use of aerosols to deliver drugs requires two essential factors: the use of a particle size that will deposit throughout the respiratory tract, and the administration of a volume of particles containing

Department of Microbiology and Immunology, Baylor College of Medicine, One Baylor Plaza, Houston, Texas 77030, USA.

enough drug to provide adequate drug therapy. Since these compounds are virustatic, their presence in infected cells must be maintained during most of the replicative cycle.

As indicated above, the deposition of aerosol in the respiratory tract is dependent on particle size. Aerosols generated from aqueous media consist of particles which undergo changes in aerodynamic mass median diameter (AMMD) in environments of different relative humidity. AMMD is the diameter of a spherical particle of unit density (1 g/cm^3) which has the same terminal settling velocity with respect to the surrounding air as the particle in question. In high relative humidity particles accrete water vapor from the air and increase in size; in low relative humidity particles lose water and shrink in size. The mass concentration of ribavirin aerosol particles produced by the Collison generator in ambient humidity is shown in Figure 1 (8). The AMMD of the particles is 1.23 μm (GSD = 2.0 μm), and a large majority are less than 5 μm in diameter. Such aqueous particles when inhaled will swell to an average diameter of about 3.4 μm during passage through the nose. In the lung they will increase to an average diameter of 4.5 μm due to the 99.5 % relative humidity at that site (9). The changes in particle size within the respiratory tract are essentially the same for infants up through adulthood because, despite differences in rate and volume of respiration, the changes in particle size in response to changes in humidity occur in less time than is required for inhalation and exhalation at any age. An example of regional deposition of inhaled aerosol is shown in Table 1 for 6-months- and

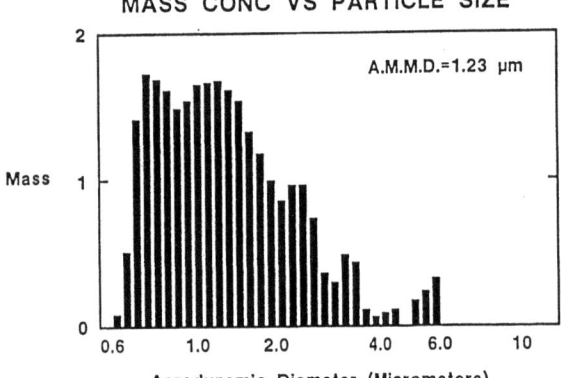

Figure 1: Mass concentration of ribavirin aerosol particles produced by the Collison nebulizer. Measured by Aerodynamic Particle Sizer, TSI, Inc., St. Paul, Minnesota (Courtesy, Mr. R. Orr, ICN Pharmaceuticals, Costa Mesa, California). Reprinted from Reference No. 8, with permission.

Table 1: Respiratory tract deposition of inhaled ribavirin small particle aerosol during normal breathing (nasal inspiration, oral expiration) and in intubated patients (nasal desposition bypassed by endotracheal tube). From Reference No. 10, with permission.

Age (years)	Type of respiration	Fraction of inhaled aerosol deposited			
		Nose	Tracheo-bronchial	Pulmonary	Total
0.5	Normal	0.507	0.207	0.035	0.749
	Intubated	–	0.574	0.052	0.626
25	Normal	0.435	0.127	0.141	0.703
	Intubated	–	0.275	0.243	0.518

dose of ribavirin aerosol deposited in patients ranging from 3 months to 25 years of age. There is little further change in dosage above 25 years of age. A sample dosage calculation is as follows. For age 6 months the dose in mg/kg of body weight/hour equals [(0.039 l, tidal volume) (36, respiratory rate/min) (60 min/hour) (0.2 mg of ribavirin/l of aerosol) (0.749, total deposition)/(7.5 kg, estimated body weight)] = 1.68 mg/kg of body weight/hour of ribavirin aerosol. Tidal volumes and respiratory rates (resting) are from a mathematical model of Hofmann (11). The aerosol concentration of ribavirin is the mean of the concentration during a 12-hour period of continuous operation (8). Body weight is taken from standard tables (10). Fever will cause an increase in ventilation and thus the dosage of aerosol will increase about 5% for each degree of fever, Fahrenheit, or 9% for each degree of fever, Celsius. Females at adolescence and beyond will have about 7% less ventilation per kg of body weight than males. The dosage for women in this age group should be reduced 7% from that shown in Figure 2. Corrections for different body weights can be made by multiplying the dosage described in Figure 2 by the actual weight of the patient, divided by the weight used in the figure for that year of age (10). The effect of pulmonary disease on deposition has not been calculated because deposition data for the various disease states are not available. It seems certain that lung disease will alter deposition of aerosol particles; however, prolonged dosage such as we employ may adequately dose areas where obstruction of airways might reduce inflow of aerosol particles.

25-year-old individuals (10). Also shown is the deposition in the tracheobronchial and pulmonary areas when the nose is bypassed in patients with endotracheal tubes in place. Overall deposition at both ages is somewhat more than 70% of inhaled air. At 6 months of age, a larger proportion is deposited in the tracheobronchial area and a smaller proportion in the pulmonary area than in the 25-year-old individual. This may be explained in part by the smaller dimensions of tracheobronchial airways in the infant which would cause greater deposition of particles. When the total input of aerosol is directed into the lung of intubated patients there is a considerable increase of deposition in these areas, although it is still somewhat less than the total deposition when the aerosol passes through the nasal area.

The dosage of drug carried in small particle aerosol can be calculated according to the age of the patient, and additional corrections for sex, body weight and fever can be made (10). Figure 2 shows the estimated

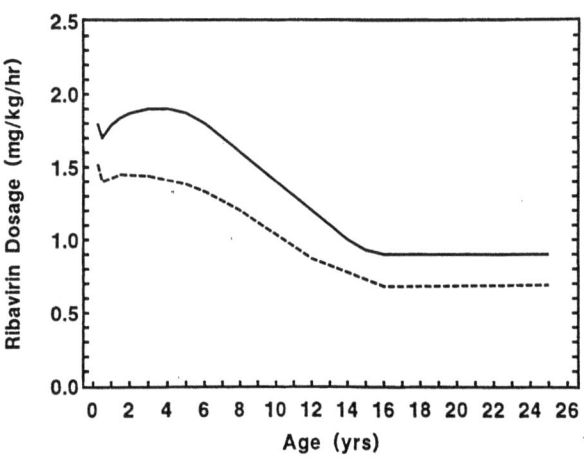

Figure 2: Respiratory tract dosage according to age in non-intubated and intubated patients. ———, non-intubated patients; – – – –, intubated patients. Calculations are for concentrations of ribavirin administered as a small particle aerosol containing 200 µg of ribavirin/l of aerosol. Reprinted from Reference No. 10, with permission.

Ribavirin Deposition and Absorption after Aerosol Administration

Conner et al. (12) found concentrations of ribavirin of 1,000 (244 µg/ml) to 7,700 (1880 µg/ml) µM in endotracheal secretions from intubated patients treated with the standard regimen in which the aerosol concentration of ribavirin averaged 200 µg/l during several hours of treatment. In other patients, plasma ribavirin concentrations increased during several treatment periods over three days from about 1 µM (0.2 µg/ml) after the first treatment to 3–6 µM (0.7 to 1.5 µg/ml) after the third day of treatment. The above values are representative of published data on this subject. The assay used employed rabbit antibody to ribavirin which detects both the nucleoside and the phosphorylated derivatives (personal communication, Dr. J. Conner). Since the phosphorylated derivatives are only produced intracellularly and transport out of the cells requires dephosphorylation, it is probable that the foregoing assays measured largely nucleoside concentrations.

Gilbert and Wyde (13) assayed ribavirin in body fluids of mice by high performance liquid chromatography following chromatographic extraction of the sample on a phenylboronate affinity column. Figure 3 shows serum, lung and brain assays of ribavirin in mice during and after a 12-hour period of aerosol treatment. The aerosol generator contained the standard dose of ribavirin used in human treatment (20 mg of ribavirin/ml), and the aerosol concentration averaged 200 µg of ribavirin/l during the inhalation period. Lung concentrations increased rapidly after start of treatment, reaching about 22 nmol/lung in one-half hour with peak concentrations (33 nmol/lung) occurring in 2–4 h. These levels were maintained for the remainder of the 12 h of treatment, but declined with a half-life disappearance time of approximately 3–4 h after treatment was stopped. Serum concentrations rose more slowly: the highest concentration of 21 µM was reached at 12 h of treatment, and 12 h later the serum concentration was still 6.7 µM. Brain concentrations rose gradually. Concentrations reached 5 nmol/brain in 12 h and were still 3.6 nmol/brain 12 h later.

Table 2 shows a comparison of the amounts of ribavirin at various sites in the mouse after 12 h of treatment. Shown in the second column are total nmoles of ribavirin detected in whole tissues. In addition, on the assumption that the drug will be principally present in interstitial fluid, the amounts of drug in lung mucus, the site of deposition of inhaled particles, and in the cerebrospinal fluid are shown. In the last column the concentrations are presented as µM or per gm of tissue. The lung had eight times more ribavirin in it than serum, and the estimated concentration of ribavirin in mucus was 56 times greater than in serum. The estimated concentration of ribavirin in the cerebrospinal fluid (118 µM) was six times that of serum (21 µM). Ribavirin enters cells in culture promptly and is phosphorylated (14, 15). To exit a cell, ribavirin triphosphate is dephosphorylated and ribavirin is transported out of the cells. From this it is reasonable to expect that in vivo concentrations of intracellular ribavirin nucleotides reach a high proportion of the extracellular concentrations of ribavirin nucleoside. Assays of ribavirin may thus be an indirect indicator of the antiviral nucleotides in the cell. More information will be available when an assay for ribavirin nucleotides in tissues is developed. These studies in mice reveal that ribavirin given by aerosol reaches high concentrations in the lung, the initial site of deposition, and that the concentration in brain fluids exceeds that in serum; moreover, clearance from the brain is much slower than clearance from serum or the lung.

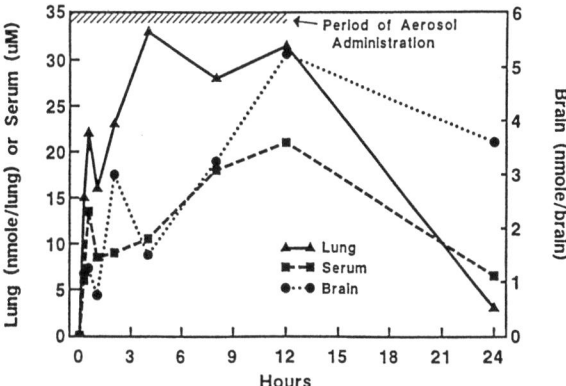

Figure 3: Pharmacokinetics of ribavirin in lung, serum, and brain tissues after a single administration by small particle aerosol for 12 h with 20 mg of drug/ml in the reservoir. Ribavirin levels were measured by high performance liquid chromatography. Values represent the means of data for three mice. Symbols: ▲, lung; ■, serum; ●, brain. Reprinted from Reference No. 13, with permission.

Table 2: Ribavirin in mouse serum, lung, lung mucus, brain and cerebrospinal fluid samples at the end of 12 h of ribavirin aerosol treatment.

Tissue (weight or volume)[a]	Ribavirin content	Ribavirin concentration
Lung (0.2 gm)	33 nmol	165 nmol/gm
Lung mucus (0.028 ml)	33 nmol	1178 µM
Brain (0.84 gm)	4.7 nmol[b]	5.6 nmol/gm
CSF (0.04 ml)	4.7 nmol[b,c]	118 µM
Serum (1.1 ml)	23 nmol	21 µM

[a] Estimate based on a 28 gm mouse (13).
[b] Reduced by approximately 10% for the estimated amount of ribavirin present in blood within the brain.
[c] Based on the assumption that ribavirin measured in the brain was mainly distributed in the CSF.

Treatment of Respiratory Syncytial Virus Infection with Ribavirin Aerosol

A number of reports (16–21) confirm the original observations of Taber et al. (22) and of Hall et al. (23) that ribavirin aerosol is an effective treatment for respiratory syncytial virus infection in infants. Figure 4 shows the results of studies by the latter authors in which infants with and without underlying disease were treated with ribavirin aerosol for about 21 h/day for periods of 3–5 days (24). There were 14 treated patients of whom six had congenital heart disease or bronchopulmonary dysplasia. Twelve patients served as controls of whom six had congenital heart disease or bronchopulmonary dysplasia. Control patients received distilled water aerosol for periods corresponding to treatment with ribavirin aerosol. Figure 4 shows the results divided into days 1–2 and days 3–4 of treatment. Patients treated with ribavirin improved almost 20% clinically in the first treatment period and a further 35% in the 3–4 day period for a total of 55% improvement during treatment. Control patients failed to improve during the 1–2 day period and improvement of only 29% was observed, during the 3–4 day period. These results demonstrate a prompt and substantial reversal of the illness early in the treatment period that was sustained in the latter half of treatment. When the patients with complicating illnesses were examined separately a significant but smaller difference between treated and control patients was observed. Virus shedding from these patients is shown in Table 3. Initial titers were similar at start of treatment with values of 2.4 and 2.0 TCID50 ($\log_{10}$, 50% tissue culture infectious dose) in treated and control patients, respectively. Among treated patients these values declined progressively to 0.8 TCID50 on day 5, while titers in control patients actually increased to 2.9 TCID50 by this time ($P < 0.02$). Coinciding with the clinical and virologic differences between treated and control patients was a more rapid return toward normal of arterial oxygen tension (Table 4). Hypoxemia is a common and serious physiological abnormality in RSV infection indicating a profound effect of the infectious lesion in the lung on oxygen diffusion. The more rapid improvement of this abnormality in treated patients coincides with the other findings indicating a benefit of treatment. Improvement in arterial oxygen tension associated with treatment was observed in an earlier study by Hall et al. (23). Studies reported by others have varied in experimental details but all have been consistent in indicating a favorable effect of aerosol treatment. A summary is presented in Table 5. There are no reports of systemic toxicity or local intolerance to the treatment.

Ribavirin Aerosol Treatment of Influenza

Influenza virus infections were the first diseases to be treated with ribavirin aerosol. The studies, conducted over a period of years in a college student population during the course of annual occurrences of influenza,

Table 3: Quantity of virus shed in the nasal wash of 26 infants with respiratory syncytial virus lower respiratory tract disease.

Treatment group (No. of patients)	Mean titer[a] (SE)[b]		
	Day 1	Day 3	Day 5[c]
Ribavirin (14)	2.4 (0.52)	1.6 (0.32)	0.8 (0.43)
Placebo (12)	2.0 (0.65)	2.2 (0.53)	2.9 (0.64)

[a] Mean titer = $\log_{10}$, 50% tissue culture infectious dose/ml.
[b] Standard error.
[c] $p < 0.02$ for Day 5.

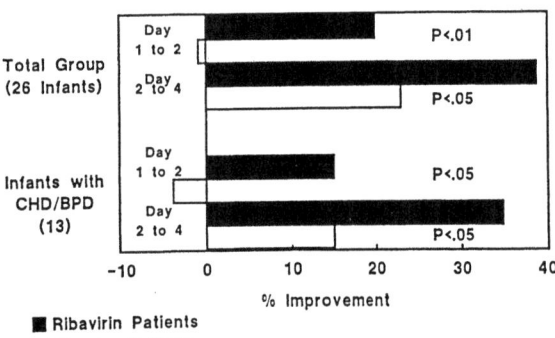

Figure 4: Percent improvement in illness severity score from day 1 to day 2 and from day 2 to day 4 in infants with respiratory syncytial virus infections who received ribavirin compared with those who received placebo for total group of infants (top bars) and for those infants with congenital heart disease (CHD) and bronchopulmonary dysplasia (BPD) (bottom bars). Modified from Reference No. 24.

Table 4: Arterial oxygen tension in respiratory syncytial virus infected children treated with ribavirin aerosol.

Treatment protocol	No. of patients	Arterial oxygen tension (mm Hg)	
		Before treatment	After treatment
Ribavirin Aerosol (6 BPD/CHD)[a]	14	50.6	72.5[b]
Water Aerosol (7 BPD/CHD)[a]	12	56.8	58.2[b]

[a] BPD = bronchopulmonary dysplasia; CHD = congenital heart disease.
[b] $p < 0.01$.

Table 5: Summary of ribavirin aerosol treatment of respiratory syncytial virus infections in infants.

Authors (Reference no.)	Year of study	Patient symptoms	No. of patients (Treated/Control) Total	Reduction Symptoms	Reduction Viral Shedding	Increased pO_2 after treatment	Some assisted ventilation	Toxicity	Positive overall evaluation
Hall et al. (23)	1983	pneumonia	16/17 33	+	+	+	–	–	+
Taber et al. (22)	1983	bronchiolitis	12/14 26	+	–	not tested	–	–	+
Gelfand et al. (19)	1983	SCID[a]	1/0 1	+	+	+	?	–	+
McIntosh et al. (20)	1984	SCID[a]	1/0 1	+	+	+	–	–	±
Hall et al. (24)	1985	BPD/CHD[b]	14/12 53	+	+	+	+	–	+
Barry et al. (16)	1986	bronchiolitis	14/12 26	+	–	not tested	–	–	±
Rodriguez et al. (18)	1987	bronchiolitis and/or pneumonia	20/10 30	+	–	+	–	–	+
Conrad et al. (17)	1987	bronchiolitis and/or pneumonia	33/97[c] 130	+	–	not tested	+	–	+

[a] SCID = severe combined immunodeficiency disease.
[b] BPD = bronchopulmonary dysplasia; CHD = congenital heart disease.
[c] Control patients were untreated infants hospitalized during epidemic period.

Table 6: Fever and virus shedding in patients treated for influenza with ribavirin aerosol. Reprinted from Reference No. 9, with permission.

Influenza virus	Year	Duration of fever in hours[a] (No. of Patients) Control	Duration of fever in hours[a] (No. of Patients) Treated	p value	Virus shedding[b] p value
A(H3N2)	1983	55.5 (3)	25.1 (2)	0.017	0.037
B	1982	55.0 (7)	36.1 (9)	0.047	0.017
A(H1N1)	1984	48.6 (20)	29.9 (18)	0.004	0.001
	1983	33.5 (14)	30.3 (13)	0.3	0.3
	1982	42.7 (11)	31.4 (8)	0.066	0.3
	1981	35.5 (17)	21.1 (14)	0.015	0.008
Mean	1981–1984	42.6 (72)	28.9 (64)		

[a] Duration of fever = start of treatment to afebrile (< 100 °F). p values for control versus treated patients were obtained from analysis of data by Student's + test, two-tailed. Student's t test for A(H1N1) data for different years: Control 1982 versus 1981 or 1983; 1981 or 1983 versus 1984, not significant. Treated 1981 versus 1982, p = 0.016; 1981 versus 1983, p = 0.032; 1981 versus 1984 and 1982 versus 1983, not significant.
[b] Virus shedding was determined 17 to 24 h after the start of treatment. p values were determined by Wilcoxon rank sum test, two-tailed.

were controlled, and untreated patients were given saline or distilled water aerosol treatments corresponding to those given to treated patients. The diagnosis of influenza was based on virus isolation and strain characterization of respiratory tract specimens from each patient. The principal criteria for evaluation were recovery from illness, height and duration of fever, and quantitative virus shedding from the respiratory tract. We previously noted that duration of fever and virus shedding agree closely as indicators of recovery and parallel other criteria of evaluation (4). Table 6 presents a summary of the duration of fever and virus shedding from treated and control patients in six outbreaks of influenza among college students during the four years of our study.

The first study was performed in 1981 when virus shedding and duration of fever in treated patients were greatly reduced in comparison to control patients (1). The etiology of the disease that year was influenza A/England/333/80 (H1N1). In 1982 and 1983 variants of this strain caused the disease, and evidence for therapeutic effect diminished progressively. In 1982, although the duration of fever was shorter in treated patients, there was only a trend toward drug effect (25). If the duration of illness was measured from onset of illness, however, fever was significantly reduced in treated patients ($P < 0.05$) (data not shown). However, virus shedding was similar in treated and control groups. In 1983, the third year of circulation of the A/England strain, there was no evidence of drug effect either by diminished fever or reduced virus shedding (27). In the following year, in a study of a new etiologic strain, A/Victoria/7/83 (H1N1), associated with greater severity of disease, fever and virus shedding were observed to be significantly reduced in treated compared to control patients (3). Height of fever and symptoms were also reduced in treated compared to control patients. No definite explanation is available for the progressive lack of drug effect in 1982 and 1983, except that the disease in those years was less severe with shorter periods of fever in control patients. With the numbers of patients available for these studies a margin of difference of 12 h or more of duration of fever between treated and control patients was required for significance. In 1982 and 1983 significant drug effects were observed during small outbreaks of influenza A (H3N2) and influenza B virus infections (4,27). In these outbreaks fever in control patients was the most prolonged of that observed in any of the studies. In summary, significant therapeutic effect was observed in four of six outbreaks of acute influenza in college students, marginal benefit was observed in one and no effect was seen in a sixth study. We believe these data provide evidence of therapeutic benefit or ribavirin aerosol in the treatment of influenza A (H1N1), A (H3N2) and influenza B virus infections.

We have also observed the treatment of six patients with influenzal pneumonia (Table 7) (1, 4, 27–28), five of which had known risk factors for this disease: four patients had underlying illnesses and one patient was pregnant (28). One patient with influenza B virus pneumonia had no known risk factor. Four of six patients required assisted ventilation. Recovery in all six within a few days was associated with 50 to 101 hours of the standard ribavirin aerosol treatment. The pregnant patient had a level of ribavirin of $4.8\,\mu M$ ($1.2\,\mu g/ml$) in her breast milk after about 6 h of therapy on day 5 of treatment. After the first 18 h of treatment her serum contained $5.8\,\mu M$ ($1.4\,\mu g/ml$) ribavirin (unpublished data, this laboratory). She was also treated with amantadine (100 mg twice daily) during acute illness. We believe these results are indicative of a favorable effect of ribavirin aerosol treatment of severe influenzal pneumonia.

Table 7: Influenzal pneumonia treated with ribavirin aerosol.

Date of admission (Viral etiology)	Age/Sex	Underlying illness	Secondary bacterial infection	Assisted ventilation required	Hours of treatment[a]	Outcome of infection	Reference
12-30-80 A/Bangkok/79 (H3N2)	61/M	acute myocardial infarction	no	yes	60.5	recovery, no sequelae	Knight et al. (1)
3-16-84 Hemadsorbing agent, A/Phillippines/2/82 (H3N2)	32/F	none	*Pseudomonas aeruginosa*	yes	101	recovery, no sequelae	Knight and Gilbert (26)
2-4-84 B/Singapore/82	33/M	pulmonary fibrosis from chemical exposure	no	no	51	recovery, no sequelae	Gilbert et al. (27)
1-1-86 B/Singapore/82	36/M	diabetes, alcoholism	Streptococcus B	yes	63	recovery, no follow-up	Knight et al. (4)
3-9-86 Influenza A	34/F	pregnant, 33 weeks	no	yes	50	recovery, 2 years	Kirshon et al. (28)
2-16-88 Influenza A/Sichuan (H3N2)-serological diagnosis	70/M	Alzheimer's disease, severe	gram-positive coccus, bacteremia	no	72	slow recovery	Knight, this report

[a] Estimated dosage to the respiratory tract, 50 mg/h.

Enviroxime Treatment of Rhinovirus Infections

Enviroxime, an anti-rhinovirus drug developed by scientists at Eli Lilly (29), is an imidazole derivative with the structural formula shown in Figure 5. In previous studies it inhibited all 83 rhinovirus types tested at extremely low concentrations of 10 to 120 ng/ml, and was also strongly inhibitory to poliovirus, Coxsackie and Echo virus replication. Phillpotts et al. (30) treated 18 volunteers challenged with rhinovirus 9 while 18 other volunteers served as controls. Intranasal spray was administered four times daily. Five doses were given before and 20 doses after viral challenge. The nasal spray dose was 568 µg q.i.d. or a total of 2272 µg. Oral dosage was 25 mg q.i.d. or 100 mg/day. Symptoms of rhinovirus infection and titer of virus in nasal wash specimens were reduced in treated patients. Levandowski et al. (31) gave a nasal spray of enviroxime at a dosage of 568 µg q.i.d. or 2272 µg/day for seven days. Several dosage schedules were used and treatments neither prevented infection nor reduced the frequency of colds. Concentrations of enviroxime in nasal secretions 12 h after the last daily dose ranged from 0 to 4,662 ng/ml. The authors suggested that those patients with higher drug concentrations showed some benefit from treatment.

Betts et al. (personal communication) did five studies in volunteers challenged with rhinovirus 13. Aerosol dosage was administered as in the described studies above. In four of their five studies treated volunteers had significantly fewer virus-positive days than control patients. Hayden and Gwaltney (32) tested enviroxime in rhinovirus 39 infection induced in volunteers. They used an aerosol dosage similar to those described above. Intranasal enviroxime begun one day before challenge and continuing for four days after did not reduce infection or illness. They were able to measure about 200 µg/ml of enviroxime in nasal secretions 5 min after the start of a single treatment, but concentrations fell rapidly over the next 30 min. Multiple sprayings gave a 43% higher concentration of enviroxime than did a single spray. Phillpotts et al. (33) administered enviroxime nasal spray to volunteers in the treatment of rhinovirus infection. The treatment regimen was like that of Hayden and Gwaltney (34). They showed earlier resolution of illness but no effect on rhinovirus shedding. Using the same preparation of enviroxime and a similar schedule as Phillpotts and Wallace (33), Miller et al. (34) found no therapeutic effect of enviroxime in natural rhinovirus infection. From the foregoing studies we judged that enviroxime possessed anti-rhinovirus activity in vivo but that its effect was limited by the difficulty of getting the drug in sufficient dosage to the site of infection. The maximum dose given by nasal spray of this may have been swallowed promptly after administration because of deposition of drug particles in the nasopharynx.

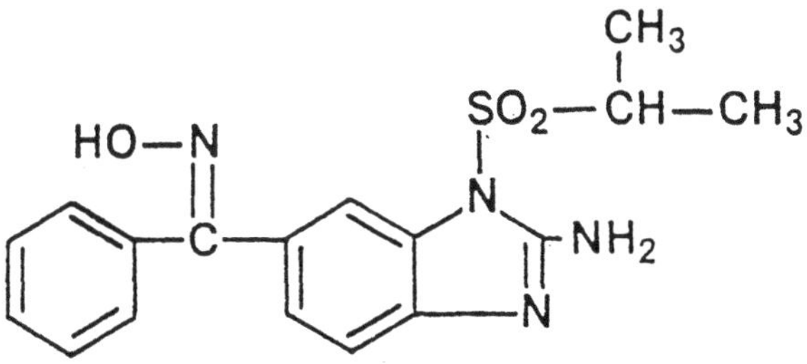

It seemed to us that if we could increase the dose and distribute the drug over a wider area of the respiratory tract, the clinical effect would be improved. To achieve this goal we proposed to incorporate enviroxime in liposomes of phosphatidylcholine, thus increasing enviroxime's solubility, and administer this preparation to the respiratory tract in a small particle aerosol. Results of investigations so far indicate the possibility of success of this effort.

Preparation and Properties of Liposomes Containing Enviroxime

Enviroxime-liposomes were prepared by adding micronized enviroxime powder to egg yolk phosphatidylcholine in chloroform (6). The liquid phase was removed by rotovaporization under vacuum. The lipid film was then dissolved in t-butanol and dried twice under vacuum. At the time of use, a lyophilized preparation of enviroxime containing 120 mg of enviroxime and 450 mg of egg yolk phosphatidylcholine (Avanti Polar Lipids, Birmingham, AL, USA) was suspended in 30 ml of distilled, pyrogen-free water. This material formed multi-lamellar liposomes as seen by electron microscopy. The particle size before and after dissemination in small particle aerosol in the Puritan-Bennett nebulizer (Model No. 1920) is shown in Table 8 (7). It is apparent that liposome particles were sheared to a uniformly small size by nebulization. The particle size distribution of aerosol droplets containing liposomes is shown in Table 9. The AMMD of particles produced by these aerosols, 2.4 µm and 3.1 µm for the Collison and Puritan-Bennett generators, respectively, are appreciably larger than that produced by aerosols of ribavirin dissolved in water (approximately 1.4 µm AMMD). The larger mean diameter of Puritan-Bennett aerosol particles is principally due to a larger number of particles 4.7 µm and greater in diameter. These larger particles would tend to deposit in the nasopharynx and the smaller par-

Figure 5: Structural formula for (E)-6[(hydroxyimino)phenylmethyl]-1-[(1-methylethyl)-sulfonyl]-1H-benzimidazol-2-amine (Enviroxime).

Table 8: Change in distribution of liposome particle size following aerosolization. Reprinted from Reference No. 7, with permission.

	Percent of particles[a] by size range (nm)			
	100–250	250–500	500–750	>750
Before aerosolization	37	40	22	1
After aerosolization	91	8	2	0

[a] Percent of total particles ⩾ 100 nm in diameter. Eight and seven photographs taken randomly before and after aerosolization, respectively, were measured. A total of 218 and 53 liposome particles before and after aerosolization, respectively, were measured.

Table 9: Particle size distribution and quantity of phosphatidycholine (calculated from phosphate determinations) recovered from liposome particles.

		Phosphatidylcholine recovered (μg)	
Impaction range of plate (μm)	Plate[a] no.	Collison nebulizer	Puritan-Bennett nebulizer (diluting air aperture closed)
4.7–>9.0	1	1440	3880
3.3–>4.7	2	1185	1230
2.1–>3.3	3	1545	1395
1.1–>2.1	4	1680	1365
0.7–>1.1	5	600	570
0.4–>0.7	6	250	375
0.0–>0.4	7	400	390
Total		7100	9205
Aerodynamic mass median diameter (μm)		2.4	3.1
Geometric standard deviation (μm)		2.8	3.1
Phospholipid output (μg/l)		113	147
Aerosol flow rate (l/min)		12–13	12–13

[a] Anderson cascade sampler plates, 5 min sample.

ticles would deposit in significant proportions in the lower respiratory tract.

Antiviral and Cell Toxicity of Enviroxime-Liposomes

The activity of enviroxime in liposomes and of enviroxime not incorporated into liposomes was essentially the same against rhinovirus 1A and rhinovirus 13 as measured by cytopathic effect and by plaque reduction (5). Fifty percent inhibitory concentrations by both methods ranged from 0.03 to 0.09 μg/ml. In contrast, cell toxicity of enviroxime was greatly reduced when it was contained in liposomes (Table 10). With the exception of one test result of enviroxime in methanol when the 50% cell toxic concentration against HeLa cells was 31 μg/ml, the decrease in toxicity in cell cultures tested with enviroxime in liposomes averaged 25-fold.

Respiratory Tract Deposition of Enviroxime in Liposomes Administered in Small Particle Aerosol

Aerosols generated in jet spray devices produce water vapor in excess of drug-containing particles leading to concentration of drug in the reservoir with continued operation of the nebulizer. This event is demonstrated for enviroxime liposomes in Figure 6. Shown is the concentration of enviroxime in the reservoir liquid and in the aerosol over a 75-min period of operation. The reservoir initially contained about 5 mg/ml of enviroxime in a 30 ml volume of enviroxime-liposomes suspended in water. After 75 min this concentration had escalated to about 40 mg/ml. At this time only a few milliliters of the original 30 ml volume of enviroxime-liposome suspension remained in the reservoir. The aerosol concentration of enviroxime showed a similar rate of increase in concentration ranging from 12 to more than 100 μg/l of air during the 75-min run. However, at one hour the concentration was only 45 μg/l. In practice, treatment periods would not exceed one hour and the average concentration of enviroxime in the aerosol over this period of time would be about 20 μg/l of aerosol.

Using this dosage of enviroxime-liposome aerosol, mice were exposed to aerosol. Lung lavage and nasal

Table 10: Effect of liposomes (phosphatidylcholine) on cell toxicity of enviroxime.

		50% cell toxic concentrations			
Preparation	Experiment no.	Percent methanol in test (μg of enviroxime/ml)			
		KB	HeLa	L929	MDCK
Methanol	1	1	1	3	3
	2	3	12	6	12
Enviroxime in methanol	1	0.1 (2)	0.5 (5)	0.4 (4)	0.7 (8)
	2	0.7 (8)	3 (31)	0.1 (1)	0.7 (8)
Enviroxime in liposomes[a]	1	(>125)	(>125)	(>125)	(>125)
	2	(>125)	(>125)	(>125)	(>125)

[a] Liposomes alone were not toxic in concentrations up to 3 mg/ml of egg yolk phosphatidylcholine.

Antiviral therapy with small particle aerosols 143

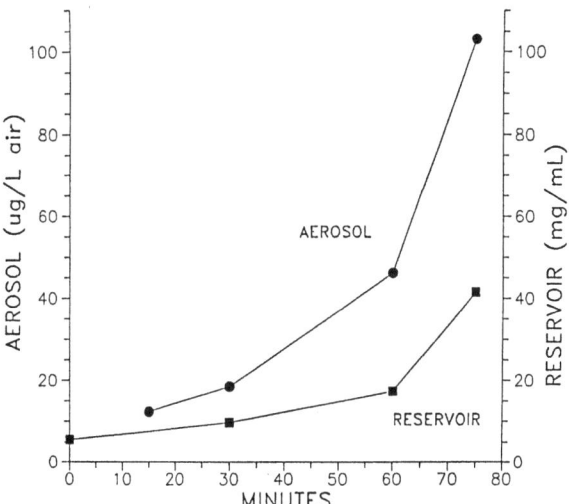

Figure 6: Kinetics of generation of aerosol of enviroxime containing liposomes. Aerosol was generated with the Puritan-Bennett nebulizer, Model No. 1920, and enviroxime was quantitated by high performance liquid chromatography assay. Symbols represent the amount of enviroxime in the aerosol (●) and reservoir (■). Reprinted from Reference No. 7, with permission.

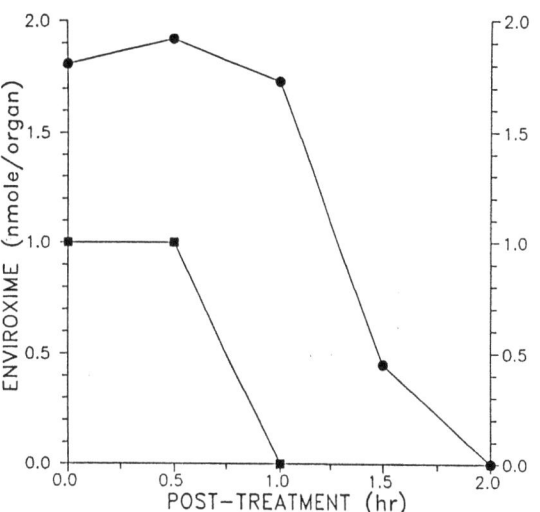

Figure 8: Levels of enviroxime in nasal washes (●) and lungs (■) of mice exposed for 20 min to small particle aerosol of liposomes containing enviroxime (reservoir concentration = 4 mg of enviroxime/ml), as determined by high performance liquid chromatography. Reprinted from Reference No. 5, with permission.

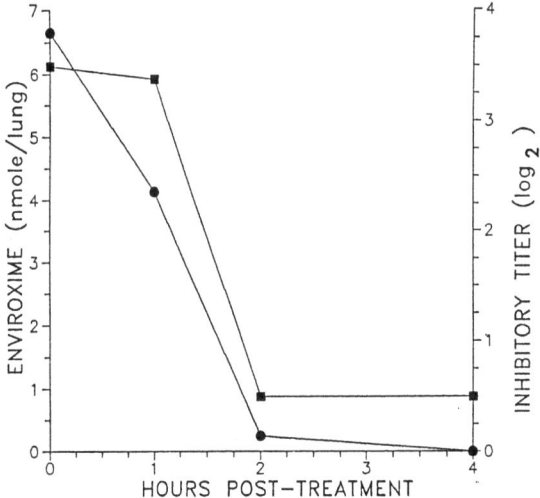

Figure 7: A comparison of the antiviral activity with levels of enviroxime in lung lavage fluids obtained from mice exposed for 90 min to small particle aerosols of liposomes containing enviroxime (reservoir concentration = 4 mg of enviroxime/ml). ●, mean enviroxime values as determined by high performance liquid chromatography; ■, geometric mean inhibitory titers ($\log_2$)/0.05 mL of lung lavage fluid. The latter test was performed in KB tissue culture cells using approximately 33 median infectious doses of rhinovirus 13 as the challenge virus. Reprinted from Reference No. 5, with permission.

wash fluids were assayed for enviroxime by inhibition of rhinovirus replication in cell culture. Figure 7 shows the presence of anti-rhinovirus activity in lung lavage fluid for periods after completion of 90 min of aerosol exposure. This correlated with the concentration of enviroxime in the lung as determined by high performance liquid chromatography. A similar study of exposure of mice to enviroxime-liposome aerosol for 20 min is shown in Figure 8. A high level of enviroxime persisted in the nose for one hour and then dropped progressively over a second hour to unmeasurable levels. Lung concentrations dropped more rapidly so that no activity was measurable one hour after stopping treatment. Although there is a major difference in absolute concentrations of drug in nose and lung, the significance of the difference is uncertain because of technical differences in the procedures for assay.

Enviroxime-Liposome Aerosol Administration to Normal Volunteers

Five male adult volunteers inhaled enviroxime-liposome aerosol through a face mask for one hour (Table 11) (7). The concentration of enviroxime in liposomes was the same as that used for animal experiments. There was no intolerance to the treatment and the only reported change was increase in a mucus-like nasal secretion occurring only during the treatment period and a feeling of opening up of air passages. Nasal secretions were obtained and enviroxime was quantitated by chemical and anti-viral assays. All samples were positive by chemical assay. Substantial amounts of drug were detected throughout the hour after treatment by both high performance liquid

Table 11: Recovery of enviroxime from nasal wash fluid of volunteers following a one-hour inhalation of enviroxime in liposome small particle aerosol.

Volunteer	Sample time after treatment (min)[a]	Enviroxime concentration μg/sample [vol]	Antiviral assay[b]
A	5	84 [3 ml]	ND
B	5	227 [1 ml]	128
C	15	750 [9 ml]	>256
D	30	159 [4 ml]	>256
E	60	612 [7 ml]	>256

[a] Aerosol treatment: 1 h inhalation of 20 μg of enviroxime/l in aerosol. Estimated dose to respiratory tract in 1 h = 8.4 mg.

[b] MIC in KB tissue culture cells challenged with approximately 100 TCID50 of rhinovirus 13. ND = not done.

chromatography analysis and bioassay. Based on this and other observations, it is our plan to proceed to clinical trials of treatment of rhinovirus infections in man with enviroxime-liposomes administered in a small particle aerosol.

Acknowledgements

This work was supported in part by funds from the Clayton Foundation for Research, Houston, Texas. Computational assistance for portions of the work was provided by the CLINFO project, funded by the Division of Research Resources of the NIH under grant #RR-00350.

References

1. Knight, V., Wilson, S. Z., Quarles, J. M., Greggs, S. E., McClung, H. W., Waters, B. K., Cameron, R. W., Zerwas, J. M., Couch, R. B.: Ribavirin small particle aerosol treatment of influenza. Lancet 1981, ii: 945–949.
2. Wilson, S. Z., Knight, V., Moore, R., Larson, E. W.: Amantadine small particle aerosol: generation and delivery to man. Proceedings of the Society for Experimental Biology and Medicine 1979, 161: 350–354.
3. Gilbert, B. E., Wilson, S. Z., Knight, V., Couch, R. B., Quarles, J. M., Dure, L., Hayes, N., Willis, G.: Ribavirin small particle aerosol treatment of infections caused by influenza virus strains A/Victoria/7/83 (H1N1) and B/Texas/1/84. Antimicrobial Agents and Chemotherapy 1985, 27: 309–313.
4. Knight, V., Gilbert, B., Wilson, S. Z.: Ribavirin small particle aerosol treatment of influenza and respiratory syncytial virus infections. In: Stapleton, T. (ed.): International Congress and Symposium series. Royal Society of Medicine Services, London, 1986, p. 37–56.
5. Wyde, P. R., Six, H. R., Wilson, S. Z., Gilbert, B. E., Knight, V.: Activity against rhinoviruses, toxicity, and delivery in aerosol of enviroxime in liposomes. Antimicrobial Agents and Chemotherapy 1988, 32: 890–895.
6. Six, H. R., Gilbert, B. E., Wyde, P. R., Wilson, S. Z., Knight, V.: Liposomes as carriers of enviroxime for use in aerosol therapy of rhinovirus infections. In: Lopez-Berestein, G., and Fidler, I. (ed.): UCLA Symposium on Molecular and Cellular Biology 1988, in press.
7. Gilbert, B. E., Six, H. R., Wilson, S. Z., Wyde, P. R., Knight, V.: Small particle aerosols of enviroxime-containing liposomes. Antiviral Research 1988, in press.
8. Knight, V., Gilbert, B. E., Wilson, S. Z.: Ribavirin aerosol treatment of influenza and respiratory syncytial virus infections. In: Knight, V., Gilbert, B. E. (ed.): Antiviral chemotherapy: infectious disease clinics of North America. W. B. Saunders Company, Philadelphia, 1986, p. 441.
9. Knight, V., Yu, C. P., Gilbert, B. E., Orr, R.: Ribavirin aerosol treatment: emerging technology and clinical summary. In: Stapleton, T. (ed.): International Congress and Symposium series. Royal Society of Medicine Services, London, 1988, in press.
10. Knight, V., Yu, C. P., Gilbert, B. E., Divine, G.: Ribavirin aerosol dosage according to age and other variables. Journal of Infectious Diseases 1988, 158: 443–448.
11. Hofmann, W.: Mathematical model for the post natal growth of the human lung. Respiratory Physiology 1982, 49: 115–129.
12. Connor, J. D., Hrutz, M., Van Dyke, R., McCormick, J. B., McIntosh, K.: Ribavirin pharmacokinetics in children and adults during therapeutic trials. In: Smith, R. A., Knight, V., Smith, J. A. D. (ed.): Clinical applications of ribavirin. Academic Press, New York, 1983, p. 107.
13. Gilbert, B. E., Wyde, P. R.: Pharmacokinetics of ribavirin aerosol in mice. Antimicrobial Agents and Chemotherapy 1988, 32: 117–121.
14. Zimmerman, T. P., Deeprose, R. D.: Mechanisms of 5-amino-1-B-D-ribofuranosyl-imidazole-4-carboxamide and related five membered heterocycles to 5'-triphosphates in human blood and L5178Y cells. Biochemical Pharmacology 1978, 27: 709–716.
15. Smee, D. F., Matthews, T. R.: Metabolism of ribavirin in respiratory syncytial virus-infected and uninfected cells. Antimicrobial Agents and Chemotherapy 1986, 30: 117–121.
16. Barry, W., Cockburn, R., Cornall, R., Price, J. F., Sutherland, G., Vardag, A.: Ribavirin aerosol for acute bronchiolitis. Archives of Diseases in Childhood 1986, 61: 593–597.
17. Conrad, D. A., Christenson, J. C., Waner, J. L., Marks, M. I.: Aerosolized ribavirin treatment of respiratory syncytial virus infection in infants hospitalized during an epidemic. Pediatric Infectious Disease Journal 1987, 6: 152–158.
18. Rodriguez, W. J., Kim, H. W., Brandt, C. D., Find, R. J., Getson, P. R., Arrobio, J., Murphy, T. M., McCarthy, V., Parrott, R. H.: Aerosolized ribavirin in the treatment of patients with respiratory syncytial virus disease. Pediatric Infectious Disease Journal 1987, 6: 159–163.
19. Gelfand, E. W., McCurdy, D., Rao, C. P., Middleton, P. J.: Ribavirin treatment of viral pneumonitis in severe combined immunodeficiency disease. Lancet 1983, ii: 732–733.
20. McIntosh, K., Kurachek, S. C., Cairns, L. M., Burns, J. D., Goodspeed, B.: Treatment of respiratory viral infection in an immunodeficient infant with ribavirin aerosol. American Journal of Diseases of Childhood 1984, 138: 305–308.
21. Rosner, I. K., Welliver, R. C., Edelson, P. J., Geraci-Ciardullo, K., Sun, M.: Effect of ribavirin therapy on respiratory syncytial virus-specific IgE and IgA responses after infection. Journal of Infectious Diseases 1987, 155: 1043–1047.

22. Taber, L. H., Knight, V., Gilbert, B. E., McClung, H. W., Wilson, S. Z., Norton, H. J., Thurson, J. M., Gordon, W. H., Atmar, R. L., Schlaudt, W. R.: Ribavirin aerosol treatment of bronchiolitis associated with respiratory syncytial virus infection in infants. Pediatrics 1983, 72: 613–618.
23. Hall, C. B., McBride, J. T., Walsh, E. E., Bell, D. N. J., Gala, C. L., Hildreth, S., Ten Eyck, L. G., Hall, W. J.: Aerosolized ribavirin treatment of infants with respiratory syncytial viral infection. New England Journal of Medicine 1983, 308: 1443–1447.
24. Hall, C. B., McBride, J. T., Gala, C. L., Hildreth, S. W., Schnabel, K. C.: Ribavirin treatment of respiratory syncytial viral infection in infants with underlying cardiopulmonary disease. Journal of the American Medical Association 1985, 254: 3047–3051.
25. Wilson, S. Z., Gilbert, B. E., Quarles, J. M., Knight, V., McClung, H., Moore, R., Couch, R.: Treatment of influenza A (H1N1) virus infection with ribavirin aerosol. Antimicrobial Agents and Chemotherapy 1984, 86: 200–203.
26. Knight, V., Gilbert, B. E.: Chemotherapy of respiratory viruses. In: Stollerman, W. J., Harrington, W. J., Lamont, J. T., Leonard, J. J., Siperstein, M. D. (ed.): Advances in internal medicine. Year Book Medical Publishers, Chicago, 1986, p. 95.
27. Gilbert, B. E., Wilson, W. Z., Knight, V.: Ribavirin aerosol treatment of influenza virus infections. In: Kendal, A. P., Patriarca, P. A. (ed.): Options for the control of influenza: UCLA symposia on molecular and cellular biology. Alan R. Liss, New York, 1986, p. 343.
28. Kirshon, B., Faro, S., Zurawin, R. K., Samo, T. C., Carpenter, R. J.: Favorable outcome after treatment with amantadine and ribavirin in a pregnancy complicated by influenzal pneumonia. Journal of Reproductive Medicine 1988, 33: 399–401.
29. DeLong, D. C., Reed, S. E.: Inhibition of rhinovirus replication in organ cultures by a potential antiviral drug. Journal of Infectious Diseases 1980, 141: 87–91.
30. Phillpotts, R. J., DeLong, D. C., Wallace, J., Jones, R. W., Reed, S. E., Tyrrell, D. A. J.: The activity of enviroxime against rhinovirus in man. Lancet 1981, i: 1342–1344.
31. Levandowski, R. A., Pachucki, C. T., Rubenis, M., Jackson, G. G.: Topical enviroxime against rhinovirus infection. Antimicrobial Agents and Chemotherapy 1982, 22: 1004–1007.
32. Hayden, G. F., Gwaltney, J. M., Jr.: Prophylactic activity of intranasal enviroxime against experimentally induced rhinovirus type 39 infection. Antimicrobial Agents and Chemotherapy 1982, 21: 892–897.
33. Phillpotts, R. J., Wallace, J., Tyrrell, D. A. J., Tagart, V. B.: Therapeutic activity of enviroxime against rhinovirus infection in volunteers. Antimicrobial Agents and Chemotherapy 1983, 23: 671–675.
34. Miller, F. D., Monto, A. S., DeLong, D. C., Exelby, A., Bryan, E. R., Srivastava, S.: Controlled trial of enviroxime against natural rhinovirus infections in a community. Antimicrobial Agents and Chemotherapy 1985, 27: 102–106.

Liposomes and Lipid Structures as Carriers of Amphotericin B

A. S. Janoff

Almost 25 years ago, Bangham noted that "smectic mesophases" formed when biological lipids were dispersed in aqueous media (1). These structures, later described as multilamellar liposomes, consisted of concentric biomolecular lamellae of lipid, each separated by an aqueous compartment. Although important as models of cellular membranes, the potential of these systems as drug carriers was not lost. It was quickly recognized that water-soluble drugs could be entrapped within the aqueous spaces of the vesicles, while hydrophobic drugs would intercalate into the lipid layers. The more recent development of preparative techniques allowing control over the size, lamellarity, trapped aqueous volume and solute distribution in the final emulsions has led to a rapid expansion in this field (2). In fact, the emergence of liposomes as drug delivery vehicles is now extensively documented (3). Liposome-dependent alterations in pharmacokinetics/pharmacodynamics have been well described for a variety of biologically active compounds. Perhaps far more remarkable, however, have been the reports that certain liposome formulations are also able to attenuate toxicities of associated drugs without substantially compromising efficacy (4). One drug affected in this manner is amphotericin B.

In the case of amphotericin B, subsequent work has led to a greater understanding of how hydrophobic drugs can interact specifically with lipid and has provided insights into how drugs are transferred to cellular membranes in general (5). These biophysical advancements notwithstanding, it must be appreciated that the impetus for the development of lipid-based alternative dosage forms of amphotericin first grew out of a need for less toxic therapies and the ability of the growing field of liposomology to adequately meet these needs.

Despite its associated toxicities, amphotericin B, remains the drug of choice for most fungal infections in humans. The mechanism of action of this compound is thought to reside in its ability to form membrane ion channels (with associated lethal permeability changes), particularly in the presence of sterols (6). The occurrence of channel formation at lower concentrations in the presence of ergosterol (the predominant sterol in fungal cell membranes) as opposed to cholesterol (the predominant sterol in mammalian cell membranes) most likely forms the basis of the selective toxicity for this compound (7). Still, in its present dosage form, which is a mixed micelle with deoxycholate, host-mediated toxicities including fever, chills, bronchospasms and renal and central nervous system involvement clearly limit its clinical utility. The poor water solubility and high lipid solubility of amphotericin, however, make it an ideal candiate for liposome encapsulation, and numerous preparations of reduced toxicity that were formulated based on this approach consistently offered the promise of clinical success, fueling the rapid development of this dosage form.

New and co-workers were the first to report that liposomes were capable of buffering amphotericin-dependent host-related acute toxicities in rodents (8). In this work amphotericin incorporated at 4 mol % of the bulk lipid in a variety of liposome preparations comprised of various phospholipids maintained good efficacy against the leishmanial parasite. Host-mediated toxicity was decreased to a greater extent if liposomes comprised of rigid lipids were employed; although the dependence of parasite clearance upon liposome composition was more difficult to assess, taken together this data clearly suggested a degree of selective transfer between the amphotericin lipid intermediate and fungal/mammalian cell membranes.

Further work by Taylor (9) and Graybill (10) confirmed that liposome-associated amphotericin B offered a dosage form of altered selective toxicity. More specifically, when incorporated into liposome preparations at low concentrations (below 5 mol % of the bulk lipid), the acute toxicities of the drug were reduced five-to ten-fold. On the other hand, efficacies regarding histoplasmosis and cryptococcosis were particularly enhanced, presumably because the reduced toxicities permitted larger than usual concentrations of amphotericin to be administered. This work was extended by Lopez-Berestein and Juliano (11, 12), who were able to demonstrate that liposomally associated amphotericin was effective and less toxic than conventional amphotericin in systemic candidiasis in mice. In these studies amphotericin concentrations were again fairly low, remaining between 5 and 10 % of the bulk lipid.

The observations regarding candidiasis were quickly reproduced by these and other authors (13–16), extending their validity and sparking the initiative

The Liposome Company, Inc., 1 Research Way, Princeton, New Jersey 08540, USA.

that brought liposomally associated amphotericin into clinical trials. The Juliano/Lopez-Berestein formulation, in which amphotericin constituted 5 mol% of a multilamellar liposome suspension comprised of dimyristoylphosphatidylcholine (DMPC): dimyristoylphosphatidylglycerol (DMPG) in a 7:3 mol ratio, was first used to treat patients with systemic candidiasis at M. D. Anderson Hospital in Houston, Texas, a number of years ago (17, 18). These trials were a realization of therapeutic promises implied in the earlier in vitro work and were eventually extended to patients with *Aspergillus* sinusitis (19). Although other liposome formulations have been used in limited clinical trials, data from only one other group, Sculier and co-workers (20), has been published. In trials designed to study the effect of a sonicated preparation of liposomes containing amphotericin ($<$ 5 mol%) and egg phosphatidylcholine, cholesterol, and stearylamine in a molar ratio of 4:3:1, patients with a variety of fungal diseases were treated. The results suggested again that liposome dispersions are capable of increasing the therapeutic index of amphotericin B, and the belief that amphotericin in a lipid-based dosage form would have wide ranging clinical utility was further reinforced.

Concomitant with the ongoing clinical successes of liposome amphotericin B formulations, work aimed at uncovering the basic mechanism inherent in the amphotericin B lipid interaction continued. The demonstration by the Juliano/ Lopez-Berestein group that the in vivo effects of liposomally associated amphotericin could be mimicked in in vitro systems suggested that fundamental molecular events must be involved (21). In these studies free but not liposomally associated amphotericin was hemolytic, but both free and liposomally associated drug showed substantially equal candicidal effects. Thus the altered selective toxicity achieved by associating amphotericin B with lipid became difficult to explain based on alterations in pharmacokinetics or drug distribution.

The ability of liposomally associated amphotericin B to discriminate between host cells and pathogens was further explored as a function of the lipid composition of the carrier state. Basically this work supported and extended the earlier work of New, in that more highly saturated or sterol-containing (rigid) lipid matrixes were found to offer the best therapeutic advantages. The in vitro transfer of amphotericin from the carrier to yeast or red blood cells as judged by the efflux of previously loaded rhubidium into these cells could be related to fluidity differences between both donor and acceptor membranes (22). More rigid carrier systems clearly offered the greatest margin of selective toxicity. Further, a systematic evaluation of the effect of lipid composition and liposome size on in vivo mammalian toxicity revealed the order of reduction of lethality to be sterol-containing liposomes $>$ solid liposomes $>$ fluid liposomes (23). In these studies small sterol-containing vesicles were generally less lethal than larger vesicles of the same composition. The 24-hour organ distribution of amphotericin was similar, whether the drug was given as the deoxycholate preparation or as a liposome preparation. In support of the bulk of the work in this area, there were no differences among any of the preparations regarding their fungicidal activity against *Candida* spp. or *Sacchromyces* spp. in vitro, despite their decreased mammalian cell toxicities.

It was against this backdrop that we became involved with amphotericin (5). To us it was not readily apparent why the toxicity of this drug should be so markedly selectively reduced by its incorporation into a liposomal as opposed to a micellar matrix. Experiments utilizing polymerizable lipids indicated that mammalian cell toxicity was not reduced when amphotericin was incorporated into liposomes of this type, suggesting the crucial nature of the amphotericin-lipid interaction (24). However, the nature of this interaction and the parameters able to modulate it were still unknown. Our work in this area has subsequently revealed that when amphotericin interacts with phospholipid in an aqueous environment, ribbon-like structures clearly distinct from liposomes result (5). At high amphotericin-to-lipid ratios, these structures become prevalent, resulting in an enhanced reduction of amphotericin-mediated mammalian cell but not fungal cell toxicity. In fact, it seems likely that these structures are responsible for the enhanced selective toxicity that has been widely reported to result from the incorporation of this drug into intact vesicles.

Our experiments began with the Juliano/Lopez-Berestein formulation. We felt this was the logical place to start, because of both the extensive in vitro work and the positive clinical experiences involving this preparation. Our initial trials revealed, surprisingly, the heterogeneous nature of the amphotericin-lipid interaction. As shown in Figure 1A, when the Juliano/Lopez-Berestein formulation (prepared by hydration of a DMPC:DMPG thin film containing 5 mol% amphotericin) was fractionated on an isopycnic sucrose density gradient, two major populations emerged: a high density amphotericin-rich population and a low density lipid-rich population. While attempts to arrive at a single homogenous population comprised of 5 mol% amphotericin B were successful (data not shown), they did not yield a reduction in mammalian lethality. In fact, these homogeneous formulations, which exhibited densities intermediate to the two populations of the Juliano/Lopez-Berestein formulation, yielded LD50 values somewhat lower than the Juliano/Lopez-Berestein formulation in Swiss Webster mice.

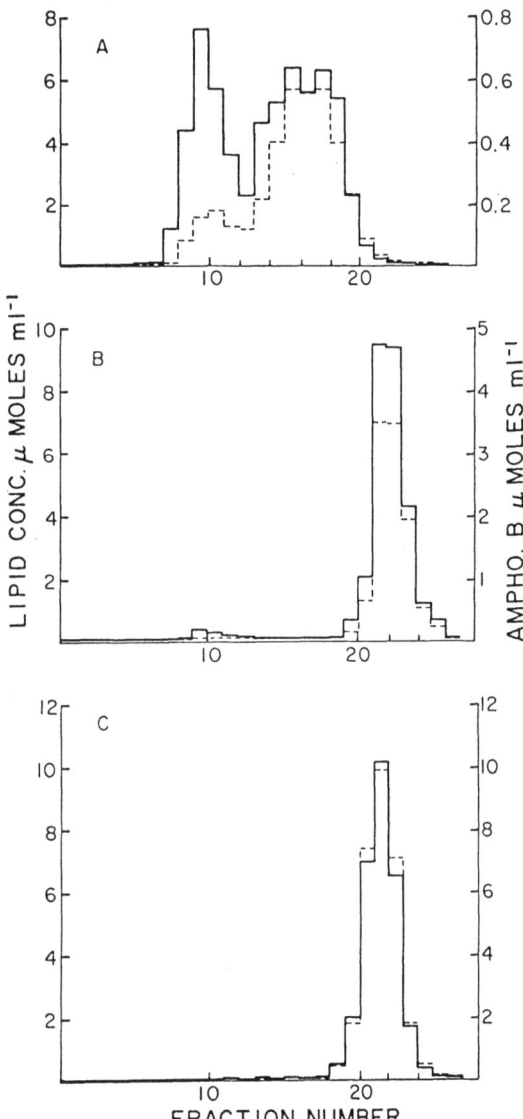

Figure 1: Isopycnic sucrose density profiles of DMPC: DMPG (7:3) lipid dispersions incorporating A) 5 mol%, B) 25 mol% and C) 50 mol% amphotericin B. The gradient ranged from 0–29 wt% sucrose for the 5 and 25 mol% samples, and from 0–41 wt% sucrose for the 50 mol% sample. Typically, 200 μl of material was layered onto a continuous sucrose gradient in 150 mm NaCl, 20 mM hepes, pH 7.4. The gradient was centrifuged for 22 h at 22 °C in an SW 60 rotor (Beckman) at 230,000 × g. Following centrifugation the gradient was fractionated in 150 μl aliquots and assayed for amphotericin B (from absorbance at 412 nm in dimethylformamide) and phospholipid (from phosphate assay following digestion).

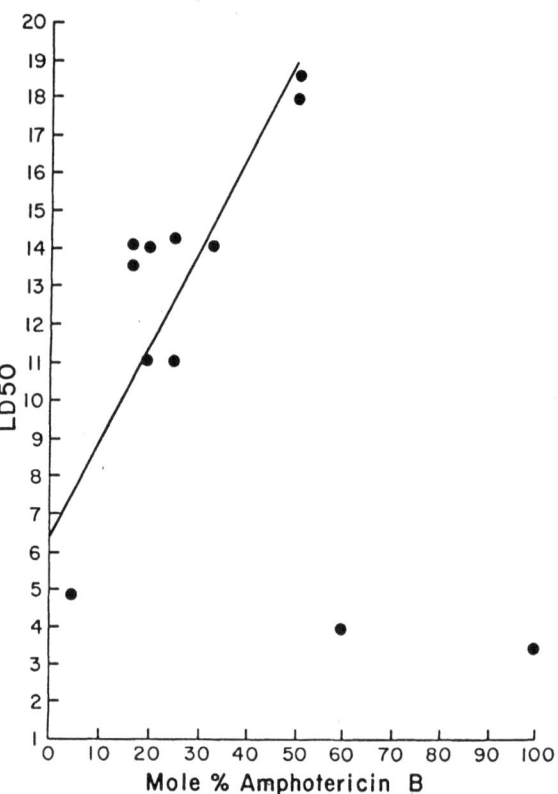

Figure 2: Ten day acute LD50 values in mice (expressed as mg of amphotericin per kg of body weight) versus the mole percentage of amphotericin incorporated into DMPC: DMPG (7:3) lipid dispersions. In these experiments lipid alone was not toxic.

The fact that these 5 mol% homogeneous formulations were more toxic than the heterogeneous Juliano/Lopez-Berestein formulation was puzzling until we separated the latter into its two major fractions and performed toxicity measurements on both. In Swiss Webster mice the high density amphotericin-rich fraction was somewhat less toxic than the lower density lipid-enriched fraction. The DMPC:DMPG ratio in the high density fraction was not different than the ratio of these two lipids in the low density fraction. The amphotericin: lipid ratio in the two fractions was, however, quite different. Following this lead we prepared and characterized formulations of varying mole percentages of amphotericin compared to the bulk lipid.

Figure 2 shows that by elevating the mole fraction of amphotericin from 5 to 50 % in DMPC:DMPG (7:3) lipid systems, a dramatic decrease in toxicity could be achieved. When the mole fraction of amphotericin exceeded 50 % of the lipid, however, its solubility in the lipid matrix was presumably exceeded and toxicities close to those determined for free amphotericin (100 mol%) were recorded. Toxicity profiles similar to that shown in Figure 2 were acquired in an in vitro hemolysis model, but efficacy as judged in an in vivo candidiasis model was comparatively unchanged by the manipulation of drug-to-lipid ratios. The finding that increasing the percentage of amphotericin in the lipid matrix would actually lead to a decrease in toxicity made clear to us the necessity of defining the biophysical nature of the amphotericin-lipid interaction in specific.

Liposomes and lipid structures as carriers of amphotericin B

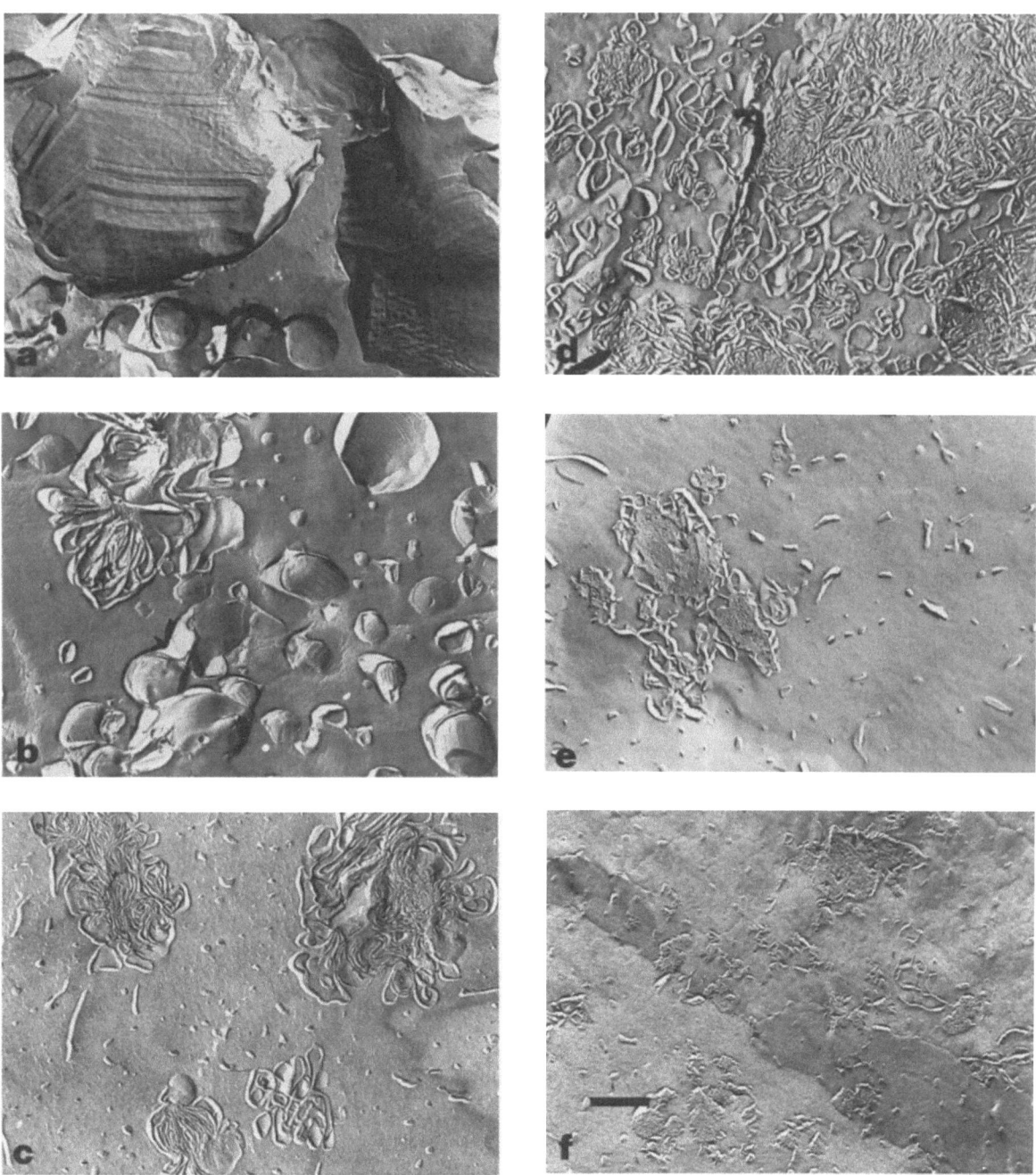

Figure 3: Freeze-etch electron micrographs of various DMPC/DMPG/amphotericin B dispersions quenched from 20 °C. All systems contained DMPC:DMPG in a molar ratio of 7:3 and an amphotericin B molar percentage (with respect to the bulk lipid) of a) 0 %, b) 5 %, c) 25 %, d) 50 % and e) 60 %. A dispersion of pure amphotericin B is also shown (f). Bar = 0.4 μm. Samples were prepared by quick freezing into liquid propane without a cryoprotectant. Replicas were viewed on a Philips 300 electron microscope at a magnification of 21,000.

Figure 3 shows the morphological parameters of this interaction as revealed by freeze-etch microscopy. Lipid dispersions free of amphotericin contained vesicles, all of which exhibited the $P\beta'$ (ripple) structure characteristic of these lipids when quenched at room temperature. When 5 mol% amphotericin was incorporated into the bulk lipid, however, a heterogeneous mixture arose, consisting of clumps of loosely packed ribbon structures and vesicles exhibiting the ripple phase. Since the ripple phase is sensitive to perturbations, it is likely that these vesicles contained little amphotericin, thus corresponding to the lipid-enriched fraction of this formulation uncovered by the isopycnic density gradient work. Increasing the amphotericin content to 25 mol% resulted in a complete loss of defined liposomal structures, as shown in Figure 3C. The predominant ribbon-like structures in this preparation seemed more tightly packed and clearly defined. Qualitatively similar ribbon structures existed in the 50 mol% samples but tended to be replaced in the 60 mol% and free amphotericin samples by more amorphous (presumably toxic), rougher-textured material.

When we examined the amphotericin lipid complex by X-ray diffraction, differential scanning calorimetry, ^{31}P nuclear magnetic resonance, and absorbance spectroscopy (5), we found that as a consequence of increasing the amphotericin-to-lipid ratio, the lipid itself became increasingly immobilized, resulting in closer amphotericin-amphotericin and amphotericin-lipid associations. Thus, as shown in Figures 1B and 1C, when amphotericin comprised 25 or 50 mol% of the bulk lipid, all of the drug was associated with all of the lipid in a single iso-dense bond. The gel phase lipid shown by the X-ray diffraction experiments to be present in these (less toxic) samples has been implicated to interact with amphotericin to a much greater extent than more fluid phase lipid (25).

Our studies in this area thus have strongly suggested that nonliposomal lipid-stabilized complexes of amphotericin are largely responsible for the lipid-mediated toxicity attenuation of amphotericin. In fact, these complexes provide a simple structural rationale for such toxicity attenuation. This rationale is based on the assumption that the aqueous diffusion of amphotericin from the complex would be limited compared to its diffusion from a micelle or liposome.

Since amphotericin binds with a tenfold greater affinity to ergosterol compared to cholesterol (26), and since amphotericin sterol interactions most likely result in target cell permeability changes in a steep, concentration-dependent fashion (27), it seems reasonable to propose that this attenuated diffusion would result in an enhanced selective toxicity. Diffusion of amphotericin monomers from the complex would be expected to be dependent on both drug-drug and drug-lipid interactions. Both types of interactions would be expected to progressively limit the release of amphotericin from the complex (resulting in enhanced differential toxicity) at higher drug-to-lipid ratios, the former due to concentration considerations (28), the latter due to the increasing immobilization of the bulk lipid (25). Thus the improved therapeutic value of amphotericin in a lipid-stabilized complexed state can be explained in purely physical terms. We believe this explanation offers both mechanistic insights into the source of the selective toxicity of the amphotericin B lipid complex and a means for the production of less toxic dosage forms.

Acknowledgement

We acknowledge the Squibb Institute for Medical Research for its support of this project.

References

1. Bangham, A. D., Standish, M. M., Watkens, J. C.: Diffusion of univalent ions across the lamellae of swollen phospholipids. Journal of Molecular Biology 1965, 13: 238–252.
2. Hope, M. J., Bally, M. B., Mayer, L. D., Janoff, A. S., Cullis, P. R.: Generation of multilamellar and unilamellar phospholipid vesicles. Chemistry and Physics of Lipids 1986, 40: 89–107.
3. Cullis, P. R., Hope, M. J., Bally, M. B., Madden, T. D., Mayer, L. D., Janoff, A. S.: Liposomes as pharmaceuticals. In: Ostro, M. J. (ed.): Liposomes from biophysics to therapeutics. Marcel Dekker, New York, 1987, p. 39–72.
4. Mayhew, E., Papahadjopoulos, D.: Therapeutic applications of liposomes. In: Ostro, M. J. (ed.): Liposomes. Marcel Dekker, New York, 1983, p. 289–341.
5. Janoff, A. S., Boni, L. T., Popescu, M. C., Minchey, S. R., Cullis, P. R., Madden, T. D., Taraschi, T., Gruner, S. M., Shyamsundh, E., Tate, M. W., Mendelsohn, R., Bonner, D.: Unusual lipid structures selectively reduce the toxicity of amphotericin B. Proceedings of the National Academy of Sciences of the USA 1988, 85: 6122–6126.
6. DeKruijff, B., Gerritsen, W. J., Oerlemans, A., Demel, R. A., Van Deenen, L. L. M.: Polyene antibiotic-sterol interactions in membranes of acholeplasma laidlawii cells and lecithin liposomes. Biochimica et Biophysica Acta 1974, 339: 30–43.
7. Croquin, A. V., Bolard, J., Chabbert, M., Gary-Bobo, C.: Differences in the interaction of the polyene antibiotic amphotericin B with cholesterol or ergosterol-containing phospholipid vesicles. A circular dichroism and permeability study. Biochemistry 1983, 22: 2939–2944.
8. New, R. R. C., Chance, M. L., Heath, J.: Antileishmanial activity of amphotericin and other antifungal agents entrapped in liposomes. Journal of Antimicrobial Chemotherapy 1981, 8: 371–381.
9. Taylor, R. L., Williams, D. M., Craven, P. C., Graybill, J. R., Drutz, D. J., Magee, W. E.: Amphotericin B in liposomes: a novel therapy for histoplasmosis. Annual Reviews of Respiratory Diseases 1982, 125: 610–611.
10. Graybill, J. R., Craven, P. C., Taylor, R. L., Williams, D. M., Magee, W. E.: Treatment of murine cryptococcosis with liposome-associated amphotericin B. Journal of Infectious Diseases 1982, 145: 748–752.
11. Lopez-Berestein, G., Mehta, R., Hopfer, R., Mehta, K., Hersh, E. M., Juliano, R.: Effects of sterols on the therapeutic efficacy of liposomal amphotericin B in murine candidiasis. Cancer Drug Delivery 1983, 1: 37–42.
12. Lopez-Berestein, G., Mehta, R., Hopfer, R. L., Mills, K., Kasi, L., Mehta, K., Fainstein, V., Luna, W., Hersh, E. M., Juliano, R. L.: Treatment and prophylaxis of disseminated infection due to Candida albicans in mice with liposome encapsulated amphotericin B. Journal of Infectious Diseases 1983, 147: 939–945.
13. Ahrens, J., Graybill, J. R., Craven, P. C., Taylor, R. L.: Treatment of experimental murine candidiasis with liposome associated amphotericin B. Sabouraudia Journal of Medical and Veterinary Mycology 1984, 22: 163–166.

14. Lopez-Berestein, G., Hopfer, R. L., Mehta, R., Mehta, K., Hersh, E., Juliano, R. L.: Prophylaxis of *Candida albicans* infection in neutropenic mice with liposome-encapsulated amphotericin B. Antimicrobial Agents and Chemotherapy 1984, 25: 366–367.
15. Hopfer, R. L., Mills, K., Mehta, R., Lopez-Berestein, G., Fainstein, V., Juliano, R. L.: In vitro antifungal activities of amphotericin B and liposome-encapsulated amphotericin B. Antimicrobial Agents and Chemotherapy 1984, 25: 287–389.
16. Tremblay, C., Barza, M., Fiore, C., Szoka, F.: Efficacy of liposome intercalated amphotericin B in the treatment of systemic candidiasis in mice. Antimicrobial Agents and Chemotherapy 1984, 26: 170–173.
17. Lopez-Berestein, G., Fainstein, V., Hopfer, R., Mehta, K., Sullivan, M. P., Keating, M., Rosenblum, M. G., Mehta, R., Luna, M., Hersh, E. M., Reuben, J., Juliano, R. L., Bodey, G. P.: Liposomal amphotericin B for the treatment of systemic fungal infections in patients with cancer: a preliminary study. Journal of Infectious Diseases 1985, 151: 704–710.
18. Lopez-Berestein, G., Bodey, G. P., Frankel, L. S., Mehta, K.: Treatment of hepatosplenic candidiasis with liposomal amphotericin B. Journal of Clinical Oncology 1987, 5: 310–315.
19. Weber, R. S., Lopez-Berestein, G.: Treatment of invasive *Aspergillus* sinusitis with liposomal amphotericin B. Larynascope 1987, 97: 937–941.
20. Sculier, J. P., Coune, A., Meunier, F., Brassinne, C., Laduron, C., Hollaert, C., Collette, N., Heymons, C., Klastersky, J.: Pilot study of amphotericin B entrapped in sonicated liposomes in cancer patients with fungal infections. European Journal of Cancer and Clinical Oncology 1988, 24: 527–538.
21. Mehta, R., Lopez-Berestein, G., Hopfer, R., Mills, K., Juliano, R.: Liposomal amphotericin B is toxic to fungal cells but not to mammalian cells. Biochiimica et Biophysica Acta 1984, 770: 220–234.
22. Juliano, R. L., Grant, C. W. M., Barber, K. R., Kalp, M. A.: Mechanism of the selective toxicity of amphotericin B incorporated into liposomes. Molecular Pharmacology 1986, 31: 1–11.
23. Szoka, F. C., Milholland, D., Barza, M.: Effect of lipid composition and liposome size on toxicity and in vitro fungicidal activity of liposome-intercalated amphotericin B. Antimicrobial Agents and Chemotherapy 1987, 31: 421–429.
24. Mehta, R., Hsu, M. J., Juliano, R. L., Kranse, H. J., Regen, S. L.: Polymerized phospholipid vesicles containing amphotericin B: evaluation of toxic and antifungal activities in vitro. Journal of Pharmaceutical Sciences 1986, 75: 579–581.
25. Bolard, J., Vertut-Croquin, A., Cybulska, B. E., Gary-Bobo, C. M.: Transfer of the polyene antibiotic amphotericin B between single-walled vesicles of dipalmitoylphosphatidylcholine. Biochemica et Biophysica Acta 1981, 647: 241.
26. Readio, J. D., Bittman, R.: Equilibrium binding of amphotericin B and its methyl ester and borate complex to sterols. Biochimica et Biophysica Acta 1982, 685: 219–224.
27. Cybulska, B., Herve, M., Borowski, E., Gary-Bobo, C. M.: Effect of the polar head structure of polyene macrolide antifungal antibiotics on the mode of permeabilization of ergosterol- and cholesterol-containing lipidic vesicles studied by ^{31}P-NMR. Molecular Pharmacology 1986, 79: 293.
28. Ghielmetti, G., Bruzzese, T., Bianchi, L., Recusani, F.: Relationship between acute toxicity in mice and polymorphic forms of polyene antibiotics. Journal of Pharmaceutical Sciences 1976, 65: 905.

Targeted Liposomes Bearing Sendai for Influenza Envelope Glycoproteins as a Potential Carrier for Protein Molecules and Genes

A. Loyter

Infection of animal cells by enveloped viruses is mediated by a membrane fusion step. Sendai virus particles introduce nucleoprotein molecules into recipient cells via fusion with the plasma membrane of the cells, while influenza viruses accomplish this via fusion with membranes of endosomes following receptor-mediated endocytosis of virus particles. Virus-membrane fusion can be observed on a quantitative basis using fluorescently labeled virus particles (bearing octadecylrhodamine B-chloride, R_{18}) and the fluorescent dequenching method. Treatment of either Sendai or influenza virus particles with the non-ionic detergent Triton X-100 results in solubilization of the virus envelopes' glycoproteins and phospholipids. Removal of the detergent leads to the formation of fusogenic reconstituted viral envelopes. Macromolecules such as SV40-DNA or Ricin A (the A subunit of the plant toxin Ricin) can be enclosed within reconstituted viral envelopes if added to the reconstitution system. With the aid of cross-linking reagents, specific non-viral binding proteins such as anti-membrane antibodies or polypeptide hormones can be attached to the viral envelopes, resulting in the formation of "targeted" fusogenic envelopes. Using these methods, reconstituted Sendai virus envelopes bearing insulin molecules and loaded with either SV40-DNA or Ricin A molecules were able to introduce their content into cultured cells from which virus receptors were removed by treatment with neuraminidase. Fusion-mediated microinjection of SV40-DNA and Ricin A was inferred from the appearance of SV40-T-antigen and the inhibitions of protein synthesis in recipient cells, respectively. Free insulin molecules completely inhibited fusion-mediated microinjection, indicating that virus-cell binding was promoted by virus-attached insulin molecules.

A membrane fusion step mediates the penetration of animal cells by all enveloped viruses and leads to introduction of the viral content directly into the recipient cell cytoplasm. Enveloped viruses fuse with either cell plasma membranes at pH 7.4 or membranes of intracellular organelles at pH 5. Solubilization of intact virus particles with various detergents followed by sedimentation of detergent-insoluble material and removal of the detergent from the clear supernatant obtained after the sedimentation step results in the formation of reconstituted viral envelopes. Such membrane vesicles contain only the viral glycoproteins and are devoid of the viral genetic material.

Reconstituted Sendai virus envelopes (RSVE) as well as reconstituted influenza virus envelopes (RIVE) are as fusogenic as intact virus particles. This has been inferred from quantitative determination of virus-membrane fusion processes using fluorescently labeled envelopes and fluorescence dequenching methods. RSVE and RIVE may be used as efficient biological carriers for the introduction of foreign macromolecules and drugs into living cultured cells. When added during the reconstituion process, protein as well as RNA and DNA molecules can be enclosed within reconstituted viral envelopes. Furthermore, attachment of anti-membrane antibodies or polypeptide hormones to such reconstituted envelopes leads to the formation of "targeted" fusogenic envelopes which bind to and fuse with cells containing the appropriate antigens or hormone receptors.

We loaded RSVE with the potent toxin Ricin A and with SV_{40}-DNA. Loaded RSVE bearing insulin molecules were able to bind to cell cultures (hepatoma tissue cultures) from which Sendai virus receptors had been removed by treatment with neuraminidase. Incubation of Ricin A-loaded viral envelopes with virus receptor depleted hepatoma cells resulted in fusion-mediated injection of the toxin as was inferred from the inhibition of protein synthesis and the decrease in cell viability in the microinjected cells. Fusion-mediated injection of SV_{40}-DNA was inferred from the appearance of SV_{40}-tumor antigen (T-antigen) in the microinjected cells. The potential use of such "targeted" fusogenic viral envelopes as biological or drug carriers is discussed.

Department of Biological Chemistry, Institute of Life Sciences, Hebrew University of Jerusalem, Jerusalem 91904, Israel.

Quantitative Determination of Virus-Membrane Fusion

Penetration of animal cells by all enveloped viruses is mediated by a membrane fusion step (1, 2). Following adsorption to specific surface receptors, most viruses are enclosed within endocytic vesicles, the low pH environment of which activates their viral fusion polypeptide. A low pH-dependent fusion of the viral envelopes with the endosomal membranes results in microinjection of the viral content into the cell cytoplasm. This pattern of behavior is characteristic of enveloped viruses belonging to the orthomyoxvirus, toga, rhabdo and herpes groups. Enveloped viruses belonging to the myoxvirus and possibly also to the retrovirus groups are able to fuse with the cell plasma membrane at pH 7.4. A low pH environment is not required to activate their fusion protein (1). Evidently, fusion with the cell plasma membrane also results in introduction of the viral content directly into the cell cytoplasm (1, 2).

Recently, it was confirmed that fluorescent probes and energy transfer methods can be used to observe fusion processes between enveloped viruses and recipient membranes on a quantitative basis (3–5). Adsorption of the hydrophobic fluorescence probe, octadecylrhodamine-B-chloride (R_{18}), to enveloped viruses resulted in it becoming self-quenched. Processes, such as virus-membrane fusion, which lead to the dilution of both the viral envelope phospholipids and the virus-associated probe, should result in fluorescence dequenching. Thus, fusion between enveloped viruses and recipient membranes can be studied on a quantitative basis by determination of R_{18} fluorescence relieved after self-quenching.

The results in Table 1 show that incubation of several fluorescently labeled enveloped viruses such as Sendai, influenza and Semliki Forest virus (SFV) with living cultured cells or human erythrocytes resulted in fluorescence dequenching. Very little fluorescence dequenching was observed following incubation of inactivated-unfusogenic viruses with the cells, emphasizing that the increase in fluorescence observed indeed reflects of process of virus-membrane fusion. The fusogenic activities of influenza and SFV were blocked by treatment with glutaraldehyde or hydroxylamine, or by incubation at a low pH or at 85 °C (3, 4). On the other hand, Sendai virions were rendered unfusogneic by either trypsinization or treatment with glutaraldehyde, phenylmethylsulfonyl fluoride (PMSF), or dithioerythrol (DTT). A low increase in fluorescence dequenching was also observed following incubation of HA_0-influenza viruses, namely viruses bearing an uncleaved HA_0-glycoprotein, and recipient

Table 1: Quantitative determination of fusion of enveloped viruses with living cultured cells and human erythrocytes.

System	pH of incubation	Fluorescence dequenching (%) of viruses incubated with:	
		Living cultured cells (Hela, lymphoma S_{49})	Human erythrocytes
Influenza treated with:			
None	5	49	47
	7.4	42	8
Glutaraldehyde	5	6	8
Hydroxylamine	5	10	7
Low pH	5	5	8
HA_0-influenza	5	8	9
	7.4	6	6
Trypsinized HA_0-influenza	5	38	38
	7.4	34	6
Sendai treated with:			
None	5	48	46
	7.4	55	60
Glutaraldehyde	7.4	8	10
Trypsin	7.4	7	11
PMSF	7.4	8	7
DTT	7.4	8	8
Semliki Forest virus	5	48	–
	7.4	16	–

For experimental details of virus preparation, culturing of cells, determination of fluorescence dequenching and inactivation of influenza and Sendai fusogenic abilities, see References No. 3–5, 9, 12 and 15. Influenza, Sendai or Semliki Forest virus were incubated at 37 °C with cultured cells or human erythrocytes as described in References No. 3–5, 9 and 12. For determination of fluorescence dequenching, human erythrocytes were hemolyzed with hypotonic buffer and fluorescence dequenching determination was performed on the human erythrocyte ghost obtained. HA_0-influenza virus particles were prepared and trypsinized as described in Reference No. 6.

cells (Table 1). It has been well established that such HA_0-influenza virions are neither fusogenic nor infective (6); mild trypsinization of influenza virions was shown to cause cleavage of the HA_0-glycoprotein with restoration of the virus fusogenic activity. The results in Table 1 show that a relatively high degree of fluorescence dequenching was obtained using trypsinized HA_0-influenza virions as opposed to the low degree of fluorescence dequenching observed with untrypsinized HA_0-virus particles. Influenza virus particles and SFV particles fused with living cultured cells at pH 5 as well as at pH 7.4. However, a high degree of fluorescence dequenching, indicating fusion of influenza virions with human erythrocytes, was observed only at pH 5. Unpublished and previous (3, 4) results have also shown that only the fluorescence dequenching observed following incubation of influenza with cultured cells at pH 7.4 was inhibited by lysosomotropic agents or reagents which cause cell ATP-depletion. Furthermore, chelators of bivalent metals such as EDTA drastically reduced the fluorescence dequenching observed at pH 7.4, but not that obtained at pH 5. Lyosomotropic agents increased the intraendosomal low pH values while reagents such as NaN_3 or EDTA blocked the endocytic process itself. These results clearly indicate that the fluorescence dequenching observed following incubation of influenza and SFV with cultured cells at pH 7.4 results from fusion with membranes of intracellular organelles such as endosomes, while that observed at pH 5 is due to fusion with the cell plasma membranes. This is consistent with the view that a low pH environment is required to activate the HA glycoprotein of influenza or the fusion protein of SFV (1).

Human erythrocytes lack the ability to enclose enveloped viruses or any other particulate material by endocytosis, and therefore at pH 5, influenza viruses are able to fuse with only the plasma membrane of the erythrocyte (Table 1). Essentially the same results were obtained when another enveloped virus was used, the vesicular stomatitis virus (VSV) (3, 4). Recent experiments showed that a relatively high degree of fluorescence dequenching was obtained upon incubation of VSV with living cultured cells at either pH 7.4 or pH 5. A different pattern was obtained following the incubation of fluorescently labeled Sendai virus particles with either cultured cells or with human erythrocytes (Table 1). A high degree of fluorescence dequenching was also observed with active, non-treated particles at both pH 5 and pH 7.4. This is not surprising since the fusogenic activity of Sendai virions is expressed at low pH as well as at neutral pH values such as pH 7.4 (1, 3, 4).

Fusogenic Liposomes Bearing Virus Glycoproteins: Reconstitution of Influenza or Sendai Envelopes and Influenza-Sendai Hybrid Vesicles

Reconstituted viral envelopes, namely liposomes bearing only viral glycoproteins and devoid of the viral nucleoproteins, can be obtained following solubilization of intact virus particles with various detergents (1, 2, 7, 8). The non-ionic detergent Triton X-100 has been used for the solubilization of intact Sendai and influenza virus particles (2, 7, 9). Centrifugation of the detergent-solubilized virus suspension resulted in sedimentation of the viral internal proteins and genetic material. Since Triton X-100 has a low critical micelle concentration (C.M.C.), simple dialysis cannot be used to remove it from the clear supernatant which contains the viral phospholipids and glycoproteins (2, 7, 9); however, its removal can be achieved by the addition of the hydropholic biobeads SM-2. Removal of the detergent resulted in the formation of resealed membrane vesicles containing only the viral envelope glycoproteins. Reconstituted influenza virus envelopes (RIVE) contained only the HA and NA (Neuraminadase) viral polypeptides while reconstituted Sendai virus envelopes (RSVE) contained the HN (Hemagglutinin/Neuraminidase) and F (Fusion) viral polypeptides. The HA glycoprotein of influenza was shown to mediate binding as well as fusion of the virus particles with recipient membranes (1, 10). The influenza NA glycoprotein possesses only neuraminidase activity, which apparently is not required for the fusion step itself (11, 12). In Sendai virus particles the viral fusogenic activity is located on the F-glycoprotein, while the viral binding and neuraminidase activities are located on a different polypeptide, the HN glycoprotein (1, 2).

Recent studies (3, 4, 9, 13) (Table 2) have shown that RIVE as well as RSVE, namely liposomes bearing only the virus envelope glycoprotein, are as fusogenic as intact virus particles. Similar to intact influenza virus particles (Table 1), RIVE were able to fuse not only with human erythrocytes at pH 5, but also with living cultured cells at pH 5 and at pH 7.4 (Table 2). On the other hand, RSVE were able to fuse with human erythrocytes and with living cultured cells at both pH 5 and pH 7.4 (Table 2). As expected, RIVE failed to fuse at pH 7.4 with living cultured cells whose endocytic activity was inhibited or whose intraendosomal low pH value was increased by lypsosomotropic agents (9).

Liposomes bearing influenza or Sendai individual glycoproteins can be prepared using ion-exchange column or affinity chromatography methods for separation of the viral polypeptides (3, 4, 9, 11–13). The influenza HA glycoprotein can be separated from the viral NA glycoprotein by ion-exchange chromatography (11, 12). Fluorescence dequenching determination has clearly demonstrated that HA-vesicles, name-

Table 2: Fusogenic properties of reconstituted envelopes bearing influenza and/or Sendai virus glycoproteins. Reconstituted influenza virus envelopes (RIVE), Reconstituted Sendai virus envelopes (RSVE) and co-reconstituted influenza-Sendai virus envelopes were prepared as described in References No. 2, 7, 9 and 18. Membrane vesicles bearing only the influenza HA (Hemagglutinin) (HA-vesicles) or NA (Neuraminidase) glycoprotein were prepared as described in Reference No. 12. Membrane vesicles bearing the Sendai F (fusion) (F-vesicles) or HN (Hemagglutinin/Neuraminidase) (HN-vesicles) or both (F-HN vesicles) were prepared as described in Reference No. 13. All other experimental conditions and fluorescence dequenching determinations were prepared as described in References No. 3 and 4.

System	pH of incubation	Fluorescence dequenching (%) of reconstituted envelopes incubated with:	
		Lymphoma S49 cultured cells	Human erythrocytes
Influenza reconstituted envelopes			
RIVE	5	46	42
	7.4	38	43
HA-vesicles	5	39	43
NA-vesicles	5	8	10
	7.4	8	7
Sendai reconstituted envelopes			
RSVE	5	43	40
	7.4	49	52
F-vesicles	7.4	6	7
HN-vesicles	7.4	8	5
F-HN-vesicles	7.4	44	46
Influenza-Sendai co-reconstituted envelopes			
RISH	5	46	44
	7.4	48	53
DTT-treated RISH	5	43	41
	7.4	34	7

ly liposomes bearing only the influenza HA glycoprotein, are highly fusogenic (Table 2). These results show that the NA glycoprotein does not play any active role in the virus-membrane fusion process. On the other hand, liposomes bearing the individual Sendai glycoproteins are not fusogenic. Only liposomes containing the Sendai HN and F polypeptide within the same membrane are fusogenic and fuse with living cultured cells as well as with human erythrocytes (3, 4). This is not because the HN glycoprotein is required to mediate binding of the reconstituted vesicles to recipient cell membranes. It has been well established that liposomes bearing only the Sendai F glycoproteins fail to fuse with recipient membranes even when the binding of these vesicles is mediated by non-viral binding proteins (14). Several lines of evidence have indicated that the Sendai virus HN glycoprotein, aside from acting as the virus binding protein, also actively participates in the membrane fusion step itself (3, 4, 13, 14).

Recently it was shown that co-reconstitution of influenza and Sendai virus glycoproteins, namely removal of Triton X-100 from a mixture containing viral glycoproteins and phospholipids from both viruses, resulted in the formation of hybrid vesicles (unpublished results). Such reconstituted influenza-Sendai hybrid vesicles (RISH) contain the influenza HA and NA and Sendai HN and F glycoproteins within the same membrane. The presence of influenza and Sendai glycoprotein within the same phospholipid bilayer was inferred mainly from immunoprecipitation experiments showing that anti-influenza antibodies were able to precipitate Sendai virus glycoproteins only when such antibodies were added to preparation of RISH. Fluorescence dequenching determinations (Table 2) demonstrated that RISH possess the fusogenic properties of influenza as well as those of Sendai virus particles. This was inferred from experiments showing that RISH were able to fuse with human erythrocytes and with living cultured cells at pH 5 as well as at pH 7.4. As can be seen, reduction of RISH by DTT (or treatment with trypsin or PMSF) caused complete inhibition of the ability of RISH to fuse with human erythrocytes at pH 7.4, but did not affect its ability to fuse with the erythrocyte membrane at pH 5. It is conceivable that the fusogenic activity which was expressed by the trypsinized or DTT-treated RISH is due to the presence of an active influenza HA-glycoprotein. Neither DTT nor trypsinization causes inhibition of influenza fusogenic activity. Complete inhibition of the RISH fusogenic activity could be achieved, however, by anti-Sendai or anti-influenza antibodies (unpublished results). These results further support the view that the RISH vesicles are liposomes bearing the influenza and Sendai envelope glycoproteins within the same membrane.

The localization and fate of fused fluorescently labeled RISH within living cells was studied with the help of a fluorescence microscope. The results showed that incubation of fluorescently labeled RISH with living cells at pH 5 caused the appearance of fluorescence rings around the cell, indicating fusion with the cell plasma membrane. On the other hand, incubation of RISH with living cultured cells at pH 7.4 led to the appearance of distinct intracellular fluorescence spots as well as fluorescence rings around the cells. These observations confirm the view inferred from the fluorescence dequenching determinations that RISH are able to fuse with cell plasma membranes and with membranes of intracellular organelles at pH 7.4.

Fusion of Enveloped Viruses with Liposomes: A Way to Insert Viral Glycoproteins into Phospholipid Vesicles

In addition to the reconstitution methods described in the previous section, fusion of enveloped viruses or their reconstituted envelopes with liposomes provides another way of obtaining fusogenic liposomes bearing viral glycoproteins. The ability of enveloped viruses from different groups to fuse with liposomes of various compositions was demonstrated by several laboratories (1, 3, 4, 15). Fluorescently labeled viruses or liposomes were used to quantitatively determine fusion of influenza and Sendai virus particles with liposomes composed of negatively charged or neutral phospholipids (3, 4, 16). Both viruses efficiently fused with liposomes composed of negatively charged phospholipids such as phosphatidylserine (PS). RIVE and RSVE also fused efficiently with PS liposomes (Table 3).

Fusion of influenza and Sendai viruses with PS liposomes is accompanied by a process of virus-induced release of the liposome content (Table 3). This was inferred from experiments showing that incubation of either of these viruses with carboxyfluoroscein- or calcein-loaded liposomes promoted increase in fluorescence. The increase is due to release of the fluorescence probes which are enclosed within the liposomes at self-quenching concentrations (3, 4, 16). It is noteworthy that both influenza and Sendai virus particles are known to be lytic viruses whose fusion with erythrocytes or living cultured cells promotes lysis and release of cell content (1, 2).

Binding and fusion of both viruses with biological membranes is absolutely dependent on the presence of virus receptors, namely sialic acid residues of glycolipids and glycoproteins. Neither virus-cell binding nor virus-membrane fusion was observed upon interaction of either Sendai or influenza virus particles (or RIVE and RSVE) with neuraminidase-treated cells (1–4). However, the results obtained in previous studies (1, 16) and those summarized in Table 3 clearly show that Sendai and influenza virus or their reconstituted envelopes fuse efficiently with negatively charged liposomes lacking virus receptors. The extent of fluorescence dequenching observed upon incubation of RIVE with PS liposomes at pH 7.4 was, as expected, significantly lower than that observed at pH 5. However, essentially the same results were obtained with RSVE, whose optimal fusogenic activity was reported to be around pH 7.4–7.8 (1, 2). In addition, RSVE as well as intact virions were able to induce lysis of loaded liposomes at pH 7.4, a

Table 3: Fusion of RIVE and RSVE with phospholipid vesicles (liposomes). Empty or carboxyfluorescein (CF) loaded liposomes of PS, PC, PC:chol/cholesterol (chol) and PC:chol:gangliosides (PC:chol:gang) were prepared and incubated with fluorescently labeled fusogenic RIVE or RSVE or unfusogenic (Hydroxylamine or DTT-treated) viral envelopes as described in References No. 3, 4, 15 and 16.

System	pH of incubation	Fluorescence dequenching (%) of liposomes composed of:			
		PS	PC	PC:chol	PC:chol:gang
Virus-liposomes fusion					
RIVE	5	48	10	32	40
	7.4	22	6	7	8
Hydroxylamine-RIVE	5	46	8	11	13
	7.4	21	8	6	8
RSVE	5	49	6	18	17
	7.4	51	8	31	36
DTT-RSVE	5	52	8	7	11
	7.4	48	8	6	9
Virus induced release liposome content (CF)					
RIVE	5	64	6	7	46
	7.4	58	5	5	8
Hydroxylamine-RIVE	5	49	5	7	13
	7.4	42	5	4	4
RSVE	7.4	63	6	7	38
DTT-RSVE	7.4	51	5	6	7

pH at which the virus is unable to express its fusogenic activity (1). Interestingly, a relatively high degree of fluorescence dequenching was also observed upon incubation of inactivated-unfusogenic RIVE or RSVE with PS-liposomes. Similar results were obtained upon incubation of intact inactivated-unfusogenic influenza or Sendai virions with PS liposomes (3, 4, 16) (Table 3). All these results led to the following conclusions: (a) Enveloped viruses fuse efficiently with and induce lysis of liposomes composed of negatively charge phospholipids; (b) Fusion with negatively charged liposomes is not dependent on the presence of specific receptors for the virus particles in the liposome bilayers; (c) Fusion with negatively charged liposomes does not reflect the virus fusogenic activity needed for penetration into living cells since a high degree of fusion was also observed with inactivated virions.

A different pattern of behavior was obtained when RIVE or RSVE as well as intact influenza in Sendai virions were incubated with liposomes composed of neutral phospholipids, such as those composed of phosphotidylcholine (PC) (3, 4). A high degree of fluorescence dequenching, indicating virus-liposome fusion, was observed only with liposomes composed of PC and cholesterol while very little if any fluorescence dequenching was observed with liposomes composed of only PC (Table 3). Thus, fusion with PC-liposomes was dependent to a large extent on the presence of cholesterol in the phospholipid vesicles, and its degree was proportionally related to the amount of cholesterol present. RIVE fused with PC/chol liposomes only at low pH values, while RSVE fused at pH 5 as well as at pH 7.4. Inactivated-unfusogenic RIVE or RSVE failed to fuse with liposomes composed of PC/chol, clearly indicating that fusion with these kind of liposomes is catalyzed by the viral fusion polypeptides. The results in Table 3 also show that fusion of the viral reconstituted envelopes is similar to fusion of intact virions with PC/chol liposomes in a non-leaky process, namely it does result in release of the liposome content. However, incorporation of virus receptors, namely gangliosides (gang), into the PC/chol liposomes render them susceptible to the virus lytic activity. Fusion of both RIVE and RSVE with PC/chol/gang liposomes induces the release of the liposome content. Inactivated-unfusogenic RIVE or RSVE did not cause any liposome leakage, again indicating that fusion and lysis of PC/chol/gang liposomes is due to the biological activity of the viruses glycoproteins.

Fusion of RIVE or RSVE (or intact virus particles) with either negatively charged or neutral phospholipid vesicles should result in the formation of liposomes bearing the viral glycoproteins (17). Such liposomes should possess fusogenic properties similar to those of reconstituted viral envelopes and should be able to fuse with isolated biological membranes of living cells. Indeed, incubation of fluorescently labeled liposomes (R_{18}-liposomes) with Hela cells in the presence of RSVE resulted in a significant increase in the degree of fluorescence (Table 4). RSVE were first incubated with the liposomes and the proteoliposomes formed were then fused with the membranes of the Hela cells. Fluorescence microscopy observations proved that the increase in fluorescence was due to fusion of liposomes containing the RSVE glycoproteins with Hela cell plasma membranes (Figure 1). This is inferred from results showing that a clear fluorescence ring appeared around the cells following incubation of R_{18}-liposomes with fusogenic-active RSVE (Figure 1A), but not when the same R_{18}-liposomes were incubated with inactive-unfusogenic RSVE (Figure 1B).

The view that the fluorescence dequenching observed is due to fusion of proteoliposomes, namely liposomes bearing viral glycoproteins with the Hela cell membranes, is supported by the results showing that very little if any fluorescence dequenching was observed when R_{18}-liposomes were incubated with RSVE in the absence of Hela cells (Table 4). A relatively high degree of fluorescence dequenching was observed when negatively charged liposomes such as those composed of PS or neutral liposomes composed

Table 4: Fusion between liposomes and Hela cultured cells mediated by Sendai virus particles. Liposomes of PC, PC : chol or PC : PE : chol were prepared and fluorescently labeled with R_{18} as described for fluorescent labeling of Sendai virions (References No. 3, 4 and 15). Incubation with Hela cells and determination of fluorescence dequenching as described in References No. 9, 16–19. Unfusogenic Sendai virus (DTT-Sendai) were prepared as described in References No 3, 4 and 7.

Composition of fluorescently labeled liposomes	Virus	Hela cells	Fluorescence dequenching (%)
PC	Sendai	present	5
PC : chol	Sendai	present	24
PC : chol	Sendai	absent	6
PC : chol	DTT-Sendai	present	8
PC : PE : chol	Sendai	present	29
PC : PE : chol	Sendai	absent	9
PC : PE : chol	DTT-Sendai	present	11

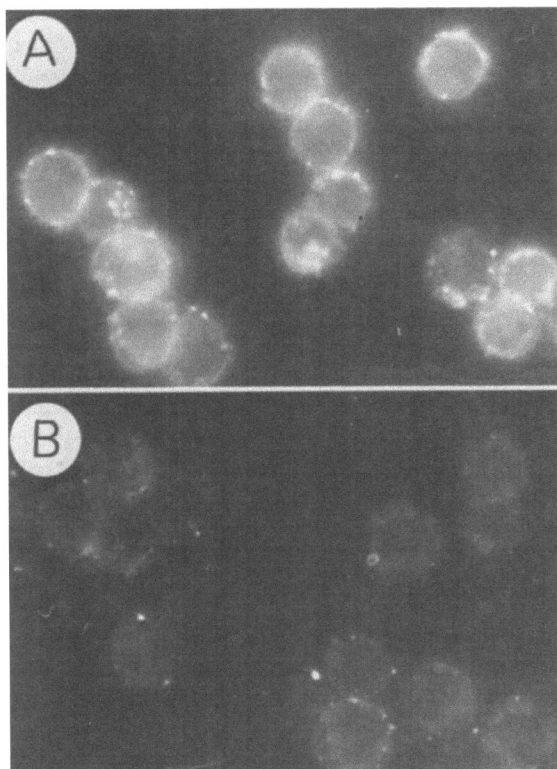

Figure 1: Fluorescence microscopy photo of fusion of proteoliposomes bearing Sendai virus glycoproteins with Hela cells. Experimental conditions as described in the legend to Table 4 and before. Fluorescently labeled liposomes composed of PC:chol were preapred as described in Reference No. 15 and incubated with fusogenic active Sendai virus particles (A) or DTT-treated virus particles (B). Following 15 min incubation at 37 °C, the proteoliposomes formed were incubated with the Hela cells (2.10^6 cells/system) and observed by fluorescence microscopy. Note that only incubation with active-fusogenic Sendai virus particles led to the appearance of fluorescence rings around the Hela cells.

of PC/chol were used. A high degree of fluorescence dequenching was also observed when liposomes containing phosphatidylethanolamine (PE) such as PC/PE/chol or PC/PE/chol/gang were employed. As expected, a low degree of fluorescence dequenching was observed when R_{18} liposomes composed only of PC were first incubated with RSVE and then with Hela cells.

Fusion Mediated Microinjection of Macromolecules into Cultured Cells: Use of Reconstituted Viral Envelopes as Efficient Biological Carriers

It has been well established that soluble macromolecules such as polypeptides (toxins or specific enzymes) or nucleic acid (RNA and DNA) can be en-closed within RSVE if added during the reconstitution process (2). Recently, it was shown that similar to RSVE, RIVE can also be loaded with molecules of large molecular weights (18). Quantitative analysis revealed that about 3–5% of added-soluble macromolecules were trapped within the viral envelopes formed by removal of the detergent from the detergent solution containing the viral phospholipids and glycoproteins (2, 18). RSVE have been used as a biological carrier for the introduction of the fragment A of Ricin and of two amine oxidase into cultured cells (19–22). Ricin is a plant toxin whose A subunit, after being transferred to cell cytoplasm by the B-subunit, causes inhibition of protein synthesis and eventually cell death. The fragment A of the toxin (Ricin A) is by itself harmless unless it is injected directly into the cytoplasm of living cells. Ricin A was enclosed within RSVE or RIVE (18, 21) by methods described above and previously (2). Incubation of loaded RSVE with Hela cells caused almost complete inhibition of protein synthesis and subsequent cell death (Table 5) (20, 21).

RIVE were less efficient as biological carriers. Preliminary results show that protein synthesis was inhibited by about 46% in cells incubated with Ricin A-loaded RIVE. Significantly less inhibition of protein synthesis or cell death was observed when the cells were incubated with inactivated-unfusogenic loaded viral envelopes or with empty viral envelopes in the presence of externally added Ricin A molecules (Table 5) (18). Inhibition of protein synthesis and cell death were due to the introduction of Ricin A fragments into the cell via the loaded fusogenic envelopes. RSVE were also used as mentioned above for fusion-mediated microinjection of the enzymes serum amine oxidase and porcine kidney diamine oxidase (19). These two enzymes are involved in the catabolism of naturally occurring polyamines. Microinjection of the above oxidases into cultured cells via loaded RSVE caused almost total arrest of protein and DNA synthesis. The microinjected enzymes probably caused oxidation of intracellular polyamines whose oxidation products promoted arrest in the synthesis process of intracellular macromolecules (19).

Fusion-mediated microinjection of nucleic acid and functional DNA molecules into cultured cells was also demonstrated by the use of loaded RSVE (2, 20–22). Introduction of poly(I)poly(C) into living animal cells via loaded RSVE was shown to cause inhibition of protein synthesis (22). Detailed analysis of the experimental systems demonstrated that inhibition of protein synthesis in microinjected L-cells was due to poly(I)poly(C) activation of the (2'–5') oligoadenylate-synthetase-RNase pathway. SV_{40}, EBV (Epstein-Barr virus)–DNA and the HSV-TK (Herpes Simplex thymidine kinase gene) were also enclosed within RSVE (2, 20, 21). Fusion-mediated micro-

Table 5: Loaded and targetted RSVE and RIVE as biological carriers: fusion-mediated microinjection of the toxin Ricin A and SV_{40}-DNA. Sendai and influenza reconstituted envelopes loaded with either Ricin A or SV_{40} were prepared as described in References No. 14 and 21. Insulin molecules were covalently attached to RSVE as described in References No. 14 and 21. Incubation with hepatoma tissue cultured cells and determination of protein synthesis or appearance of SV_{40}-T-antigen was performed as described in References No. 14 and 21. Virus receptors were removed from hepatoma tissue cultured cells by treatment with neuraminidase (desialized cells) as described in Reference No. 21. RSVE (Ricin A) and RIVE (Ricin A) were Sendai and influenza viral envelopes loaded with Ricin A, respectively. RSVE + Ricin A and RIVE + Ricin A were viral envelopes with externally added Ricin A molecules. RSVE-insulin (SV_{40}-DNA) and RSVE-insulin + SV_{40}-DNA were RSVE bearing covalently attached insulin molecules with enclosed and externally added insulin molecules, respectively.

Microinjection of Ricin A	Inhibition of protein synthesis in hepatoma tissue cultured cells (% of total)	
	Nontreated	Desiliazed
(A) RSVE (Ricin A)	94	12
RSVE + Ricin A	10	9
RSVE-insulin (Ricin A)	96	95
RSVE-insulin (Ricin A) + free insulin	N.D.	6
RSVE-insulin Ricin A	11	8
(B) RIVE (Ricin A)	46	N.D.
RIVE + Ricin A	16	N.D.

Microinjection of SV_{40}-DNA	T-antigen positive hepatoma tissue cultured cells (% of total)	
	Nontreated	Desialized
RSVE (SV_{40}-DNA)	52	0
RSVE + SV_{40}-DNA	3	N.D.
RSVE-insulin (SV_{40}-DNA)	48	38
RSVE-insulin (SV_{40}-DNA) + free insulin	41	0
RSVE-insulin + SV_{40}-DNA	3	0

injection of SV_{40}-DNA into several cultured cells lines resulted in the appearance of the SV_{40} T-antigen (20, 21). The results in Table 5 show that 40–50% of hepatoma cultured cells expressed SV_{40}-T-antigen following fusion with SV_{40}-DNA loaded RSVE. Introduction of HSV-TK into LTK$^-$ cells resulted in the appearance of LTK$^+$ cells with relatively high efficiency (20).

Recently, experiments by Kaneda (17) and colleagues have shown that proteoliposomes bearing Sendai virus glycoproteins can serve as an efficient vehicle for fusion-mediated microinjection of HSV-TK into LTK$^-$ cells (Table 5). The HSV-TK gene was first enclosed with high efficiency within liposomes by using conventional methods (17). Loaded liposomes were then fused with Sendai virus particles and the proteoliposomes obtained were then incubated with LTK cells. Quantitative analysis of the results revealed that the HSV-TK genes were transferred into LTK$^-$ cells with extremely high efficiency. This was inferred from the transient expression of the thymidine kinase gene and from the stable appearance of LTK$^+$ cells.

Reconstitution of Targetted RSVE: Fusion-Mediated Microinjection of Macromolecules into Virus-Receptor Depleted Cultured Cells

Loaded RIVE, RSVE or RISH, namely hybrid envelopes containing viral glycoproteins of both viruses, may offer an excellent drug delivery system for introduction of macromolecules into cultured cells and for in vivo use after some modification. RSVE, as was demonstrated previously (2) and in the present work, fuse with cell plasma membranes mainly at pH 7.4 and consequently introduce their content directly into cytoplasm of recipient cells. Introduction of RIVE content into cell cytoplasm is due to its fusion at pH 5 with membranes of intracellular organelles following receptor-mediated endocytosis of cell-associated RIVE. RISH were shown to possess the fusogenic properties of both viruses (Table 2) and therefore loaded RISH should introduce their content via fusion with cell plasma membranes as well as with membranes of intracellular organelles. Preliminary experiments verify this assumption (M. Lapidot, unpublished results). Due to the presence of influenza and Sendai binding and fusion proteins, RISH may theoretically be the most efficient biological carrier. It should be emphasized, however, that any fusogenic liposomes bearing viral glycoproteins will not possess specific binding properties and will bind to and fuse with any biological membrane containing sialic acid residues. An important feature of an ideal delivery system should be its ability to bind to and subsequently to fuse with a limited, specific number of cells. This is not a characteristic feature of influenza and Sendai virus particles nor of any liposomes which carry their binding proteins, namely the HA of influenza and the HN of Sendai. Due to the fact that sialoglycolipids or sialoglycoproteins are present in almost any animal cell line, these viruses fuse with a wide range of cells (1, 2).

Substituting the Sendai HN glycoproteins (and probably the HA_1-glycoproteins of influenza virions) with another non-viral binding polypeptide such as specific antibodies or lectins should result in the formation of targetted fusogenic membrane vesicles. Binding of such vesicles with recipient cells should be mediated by the added non-viral binding protein, and fusion should be mediated by the viral F (fusion) protein. However, as mentioned above and reported before (2, 4, 23), the Sendai HN glycoprotein, besides serving as the virus binding protein, also plays an active role in the membrane fusion step itself and therefore has to be present in any fusogenic vesicle bearing Sendai glycoproteins. This was inferred mainly from experiment showing that liposomes bearing only the Sendai F-glycoprotein possessed no fusogenic activity, neither toward biological membranes nor to PC/chol liposomes. Furthermore, even when binding of such F vesicles to living cells was mediated by non-viral binding proteins such as specific membrane antibodies or plant lectins, they still possessed no fusogenic activity (3, 4, 23). Thus, due to the presence of the HN polypeptide, the interaction of fusogenic vesicles bearing Sendai virus glycoproteins with sialic acid residues of biological membranes cannot be avoided. This means that construction of targetted fusogenic vesicles containing viral envelope glycoprotein is a more complex process than construction of targetted pure liposomes.

Targetted reconstituted fusogenic vescicles will be required for in vivo experiments for use as drug carriers after intravenous injection. In in vitro experiments, it has been demonstrated that interaction of enveloped viruses and especially of Sendai and influenza virus with cultured cells is inhibited by the addition of relatively low amounts of serum. It is conceivable that serum glycoprotein competitively blocks interaction between the viral binding proteins and their appropriate membrane receptors. A similar inhibition is expected to occur following intravenous injection of fusogenic liposomes bearing viral glycoproteins. Several glycoproteins may strongly mask the interaction of such fusogenic vesicles with either cells in the blood or cells of the reticuloendothelial system (RES). This inhibition may be overcome by the use of targetted vesicles whose binding to recipient membranes will be mediated by specific non-viral binding proteins.

Two methods have been developed for the construction of targetted RSVE, namely RSVE whose binding to cells is mediated by non-viral ligands such as specific anti-membrane-antibodies or polypeptide hormones (14, 21, 23). In order to study the binding and the fusogenic activity of such targetted RSVE, their interaction with neuraminidase treated cells was used as a model system. Preliminary experiments have shown that the same methods can be employed for the construction of targetted RIVE or RISH. However, since results with these reconstituted vesicles are very preliminary, the present work describes data obtained only with RSVE.

In the first method, protein molecules such as anti-human erythrocyte antibodies or polypeptide hormones (insulin) were covalently attached to the thio-containing paraffin, dodecanethiol, by the use of the cross-linking agent succinimidyl-4-(P-maleimidophenyl)–butyrate (SMPB). The product formed, dodecanethiol-MPB (malemilophenylbutyrate)-antibody (or other polypeptides), was added to the viral reconstitution system, namely to the detergent solution of the viral phospholipids and glycoproteins. Removal of the detergent resulted in the formation of membrane vesicles (liposomes) bearing the Sendai virus glycoproteins and the complex dodecanethiol-MPB-antibody. RSVE bearing antibodies raised against the human erythrocyte membranes were able to interact and fuse with human erythrocytes lacking virus receptors (14, 21, 23).

An alternative method for the construction of targetted RSVE is to covalently attach specific antibodies or other polypeptides directly to the Sendai virus glycoproteins. Experiments have shown that covalent attachment of insulin molecules to Sendai envelope glycoproteins using the cross-linking reagent SMPB caused complete inactivation of the envelope biological activities (14, 23). However, fusogenic active targetted RSVE were obtained following co-reconstitution of the modified viral glycoproteins bearing insulin molecules with untreated active glycoproteins. Targetted RSVE obtained by this method were able to ineract with and microinject their content into cultured cells lacking virus receptors (Table 5). RSVE loaded with SV_{40}-DNA and bearing insulin molecules were able to efficiently attach to neuraminadase-treated hepatoma tissue cultured cells. Furthermore, the results showed that such loaded-targetted RSVE were able to induce the synthesis of SV_{40}-T-antigen in the recipient hepatoma tissue cultured cells, indicating fusion-mediated transfer of the RSVE content. A very low degree of virus-cell binding as well as induction of T-antigen synthesis was observed when non-targetted RSVE were incubated with desialized cells. The results further showed that binding of the targetted RSVE was mediated by the virus-associated insulin molecules. The fusion-mediated microinjection process was mediated by the viral envelope glycoproteins. This was inferred from experiments which showed that addition of excess free insulin molecules prior to incubation with the loaded RSVE caused strong inhibition of RSVE binding and T-antigen appearance (Table 5) (14, 21). On the other hand, a high degree of RSVE cell-binding but no induction of T-antigen synthesis was observed following incubation of unfusogenic loaded targetted RSVE with desialized hepatoma tissue cultured cells.

Essentially the same results were obtained when targetted RSVE loaded with Ricin A were incubated with desialized hepatoma tissue cultured cells. Complete inhibition of protein synthesis in cultured hepatoma tissue cultured cells was observed upon incubation with active-targetted RSVE but not with inactivated-unfusogenic targetted RSVE (Table 5). No inhibition of protein synthesis in the recipient hepatoma tissue cultured cells was observed upon incubation with empty RSVE, or with empty RSVE in the presence of empty RSVE and externally added Ricin A molecules. In addition, protein synthesis in hepatoma tissue cultured cells was not inhibited when free insulin molecules were added to the cell suspension before RSVE, again supporting the view that binding is mediated by virus-associated insulin molecules.

Conclusion

Investigations during the past few years have clearly demonstrated enclosure of macromolecules such as polypeptides or oligonnucleotides within reconstituted viral envelopes such as those obtained from Sendai or influenza virus particles. Non-viral membrane components can also be inserted into the viral envelopes if added to the viral envelope reconstitution system. Fusion of such loaded or hybrid reconstituted envelopes with cultured cells results in transfer of the viral envelope content into the recipient cell cytoplasm or plasma membranes.

In spite of these achievements, the value of the use of liposomes bearing viral glycoproteins for the delivery of drugs or macromolecules in vivo is still questionable for the following reasons: (1) Due to the presence of viral glycoproteins, repeated injection of RSVE will raise immunological response in the injected organism. This will obviously nullify their continuous injection into any particular animal. (2) The use of reconstituted viral envelopes as biological carriers for the delivery of certain macromolecules or drugs will necessitate the growth and production of huge numbers of viruses. This may also raise problems, thus limiting their commercial use.

Once these two obstacles are overcome, fusogenic reconstituted viral envelopes may become a very efficient drug delivery system, having several crucial advantages over the use of liposomes. Such envelopes will fuse with membranes of recipient cells, either with the cell plasma membrane or with the membranes of intracellular organelles, thus introducing their content directly into the cell cytoplasm. As biological carriers they may be highly efficient and therefore their use may permit low doses and perhaps only a few injections. Proteoliposomes bearing small amounts of viral glycoproteins may offer another way for the preparation of highly fusogenic biological carriers. Such fusogenic liposomes are of high enclosure efficiency and minimum antigen activity. Experiments testing the fate of intravenously injected viral envelopes and their immunological potential are still lacking. Studies to investigate the events following viral envelope injection into laboratory animals are currently underway using various methods involving immunoprecipitation and electron microscopy techniques.

References

1. **White, J., Kielian, M., Helenius, A.:** Membrane fusion proteins of enveloped animal viruses. Quarterly Review of Biophysics 1983, 16: 151–195.
2. **Loyter, A., Volsky, D. J.:** Reconstituted Sendai virus envelopes as carriers for the introduction of biological materials into animal cells. In: Poste, G., Nicolson, G. L. (ed.): Membrane reconstitution. Biomedical Press, Amsterdam, 1982, p. 215–266.
3. **Loyter, A., Citovsky, V., Blumenthal, R.:** The use of fluorescence dequenching methods to follow viral membrane fusion events. In: Glick, D. (ed.): Methods of biochemical analysis 1988, p. 129–164.
4. **Chejanovsky, N., Nussbaum, O., Loyter, A., Blumenthal, R.:** Fusion of enveloped viruses with biological membranes: fluorescence dequenching studies. In: Hildenson, H. (ed.): Subcellular biochemistry. Plenum Press, London, 1988, (in press).
5. **Hoekstra, D., de Boer, T., Klappe, K., Wilschut, J.:** Fluorescence method for measuring the kinetics of fusion between biological membranes. Biochemistry 1984, 23: 5675–5681.
6. **Klenk, H. D., Rott, R., Orlich, M., Blodorn, J.:** Activation of influenza A viruses by trypsin treatment. Virology 1975, 68(2): 426–439.
7. **Vainstein, A., Hershkovitz, M., Israel, S., Rabin, S., Loyter, A.:** A new method for reconstitution of highly fusogenic Sendai virus envelopes. Biochimica et Biophysica Acta 1984, 773: 181–188.
8. **Melsikko, K., van Meer, G., Simons, K.:** Reconstitution of fusogenic activity vesicular stomatitis virus. EMBO journal 1986, 5: 3429–3435.
9. **Nussbaum, O., Lapidot, M., Loyter, A.:** Reconstitution of functional influenza virus envelopes and fusion with membrane and liposomes lacking virus receptors. Journal of Virology 1987, 61: 2245–2252.
10. **Ruigrok, R. W., Martin, S. R., Wharton, S. A., Skehel, J. J., Bayley, P. M., Wiley, D. C.:** Conformational changes in the hemagglutinin of influenza virus which accompany heat-induced fusion of virus with liposomes. Virology 1986, 155(2): 484–497.

11. Wharton, S. A., Skehel, J. J., Wiley, D. L.: Studies of influenza haemagglutinin-mediated membrane fusion. Virology 1986, 144: 27–35.
12. **Lapidot, M., Nussbaum, O., Loyter, A.**: Fusion of membrane vesicles bearing only the influenza hemagglutinin with erythrocytes, living cultured cells and liposomes. Journal of Biological Chemistry 1987, 262: 13736–13741.
13. **Citovsky, V., Yanai, P., Loyter, A.**: The use of circular dichroism to study conformational changes induced in Sendai viral envelope glycoproteins: a correlation with the viral fusogenic activity. Journal of Biological Chemistry 1986, 261: 2235–2239.
14. **Loyter, A., Gitman, A. G., Chejanovsky, N., Nussbaum, O.**: Fusion-mediated microinjection of macromolecules into living cultured cells by "targetted" Sendai virus envelopes. In: Celis, J. E., Graessmann, A., Loyter, A. (ed.): Microinjection and organelle transplantation. Academic Press, New York, 1986, p. 135–155, 179–197.
15. **Citovsky, V., Blumenthal, R., Loyter, A.**: Fusion of Sendai virions with phosphatidylcholine-cholesterol liposomes reflects the viral activity required for fusion with biological membranes. FEBS Letters 1985, 193: 135–140.
16. **Amselem, S., Loyter, A., Lichtenberg, D., Barenholtz, Y.**: The interaction of Sendai virus with negative charged liposomes: virus induced lysis of carboxyfluorescein-loaded small unilamellar vescicles. Biochimica et Biophysica Acta 1985, 820: 1–10.
17. Kaneda, Y., Uchida, T., Kim, J., Ishiura, M., Okada, Y.: The improved efficient method of introducing macromolecules into cells using HVJ (Sendai Virus) liposomes with gangliosides. Experimental Cell Research 1987, 173: 56–69.
18. **Loyter, A., Lapidot, M.**: Reconstituted influenza virus envelopes as potential carriers for fusion-mediated microinjection of macromolecules into living cells. In: Gregoriadis, G. (ed.): Targetting of drugs. Plenum Press, London, 1988, (in press).
19. **Loyter, A., Citovsky, V., Ballas, N.**: Sendai virus envelopes as a biological carrier: Reconstitution, targetting and application. In: Wilschut, J., Hoekstra, D. (ed.): Cellular Membrane fusion: fundamental mechanisms and application of membrane fusion techniques. Dekker, New York, 1988, (in press).
20. **Vainstein, A., Razin, A., Graessman, A., Loyter, A.**: Fusogenic reconstituted Sendai virus envelopes as a vehicle for introducing DNA into viable mammalian cells. Methods in Entymology 1983, 101: 492–512.
21. **Gitman, A. G., Graessmann, A., Loyter, A.**: Targetting of loaded Sendai virus envelopes by covalently attached insulin molecules to virus receptor-depleted cells: fusion mediated microinjection of Ricin A and Simian Virus 40-DNA. Proceedings of the National Academy of Sciences, USA 1985, 82: 7309–7313.
22. **Arad, G., Hershkovitz, M., Panet, A., Loyter, A.**: Use of reconstituted Sendai virus envelopes for fusion-mediated microinjection of double-stranded RNA: inhibition of protein synthesis in interferon-treated cells. Biochimica et Biophysica Acta 1986, 859: 88–94.
23. **Gitman, A. G., Khanae, I., Loyter, A.**: Use of virus-attached antibodies or insulin molecules to mediate fusion between Sendai virus envelopes and neuraminidase-treated cells. Biochemistry 1985, 24: 2762–2768.

Host Determinants
in Anti-Infective Chemotherapy

Cell Mediated Immunity, Immunodeficiency and Microbial Infections

S. H. E. Kaufmann*, I. E. A. Flesch

Mycobacterium tuberculosis, Listeria monocytogenes and *Cryptococcus neoformans* are frequent infectious agents of the immunocompromised host. Mycobacteria and listeriae are intracellular bacteria capable of residing inside macrophages, whereas cryptococci are extracellular fungi which evade phagocytosis. Host defence against these microbes depends on macrophages and T lymphocytes. Recent studies suggest that besides interferon-γ, interleukin 4 and interleukin 5 are also capable of activating antimicrobial macrophage functions, and that besides interleukin secreting helper T lymphocytes, cytolytic T lymphocytes also contribute to resistance. This treatise discusses possible interactions between helper T cells, cytolytic T cells, and macrophages in mechanisms of host resistance to microbial pathogens. Furthermore, possible consequences of immunodeficiencies on infections with these agents are examined.

A major challenge for the immune system is the combat of infectious agents. While many microorganisms are eliminated by humoral immunity, others have selected intracellular niches as their habitat to evade humoral effector mechanisms (1, 2). Often these intracellular microorganisms are of low toxicity and form a parasitic relationship with the host. A major target for these pathogens is the mononuclear phagocyte. After interaction with specific T lymphocytes, however, the very same cell type becomes the prime effector cell in host resistance against intracellular microbes. Infected mononuclear phagocytes yielding microbial antigens in the context of self molecules encoded by the major histocompatibility complex (MHC) stimulate specific T lymphocytes, which after a second encounter with antigen-presenting mononuclear phagocytes induce granuloma formation at the site of microbial colonization, where mononuclear phagocytes and T cells initiate protective immune mechanisms.

The crucial role of T lymphocytes in the control of these intracellular pathogens is perhaps best revealed by the high incidence of infections in patients with a compromised T-cell system. This is particularly true for patients suffering from the acquired immunodeficiency syndrome (AIDS) (3). This disease is caused by the human immunodeficiency virus (HIV), which primarily affects CD4 T lymphocytes, the central regulators of cellular immunity. The purpose of this treatise is to first describe experiments concerned with the principle mechanisms underlying cellular immunity to mycobacteria, *Listeria monocytogenes* and *Cryptococcus neoformans*, which cause frequent secondary infections in immunocompromised patients. Then, possible consequences arising from deficiencies in the cellular immune system for host defence against these microbes will be discussed.

The T-Cell Response

On the basis of their phenotype and antigen recognition pattern, T lymphocytes segregate into two distinct subpopulations, namely MHC class II-restricted CD4 T cells and MHC class I-restricted CD8 T cells (4). Because CD4 T cells have the capacity to activate a variety of target cells they are often called helper T cells. Activation is mediated by soluble factors called interleukins, which are produced by CD4 T cells after antigenic stimulation. Therefore, virtually all cells of the immune system are under the control of CD4 T lymphocytes and their interleukins. The CD4 molecule is the receptor for HIV, whose prime target therefore is the CD4 T lymphocyte. Many nonlymphoid cells including mononuclear phagocytes, astrocytes, oligodendrocytes and Langerhans cells also express the CD4 molecule and hence can be infected by HIV as well. Although direct effects on these cells — without doubt — are responsible for many pathogenic aspects of AIDS, interference with CD4 T-cell func-

---

Department of Medical Microbiology and Immunology, University of Ulm, Oberer Eselsberg, D-7900 Ulm, FRG.

tions is of great importance for the high susceptibility to secondary infections. In addition, HIV infection of mononuclear phagocytes may affect antimicrobial resistance to a greater degree than currently appreciated.

Recent observations indicate that two types of helper T cells which produce different interleukins may exist (5). However, this separation is not absolute and overlapping may occur. So-called TH1 cells secrete interleukin 2 (IL-2), which induces differentiation and activation of cytolytic T lymphocytes (6); tumor necrosis factor-β (TNF-β), which induces destruction of appropriate target cells (7); and interferon-γ (IFN-γ), which activates macrophages and induces MHC class II expression on a variety of host cells (8). TH2 cells produce the B-cell stimulatory factors interleukin 4 (IL-4) and interleukin 5 (IL-5) (9, 10). IL-4 also induces differentiation of mast cells and IL-5 differentiation of eosinophils. Both TH1 and TH2 cells secrete interleukin 3 (IL-3) (multi-colony-stimulating factor), which acts on bone marrow precursor cells (11). According to this scheme, the T lymphocytes, which are responsible for cell-mediated immunity, should reside primarily in the TH1 cell population whereas those responsible for humoral immunity should bear the TH2 phenotype.

CD8 T cells have the capacity to lyse their targets by direct cell contact and hence are commonly termed cytolytic T lymphocytes. Their major role in host defence against infectious agents is thought to be one of mediation of antiviral immunity, and commonly they are not associated with protection against bacteria, fungi or protozoa. Results from our experimental studies indicate that not only TH1 cells but also TH2 cells and cytolytic T lymphocytes are required for resistance against intracellular microbial infections.

The Pathogens

Mycobacteria. Mycobacteria are acid-fast bacilli which include pathogenic species, e.g. *Mycobacterium tuberculosis* and *Mycobacterium bovis* as well as opportunistic species, e.g. *Mycobacterium avium, Mycobacterium intracellulare* and *Mycobacterium kansasii* (12). Although tuberculosis is still a major health problem worldwide, its incidence in developed countries has declined. However, due to the increasing numbers of immunodeficient patients in many developed countries, this situation is changing. This is particularly true for AIDS patients in whom mycobacteria together with *Pneumocystis carinii* and cytomegalovirus are the major causes of secondary infections (13). Tubercle bacilli and nontuberculous mycobacteria of the *Mycobacterium avium/intracellulare* (MAI)-complex are primarily responsible for mycobacterial infections in AIDS patients. Tubercle bacilli are often capable of persisting even in activated mononuclear phagocytes without causing clinical signs of disease (2). It can be assumed that the number of individuals infected with *Mycobacterium tuberculosis* is 10- to 100-fold higher than the number of patients suffering from active tuberculosis. As long as an efficient immune response exists, tubercle bacilli are contained in discrete primary lesions. However, subtle changes in the cellular immune response may result in mycobacterial growth and development of disease. In AIDS patients, therefore, tuberculosis will frequently develop through reactivation of existing foci rather than by primary infection. Accordingly, in AIDS patients suffering from tuberculosis discrete granulomas can still be identified, probably because they had been formed before development of the immunodeficient state.

MAI are of low virulence, i.e. they can be eradicated effectively by mononuclear phagocytes even of low activation level. Accordingly, in the normal host, cellular immune mechanisms will easily eradicate invading organisms of the MAI-complex. However, these microbes are widespread throughout nature and highly resistant to conditions that are harmful to many pathogens. For example, MAI have been identified in the water supply of several hospitals in Boston (14). Therefore, the risk of contact with MAI is high. Only in the immunocompromised host, however, will contact result in disease. Accordingly, MAI infections in AIDS patients are normally disseminated and granulomas are missing. It is therefore reasonable to assume that depending on the prevalence of tuberculosis in the population and the distribution of MAI in the environment, either *Mycobacterium tuberculosis* or MAI infection will dominate in AIDS patients.

Listeria monocytogenes is a gram-positive rod which is widely distributed in nature (15). Cases of human listeriosis are rare and mostly restricted to immunocompromised hosts. Individuals suffering from Hodgkin's lymphoma and renal transplant patients are at increased risk. Furthermore, the risk of disease is high in the perinatal and neonatal stages of life; listeriosis is one of the major causes for stillbirth due to infectious agents. Surprisingly, listeriosis in AIDS patients is extremely rare. In neonates as well as in immunocompromised adults, meningoencephalitis is the most common clinical form of listerial infection. Recent epidemics in the USA have revealed that *Listeria monocytogenes* is a frequent contaminant of dairy products and have pointed to listeriosis as a foodborne disease.

Cryptococcus neoformans is an encapsulated yeast-form fungus which is widespread throughout nature (16). It causes pulmonary and meningeal infections, primarily in immunocompromised hosts. Cryptococcosis has been found in 2–10% of AIDS patients in the Western world (13). Hodgkin's disease patients are also often susceptible to *Cryptococcus neoformans* infections. Specific polysaccharides in the capsule of *Cryptococcus neoformans* protect the fungus from adherence to phagocytes and subsequent phagocytosis. Hence these antiphagocytic capsular polysaccharides are an important virulence factor. Although the fungus resides in the extracellular milieu, it appears that cell-mediated immunity plays a major role in defence, probably by activation of extracellular killer mechanisms in mononuclear phagocytes.

Interleukins in Antimicrobial Host Defence

Using recombinant molecules we have assessed the capacity of IFN-γ, IL-4, and IL-5 to activate antimicrobial macrophage functions.

Mycobacteria. Although the concept of macrophage activation had originally evolved from studies in experimental mycobacterial infections, only few experiments have dealt with the in vitro activation of antimycobacterial macrophage functions (2). This is due at least in part to the marked variation of tissue macrophages in their activation stage. Bone marrow-derived macrophages (BMMφ) cultured for 9 days in serum-free medium yielded a highly quiescent homogeneous population of mononuclear phagocytes (17). These BMMφ were activated with IFN-γ, IL-4, or IL-5, respectively, and after 24 h were infected with viable *Mycobacterium bovis* organisms. After 4–5 days surviving intracellular bacteria were determined by measuring ^{3}H-uracil uptake or by counting colony-forming units (CFU). Under these circumstances, IL-4 and IL-5 failed to activate tuberculostatic macrophage functions. In contrast, IFN-γ induced marked inhibition of mycobacterial growth (Table 1). A different picture emerged when BMMφ were first infected with mycobacteria and subsequently stimulated with interleukins. Under these conditions IFN-γ induced lower but still significant tuberculostasis. More importantly, IL-4 and IL-5 were potent inhibitors of mycobacterial growth (Table 2). Thus, in addition to IFN-γ the TH2 cell-derived B-cell stimulatory factors expressed macrophage activating capacity. However, they acted only on mononuclear phagocytes that were already infected and hence seem to function differently from IFN-γ.

Listeria monocytogenes. Currently, the role of IFN-γ in host defense against *Listeria monocytogenes* is a matter of debate (18). Administration of IFN-γ has been shown to protect mice against subsequent infection with *Listeria monocytogenes* (19) and antibodies against IFN-γ exacerbate listeriosis in mice (20). On the other hand, evidence has been presented showing that inflammatory phagocytes are already highly listericidal and not further stimulated by IFN-γ (21). The listericidal capacity of BMMφ after interleukin activation was therefore analyzed. For these studies a temperature-sensitive strain of *Listeria monocytogenes* was used in order to avoid possible growth of bacteria during the assay period. BMMφ were infected for 2 h with viable *Listeria monocytogenes* and subsequently stimulated with interleukins for 18 h at 37 °C. Afterwards, BMMφ were lysed and viability of *Listeria monocytogenes* was assessed by ^{3}H-uracil uptake for 90 min at room temperature. IL-4, IL-5 and IFN-γ were all capable of drastically reducing listerial growth, with IFN-γ being the least effective factor (Table 3). Preliminary evidence indicates that prior infection is a prerequisite for stimulation of listericidal activities by interleukins. Thus, the findings support the notion that IFN-γ is capable of inducing anti-listerial mechanisms which may not be detectable in mononuclear phagocytes which have already undergone certain steps of activa-

Table 1: Effect of recombinant interleukins on the growth inhibition of *Mycobacterium bovis* by bone marrow-derived macrophages (BMMφ). BMMφ (1×10^5/assay) were stimulated with interleukins for 24 h, washed, and infected with 1×10^6 viable *Mycobacterium bovis* organisms. Viability of intracellular bacteria was determined after 4 days by ^{3}H-uracil incorporation. Percent inhibition = (1-^{3}H-uracil uptake after culture with interleukin-activated BMMφ/^{3}H-uracil uptake after culture with nonactivated BMMφ) × 100.

Interleukin	Concentration (U/ml)	Inhibition (%)
IFN	500	64
	2500	88
IL-4	5	0
	50	0
	100	0
	500	0
IL-5	25	0
	250	0
	500	0
	2500	15

Table 2: Effect of interleukins on the tuberculostatic activity of infected BMMφ. BMMφ (1×10^5/assay) were infected with 1×10^6 viable *Mycobacterium bovis* organisms. After removal of extracellular bacteria, interleukins were added for 40 h. Viability of intracellular bacteria was determined by ^{3}H-uracil incorporation. Percent inhibition was calculated as indicated in Table 1.

Interleukin	Concentration (U/ml)	Inhibition (%)
IFN-γ	50	40
	500	50
IL-4	5	60
	50	37
	500	80
IL-5	5	26
	50	64
	500	81

tion. Again this study indicates the potent macrophage activating capacity of the B-cell-stimulating factors IL-4 and IL-5 in intracellular bacterial infections.

1,25-dihydroxyvitamin D3. Evidence has been presented that 1,25-dihydroxyvitamin D3 is capable of activating different functions in human blood monocytes (22). Peripheral blood monocytes from healthy individuals were stimulated with 1,25-dihydroxyvitamin D3 and afterward infected with *Mycobacterium bovis*. Alternatively, monocytes were first infected and afterward stimulated with 1,25-dihydroxyvitamin D3. Monocytes from many donors expressed spontaneous tuberculostatic activity which could not be further increased by exogenous factors (unpublished observation). However, monocytes which lacked spontaneous tuberculostatic activity could be activated by 1,25-dihydroxyvitamin D3 by about 50%, as was shown when pre-infected or non-infected macrophages were stimulated (Table 4). This finding confirms earlier data by Rook et al. (23) and Crowle et al. (24). 1,25-dihydroxyvitamin D3 is the most active metabolite of vitamin D3. The circulating precursor, 25-hydroxyvitamin D3, has only low biological activity. It has been shown recently that human mononuclear phagocytes possess 1α-hydroxylase activity (22). Therefore IFN-γ activation of mononuclear phagocytes at the site of mycobacterial growth could result in the formation of 1,25-dihydroxyvitamin D3 from 25-hydroxyvitamin D3 in the circulation, which then could activate tuberculostatic macrophage functions locally. This scheme is illustrated in Figure 1. Since vitamin D3 is produced in the skin under the influence of light, this finding might explain the beneficial effects on tuberculosis of the sanatory cures practiced in preantibiotic days.

Cryptococcus neoformans. IFN-γ not only activates macrophages to suppress growth of intracellular pathogens but also enables them to kill the extracellular fungus *Cryptococcus neoformans* (25). As shown in Table 5, BMMφ stimulated with IFN-γ were able to suppress growth of *Cryptococcus neoformans* significantly. The effect of IFN-γ was augmented by lipopolysaccharide (LPS). Killing of *Cryptococcus neoformans* was also achieved by supernatants from BMMφ activated with IFN-γ plus LPS. Recently it was found that killing of *Cryptococcus neoformans* is mediated by a fungicidal protein of apparent molecular weight of 17,000, which is secreted by activated BMMφ and distinct from TNF-α (I.E.A. Flesch, G. Schwamberger, S.H.E. Kaufmann, unpublished re-

Table 3: Effect of interleukins on the growth inhibition of a temperature-sensitive strain of *Listeria monocytogenes* by BMMφ. BMMφ (1×10^5/assay) were infected with a temperature-sensitive strain of *Listeria monocytogenes* (1×10^6/assay) for 2 h. Extracellular bacteria were washed off and cells were incubated with interleukins for 18 h at 37 °C. Viability of intracellular bacteria was determined by ^{3}H-uracil uptake for 90 min at room temperature. Percent inhibition was calculated as indicated in Table 1.

Interleukin	Concentration (U/ml)	Inhibition (%)
IL-4	10	90
	100	92
IL-5	10	96
	100	97
IFN-γ	10	75
	100	60

Table 4: Effect of 1,25-dihydroxyvitamin D3 on the tuberculostatic activity of human monocytes.

Concentration (ng/ml)	Inhibition (Stimulation – Infection)[a] (%)	Inhibition (Infection – Stimulation)[b] (%)
50	52	25
100	62	61

[a] Human monocytes were stimulated with 1,25-dihydroxyvitamin D3 for 3 days and subsequently infected with 1×10^6 viable *Mycobacterium bovis* organisms. Viability of intracellular bacteria was determined by ^{3}H-uracil uptake after 3 days.
[b] Human monocytes were infected with 1×10^6 viable *Mycobacterium bovis* organisms and subsequently stimulated with 1,25-dihydroxyvitamin D3. Viability of intracellular bacteria was determined by ^{3}H-uracil uptake after 40 h. Percent inhibition was calculated as indicated in Table 1.

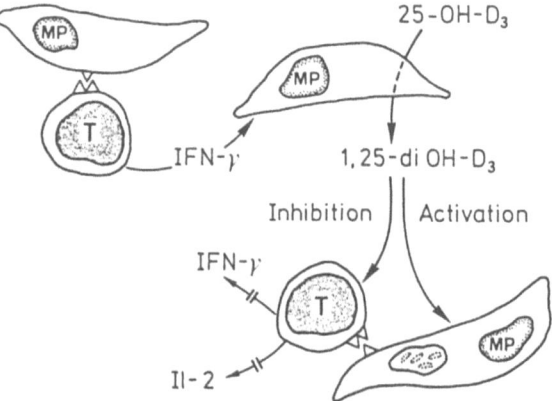

Figure 1: Hypothetical scheme of local activation of tuberculostatic mononuclear phagocytes. Infected mononuclear phagocytes expressing mycobacterial antigens stimulate T lymphocytes to secrete IFN-γ, which activates 1α-hydroxylase activity in mononuclear phagocytes. IFN-γ-activated macrophages convert circulating 25-hydroxyvitamin D3 into 1,25-dihydroxyvitamin D3. 1,25-dihydroxyvitamin D3 activates tuberculostatic macrophage functions and at the same time inhibits T-cell functions.

sults). Fungicidal macrophage activities after IFN-γ stimulation were also described for other fungi (16), and it remains to be established whether the same protein is involved in the killing of these pathogens as well.

Table 5: Growth inhibition of *Cryptococcus neoformans* by murine BMMφ. BMMφ (1 × 10⁵/assay) were stimulated with 500 U/ml IFN, either alone or in combination with LPS (50 ng/ml). After 24 h, 2.5 × 10³ viable *Cryptococcus neoformans* organisms were added. Viability of *Cryptococcus neoformans* was determined by CFU after 24 h. Percent inhibition = (1 − number of CFU after culture with activated BMMφ/number of CFU after culture with nonactivated BMMφ) × 100.

Culture condition	Inhibition %
BMMφ + IFN-γ	53
BMMφ + IFN-γ + LPS	79

Killer Cells in Antimicrobial Host Defence

According to the current view, microbial antigens can only be presented in the context of MHC class II molecules (4). Hence, in microbial infections CD8 T cells should not be generated. However, recent data from different laboratories indicate that CD8 cytolytic T lymphocytes with specificity for microbial antigens exist (26).

Cytolytic T Lymphocytes, Mycobacteria and Listeriae.
T-cell lines established from mice infected with viable *Listeria monocytogenes* were capable of lysing BMMφ expressing listerial antigens (27) (Figure 2). These cytolytic T lymphocytes expressed the CD8 phenotype and some though not all of the lines were MHC class I restricted (28) (Figure 2). Even in cases when MHC class I restriction was not demonstrable, target cell recognition was antigen-specific and mediated by the T-cell receptor (28). After adoptive transfer these cytolytic T lymphocytes conferred a marked degree

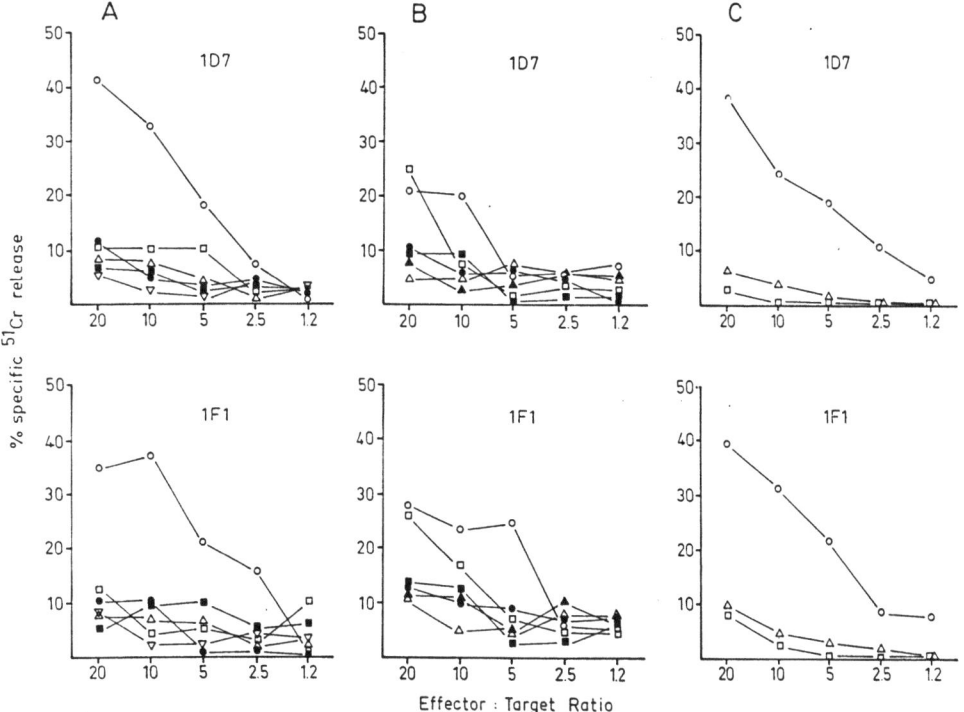

Figure 2: Cytolytic activities of cloned *Listeria monocytogenes*-specific CD8 T-cell lines. Clones 1D7 and 1F1 were tested for their cytolytic activity against different ⁵¹Cr labelled target cells. A: (○) peritoneal cells from *Listeria monocytogenes*-infected C57Bl/6 mice; (●) peritoneal cells from untreated C57Bl/6 mice; (□) peritoneal cells from *Listeria monocytogenes*-infected DBA/2 mice; (■) peritoneal cells from untreated DBA/2 mice; (△) YAC-1; (▽) P815. B: (○) peritoneal cells from *Listeria monocytogenes*-infected C57Bl/6 mice; (●) peritoneal cells from untreated C57Bl/6 mice; (△) peritoneal cells from *Listeria monocytogenes*-infected B6.C-H2bm1 mice; (▲) peritoneal cells from untreated B6.C-H2bm1 mice; (□) peritoneal cells from *Listeria monocytogenes*-infected B6.C-H2bm12 mice; (■) peritoneal cells from untreated B6.C-H2bm12 mice. C: (○) *Listeria monocytogenes*-infected C57Bl/6 BMMφ; (□) *Mycobacterium bovis*-infected C57Bl/6 BMMφ; (△) uninfected C57Bl/6 BMMφ. Data adopted from Reference No. 27 with permission.

of protection against infections with *Listeria monocytogenes*. CD8 T-cell lines from mice immunized with killed *Mycobacterium tuberculosis* in Freund's adjuvant or viable *Mycobacterium bovis* expressed similar activities (29). Interestingly, in vitro these cells were capable of inhibiting the intracellular growth of *Mycobacterium bovis* in BMMφ. First, they did so by secreting IFN-γ in the presence of exogenous IL-2 similarly as described above (data not shown). Second, they induced tuberculostasis via an IFN-γ independent mechanism (Figure 3). BMMφ infected with mycobacteria for 4 days were cocultured with cytolytic T lymphocytes for 18 h. Afterward mycobacterial growth was assessed by ^{3}H-uracil uptake for 8 h. The significant reduction of ^{3}H-uracil uptake seen under these conditions was probably related to lysis of infected BMMφ. Thus, lysis of mycobacteria-infected macrophages might contribute to protection.

Direct Effects of Killer Cells on *Cryptococcus neoformans*

Among the cytolytic T lymphocyte clones with reactivity to *Listeria monocytogenes* or to mycobacteria, some clones were capable of lysing YAC-1 cells, indicating that they possessed natural killer activity in addition to their antigen-specific cytolytic T lymphocyte activity. It has been shown earlier that natural killer cells are capable of inhibiting the growth of *Cryptococcus neoformans* in vitro (30). Furthermore, beige mice with a deficient natural killer system suffer from impaired resistance to cryptococcosis (31). Different T-cell lines were cocultured with *Cryptococcus neoformans* organisms for 18 h and afterwards survival of the latter was determined by counting CFU. In parallel, natural killer activity of the cytolytic T lymphocyte lines was assessed using YAC-1 cells as targets. It was found that cytolytic T lymphocytes of different specificity, independent of their natural killer activity, were capable of inhibiting the growth of *Cryptococcus neoformans*. Results from two representative subclones with reactivity to *Listeria monocytogenes* are shown in Table 6. These findings show that *Cryptococcus neoformans* is susceptible to the killing by cytolytic T lymphocytes with distinct specificity, independent of YAC-1 cell killing. Although the exact mechanisms of killing remain unclear, it appears that cell contact occurred independent of the natural killer and the T-cell-receptor and via an as yet unknown structure. In any case these findings indicate that *Cryptococcus neoformans* is susceptible to the killer machinery existent in cytolytic T lymphocytes. Thus, activated mononuclear phagocytes, and natural killer cells could all contribute to the elimination of *Cryptococcus neoformans* in the normal host. In AIDS patients, natural

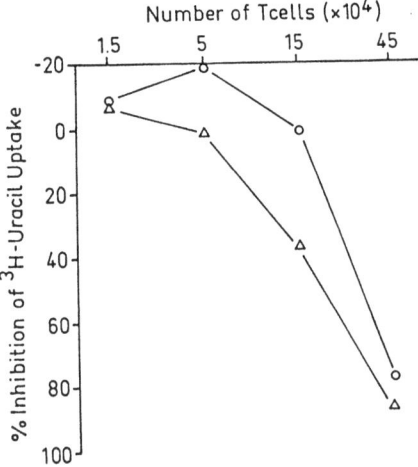

Figure 3: Inhibition of mycobacterial growth in BMMφ by mycobacteria-reactive CD8 T-cells. BMMφ were infected with viable *Mycobacterium bovis* organisms and graded numbers of *Mycobacterium tuberculosis* reactive CD8 T cells were added 4 days later. On the next day, surviving mycobacteria were determined by ^{3}H-uracil uptake and percent of growth inhibition was calculated. (○), T-cell clone; (△), short-term cultured T-cell line. Data adopted from Reference No. 29 with permission.

Table 6: Growth inhibition of *Cryptococcus neoformans* by cytolytic T lymphocytes expressing or lacking natural killer activity.

Clone	Percent growth inhibition of *Cryptococcus neoformans* at effector to target ratio:			Percent specific killing of YAC-1 cells at effector to target ratio		
	300 : 1	100 : 1	30 : 1	80 : 1	40 : 1	20 : 1
28-1	85	72	26	64	43	30
28-2	83	40	18	4	0	0

CD8 cytolytic T lymphocytes with specificity for *Listeria monocytogenes* were cocultured with 2.5×10^3 *Cryptococcus neoformans* for 18 h or with 2×10^3 ^{51}Cr-labeled YAC-1 cells for 4 h. Growth inhibition of *Cryptococcus neoformans* was determined by counting CFU and natural killer activity by ^{51}Cr-release.

killer cells circulate in normal numbers, but their killer capacity is reduced due to their dependence on interleukins from CD4 T lymphocytes. Thus, the high incidence of cryptococcosis in AIDS patients could best be explained by the lack of appropriate signals from CD4 T cells, which are crucial for the expression of functional activities in cytolytic T lymphocytes, mononuclear phagocytes and natural killer cells.

In Vivo Studies

The in vitro data described thus far strongly suggest that both CD4 and CD8 T cells contribute to protection against many intracellular microbial infections. While the relevance of CD4 T lymphocytes in the combat of these pathogens is illustrated by the severity of these infections in AIDS patients, selective deficiencies in the CD8 T cell compartment are extremely rare in humans. However, in the murine model selective deficiencies of CD4 and CD8 T cells can be generated by administration of certain monoclonal antibodies with specificity for the CD4 and CD8 molecule. Using these monoclonal antibodies mice deficient in CD4, CD8, or both T-cell populations were generated. After infection with *Mycobacterium tuberculosis* not only CD4 deficient but also CD8 deficient mice suffered from exacerbated tuberculosis with more severe effects observed in CD4 deficient mice (32) (Figure 4). Similar though less dramatic effects were seen in *Listeria monocytogenes*-infected animals (data not shown). These in vivo studies enlighten the importance of both T-cell populations for host defence against intracellular bacteria.

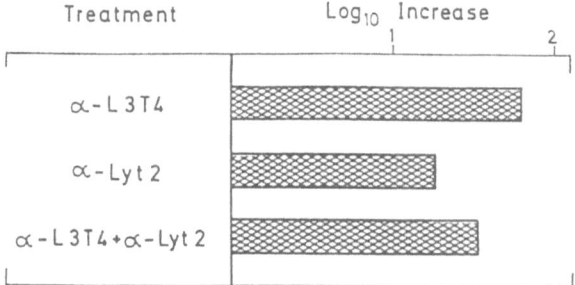

Figure 4: Effects of in vivo application of anti-Lyt2 or anti-L3T4 monoclonal antibodies on tuberculosis. Thymectomized mice were injected twice with anti-Lyt2 (CD8) or anti-L3T4 (CD4) monoclonal antibodies. Afterward they were infected with viable *Mycobacterium tuberculosis* H37Rv and 20 days later, CFU in spleens were determined by plating aliquots of spleen homogenate on Middlebrook Dubos agar plates. Data adopted from Reference No. 32 with permission.

Discussion

In the normal host intracellular bacteria including mycobacteria and listeria are contained in granulomatous lesions. These lesions are composed of different mononuclear phagocytes including macrophages, monocytes and multinucleated giant cells as well as CD4 and CD8 T lymphocytes (26). CD4 T cells are dispersed throughout the granuloma whereas CD8 T cells are located in a surrounding mantle.

Mononuclear phagocytes infected with mycobacteria can be activated by interleukins from CD4 T cells. The in vitro data presented here indicate that IL-4 and IL-5 as well as IFN-b can perform this task. In addition, it appears that 1,25-dihydroxyvitamin D3 is involved in the activation of mononuclear phagocytes in humans. Recently, IL-4 has been shown to induce giant cell formation from mononuclear phagocytes (33). It therefore appears that interleukin activation plays a dominant role in local resistance in the granuloma. However, at least part of the mononuclear phagocytes within the granuloma may not be able to eliminate their intracellular parasites. Rather, their main function may be to contain bacteria within discrete foci and to prevent them from dissemination. It is therefore important for the host to ensure that immigrant blood monocytes of high antimicrobial potential have access to these persisting microbes. This step could be afforded by the lysis of infected host cells by CD8 CTL. Immigrant monocytes could be activated by IFN-γ (perhaps via 1,25-dihydroxyvitamin D3) whereas IL-4 and IL-5 appear to be unable to activate noninfected mononuclear phagocytes. Activated blood-borne phagocytes could take up microorganisms released from less efficient granuloma mononuclear phagocytes and then eliminate them. In addition, lysis of infected macrophages may exert direct microbicidal effects. Thus, release of mycobacteria into the hypoxic necrotic centre could lead to death of these obligate aerobic bacilli. On the other hand, target cell lysis could allow microbial dissemination to secondary tissue sites via the bloodstream or the spread to other individuals via the bronchioalveolar tree. In addition, target cell lysis by CD8 T cells or by tumor necrosis factor could contribute to tissue destruction and granuloma caseation. It has been shown recently that tumor necrosis factor in combination with LPS induces marked necrotic lesions in mice (34), and recently we found that mycobacteria and listeriae synergize with tumor necrosis factor in a similar fashion. Possible interactions between TH1 cells, TH2 cells, killer cells and mononuclear phagocytes within a granuloma are illustrated in Figure 5 (35).

Due to the central role of CD4 T cells and mononuclear phagocytes in the different effector pathways that contribute to antimicrobial protection, any interference with these important cell types should have

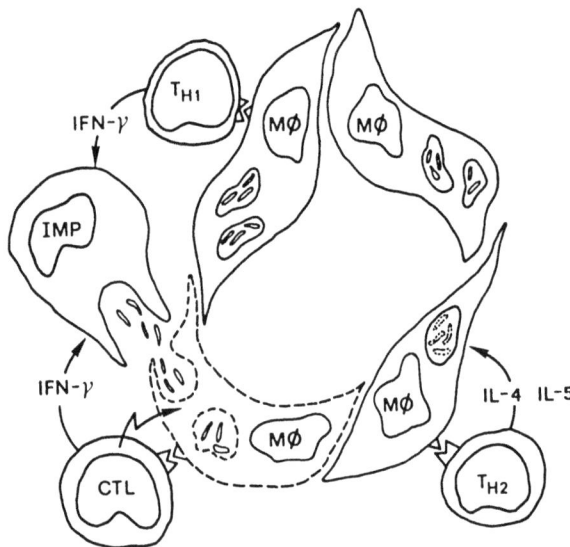

Figure 5: Hypothetical scheme of T-cell-mononuclear phagocyte interactions in a granuloma. T_{H2} cells secrete IL-4 and IL-5 which act only on pre-infected granuloma macrophages (Mϕ). Although some activated Mϕ may be capable of killing intracellular microorganisms, their principal function is microbial containment in the granuloma. Cytolytic T lymphocytes (CTL) lyse infected Mϕ with low antimicrobial potential. Lysis has two harmful sequelae: tissue destruction and bacterial dissemination. As a beneficial consequence for the host, bacteria become accessible to inflammatory mononuclear phagocytes (IMP). These can be activated by IFN to kill microorganisms with high efficiency. Note that in humans 1,25-dihydroxyvitamin D3 may be interposed as described in Figure 1.

momentous consequences for the host. This is indeed the case in AIDS patients. Still, although the principle mechanisms can be explained by now, the detailed role of the cellular populations and mechanisms operative in antimicrobial resistance remains unclear. Thus, the question as to why listeriosis is so rare in AIDS patients and occurs so frequently in other immunodeficiencies while MAI and not *Mycobacterium kansasii* occurs so frequently in AIDS patients cannot be explained as yet.

The findings that IL-4, IL-5, IFN-γ and 1,25-dihydroxvitamin D3 are capable of activating tuberculostatic macrophage functions could be considered as supportive evidence for using these factors in the therapy of T-cell deficient individuals such as AIDS patients. Indeed, this type of treatment could bypass the CD4 T-cell dependence of many effector functions. However, there is an important caveat. Recently, it has been shown that interleukin activation of certain mononuclear phagocyte lines latently infected with HIV in vitro not only activates these cells but also increases expression of HIV, probably by a transactivation event (36). Hence, treatment of AIDS patients with activating factors could worsen the disease.

Recent epidemiological studies by Mann et al. (37) have revealed that in Kinshasa approximately 1 % of the adult population suffers from tuberculosis and 6 % to 8 % are infected with HIV. In contrast, in tuberculosis patients the percentage of HIV infection is as high as 33 %. In light of the findings that (i) chronic infection with *Mycobacterium tuberculosis* results in a constant activation stage of the mononuclear phagocyte and (ii) that activation of the mononuclear phagocyte can result in increased HIV expression, the question arises whether tuberculosis is not only an important secondary infection in AIDS patients but also serves as a predisposing factor for AIDS.

Acknowledgements

Work from the authors' laboratory described in the text received financial support from the UNDP/ World Bank/WHO Special Program for Research and Training in Tropical Diseases, the WHO Program for Vaccine Development, the German Leprosy Relief Association and the A. Krupp award for young professors to S.H.E.K. The excellent secretarial help of R. Mahmoudi is gratefully acknowledged. R-IL-2 and 1,25 dihydroxyvitamin D3 were kindly supplied by Hoffmann-La Roche, Basel; r-IFN-γ was produced by Genentech Inc. and kindly provided by Boehringer, Ingelheim. R-IL-4 and r-IL-5 were a kind gift of A. Rolink and F. Melchers, Basel.

References

1. Moulder, J.W.: Comparative biology of intracellular parasitism. Microbiological Reviews 1985, 49: 298–337.
2. Hahn, H., Kaufmann, S.H.E.: Role of cell-mediated immunity in bacterial infections. Review of Infectious Diseases 1981, 3: 1221–1250.
3. Fauci, A.S.: The human immunodeficiency virus: infectivity and mechanism of pathogenesis. Science 1988, 239: 617–622.
4. Fitch, F.W.: T-cell clones and T-cell receptors. Microbiological Reviews 1986, 50: 50–69.
5. Mosmann, T.R., Coffman, R.L.: Two types of mouse helper T-cell clones. Implications for immune regulation. Immunology Today 1986, 8: 223–227.
6. Smith, K.A.: Interleukin 2. Annual Review of Immunology 1984, 2: 319–333.
7. Ruddle, N.H.: Tumor necrosis factor and related cytotoxins. Immunology Today 1987, 8: 129–130.
8. Vilcek, J., Gray, P.W., Rinderknecht, E., Sevastopopoulos, C.G.: Interferon-γ: a lymphokine for all seasons. In: Pick, E. (ed.): Lymphokines. Academic Press, Orlando, 1985, p. 1–32.
9. Paul, W.E., Ohara, J.: B-cell stimulatory factor-1/interleukin 4. Annual Review of Immunology, 1987, 5: 429–459.
10. Takatsu, K., Tominaga, A., Harada, N., Mita, S., Matsumoto, M., Takahashi, T., Kikuchi, Y., Yamaguchi, N.: T-cell replacing factor (TRF)/interleukin 5 (IL-5): molecule and functional properties. Immunological Reviews 1988, 102: 107–135.
11. Cosman, D.: Colony-stimulating factors in vivo and in vitro. Immunology Today 1988, 9: 97–98.
12. Schlossberg, D. (ed.): Clinical topics in infectious disease. Tuberculosis, Springer-Verlag, New York, 1988, p. 227.

13. Clumeck, N., Hermans, P., DeWit, S.: Current problems in the management of AIDS patients. European Journal of Clinical Microbiology and Infectious Diseases 1988, 7: 2–10.
14. DuMoulin, G.C., Stottmeier, K.D.: Waterborne mycobacteria: an increasing threat to health. ASM News 1986, 52: 525–529.
15. Kaufmann, S.H.E.: Listeriosis: new findings – current concern. Microbial Pathogenesis, (in press).
16. Fukazawa, Y., Kagaya, K.: Host defence mechanisms against fungal infection. Microbiological Sciences 1988, 5: 124–127.
17. Flesch, I., Kaufmann, S.H.E.: Mycobacterial growth inhibition by interferon-γ-activated bone marrow macrophages and differential susceptibility among strains of *Mycobacterium tuberculosis*. Journal of Immunology 1987, 138: 4408–4413.
18. Campbell, P.A.: Are inflammatory phagocytes responsible for resistance to facultative intracellular bacteria? Immunology Today 1986, 7: 70–72.
19. Kiderlen, A.F., Kaufmann, S.H.E., Lohmann-Matthes, M.-L.: Protection of mice against the intracellular bacterium *Listeria monocytogenes* by recombinant immune interferon. European Journal of Immunology 1984, 14: 964–967.
20. Buchmaier, N.A., Schreiber, R.D.: Requirement of endogenous interferon-γ production for resolution of *Listeria monocytogenes* infection. Proceedings of the National Academy of Science USA 1985, 82: 7404–7408.
21. Czuprynski, C.J., Henson, P.M., Campbell, P.A.: Killing of *Listeria monocytogenes* by inflammatory neutrophils and mononuclear phagocytes from immune and nonimmune mice. Journal of Leukocyte Biology 1984, 35: 193–208.
22. Rigby, W.F.C.: The immunobiology of vitamin D. Immunology Today 1988, 9: 54–58.
23. Rook, G.A.W., Steele, J., Fraher, L., Barker, S., Karmali, R., O'Riordan, J.: Vitamin D3, gamma interferon, and control of proliferation of *Mycobacterium tuberculosis* by human monocytes. Immunology 1986, 57: 159–163.
24. Crowle, A.J., Ross, E.J., May, M.H.: Inhibition by 1,25-$(OH)_2$-vitamin D3 of the multiplication of virulent tubercle bacilli in cultured human macrophages. Infection and Immunity 1987, 55: 2945–2950.
25. Diamond, R.D.: Effects of stimulation and suppression of cell-mediated immunity on experimental cryptococcosis. Infection and Immunity 1977, 17: 198–194.
26. Kaufmann, S.H.E.: $CD8^+$ T lymphocytes in intracellular microbial infections. Immunology Today 1988, 9: 168–174.
27. Kaufmann, S.H.E., Hug, E., DeLibero, G.: *Listeria monocytogenes* reactive T lymphocyte clones with cytolytic activity against infected target cells. Journal of Experimental Medicine 1986, 164: 363–368.
28. Kaufmann, S.H.E., Rodewald, H.R., Hug, E., DeLibero, G.: Cloned *Listeria monocytogenes*-specific non-MHC-restricted $Lyt2^+$ T cells with cytolytic and protective activity. Journal of Immunology 1988, 140: 3173–3179.
29. DeLibero, G., Flesch, I., Kaufmann, S.H.E.: Mycobacteria reactive $Lyt-2^+$ T-cell lines. European Journal of Immunology 1988, 18: 59–66.
30. Murphy, J.W., McDaniel, D.O.: In vitro reactivity of natural killer (NK) cells against *Cryptococcus neoformans*. Journal of Immunology 1982, 128: 1577–1583.
31. Hidore, M.R., Murphy, J.W.: Natural cellular resistance of beige mice against *Cryptococcus neoformans*. Journal of Immunology 1986, 137: 3624–3631.
32. Müller, I., Cobbold, S.P., Waldmann, H., Kaufmann, S.H.E.: Impaired resistance against *Mycobacterium tuberculosis* infection after selective in vivo depletion of $L3T4^+$ and $Lyt2^+$ T-cells. Infection and Immunity 1987, 55: 2037–2041.
33. McInnes, A., Rennick, D.M.: Interleukin-4 induces cultured monocytes/macrophages to form giant multinucleated cells. Journal of Experimental Medicine 1988, 167: 598–611.
34. Rothstein, J.L., Schreiber, H.: Synergy between tumor necrosis factor and bacterial products causes hemorrhagic necrosis and lethal shock in normal mice. Proceedings of the National Academy of Science USA 1988, 85: 607–611.
35. Kaufmann, S.H.E., Flesch, I.E.A.: The role of T-cell-macrophage interactions in tuberculosis. Springer Seminars of Immunopathology, (in press).
36. Folks, T.M., Justement, J., Kinter, A., Dinarello, C.A., Fauci, A.S.: Cytokine-induced expression of HIV-1 in a chronically infected promonocyte cell line. Science 1987, 238: 800–802.
37. Mann, J., Snider, D., Francis, H.: Association between HTLV III/LAV infection and tuberculosis in Zaire. Journal of the Americal Medical Association 1986, 256: 346.

Neutropenia: Antibiotic Combinations for Empiric Therapy

L. S. Young

> During the last two decades the mortality from gram-negative septicemia in neutropienic patients with serious underlying disease has declined from 85 % to less than 20 %. Many factors seem responsible for this trend: (a) the development of potent broad-spectrum antimicrobial agents. (b) aggressive clinical approaches to empiric therapy entailing the use of antibiotics before results of cultures are known. (c) better supportive care, (d) improved treatment of underlying disease. Controversy persists about the choice of "optimum" regimens: clinical studies to date show major differences in evaluation criteria, particularly in the definition of "response". The largest and most convincing studies of gram-negative bacteremia still favor the use of antibiotic combinations in patients with profound, persistent neutropenia.

Since the advent of intensive antineoplastic chemotherapy there has been widespread recognition of the association between neutropenia and the risk of acute bacterial infection (1, 2). In general, there has been an inverse relationship between the circulating absolute neutrophil count and the risk of serious bloodstream infections. Where the exact boundaries are between a reduced neutrophil count and levels that place the patient at increased risk has been a matter of some debate. Most authorities place the "danger zone" between 500 and 1,000 cells/μl, but it is clear that patients who are at greatest risk of developing overwhelming, acute bacterial infection have circulating levels of neutrophils of less than 100/μl. Figures in this range have been widely quoted, but another factor to consider is the rate at which the neutrophil count declines. There are many patients who have "stable" white cell counts, with neutrophils in the 300–700 μl range, and these patients may be able to avoid serious bacterial infections. When intensive conditioning regimens are delivered prior to bone marrow transplantation, the rapid decline in the white cell count, even more than absolute circulating levels, may accurately predict the onset of the serious life-threatening infectious complications.

Since the early 1960s the infectious disease literature has focused on gram-negative bacteremia as the most serious problem readily identified as causing fever and infection in the neutropenic patient. It may be important to distinguish organisms readily cultivated from blood cultures versus those organisms isolated at autopsy from patients with end-stage disease, because examples of the latter may have relatively untreatable infectious complications, such as those due to viruses and fungi.

Some of the early and often-quoted studies of gram-negative septicemia (3–5) evaluated the outcome of bloodstream infections due to gram-negative bacilli in terms of severity of underlying disease. "Appropriate antimicrobial therapy" was the term applied to the clinical situation in which the patient received at least one agent which inhibited the organism in vitro. By the McCabe and Jackson classification, those patients with rapidly fatal underlying disease were often those who had hematologic malignancies and were neutropenic (3). Unless hematologic remission was achieved, patients in this group faced an extremely poor prognosis. In the analyses of these studies (3–5), the mortality with appropriate antimicrobial therapy was 84 %, compared with an 85 % mortality with inappropriate treatment (5). Obviously there was no significant difference between appropriate versus inappropriate therapy.

Survival may well have been related not only to the availability of antimicrobial agents which were available prior to 1970, but to the types of supportive care and the nature of the treatment of the underlying disease (e.g. cancer chemotherapy). Since the beginning of the 1970s, however, there have been major changes in therapeutic approaches, first in terms of the philosophy with which patients are now treated, and secondly, in terms of the types of agents which are available to treat gram-negative bacteremia. With regard to treatment philosophy, several groups pointed out that death following *Pseudomonas aeruginosa* bacteremia in leukemic patients often occurred within a matter of days after the first positive blood cultures were drawn (6, 7). Clearly, the clinician had very little time with which to act in the treatment of septic patients. Thus, a new philosophy evolved (6, 7), involving the administration of empiric therapy which was initiated with broad-spectrum agents prior to the identification of the infecting pathogens.

Organisms associated with high mortality from bacteremia include lactose-negative, gram-negative bacili such as *Pseudomonas aeruginosa* and members of the *Klebsiella-Enterobacter-Serratia* group. The advent of two groups of agents in the early 1970s appeared to make an important difference in the outcome of sepsis. These agents included the aminoglycosides with anti-pseudomonal activity, such as gentamicin, tobramycin, amikacin and netilmicin. The other group of agents consisted of the beta-lactam compounds, including the semisynthetic anti-pseudomonal penicillin, carbenicillin. More recent congeners in this group include ticarcillin, mezlocillin, azlocillin and piperacillin.

In studies carried out with colleagues at the University of California, Los Angeles, (UCLA), we analyzed the outcome in several hundred cases of gram-negative bacteremia with respect to the use of combination therapy and whether such therapy inhibited the infecting bacteremic isolate synergistically. We found that if patients received at least one appropriate antibiotic and had a nonfatal underlying disease, there was clearly no difference in outcome between the use of synergistic versus nonsynergistic combinations. On the other hand, patients who were neutropenic, in shock, had *Pseudomonas aeruginosa* bacteremia, or had rapidly or ultimately fatal underlying disease who were treated with two agents that inhibited the infecting strain synergistically experienced a significantly better outcome than if they were treated with two agents that did not interact synergistically (8). We recognized that there is no way that one could confidently predict synergistic interactions, but these interactions were more likely to occur if the combination included an aminoglycoside and a penicillin or cephalosporin.

In the study just cited, the organisms isolated from specific bacteremic infections were tested against the actual combination regimen that was employed. That study was followed by a randomized prospective study; for one type of analysis we compared our results with those reported by the University of Maryland group (9, 10). Both of the centers, while independent and using slightly different protocols, evaluated the efficacy of an aminoglycoside plus an anti-pseudomonal penicillin in the empiric therapy of fever in neutropenic patients. The results in terms of outcome focused on gram-negative bacillary infections. At UCLA the randomization was carried out between the aminoglycosides gentamicin and amikacin, and the anti-pseudomonal penicillin used in both components of the study was carbenicillin. In Baltimore the anti-pseudomonal penicillin was either carbenicillin or ticarcillin. When the organism cultured from blood was susceptible to both antimicrobial agents initially used, over 80 % of the patients responded clinically: they survived, improved or temporarily improved. While the category of "temporary improvement" is not a satifactory study criterion, it is one way of evaluating the early response to a therapeutic regimen. When only one of the two drugs used in the combination was active in vitro against the invading pathogen, the response rate declined to 59 %. When none of the agents was effective, the response rate was only 20 %. In the UCLA study we analyzed specific synergistic interactions, testing the organism against the actual combination that was employed. On the basis of individual tests of in vitro synergism we found that synergistic activity was superior to additive activity (10).

During the 1980s we have had the advent of compounds in the cephalosporin class with greatly augmented activity (particularly against *Pseudomonas aeruginosa*) as well as agents in the beta-lactam group that also have a markedly augmented in vitro effect against gram-negative bacilli (imipenem and aztreonam). The cephalosporin group has clearly been the one that has seen the greatest development in terms of numbers of new compounds. However, treatment with the first of the so-called "third generation agents" in a protocol reported by the European Organization for the Research and Treatment of Cancer (EORTC) revealed that the combination of cefotaxime with an aminoglycoside was inferior to the combination of an anti-pseudomonal penicillin (azlocillin) plus an aminoglycoside (11). Another important and interesing study carried out by the EORTC failed to demonstrate that a three-drug combination (cefazolin, carbenicillin and amikacin) was superior to a two-drug combination consisting of carbenicillin and amikacin (12).

The advent of new, highly potent, single agents has raised the potential for monotherapy in the treatment of the neutropenic patient. Drugs such as ceftazidime, imipenem, and perhaps some of the new quinolones that can be administered intravenously offer broad-spectrum activity against gram-negative bacilli and variable activity against gram-positive organisms. Pizzo and colleagues at the National Cancer Institute in the USA compared initial monotherapy with ceftazidime with a triple-drug combination (so-called standard therapy) consisting of cephalothin, gentamicin and carbenicillin (13). This study has been published with an extensive commentary (14) and follow-up correspondence. Pizzo and colleagues found that ceftazidime as initial monotherapy appeared to be as satisfactory in febrile neutropenic patients as the triple-drug regimen. However, part of the analysis of this study included the controversial categorization of patients as being a treatment "success with modification." If a patient had been started on one regimen and therapy was altered — even if the regimen was changed and the patient did well — the treatment trial was scored as a success. However, it is interesting to observe that half of the patients with proven bacterial infections had therapy modified within 72 hours. Many authorities would have waited longer before deeming a treatment trial to be a failure and requiring "modification". In patients with documented infection there did appear to be a slight difference in favor of combination therapy. Overall, while the Pizzo study was an ambitious one and entered many hundreds of patients into a comparative trial, there were relatively few documented bacterial infections of the bloodstream due to gram-negative organisms. No information was provided regarding the clinical response rate in patients with profound persistent neutropenia (as defined by a circulating neutrophil count of less than 100 cells/μl).

In contrast to the study by Pizzo and colleagues, the fourth major collaborative trial reported by the EORTC supports the use of combination treatment (15). This represents the largest multicenter clinical trial of empiric antimicrobial therapy in cancer patients and includes the largest number of documented cases of single gram-negative bacteremia in a clinical trial reported to date. Azlocillin or ceftazidime was randomly paired with an aminoglycoside (amikacin). However, the ceftazidime trial consisted of a pairing of the cephalosporin with only a three-day course of the aminoglycoside versus a minimum of nine days of the aminoglycoside. The long course of the aminoglycoside treatment was found to be therapeutically superior in terms of response to the initial treatment, death from infection, and defervescence. It must be kept in mind that in the EORTC-IV trial a "modification" in treatment was considered a clinical failure. Thus, differences in evaluation criteria must enter into the interpretation of clinical studies.

What the EORTC-IV suggests was that a potent combination regimen-namely ceftazidime and amikacin (given for at least nine days) – was most likely to be efficacious in documented gram-negative bacteremia in neutropenic patients and was associated with a better than 80 % initial response rate. Using the concept of "success with modification" it is possible to make any regimen appear as good as another. Differences in the criteria for the interpretation of clinical trials have led many investigators to seek more common grounds in terms of entry criteria and methods for scoring clinical response. An international consensus panel was formed and convened at the most recent Immunocompromised Host Society Meeting in the Netherlands; a summary of these guidelines will be published in the near future.

While the focus of treatment has clearly been on aminoglycoside-beta-lactam combinations, it is fair to mention that other therapeutic approaches have been carefully considered. Since several important agents in cancer chemotherapy are nephrotoxic and other antibiotics can cause renal damage, there is a clear-cut interest in using drug treatments that can avoid nephrotoxicity. The so-called double beta-lactam regimens have been evaluated by ourselves and other workers in this field (16, 17). There may be some drawbacks to the use of double beta-lactam regimens such as moxalactam plus piperacillin for *Pseudomonas* spp. infections. In other regards, however, this double beta-lactam regimen appeared to be quite satisfactory. Caution must be expressed against the routine use of this regimen in individuals with documented *Pseudomonas* spp. infection.

Furthermore, there is some concern that double beta-lactam regimens may be associated with delayed recovery of the circulating neutrophil count. In view of the clinical problems with moxalactam, it should probably be replaced by ceftazidime in a double beta-lactam regimen.

What is our final conceptual assessment of the approach to the neutropenic patient? Perhaps the greatest insight has been provided by the analysis from deJongh and colleagues at the University of Maryland in Baltimore (18). These investigators assessed the outcome of gram-negative bacteremia occurring in neutropenic patients in terms of the use of one or two antimicrobial agents. These investigations again showed that the use of two appropriate agents seemed to be better overall than one. However, the subset analysis of their patients may be perhaps more meaningful. In their patients who had profound persistent neutropenia (neutrophil count less than a 100/μl), the only individuals who responded were those who received two appropriate drugs. The responses were equally good for patients who had been given one effective agent and those given two effective agents *if* the circulating neutrophil count rose from levels less than 100 μl to levels greater than 100 μl. Clearly, however, the fact that the white cell count does or does not rise can only be determined *after* this occurs. One cannot always predict which patients are likely to experience a rise in their white cell count. Therefore, it still seems prudent that one should begin initial empiric therapy in neutropenic patients with two appropriate agents.

On the basis of the nature of the organism and in vitro susceptibility results, subsequent therapeutic adjustments are possible. It is our view that if the organism is identified as *Pseudomonas aeruginosa* or one of the more resistant gram-negative bacilli (*Acinotobacter* spp., *Pseudomonas aeruginosa*), then it would be prudent to continue combination treatment until the neutrophil count has peaked above 500/μl. If the organism is an exquisitely susceptible gram-negative bacillus, then monotherapy with a potent beta-lactam compound could be deemed appropriate.

This still begs the issue of whether combination therapy can limit the emergence of resistance; it seems likely that combinations (such as those including an aminoglycoside) may still be important for long courses of treatment (19).

The selection of a monotherapeutic agent in modern times should probably be restricted to those compounds with the broadest in vitro spectrum which can be administered via the intravenous route. While the quinolones are attractive because of their excellent activity against gram-negative organisms, there are certain obvious weaknesses such as limited antistreptococcal activity. Therefore, combinations with agents that do not completely overlap in their activity (vancomycin with a quinolone or a beta-lactam agent) are being used increasingly as empiric therapy. However, this has spurred debate as to whether an agent such as vancomycin should be considered an essential part of an initial therapeutic regimen. Many have expressed the view that vancomycin treatment should be reserved only for infections caused by documented gram-positive organisms such as those due to methicillin-resistant *Staphylococcus epidermidis* or *Staphylococcus aureus* with a similar susceptibility pattern.

In the final analysis the patient's ability to recover from neutropenia seems related not so much to the selection of appropriate antibiotic therapy but to the ability to control the underlying disease. We have long emphasized that aggressive antibacterial treatment is but a holding action in patients with acute leukemia until treatment eliminates abnormal or malignant cells and the patient has some improvement in the status of his bone marrow. The currently available therapy may be viewed as "keeping the patient alive" through a period of bone marrow aplasia until the underlying disease can improve. Prognosis remains poor in patients who are persistently neutropenic.

In the history of clinical investigation there have clearly been some conceptual approaches that have been very promising but have not been supported by subsequent clinical trials. The one area that comes to mind immediately has been the therapeutic use of granulocyte transfusions, a subject that has been debated and reviewed (20). Because of the complications in the technique and the limitations about delivering adequate numbers of cells, the use of granulocyte transfusions has progressively declined in recent years. However, the concept that neutrophils are beneficial to the host remains firmly established. Currently being evaluated are approaches at hastening the recovery of the bone marrow, such as with some of the new recombinant cytokines that belong to the class of colony stimulating factors (21). Such approaches, coupled with the judicious use of broad-spectrum antibiotics, may represent the combination therapy of the future.

L. S. Young

Kuzell Institute for Arthritis and Infectious Diseases, 2200 Webster Street, San Francisco, California 94415, USA.

References

1. Young, L. S.: Management of infections in leukemia and lymphoma. In: Rubin, R. H., Young, L. S. (ed.): The clinical approach to infection in the compromised host. Plenum Press, New York, 1988, p. 467–524.
2. Bodey, G. P., Buckley, M., Sathe, Y. S., Freireich, E. J.: Quantitative relationships between circulating leukocytes and infections in patients with acute leukemia. Annals of Internal Medicine 1966, 64: 328–340.
3. McCabe, W. R., Jackson, G. G.: Gram-negative bacteremia. II. Clinical, laboratory, and therapeutic observations. Archives of Internal Medicine 1962, 110: 856–864.
4. Freid, M. A., Vosti, K. L.: Importance of underlying disease in patients with gram-negative bacteremia. Archives of Internal Medicine 1968, 121: 418–423.
5. Bryant, R. E., Hood, A. F., Hood, C. E., Koenig, M. G.: Factors affecting mortality of gram-negative rod bacteremia. Archives of Internal Medicine 1971, 127: 120–128.
6. Armstrong, D., Young, L. S., Meyer, R. D., Blevins, A.: Infectious complications of neoplastic disease. Medical Clinics of North America 1971, 55: 729–745.
7. Bodey, G. P., Jadeja, L., Elting, L.: Pseudomonas bacteremia: retrospective analysis of 410 episodes. Archives of Internal Medicine 1985, 145: 1621–1629.
8. Anderson, E. T., Young, L. S., Hewitt, W. L.: Antimicrobial synergism in the therapy of gram-negative rod bacteremia. Chemotherapy 1978, 24: 45–54.
9. Love, L. J., Schimpff, S. C., Schiffer, C. A., Wiernik, P. H.: Improved prognosis for granulocytopenic patients with gram-negative rod bacteremia. American Journal of Medicine 1980, 68: 643–648.
10. Young, L. S., Meyer-Dudnik, D., Hindler, J., Martin, W. J.: Aminoglycosides in treatment of bacteremic infections in the immunocompromised host. Journal of Antimicrobial Chemistry 1981, 8 (Supplement A): 121–132.
11. Klastersky, J., Glauser, M. P., Schimpff, S. C., Zinner, S. H., Gaya, H.: Prospective randomized comparison of three antibiotic regimens for empirical therapy of suspected bacteremia infection in febrile granulocytopenic patients. Antimicrobial Agents and Chemotherapy 1986, 29: 263–270.
12. International Antimicrobial Therapy Project Group of the European Organization for Research and Treatment of Cancer. Combination of amikacin and carbenicillin with or without cefazolin as empirical treatment of febrile neutropenic patients. Journal of Clinical Oncology 1983, 1: 597–603.
13. Pizzo, P. A., Hathorn, J. W., Hiemenz, J., Brown, M., Commers, J., Cotton, D., Gress, J., Longo, D., Marshall, D., McKnight, J., Rubin, M., Skelton, J., Thaler, M., Wesley, R.: A randomized trial comparing ceftazidime alone with combination antibiotic therapy in cancer patients with fever and neutropenia. New England Journal of Medicine 1986, 315: 552–558.
14. Young, L. S.: Empirical antimicrobial therapy in the neutropenic host. New England Journal of Medicine 1986, 315: 580.
15. EORTC Antimicrobial Therapy Project Group: Ceftazidime combined with a short or long course of amikacin for empirical therapy of gram-negative bacteremia in cancer patients with granulocytopenia. New England Journal of Medicine 1987, 317: 1692–1698.
16. Young, L. S.: Double beta-lactam therapy in immunocompromised host. Journal of Antimicrobial Chemotherapy 1985, 16: 4–6.
17. Winston, D. J., Barnes, R. C., Ho W. G., Young, L. S., Champlin, R. E., Gale, R. P.: Moxalactam plus piperacillin versus moxalactam plus amikacin in febrile granu-

locytopenic patients. American Journal of Medicine 1984, 77: 442–450.

18. de Jongh, C. A., Joshi, J. H., Newman, K. A., Moody, M. R., Wharton, R., Standiford, H. C., Schimpff, S. C.: Antibiotic synergism and response in gram-negative bacteremia in granulocytopenic cancer patients. American Journal of Medicine 1986, 80, Supplement 8C: 96–111.

19. Young, L. S.: Combination or single drug therapy for gram-negative sepsis. In: Remington, J. S., Swartz, M. N. (ed.): Current clinical topics in infectious diseases. McGraw-Hill, New York, 1982, p. 177–205.

20. Young, L. S.: Role of granulocyte transfusions in treating and preventing infection. Cancer Treatment Report 1983, 67: 109–111.

21. Brandt, S. J., Peters, W. P., Atwater, S. K., Kurtzberg, J., Borowitz, M. J., Jones, R. B., Shpall, E. J., Bast, R. C., Gilbert, C. J., Ortte, D. H.: Effect of recombinant human granulocyte-macrophage colony-stimulating factor on hematopoietic reconstitution after high-dose chemotherapy and autologous bone marrow transplantation. New England Journal of Medicine 1988, 318: 869–876.

Modulation of the Host Flora

R. van Furth, H. F. L. Guiot

Modulation of the bacterial flora of patients with a high risk of acquiring an infection can be achieved in several ways. The approach used in the Leiden University Hospital is based on selective elimination of the aerobic bacteria in the oropharyngeal cavity and intestinal tract, leaving the anaerobic flora intact. This kind of selective modulation of the host flora has an advantage in that it does not affect the colonization resistance provided by bacterial antagonism, which prevents colonization by resistant but potentially pathogenic bacteria or fungi. The elimination of aerobic bacteria combined with nursing in protective isolation and consumption of food with few bacteria has led to a significant reduction of the incidence of major and fatal infections in patients during episodes of severe granulocytopenia. From these results it may be concluded that the objective of selective antibiotic modulation, namely, the prevention of infections, can be achieved with this approach.

The human oropharyngeal cavity and gastrointestinal tract are colonized by bacteria and yeasts. Treatment with antimicrobial drugs often alters the composition of this microbial flora (1). The extent of this change is dependent on the antimicrobial properties and pharmacokinetic characteristics of the drug in question, and the route of administration. After oral administration and poor resorption, a relatively large amount of the drug will remain in gut, and after parenteral administration, antimicrobial drugs may reach the intestinal tract via hepato-biliary excretion. In both cases the numbers of aerobic and anaerobic bacteria sensitive to the drug in question may decrease. The decrease of the number of bacteria in the intestinal tract, particularly the anaerobic bacteria in the large intestine, promotes an increase of the number of resistant bacteria and yeasts acquired via the oral route. On the basis of findings in mice and monkeys treated with antibiotics, van der Waaij (2–4) formulated the principle of colonization resistance, which concerns the barriers microorganisms must overcome before they can colonize the surfaces of the body.

Initially it was thought that the anaerobic flora of the digestive tract constituted the main determinant of colonization resistance by forming various factors that check the proliferation of aerobic bacteria (5, 6). However, our studies have shown that a change in the pH and the concentration of volatile fatty acids in the cecum of rats does not affect the number of aerobic and facultative anaerobic bacteria in the cecum nor the growth rate of *Escherichia coli* injected into the cecum of live rats (7). Later studies showed that competition for the substrate needed for the growth of bacteria (9) is one of the main factors responsible for the antagonism between anaerobic and aerobic bacteria in the gut. This is illustrated by experiments with *Escherichia coli* embedded in agar slices. After preincubation of these slices in cecal contents of rats or human feces, growth of *Escherichia coli* depends on the nutrients which penetrated the agar slices during preincubation. Various control experiments demonstrated that both the maximal growth rate (k_{max}) and the yield of colony forming units of *Escherichia coli* depends on the quantity and the quality of the nutrients available within the agar slices (Table 1, Figure 1). The results of these experiments imply that a decrease of the large number of anaerobic bacteria in the large intestine (10^{12} organisms per gram feces) means that relatively more nutrients become available to the aerobic bacteria. When the colonization resistance decreases during treatment with antimicrobial drugs, bacteria which are resistant to these drugs and already present in the intestinal tract or taken in together with food can proliferate unlimited. Similar conditions also promote the dissemination of aerobic bacteria and yeasts to mesenteric lymph nodes and other organs (10–12).

In a broader sense, colonization resistance would include all factors that hamper the colonization of microorganisms. For the gastrointestinal tract, colonization resistance would then include the low pH of the gastric contents and the peristaltic movements of the gut; for the respiratory tract, the mucociliary activity and expulsion by coughing; and for

Department of Infectious Diseases, University Hospital, Building 1, C5-P, P. O. Box 9600, 2300 RC Leiden, The Netherlands.

Table 1: Growth characteristics of Escherichia coli embedded in agar slices after pre-incubation in cecal contents of rats or human feces and then incubated in various media.

Experimental details[a]		Results		
Pre-incubation (2 hours) material	Incubation (18 hours) medium	Lage phase (hours)	k_{max} (gen.h^{-1})	Yield (CFU/agar slice)
None[b]	saline	1	2.3	$10^{9.2}$
BHI broth	saline	3	2.3	$10^{8.4}$
Cecal contents of rats	BHI broth	5	2.3	$10^{9.0}$
Cecal contents of rats	saline	8	1.2	$10^{7.3}$
Cecal contents of antibiotic-treated rats	saline	6	1.7	$10^{8.0}$
Cecal contents of rats	anaerobic saline	8	0.7	$10^{6.4}$
Cecal contents of rats	anaerobic saline + $NaNO_3$	8	1.4	$10^{7.6}$
Cecal contents of rats	anaerobic BHI broth	8	2	$10^{8.8}$
Human feces	BHI broth	4.5	2.3	$10^{9.0}$
Human feces	saline	7	1.2	$10^{7.3}$

[a] 3×10^5 Escherichia coli were embedded in agar slices (0.4 gram) prepared with saline.
[b] No pre-incubation, agar slices prepared with brain-heart infusion broth (BHI).

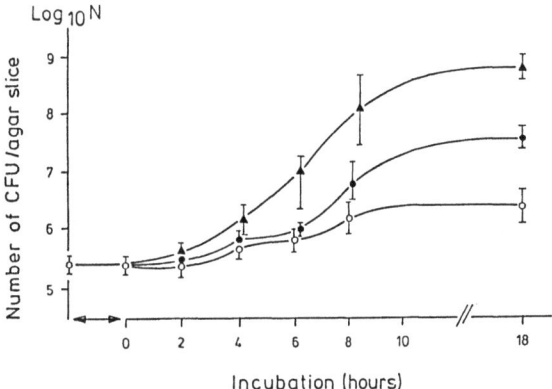

Figure 1: Growth of $10^{5.5}$ Escherichia coli in agar slices that were pre-incubated for 2 h (←→) in cecal contents of rats and then incubated under anaerobic conditions in the presence of various media. ○ = anaerobic saline. ▲ = anaerobic brain-heart infusion broth. ● = anaerobic saline with $NaNO_3$, which serves as oxygen source for bacteria (from Reference No. 8).

the skin, the bactericidal action of the long-chain fatty acids in the secretions of the sebaceous glands. We favour this broader view of colonization resistance, and use the term "bacterial antagonism" to denote the growth-controlling effect of the anaerobic flora on aerobic bacteria.

Prevention of Infection During Decreased Host Resistance

The intensive chemotherapy currently used to treat malignant diseases, e.g., leukaemia and lymphoma, and the conditioning used to prepare for bone-marrow transplantation lead to severe granulocytopenia. Damage done to the mucous membranes of the oral cavity and intestinal tract by chemotherapy promotes the penetration of bacteria that can cause a local or disseminated infection in patients with granulocytopenia. A sharp increase in the incidence of disseminated infections occurs when the number of circulating granulocytes drops below $0.1 \times 10^9 \cdot l^{-1}$ (13, 14). A number of measures can be taken to prevent infections in patients at high risk, the most effective being modulation of the microbial flora. Two approaches are available: total decontamination of the patient (removal of all aerobic and anaerobic bacteria from the oral cavity, the gastrointestinal tract, and the skin) and selective decontamination (elimination or reduction of the number of potentially pathogenic aerobic microorganisms only).

Total Decontamination

Total decontamination means elimination of all microorganisms borne by the patient. This can be achieved by oral administration of a combination of non-absorbable antimicrobial drugs against both aerobic and anaerobic bacteria and yeasts, accompanied by topical application of the antimicrobial drugs or an antiseptic agent to the mucous membrane of the naso-oropharyngeal region and the area of the prepuce or vulva. At the same time the number of bacteria on the skin must be lowered by disinfection. Because this kind of treatment severely decreases the colonization resistance, the patients must be nursed in protective isolation and the food must be sterile. A state of total decontamination proved to be difficult to achieve (15–19), expensive, and very stressful for the patient. Furthermore, poor compliance with or discontinuation of the regimen involves the risk of patients with decreased or no colonization resistance acquiring potential pathogens that can easily multiply and cause an overwhelming infection. In any case, total decontamination must be monitored by an extensive program of surveillance cultures.

Total decontamination is considered to be of importance primarily in patients who have undergone bone marrow transplantation and for whom the risk of acquiring an infection after transplantation is very high. The decrease in host resistance of these patients is caused not only by the pre-transplantation treatment with cytotoxic drugs and/or irradiation, which leads to breached body barriers and granulocytopenia, but also by the graft-versus-host disease, which affects the intestinal tract. It is not clear whether total decontamination improves the quality of life in the post-transplantation period and the ultimate survival of the patients (20–22). Reports on studies performed to compare total decontamination with selective or no decontamination describe the failure of attempts to reach total elimination of all bacteria and fungi (15–19). The dangers associated with total decontamination must never be underestimated, because failure to prevent bacterial contamination of these patients without adequate colonization resistance will inevitably result in colonization and a probably fatal infection.

Selective Antibiotic Modulation

Selective antibiotic modulation (SAM) (23) was formerly called partial antibiotic decontamination (PAD) (24) and is now often called selective decontamination or selective gut decontamination. The principle underlying the Leiden approach for of infection during the period of decreased host resistance is to eliminate all potentially pathogenic aerobic bacteria and yeasts from the oropharyngeal cavity and intestinal tract without reducing the number of anaerobic bacteria (25). Experience gained during the last twenty years has shown (26, 27) that anaerobic bacteria rarely cause infections in granulocytopenic patients; most of the infections in such patients are caused by the endogenous aerobic bacterial flora, usually members of the *Enterobacteriaceae* family (e.g., *Escherichia coli, Enterobacter* spp., and *Klebsiella pneumoniae*), *Pseudomonas aeruginosa*, coagulase-positive and -negative staphylococci, yeasts (e.g., *Candida albicans*), or fungi (e.g., *Aspergillus* spp.). Preservation of the anaerobic bacteria implies that colonization resistance, and particularly the bacterial antagonism, will remain intact and prevent enteric colonization by potential pathogens.

In Leiden, selective decontamination is achieved using oral treatment with antimicrobial drugs that are either not absorbed or do not reach an effective plasma level after absorption because renal excretion is so rapid (e.g., some of the older quinolones) (28), making them useless for the treatment of systemic infections. This means that the drugs suitable for selective decontamination are not in general use in hospitals, which reduces the chance of resistance development. In this respect amphotericin B is an exception. This antibiotic is not adsorbed when given orally, has strong antifungal activity without toxicity, and is more effective than other antifungal drugs that can be administered orally. For selective decontamination in adults, the present dosage used is 250 mg neomycin, 100 mg polymyxin B, and 250 mg amphotericin B, all given 4 times daily, and 400 mg pipemidic acid (formerly 1000 mg nalidixic acid) given twice daily (23, 24, 29). Patients undergoing bone marrow transplantation receive Orabase® containing 3 % amphotericin B, 3 % neomycin, and 3 % polymyxin B, to reduce the numbers of bacteria and yeasts in the oral cavity (30). This regimen is supplemented with disinfection of the skin using povidone-iodine soap or water containing 0.02 % chlorhexidine, consumption of food with few bacteria, and nursing in a protected environment, i.e., in laminar flow rooms or in a single room with a sluice and air conditioning for protective isolation (30). Once or twice each week during the period of selective decontamination, samples of feces and urine are taken for surveillance cultures, as are swabs from the nose, oropharynx, axilla, groin, and prepuce or vagina (29). Culture is performed according to standard bacteriologic methods. During periods of fever (axillary temperature above 38 °C) at least two blood samples are cultured daily both aerobically and anaerobically.

Results of Selective Decontamination

During the initial study, selective decontamination was effective for the elimination of potentially pathogenic microorganisms and reduction of the incidence of major infections (23, 25, 29). Microbiologic studies showed that in the majority of the patients who were not infected when admitted, most of the potentially pathogenic aerobic bacteria were eliminated within a week after selective decontamination was started (Table 2). This was not the case for patients with an infection at the time of admission, in whom the species of microorganisms involved tended to persist (Table 2). Patients without an infection at admission and whose potential pathogens were eliminated within one week after the start of selective decontamination had significantly

Table 2: The effect of selective decontamination on potentially pathogenic aerobic bacteria, as indicated by clinical results from a study of 39 patients with severe granulocytopenia ($< 0.1 \times 10^9$ cells. l^{-1}); from Reference No. 25.

	Time needed to eliminate potentially pathogenic aerobic microorganisms	
	< 1 week	> 1 week
At admission		
Minor infection	3	4
Major infection	0	5
No infection	20	7
During hospitalization		
Major infection[a]	3	5
Fatal infection	0	4
No major infection	20 ($p = 0.0037$)	6

[a] Either due to deterioration of minor infection already present at admission or newly acquired.

Table 4: Effect of selective decontamination on the number of anaerobic bacteria in the feces, as indicated by data obtained from a study of 39 patients with severe granulocytopenia given selective decontamination, and 21 healthy individuals (controls) without selective decontamination; from Reference No. 25.

Bacteria	Log_{10} CFU of bacteria per gram (wet weight) feces	
	Patients	Controls
All anaerobic species	10.5	10.3
Bacteroides spp.	10.2	10.0
Eubacterium spp.	9.9	9.7
Bifidobacterium spp.	10.0	9.5
Peptococcaceae	< 8.0	< 8.0
Clostridium spp.	< 8.0	< 8.0
Propionibacteriaceae	< 8.0	< 8.0

fewer major infections than patients in whom these pathogens were eliminated much later or not at all (Table 2).

Analysis of the results of the surveillance cultures showed that in patients with severely decreased host defense mechanisms, a majority of the aerobic bacteria were eliminated within one week from patients on the regimen of selective decontamination (Table 3), the exceptions being *Staphylococcus epidermidis* and *Streptococcus* spp., because they are intrinsically resistant to the SAM regimen, and those aerobic gram-negative rods already involved in infection at admission (e.g. *Pseudomonas aeruginosa*). *Candida albicans* was not eliminated despite the inclusion of amphotericin B, whose main effect is the prevention of proliferation of *Candida* spp. Swabs from the oral cavity (especially material from suspected plaques) and fecal samples were checked microscopically for *Candida albicans* with pseudohyphae, because this is a sign of local growth; if these were found, amphotericin B lozenges were given additionally. Preservation of the anaerobic flora during selective decontamination was demonstrated by the results of the quantitative anaerobic culture of feces (Table 4) (25). On the basis of these results, which were confirmed by later studies (not published), surveillance cultures of the anaerobic bacterial flora are no longer performed routinely during selective decontamination in Leiden.

Table 3: Course of infection with species of potentially pathogenic aerobic bacteria during selective decontamination, as indicated by clinical results from a study of 39 patients with severe granulocytopenia ($< 0.1 \times 10^9$ cell. l^{-1}); from Reference No. 25.

	Number of patients with microorganisms		
	Present at admission	Persisting for one week	Persisting and involved in major infection
Escherichia coli	39	6	3
Klebsiella spp.	15	3	2
Proteus spp.	14	3	2
Enterobacter spp.	9	1	1
Citrobacter spp.	6	0	0
Serratia spp.	1	0	0
Pseudomonas aeruginosa	5	4	4
Alcaligenes bronchisepticus	1	1	0
Haemophilus spp.	6	0	0
Staphylococcus aureus	19	4	2
Streptococcus pneumoniae	8	1	0
Staphylococcus epidermidis	39	39	0
Streptococcus faecalis	39	39	0
Streptococcus spp.	39	39	0
Candida albicans	39	39	0

Table 5: Septicaemia in selectively decontaminated patients during severe granulocytopenia following chemotherapy or bone marrow transplantation.

	Numbers of infections and causative microorganisms				
	1983	1984	1985	1986	1987
Number of infections[a] per number of episodes of granulocytopenia	14/106	35/93	40/79	28/85	24/60
Percentage of infections	13.2	37.6	50.6	32.9	40
Enterobacteriaceae	8	7	3	5	2
Pseudomonas aeruginosa	5	3	2	4	5
α Haemolytic streptococci	16	17	26	5	9
Enterococci	6	7	4	2	3
Coagulase-positive staphylococci	4	5	0	4	1
Coagulase-negative staphylococci	7	3	12	8	7
Candida spp.	0	1	1	1	2
Aspergillus spp.	0	1	1	1	2
Miscellaneous	4	3	4	0	0

[a] In some instances two or more microorganisms were involved.

The regimen for selective decontamination described above was adequate until chemotherapy for leukaemia and the conditioning performed before transplantation were intensified. After 1982, the use of intermediate and high-dose cytosine arabinoside and amsacrine (31) led to a gradual increase of the incidence of streptococcal infections from 4 % (23, 29) to 38 % (Table 5), and by 1985 this type of infection predominated (32). Almost all of the infections acquired in the hospital were septicaemias caused by α haemolytic streptococci originating in all probability from the oral cavity. In 1986, to prevent these infections, a short course of prophylactic systemic treatment was added to the regimen for selective decontamination: beginning prior to day 3 and continuing until day 11 after transplantation, or for 14 days starting on the last day of treatment with cytosine arabinoside, the patients receive either 4×10^6 U penicillin G intravenously (33), or, for those with penicillin allergy, cotrimoxazole. This has significantly decreased the incidence of streptococcal septicaemias (Table 5). Between 1983 and 1987, the incidence of septicaemia due to gram-negative rods and coagulase-positive and -negative staphylococci remained constantly low and the number of fungal infections was very low (Table 5), which confirmed the continuing adequacy of the regimen of selective decontamination with respect to the control of infections with Enterobacteriaceae, Pseudomonas aeruginosa, staphylococci, and fungi.

Other Combinations of Antimicrobial Drugs Used to Modulate the Host Flora

Elimination of the potentially pathogenic bacteria while leaving the aerobic flora intact can also be achieved with other antimicrobial drugs. Cotrimoxazole, which was initially used alone (34) but is currently combined with polymyxin B or colistin and amphotericin B, effectively reduces the number of Enterobacteriaceae, Pseudomonas spp., and yeast (35). However, because cotrimoxazole is absorbed, it is active both locally in the lumen of the intestinal tract and systemically. The development of resistance by bacteria due to selection has restricted the large-scale use of cotrimoxazole for prophylaxis. This problem can be partially solved by the addition of polymyxin B or colistin to the regimen, but because absorbed cotrimoxazole is excreted in low concentration in, for example, saliva and the exudate of wounds, local conditions become suitable for colonization by resistant bacteria. For these reasons cotrimoxazole is used prophylactically on a limited basis in Leiden, as discussed above.

Another recent trend concerns the prophylactic use of ciprofloxacin (36) in this context. Unlike the quinolone (formerly nalidixic acid and now pipemidic acid) chosen for use in Leiden, ciprofloxacin gives therapeutically adequate plasma levels when administered orally. This means that prophylaxis with ciprofloxacin provides not only elimination of bacteria from the intestinal tract but also systemic treatment. The secretion of resorbed ciprofloxacin at any mucosal surface is accompanied by the danger of emergence of resistant bacteria due to either selection or mutation (37, 38). For all of these reasons we prefer not to use ciprofloxacin for prophylaxis. If for some reason it is given prophylactically, it must be combined with an other antibiotic, for example, polymyxin B, to avoid the emergence of resistant bacteria in the intestinal tract.

One objectionable aspect of the Leiden regimen of selective decontamination is the great bulk of the drugs to be swallowed by the patients. However, where ciprofloxacin is used the daily dose must be 1600 mg, which, combined with 400 mg polymyxin B and 1000 mg amphotericin B, adds up to roughly the same amount and bulk as the 3200 mg for the combination used in Leiden.

Some groups do not use antibiotic prophylaxis during chemotherapy in leukaemic patients or for bone marrow transplantation, but start treatment with a combination of antimicrobial drugs as soon as a patient shows any sign of infection such as fever. The initial choice is based on empery, but after isolation of the causative microorganism the therapy is adjusted if necessary. According to these authors, in the long run their rates of morbidity and mortality due to infections are similar to those obtained in patients given partial decontamination (39, 40). In the absence of comparative studies we question the validity of this conclusion. Especially the enormous decrease of the incidence of severe infections with gram-negative bacteria or streptococci and the almost total elimination of infections with fungi (e.g., *Candida* spp.) have strengthened our conviction that selective decontamination deserves a place in the supportive care of patients with severely impaired host resistance.

Acknowledgement

This study was supported by the J. A. Cohen Institute of Radiopathology and Radiation Protection, Leiden, The Netherlands.

References

1. **Gorbach, S. L., Barza, M., Giuliano, M., Jacobus, N. V.:** Colonization resistance of the human intestinal microflora: testing the hypothesis in normal volunteers. European Journal of Clinical Microbial Infectious Diseases 1988, 7: 98–102.
2. **van der Waaij, D., de Vries Berghuis, J. M., Lekkerkerk van der Wees, J. E. C.:** Colonization resistance of the digestive tract in conventional and antibiotic-treated mice. Journal of Hygiene 1971, 69: 405–411.
3. **van der Waaij, D., de Vries Berghuis, J. M., Lekkerkerk van der Wees, J. E. C.:** Colonization resistance of the digestive tract in mice during systemic antibiotic treatment. Journal of Hygiene 1972, 70: 605–610.
4. **van der Waaij, D., Berghuis-de Vries, J. M.:** Selective elimination of *Enterobacteriaceae* species from the digestive tract in mice and monkeys. Journal of Hygiene 1974, 77: 205–211.
5. **Bergeim, O., Hanszen, A. H., Pincussen, L., Weiss, E.:** Relation of volatile fatty acids and hydrogen sulphide to the intestinal flora. Journal of Infectious Diseases 1941, 69: 155–166.
6. **Bohnhoff, M., Miller, C. P., Martin, W. R.:** Resistance of the mouse's intestinal tract to experimental *Salmonella* infection. I. Journal of Experimental Medicine 1964, 120: 805–816.
7. **Guiot, H. F. L.:** Volatile fatty acids and the selective growth inhibition of aerobic bacteria in the gut of rats. In: Sasaki, S., Ozawa, A., Hashimoto, K. (ed.): Recent advances in germfree research. Tokai University Press, Tokyo, 1981, p. 219–221.
8. **Guiot, H. F. L.:** Role of competition for substrate in bacterial antagonism in the intestines. Infection and Immunity 1982, 38: 887–892.
9. **Freter, R., Brickner, H., Fekete, J., Vickerman, M. M., Carey, K. E.:** Survival and implantation of *Escherichia coli* in the intestinal tract. Infection and Immunity 1983, 39: 686–703.
10. **van der Waaij, D., Berghuis-de Vries, J. M., Lekkerkerk van der Wees, J. E. C.:** Colonization resistance of the digestive tract and the spread of bacteria to the lymphatic organs in mice. Journal of Hygiene 1972, 70: 335–342.
11. **Berg, R. D., Garlington, A. W.:** Translocation of certain indigenous bacteria from the gastrointestinal tract to the mesenteric lymph nodes and other organs in a gnotobiotic mouse model. Infection and Immunity 1979, 23: 403–404.
12. **Steffen, E. K., Berg, R. D.:** Relationship between cecal population levels of indigenous bacteria and translocation to the mesenteric lymph nodes. Infection and Immunity 1983, 39: 1252–1259.
13. **Bodey, G. P., Buckley, M., Sathe, Y. S., Freireich, E. J.:** Quantitative relationship between circulating leukocytes and infections in patients with acute leukemia. Annals of Internal Medicine 1966, 64: 328–340.
14. **van der Meer, J. W. M., Boekhout, M., Alleman, M.:** Infectious episodes in severely granulocytopenic patients. Infection 1979, 7: 171–175.
15. **Bodey, G. P., Rosenbaum, B.:** Effect of prophylactic measures of the microbial flora of patients in protected environment units. Medicine 1974, 53: 209–228.
16. **Bodey, G. P.:** Current status of prophylaxis of infection with protected environments. American Journal of Medicine 1984, 76: 678–684.
17. **Schimpff, S. C.:** Infection prevention during profound granulocytopenia. New approaches to alimentary canal microbial suppression. Annals of Internal Medicine 1980, 93: 358–361.
18. **Ribas-Mundo, M., Graneda, A., Rozman, C.:** Evaluation of a protective environment in the management of granulocytopenic patients: a comparative study. Cancer 1981, 48: 419–424.
19. **Kurrle, E., Abt, C., Bhaduri, S., Heimpel, H., Krieger, D., Vanek, E., Kubanec, B.:** Possibilities and problems of protective isolation and antimicrobial decontamination in man. Zentralblatt für Bakteriologie 1979, (A) 7 (Supplement): 63–66.
20. **Guiot, H. F. L., van der Meer, J. W. M., Fibbe, W. E., de Planque, M. M., Zwaan, F. E., Biemond, I.:** The effects of the intestinal microflora of selective decontamination in patients undergoing allogeneic bone marrow transplantation. Experimental Hematology 1985, (Supplement 17) 13: 108–109.
21. **Guiot, H. F. L.:** The effect of the intestinal microflora of selective decontaminated patients on the severity of acute graft-versus-host disease. In: Gnotobiology and its applications. Proceedings of the IXth International Symposium on Gnotobiology, Versailles, France. Edition Fondation Marcel Mérieux, Lyon, 1987, p. 128–130.
22. **Petersen, F. B., Buckner, C. D., Clift, R. A., Nelsen, N., Counts, G. W., Meyers, J. D., Thomas, E. D.:** Infectious complication in patients undergoing marrow transplantation: a prospective randomized study of the additional effect of decontamination and laminar air flow isolation among patients receiving prophylactic systemic antibiotics. Scandinavian Journal of Infectious Diseases 1987, 19: 559–567.

23. Guiot, H. F. L., van den Broek, P. J., van der Meer, J. W. M., van Furth, R.: Selective antimicrobial modulation of the intestinal flora of patients with acute non-lymphocytic leukemia: a double-blind, placebo-controlled study. Journal of Infectious Diseases 1983, 147: 615–623.
24. Guiot, H. F. L., van Furth, R.: Partial antibiotic decontamination. British Medical Journal 1977, 1: 800–802.
25. Guiot, H. F. L., van der Meer, J. W. M., van Furth, R.: Selective antimicrobial modulation of human microbial flora: infection prevention in patients with decreased host defense mechanisms by selective elimination of potentially pathogenic bacteria. Journal of Infectious Diseases 1981, 143: 644–654.
26. van Furth, R., Nauta, E. H.: Principles of antibiotic treatment. In: Elkerbout, F., Thomas, P., Zwaveling, A. (ed.): Cancer chemotherapy. Leiden University Press, Leiden, 1971, p. 387–394.
27. Bodey, G. P., Rodriquez, V., Chang, H., Narboni, G.: Fever and infection in leukemic patients. Cancer 1978, 41: 1610–1621.
28. McChesney, E. W., Froelich, E. J., Lesher, G. Y., Crain, A. V. R., Rosi, D.: Absorption, excretion, and metabolism of a new antibacterial agent, nalidixic acid. Toxicology and Applied Pharmacology 1964, 6: 292–309.
29. Guiot, H. F. L., Helmig-Schurter, A. V., van der Meer, J. W. M., van Furth, R.: Selective antimicrobial modulation of the intestinal microbial flora for infection prevention in patients with hematologic malignancies. Evaluation of clinical efficacy and the value of surveillance cultures. Scandinavian Journal of Infectious Diseases 1986, 18: 153–160.
30. van der Meer, J. W. M., Guiot, H. F. L., van den Broek, P. J., van Furth, R.: Infections in bone marrow transplant recipients. Seminars in Hematology 1984, 21: 123–140.
31. Willemze, R., Peters, W. G., van Hennik, M. B., Fibbe, W. E., Kootte, A. M. M., van Berkel, M., Lie, R., Rodenburg, C. J., Veltkamp, J. J.: Intermediate and high-dose ARA-C and m-AMSA (or daunorubicin) as remission and consolidation treatment for patients with relapsed acute leukaemia and lymphoblastic non-Hodgkin's lymphoma. Scandinavian Journal of Haematology 1985, 34: 83–87.
32. Peters, W. G., Willemze, R., Colly, L. P., Guiot, H. F. L.: Side effects of intermediate- and high-dose cytosine arabinoside in the treatment of refractory or relapsed acute leukaemia and non-Hodgkin's lymphoma. Netherlands Journal of Medicine 1987, 30: 64–74.
33. Guiot, H. F. L., van den Broek, P. J., van der Meer, J. W. M., Peters, W. G., Willemze, R., van Furth, R.: The association between streptococcal infection and interstitial pneumonia in chemotherapy and BMT. Bone Marrow Transplantation 1988, (Supplement 1) 3: 274.
34. Dekker, A. W., Rozenberg-Arska, M., Sixma, J. J., Verhoef, J.: Prevention of infection by trimethoprim-sulfamethoxazole plus amphotericin B in patients with acute non-lymphocytic leukemia. Annals of Internal Medicine 1981, 95: 555–559.
35. Rozenberg-Arska, M., Dekker, A. W., Verhoef, J.: Colistin and trimethoprim-sulfamethoxazole for the prevention of infection in patients with acute non-lymphocytic leukaemia. Decrease in the emergence of resistant bacteria. Infection 1983, 11: 167–169.
36. Dekker, A. W., Rozenberg-Arska, M., Verhoef, J.: Infection prophylaxis in acute leukemia: a comparison of ciprofloxacin with trimethoprim-sulfa methoxazole and colistin. Annals of Internal Medicine 1987, 106: 7–12.
37. Piddock, L. J. V., Wijnands, W. J. A., Wise, R.: Quinolone/ureidopenicillin cross-resistance. Lancet 1987, ii: 907.
38. Sanders, C. C.: Ciprofloxacin: in vitro activity, mechanism of action, and resistance. Reviews of Infectious Diseases 1988, 10: 516–527.
39. Armstrong, D.: Protected environments are discomforting and expensive and do not offer meaningful protection. American Journal of Medicine 1984, 76: 685–689.
40. Young, L. S.: Antimicrobial prophylaxis in the neutropenic host: lessons of the past and perspectives for the future. European Journal of Clinical Microbiology and Infectious Diseases 1988, 7: 93–97.

Enhancement of Host Resistance by Control of Fungal Growth

D. Pappagianis

Efforts to contravene pathogenesis by zoopathogenic fungi are hampered because, with the exception of toxinogenic mushrooms and molds, little is clearly known about the precise properties of pathogenic fungi that permit them to cause disease. The polysaccharide capsule of *Cryptococcus neoformans* represents an aggressin; the formation of a putative invasive filamentous form (and perhaps acid proteinase) by *Candida albicans* contributes to the development of candidiasis; and the morphologic changes of *Blastomyces dermatitidis, Coccidioides immitis* and *Histoplasma capsulatum* that occur when they enter the host are associated with virulence factors not yet well defined. Pathogenesis by *Paracoccidioides brasiliensis* has been associated with the presence of abundant α-glucan, with antiphagocytic action occurring only after the organism assumes its parasitic yeast form (1). Enhancement of resistance to pathogenic fungi can be obtained by intervention with chemotherapeutic substances, by promotion of the host immune mechanisms for retardation of fungal growth and/or effects of fungal products, and by reduction of damaged tissue harboring infecting fungi by surgical means. While no further attention will be given to the last item, it should be emphasized that it is sometimes the sole curative modality.

Chemotherapeutic intervention obviously should take advantage of some selective means of inhibiting fungi. This poses something of a dilemma, because, like mammalian host cells, fungal cells are eukaryotic. With the exception of a capsule and the cell wall, the fungal cell contains internal organelles resembling those of other eukaryotic cells (Figure 1). The aim of chemotherapeutic intervention, therefore, is to affect differentially the fungal cells while minimizing effects on the host.

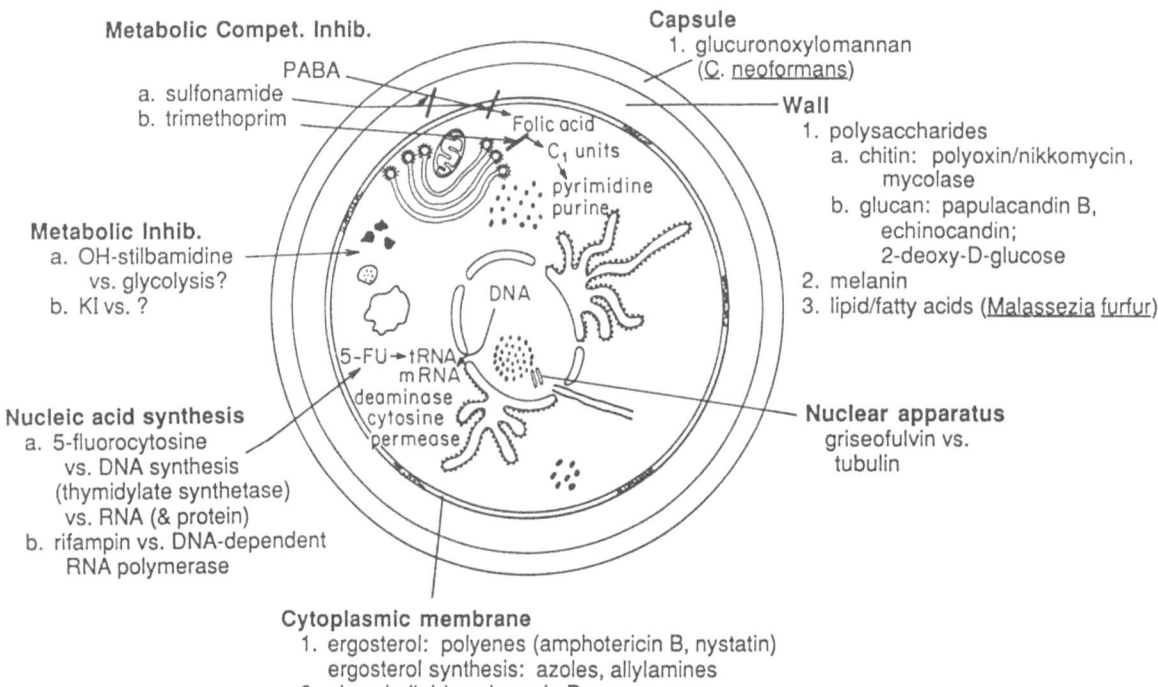

Figure 1: A representative zoopathogenic fungal cell with sites of action of antifungal agents (Fungal cell diagram based on one prepared by G. Kobayashi).

It may be asked whether the production of D-arabinitol by *Candida* spp. contrasted with the exclusive production of L-arabinitol by mammalian hosts represents a sufficient difference in metabolism that can be exploited for chemotherapy (2). Furthermore, the recent successful use of cyclosporin A against coccidioidal (3) and cryptococcal infections (4) in mice may point to yet another as yet unidentified target of selectivity. Also shown in Figure 1 are sites where presently used antifungal agents appear to act and where there are potentially useful other targets for inhibition. (This diagram was adapted slightly for use by Ryley et al. (5, 6), and a similar depiction was offered by Drouhet and Dupont (7).) Some of these compounds appear to have restricted usefulness. For example, the sulfonamides appear to act against paracoccidioidomycosis (perhaps against histoplasmosis), potassium iodide against sporotrichosis, while others affect several fungi.

Capsular Polysaccharide

Based on the presumption that the capsule of *Cryptococcus neoformans* is important in pathogenesis (acapsular mutants are non-virulent), attempts should be made to damage the capsule or inhibit its synthesis. From the extensive work of Cherniak (8), Bhattacharjee, Merrifield and their colleagues, it appears that soluble *Cryptococcus neoformans* capsular polysaccharide consists of at least three polymers: glucuronoxylomannan, galactoxylomannan and mannoprotein. The five serotypes A, B, C, D and A–D produce polysaccharides that contain glucuronic acid, xylose and mannose in different ratios. These glucuronoxylomannans possess a "backbone" consisting of $1 \rightarrow 3\alpha$ D-mannose and have lateral attachments of $1 \rightarrow 2$ linked xylose and glucuronic acid. The xylose may be essential for the aggressive (anti-host) integrity of the capsular polysaccharide. If so, it may be possible to design mimics of the xylose or its carrier that could block incorporation of this pentose into the polysaccharide.

Melanins

These pigments are large molecules, usually dark brown or black. They are produced by oxidative polymerization of phenolic compounds such as tyrosine via 3,4-dihydroxyphenylalanine to give DOPA melanins, via 1,8-dihydroxynaphthalene to give DHN melanins, and from catechols (9) (Figure 2).

The DOPA pathway is utilized in humans and other animals and in some zoopathogenic fungi, e.g. *Cryptococcus neoformans* and opportunistic *Aspergillus* spp. *Cryptococcus neoformans* appears able to make use of other substrates, e.g. indoles with a hydroxyl or amino group on the phenyl ring. The DHN pathway is found in the human pathogen *Wangiella dermatitidis*, and in others associated with chromoblastomycosis and related diseases affecting cutaneous and subcutaneous tissues. It is also present in *Phaeoannelomyces werneckii (Exophiala werneckii)*, the causative agent of tinea nigra, a black mycosis affecting only the stratum corneum.

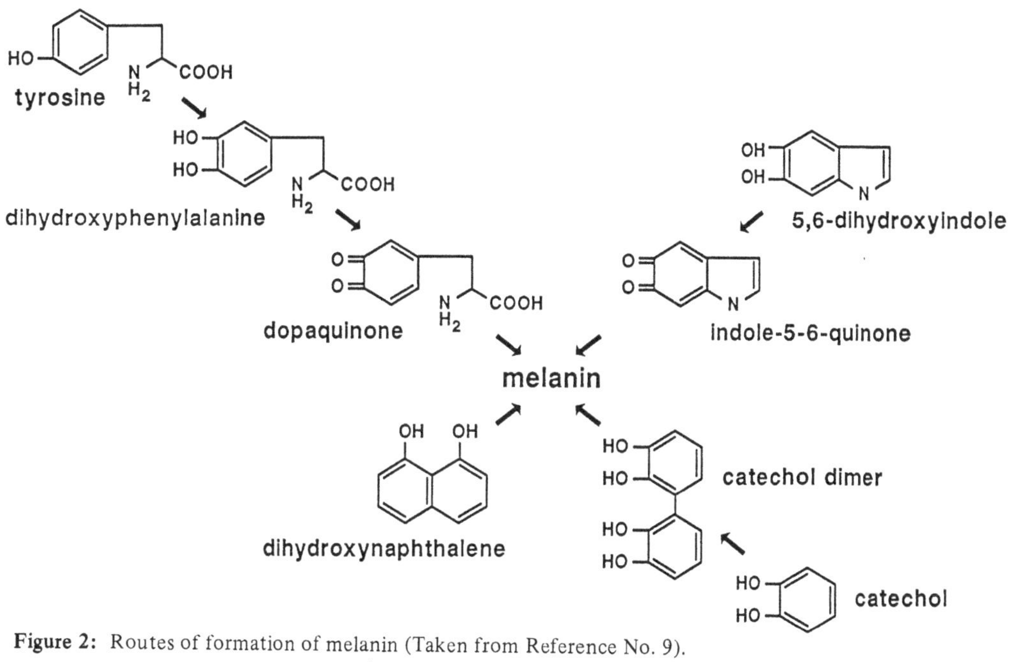

Figure 2: Routes of formation of melanin (Taken from Reference No. 9).

Melanin in fungi may be found in cell walls, in fibrillar arrays around the cell wall, or as extracellular polymers. In *Cryptococcus neoformans*, melanin has been demonstrated in the cell wall to which the polyphenoloxidase appears to be bound; however, some work also indicates the presence of melanin in intra- and extracellular sites. The precise role and importance of melanin pigmentation in human fungal pathogens has not been clarified. In studies with *Cryptococcus neoformans*, mutants that lacked the polyphenoloxidase and, therefore, the melanin synthesizing activity, had diminished virulence for mice even in the presence of normal polysaccharide encapsulation (10). This association of melanin formation and virulence was not complete, however, because, rarely, encapsulated but polyphenoloxidase-deficient yeasts were virulent. Studies with *Wangiella dermatitidis* showed that in an acute model (observation for 21 days), 100 % mortality followed intravenous injection of melanin producing wild-type strains, but there were no deaths with an albino mutant (11).

The means by which melanins contribute to virulence of human pathogens is not clear. The presence of melanin in some plant pathogens has been associated with the following properties (9): Impermeability to certain solutes, e.g. sucrose; penetration through polysaccharide plant cell walls and plant epidermis; resistance to ultraviolet radiation; and resistance to lytic carbohydrases such as chitinase and glucanases. Perhaps only the last property would apply to zoopathogenic fungi, increasing the resistance to phagocytic enzymes that is provided by capsules or cell wall polysaccharides. It is also possible that the barrier role, for example, impermeability to certain solutes, may preclude entry of some potentially damaging molecules.

Some inhibitors of melanin synthesis, e.g. tricyclazole, fthalide (Figure 3), coumarin and others, inhibit the penetration of host epidermis by some plant pathogens (9). It is proposed that compounds which can inhibit synthesis of melanin in human pathogens, e.g. *Cryptococcus neoformans*, may provide another modality of therapy. Thus, analogs of DOPA that inhibit the function of cryptococcal polyphenoloxidase should be studied. Such compounds would have to be free of inhibitory action against tyrosinase, which is required for the production of DOPA essential in neural function and normal pigmentation of humans and other mammals. It would be of further interest to learn whether any difference exists in susceptibility to *Cryptococcus neoformans* of patients with Parkinsonism and presumed deficiency of DOPA. Perhaps some of the street drugs such as MPTP (1-methyl-4-phenyl-1,2,3,6-tetrahydropyridine) that have led to Parkinsonlike disease could be modified to affect fungi rather than mammalian DOPA synthesis.

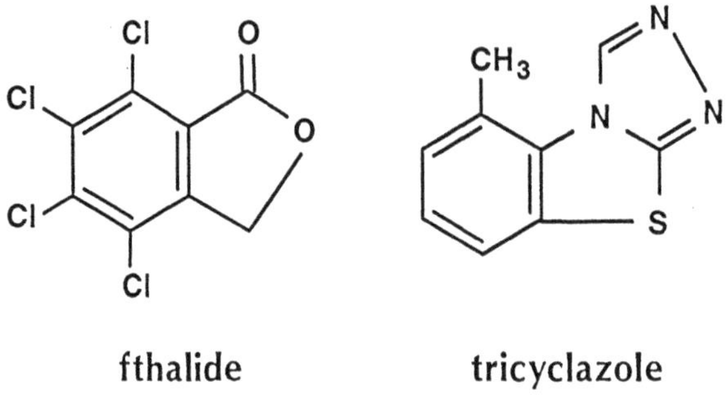

fthalide   **tricyclazole**

Figure 3: Examples of inhibitors of melanin synthesis in phytopathogenic fungi.

It should be pointed out that the systemic pathogens, *Histoplasma capsulatum* and *Coccidioides immitis*, develop brown pigments. B or brown strains of *Histoplasma capsulatum* reportedly show greater virulence in mice than the A albino form (12). The chemical nature of the brown pigment has not been explored nor clearly associated with virulence. The question arises whether the pigment could contribute to virulence by inhibiting alien (host) enzymes.

Polysaccharides

Chitin has long been recognized as a component of the cell walls of many fungi. Chitin is a polymer of N-acetylglucosamine (Figure 4). The presence of chitin has been demonstrated by X-ray crystallographic examination of fungal walls, including those of *Coccidioides immitis*. Furthermore, availability of a streptomyces chitinase permitted the demonstration over 30 years ago of the enzymatic release of N-acetylglucosamine from the walls of *Coccidioides immitis* (13, 14). In 1947, plumbagin, a product of the plant *Plumbago capensis*, was shown to inhibit growth of the mycelial phase of *Coccidioides immitis* and other fungi (15). In the late

Chitin (chitobiose) repeating unit

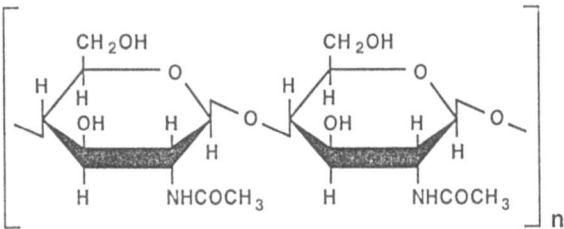

Figure 4: N-acetylglucosamine components of chitin as chitobiose repeating units.

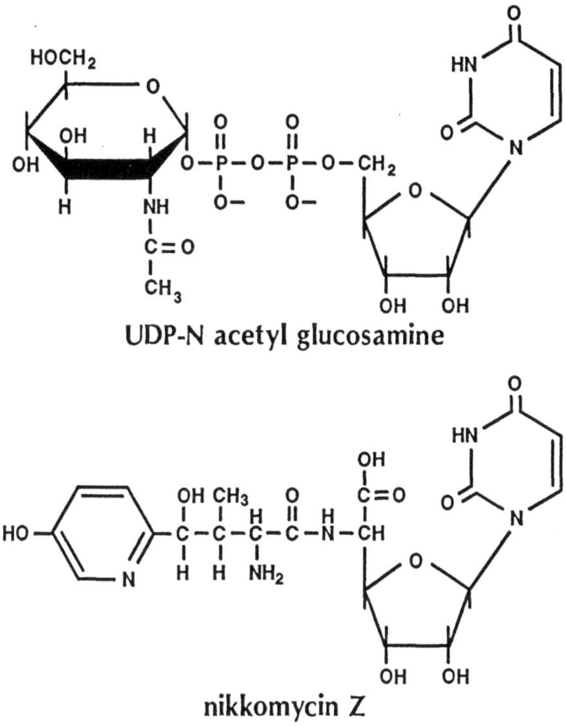

UDP-N acetyl glucosamine

nikkomycin Z

Figure 5: Similarity of structures of nikkomycin Z and uridine diphosphate N-acetylglucosamine.

1960s some products termed polyoxins in culture filtrates of certain *Streptomyces* spp. were found to inhibit synthesis of chitin (16). This action along with that of plumbagin was shown to be directed against the enzyme chitin synthetase, an action detrimental to insects as well as to fungi. The action of the chitin synthetase inhibitor that will be discussed further appears to come about through its mimicry of and interference with UDP-N acetylglucosamine, which builds the N-acetylglucosamine into the polysaccharide chain (Figure 5).

Availability of one of the compounds, polyoxin D, in 1974 permitted M. Collins, R. Hector and D. Pappagianis to demonstrate inhibition of growth of the mycelial phase of *Coccidioides immitis* in vitro. Indeed, Hector subsequently showed by electron micrography that polyoxin D inhibited the synthesis of chitin in the spherule (so-called parasitic) form of *Coccidioides immitis* cultured in vitro, but had a lesser effect on the hyphal form of the organism (17). There was not sufficient polyoxin D available at the time for in vivo studies. However, related compounds, neopolyoxins or nikkomycins, also derived from *Streptomyces* spp., became available later. Hector and co-workers tested nikkomycins in mice infected with the systemic pathogenic fungi *Coccidioides immitis*, *Blastomyces dermatitidis* and *Histoplasma capsulatum*. Nikkomycins X and Z were

tested and the latter proved more active. Indeed, the effects were impressive: at doeses of 20 to 70 mg/kg given orally b.i.d., mice were protected against otherwise lethal doses of *Coccidioides immitis* and *Blastomyces dermatitidis* (Figures 6, 7). The response of mice infected with *Histoplasma capsulatum*, although successful in some experiments, was less consistent and impressive than with the other two systemic pathogens (18).

The effect of intravenous nikkomycins against *Candida albicans* in mice appeared less impressive, but the dosage was small (8 mg/kg) (19). The lesser effectiveness against *Candida albicans* (and perhaps *Histoplasma capsulatum*) may be related to the localization and concentration of chitin. In *Candida albicans* some chitin is distributed in the entire cell wall, but is particularly concentrated at the septum and bud scar (where the bud has separated from the parent cell). By contrast, *Coccidioides immitis*, *Blastomyces dermatitidis* and *Paracoccidioides brasiliensis* have substantial chitin throughout the cell

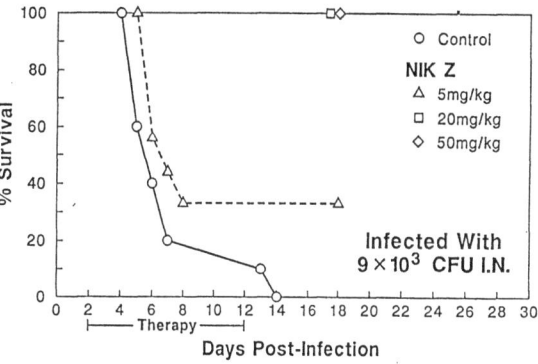

Figure 6: Survival of mice infected with *Coccidioides immitis* and treated with nikkomycin Z (Taken from Reference No. 18).

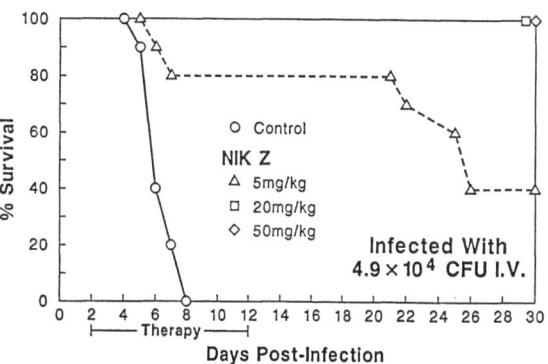

Figure 7: Survival of mice infected with *Blastomyces dermatitidis* and treated with nikkomycin Z (Taken from Reference No. 18).

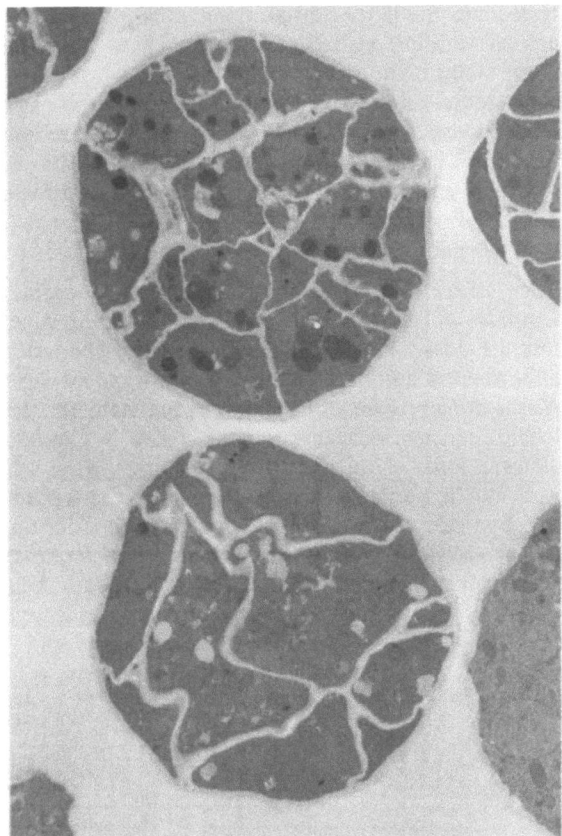 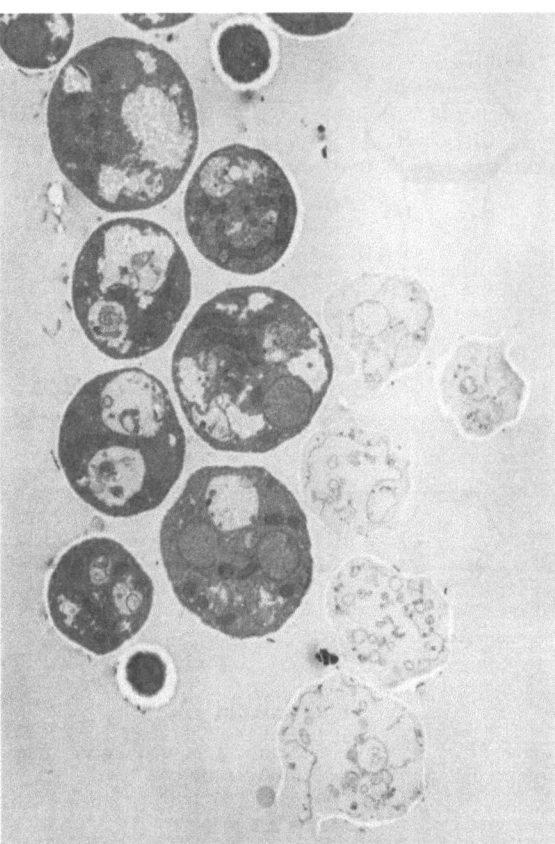

Figure 8: Transmission electron micrograph of untreated 33-hour-old spherules (left) and of spherules of the same age after exposure to 2 µg/ml of nikkomycin Z for 24 h (right). Note the relative decrease in size, the thinness of walls, and the collapse of cells treated with nikkomycin Z (Both micrographs taken at X 7,300).

wall, at least in some stage of development. With *Coccidioides immitis* this chitin is synthesized during the formation of the mature spherules, which cleave internally to form endospores (Figure 8). The addition of nikkomycin Z to early stages of conversion from endospore to mature spherule leads to impairment of growth and to alterations (thinning) of the wall, leading to degeneration in which the cell appears to lose most of its internal structure, including cleavage lines, with retraction of the cytoplasm and loss of viability (Figure 8). Compared with mature spherules the nikkomycin-altered cells are much smaller.

Glucans and Mannans

Additional cell wall polysaccharides differing from structures in the mammalian host are the glucans and the mannans. Inhibitors of beta-glucan synthesis studied thus far include the natural compounds aculeacin A, papulacandin B (Figure 9) (20), and echinocandin B (ECB), and the semisynthetic analog of the latter, LY121019 (= N-p-n-ocytyloxy-benzyol-ECB) (21). LY121019 caused severe damage to the *Candida albicans* cell wall, and when orally administered in subtoxic doses (50 and 100 mg/kg), eliminated *Candida albicans* from the gastrointestinal tract of infected mice and was effective against vaginal candidiasis in the rat as shown by Gordee et al. (21). Apparently, few studies have been carried out with this group of compounds against systemic pathogenic fungi. This is an inviting area for testing, particularly in light of the important observations of Hector and Braun (22) showing synergism between papulacandin B and the chitin synthetase inhibitors nikkomycin Z or X in the in vitro inhibition of *Candida albicans*.

Promotion of Immune Mechanism in the Immunocompromised Host for Retardation of Fungal Growth

Considering that the effect of currently used antifungal chemotherapeutic agents is largely fungistatic rather than fungicidal, a successful immunologic

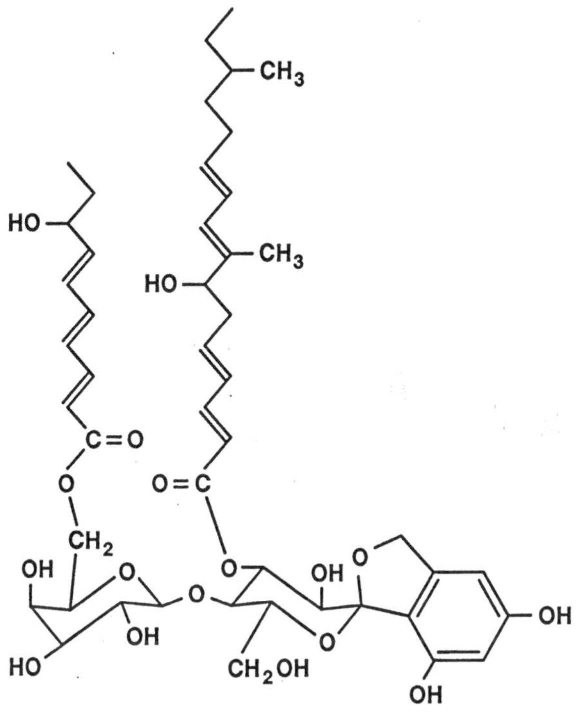

Papulacandin B

Figure 9: Structure proposed for papulacandin B (Taken from Reference No. 20). Note the disaccharide base from which fatty acids project.

Table 1: Cases of coccidioidomycosis in humans after vaccination with killed whole *Coccidioides immitis* spherules or placebo. (From D. Pappagianis, 26th Interscience Conference on Antimicrobial Agents and Chemotherapy, New Orleans, 1986, Abstract No. 784.)

	No. of cases	No. of suspected cases
Vaccine	9	9
Placebo	12	13
Total	21	22

response of the host appears essential to the ultimate arrest of fungal pathogens. This arrest may be illusory, however, as recrudescence of disease has occurred when some antifungal agents, e.g. azoles, have been discontinued too soon. Unfortunately, it is not always clear when it is appropriate to discontinue therapy. The exacerbation of previously (presumably) healed coccidioidomycosis and other fungal diseases in patients with AIDS or other immunosuppressive states clearly indicates that viable organisms can remain latent for long periods in the apparently well person. Cell mediated immunity has been regarded as a (the?) major host response necessary for the arrest of fungal growth. Without such cell mediated immunity, progression of disease seems likely to occur. However, other aspects, some related, some unrelated to cell mediated immunity, are being explored: the role of natural killer cells in cryptococcosis, the effect of γ-interferon in experimental coccidioidomycosis (23), and the role of polymorphonuclear leukocytes in systemic fungal diseases other than candidiasis.

Finally, it may be asked whether active immunization could be used to control fungal growth. Although immunity could be shown in laboratory animals vaccinated with a killed *Coccidioides immitis* whole cell vaccine, the one such vaccine field trial in humans unfortunately showed no significant protection (Table 1) (D. Pappagianis et al., 26th Interscience Conference on Antimicrobial Agents and Chemotherapy, New Orleans, 1986, Abstract No. 784). It is likely that the whole cell vaccine may need to be made into a subcellular, even soluble preparation to be tolerated by humans.

Additional means of counteracting the fungi may be considered; for example, inhibition of certain activities that may contribute to pathogenesis. Proteolytic enzymes are released by many fungi; their significance in pathogenesis remains to be elucidated. *Cocidioides immitis*, for example, liberates a serine protease elastase into the medium surrounding the spherule-endospore growth form (Figure 10) (24, 25). Perhaps such an elastase could cause damage in the lungs or other tissues. Indeed, perhaps such proteolytic enzymes themselves damage enzymes of phagocytic cells, such as human granulocyte elastase, by some component of *Streptococcus pneumoniae* (26). It may be possible to develop antibody or proteinase inhibitor with a neutralizing activity against such elastase for protection.

Antibody to cryptococcal polysaccharide appears quantitatively related to improved host response to *Cryptococcus neoformans* (Figure 11); conversely, the more soluble polysaccharide found in the cerebrospinal fluid and the serum, the worse the prognosis (Table 2) (27, 28). This may be related to the antiphagocytic effect of the capsular polysaccharide. Indeed, a relationship has been shown in experimental coccidioidomycosis between excessive coccidioidal antigen and depression of cell mediated immunity (29, 30). In coccidioidomycosis in humans, an increasing titer of serum complement fixing antibody is related to a worsening of the disease (31). It is possible that such a rising titer accompanies a rising level of circulating antigen and therefore of antigen-antibody complexes affecting cell mediated immunity. In mice infected intranasally with *Histoplasma capsulatum*, antigen levels in serum and tissues continued to rise in nude (nu/nu) mice as the disease progressed to a lethal outcome, whereas in immuno-

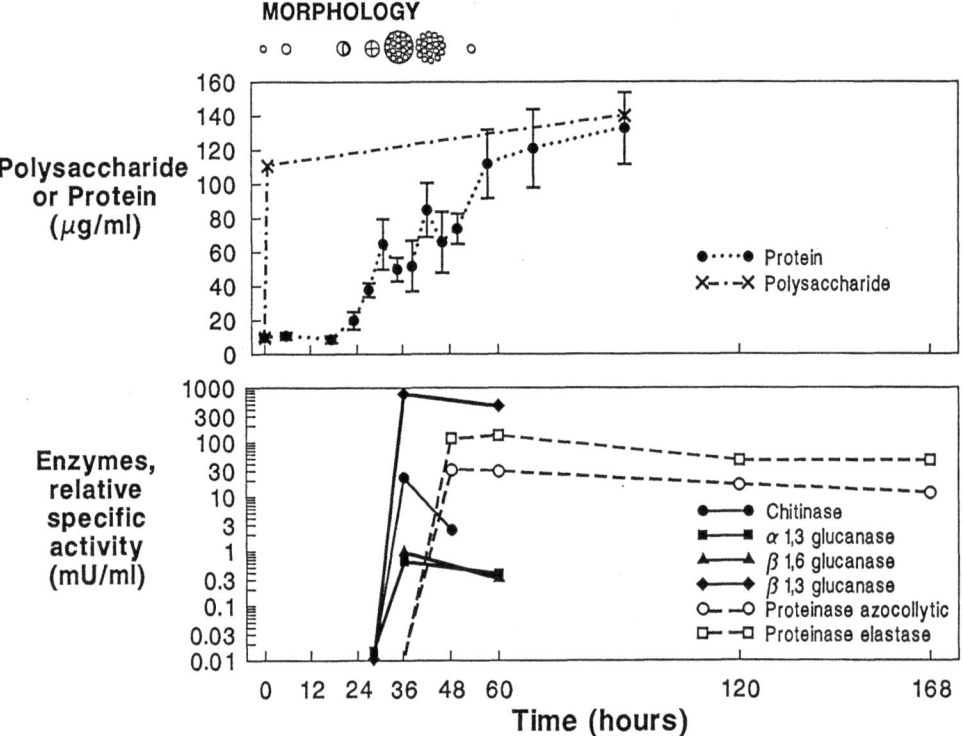

Figure 10: Enzymatic activity, including proteolytic, in culture filtrates of the spherule/endospore phase of *Coccidioides immitis* in vitro (Taken from References No. 24 and 34; R. F. Hector et al., 85th Annual Meeting of the American Society for Microbiology, Las Vegas, 1985, Abstract F61; B. L. Zimmer, D. Pappagianis, 87th Annual Meeting of the ASM, Atlanta, 1987, Abstract F48).

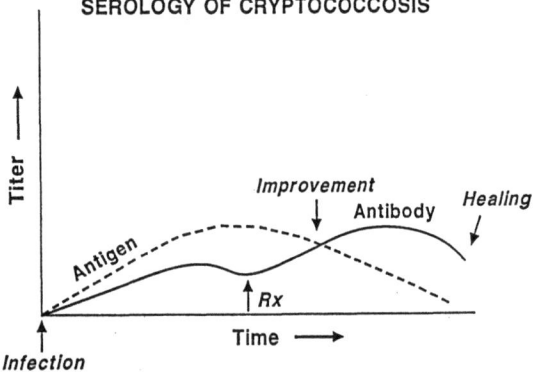

Figure 11: Diagrammatic representation of increased concentration of cryptococcal antigen in body fluids with progression of cryptococcosis, fall in concentration of antigen, and rise in titer of antibody with improvement, e.g., after chemotherapy.

Table 2: Relationship of antigen titer in body fluid with outcome of cryptococcosis. Taken from Reference No. 28.

Outcome of illness	No. of patients with:		Reciprocal of antigen titer; latex agglutination mean (range)
	Predisposing condition	Meningitis	
Fatal (n = 23)	18	22	275 (8–1200)
Non-fatal (n = 22)	14	16	39 (0–256)

logically intact (nu/+) mice an initial rise in antigen level was followed by decline of antigen and recovery of mice (32). Perhaps antigenemia in aspergillosis could lead to saturation of the lectin-like attachment sites shown on murine pulmonary alveolar macrophages to depress phagocytic activity toward aspergillus cells (33).

Whether the increase in antigen is the cause or the effect of depressed host response, plasmapheresis or immunoaffinity hemadsorption should be tested to remove cryptococcal polysaccharide, coccidioidal-antigen, antigen-antibody complexes or other fungal products from the blood to permit renewed activity of host cellular antifungal activities.

Conclusion

Several antifungal agents directed at several different targets in the fungal cell are available and have been used in one regimen or another with varying success. In at least some circumstances the antifungal activity of combinations of the antifungal agents, e.g. flucytosine and amphotericin B, has proved useful. However, other such combinations have not been adequately tested. For example, perhaps sulfonamides given in combination with amphotericin B in the treatment of paracoccidioidomycosis would permit lower and less toxic doses of amphotericin B to be given. Or, maybe multiple drug therapy directed at ergosterol (amphotericin B or azoles), at cell wall glucan (papulacandin, etc.), and at cell wall chitin (nikkomycin) would provide an even more effective, less toxic combination. Finally, perhaps immunotherapy, e.g. reduction of fungal antigenemia, combined with chemotherapy would hasten the favorable immune response of the immunocompromised host.

D. Pappagianis

Department of Medical Microbiology and Immunology, School of Medicine, University of California, Davis, California 95616, USA.

References

1. San Blas, G.: The cell wall of fungal human pathogens: its possible role in host-parasite relationship. Mycopathologia 1982, 79: 159–184.
2. Wong, B., Brauer, K. L.: Enantioselective measurement of fungal D-arabinitol in the sera of normal adults and patients with candidiasis. Journal of Clinical Microbiology 1988, 26: 1670–1674.
3. Kirkland, T. N., Fierer, J.: Cyclosporin A inhibits *Coccidioides immitis* in vitro and in vivo. Antimicrobial Agents and Chemotherapy 1983, 24: 921–924.
4. Mody, C. H., Toews, G. B., Lipscomb, M. F.: Cyclosporin A inhibits the growth of *Cryptococcus neoformans* in a murine model. Infection and Immunity 1988, 56: 7–12.
5. Ryley, J. F., Wilson, R. G., Gravestock, M. B., Poyser, J. P.: Experimental approaches to antifungal chemotherapy. Advances in Pharmacology and Chemotherapy 1981, 18: 49–176.
6. Ryley, J. F., Rathmell, W. G.: Discovery of antifungal agents: In vitro and in vivo testing. In: Trinci, A. P. J., Ryley, J. F., (ed.): Mode of action of antifungal agents. Cambridge University Press, Cambridge, 1984, p. 63–87.
7. Drouhet, E., Dupont, B.: Evolution of antifungal agents; past, present and future. Reviews of Infectious Diseases 1987, 9 (Supplement 1): S4–S14.
8. Cherniak, R.: Soluble polysaccharides of *Cryptococcus neoformans*. Current Topics in Medical Mycology 1988, 2: 40–54.
9. Wheeler, M. H., Bell, A. A.: Melanins and their importance in pathogenic fungi. Current Topics in Medical Mycology 1988, 2: 338–387.
10. Kwon-Chung, K. J., Rhodes, J. C.: Encapsulation and melaning formation as indicators of virulence in *Cryptococcus neoformans*. Infection and Immunity 1986, 51: 218–223.
11. Dixon, D. M., Polak, A., Szaniszlo, P. J.: Pathogenicity and virulence of wild-type and melanin-deficient *Wangiella dermatitidis*. Journal of Medical and Veterinary Mycology 1987, 25: 97–106.
12. Tewari, R. P., Berkhout, F. J.: Comparative pathogenicity of albino and brown types of *Histoplasma capsulatum* for mice. Journal of Infectious Diseases 1972, 125: 504–508.
13. Pappagianis, D.: Factors associated with virulence of *Coccidioides immitis*. Ph. D. dissertation, University of California, Berkeley, 1955.
14. Pappagianis, D., Kobayashi, G. S.: Approaches to the physiology of *Coccidioides immitis*. Annals of the New York Academy of Sciences 1960, 89: 109–121.
15. deSaint-Rat, L., Luteraan, P.: Action antibiotique in vitro du plumbagol, a l'egard de champignons pathogenes pour l'Homme. Compte rendus. Académie des Sciences 1947, 224: 1587–1589.
16. Endo, A., Kakiki, K., Misato, T.: Mechanism of action of the antifugal (sic) agent polyoxin D. Journal of Bacteriology 1970, 104: 189–196.
17. Hector, R. F., Pappagianis, D.: Inhibition of chitin synthesis in the cell wall of *Coccidioides immitis* by polyoxin D. Journal of Bacteriology 1983. 54: 488–498.
18. Hector, R. F., Zimmer, B. L., Pappagianis, D.: Use of chitin synthase inhibitor nikkomycin Z in murine models of coccidioidomycosis, blastomycosis and histoplasmosis (abstract 0–5). Revista Iberica de Micologia 5 1988, Supplement 1: 12.
19. Becker, J. M., Marcus, S., Tullock, J., Miller, D., Krainer, E., Khare, R. K., Naider, F.: Use of the chitin-synthesis inhibitor nikkomycin to treat disseminated candidiasis in mice. Journal of Infectious Diseases 1988, 157: 212–214.
20. Traxler, P., Tosch, W., Zak, O.: Papulacandins – synthesis and biological activity of papulacandin B derivatives. Journal of Antibiotics 1987, 40: 1146–1164.
21. Gordee, R. S., Zeckner, D. J., Ellis, L. F., Thakkar, A. L., Howard, L. C.: In vitro and in vivo anti-candida activity and toxicology of LY121019. Journal of Antibiotics 1984, 37: 1054–1065.
22. Hector, R. F., Braun, P. C.: Synergistic action of nikkomycins X and Z with papulacandin B on whole cells and regenerating protoplasts of *Candida albicans*. Antimicrobial Agents and Chemotherapy 1986, 29: 389–394.
23. Beaman, L.: Fungicidal activation of murine macrophages by recombinant gamma interferon. Infection and Immunity 1987, 55: 2951–2955.
24. Resnick, S., Pappagianis, D., McKerrow, J. H.: Proteinase production by the parasitic cycle of the pathogenic fungus *Coccidioides immitis*. Infection and Immunity 1987, 55: 2807–2815.
25. Yuan, L., Cole, G. T.: Isolation and characterization of an extra cellular proteinase of *Coccidioides immitis*. Infection and Immunity 1987, 55: 1970–1978.
26. Dal Nogare, A. R., Vial, W. C., Toews, G. B.: Bacterial species-dependent inhibition of human granulocyte elastase. American Review of Respiratory Disease 1988, 137: 907–911.
27. Gordon, M. A., Vedder, D. K.: Serologic tests in diagnosis and prognosis of cryptococcosis. Journal of the American Medical Association 1966, 197: 961–967.

28. Hay, R. J., MacKenzie, D. W. R., Campbell, C. K., Philpot, C. M.: Cryptococcosis in the United Kingdom and the Irish Republic: An analysis of 69 cases. Journal of Infection 1980, 2: 13–22.
29. Ibrahim, A. B., Pappagianis, D.: Experimental induction of energy to coccidioidin by antigens of *Coccidioides immitis*. Infection and Immunity 1973, 7: 786–794.
30. Cox, R. A., Kennell, W.: Suppression of T-lymphocyte response by *Coccidioides immitis* antigen. Infection and Immunity 1988, 56: 1424–1429.
31. Smith, C. E., Saito, M. T., Simons, S. A.: Pattern of 39,500 serologic tests in coccidioidomycosis. Journal of the American Medical Association 1956, 160: 546–552.
32. Graybill, J. R., Patino, M. M., Gomez, A. M., Ahrens, J.: Detection of histoplasmal antigens in mice undergoing experimental pulmonary histoplasmosis. American Review of Respiratory Disease 1985, 132: 752–756.
33. Kan, V. L., Bennett, J. E.: Lectin-like attachment sites on murine pulmonary alveolar macrophages bind *Aspergillus fumigatus* conidia. Journal of Infectious Diseases 1988, 158: 407–414.
34. Zimmer, B. L., Pappagianis, D.: Taxonomic and physiologic characteristics of *Coccidioides immitis*. Microbiology 1986. American Society for Microbiology, Washington, DC, 1986, p. 165–168.

Nonvaccine Immunoalteration of the Host

Passive Immunotherapy of Infectious Diseases: Lessons from the Past, Directions for the Future

J. E. Pennington

> Passive transfer of antibodies as treatment of infection is an historically important concept. Long before antimicrobial chemotherapy was available, high-titered animal sera were employed successfully to treat pneumococcal infections. Early clinical lessons regarding passive immunotherapy included the necessity for accurate serodiagnosis, the need for administration of antibody early in the course of illness and the risk of side effects. Development in recent years of human plasma-derived immunoglobulins rendered safe for high-dose intravenous infusions, and the preparation of immunoglobulins with high antibody titers directed against specific infectious agents, offer the possibility that passive immunotherapy may be combined with chemotherapy to achieve additional or synergistic therapy of infection. Furthermore, the emerging availability of anti-infective monoclonal antibodies for clinical use offers the prospect of a more plentiful supply of anti-infective immunotherapeutics which may be clinically active when used in extremely small protein doses.

For several decades, discussions about therapy of infections have focused primarily upon antibiotics and antimicrobial chemotherapy. In this paper, a considerably older therapeutic strategy will be addressed, that of immunotherapy. The hypothesis to be examined is that recent advances in the methodology of preparation of antibodies against infectious agents will provide new immunotherapeutic agents useful for the treatment of infectious diseases. For purposes of the present discussion, the term 'immunotherapy' will refer exclusively to passive transfer of antibody-containing preparations. Admittedly, future discussions of this subject might include the use of cytokines as well.

Lessons from the Past

An extensive literature documents the usefulness of immunotherapy of infections in the pre-antibiotic era. Rather than review this experience in detail, several useful clinical lessons learned during these early trials will be highlighted.

In 1930, Maxwell Finland reported the clinical experience of using equine serum to treat pneumococcal pneumonia from 1919 through 1929 at Boston City Hospital (1). Several modifications of the sera were made during this period, which resulted in preparations containing more concentrated antibodies. Acute febrile reactions were observed with some of the early lots employed, and serum sickness occurred in up to 73% of the survivors receiving early lots. Later use of Felton's antibody preparation reduced the frequency of serum sickness to 12%. Despite these adverse reactions, the impression was that serum therapy resulted in improved survival rates in patients with pneumonia. However, efficacy of immunotherapy was dependent upon two conditions. Firstly, an accurate microbiologic diagnosis, including serotyping, was necessary. Secondly, serum therapy had to be administered early in the course of infection (Table 1). Obviously, these two conditions might have resulted in antagonistic activities as witnessed by numerous "therapeutic failures" which later could be ascribed to serotyping errors during the rush of events occurring immediately after admission to the hospital. All in all, Finland's report highlights several clinical rules of immunotherapy which remain valid and useful guides today (Table 2).

The following decade was one of refinement of the principles and practice of immunotherapy. For example, considerable attention was given to the standardization of serum preparations for their antibody content; along with this came dose range finding and refinement of the concepts of 'adequate dose' and 'optimal dose' of serum. Using a murine model of pneumococcal peritonitis, Goodner and Miller demonstrated that too little, and importantly, too much serum therapy could be given (2). Underdosing with antibodies was not surprising or difficult to under-

---

Clinical Research Department, Cutter Laboratories, 4th and Parker Streets, P.O. Box 1986, Berkeley, California 94701, and Department of Medicine, University of California, San Francisco, California 94143, USA.

Table 1: Percent mortality from Type I pneumococcal pneumonia.

	All cases	Admitted after ≤ 3 days of illness	Admitted after ≥ 3 days of illness
Control patients (n = 70)	31.4	37.5	29.6
Treated patients (n = 80)	21.3	9.5	34.2

Adapted from Finland (reference 1).

Table 2: Early lessons from pneumococcal serum therapy trials.

1. Immunotherapy can reduce mortality and morbidity of infection.
2. Timing of therapy is critical.
3. Early and specific diagnosis is necessary.
4. Side effects (sometimes serious) may occur.

stand. However, the reduced survivals associated with escalating doses above a certain amount deserved careful attention. The mechanism for this phenomenon, called "prozoning" by the authors, was not clearly defined. However, it was speculated that harmful contaminants in the antibody preparation could account for the prozoning effect. In any event, an optimal dose concept was established and reduced efficacy at higher doses of antibodies remains a concern today. Whether this effect is due to blockage of Fc receptors on white cells by immunoglobulins, or simply to in vivo physical interactions of IgG molecules in high concentrations is unknown, but remains under investigation (3, 4).

Clinical trials also established a dose response in humans for anti-pneumococcal immunotherapy. In one report, the adequate dosage of serum was related not only to amount given, but also to the timing of therapy and the severity of infection (5). For example, based upon clinical observations, it was determined that in early (less than five days of illness) and uncomplicated (sterile blood culture, single lobe involvement) pneumococcal pneumonia, 75,000 units of serum was adequate. For increasingly severe cases, 150,000 units were required. For cases diagnosed after five days of illness, serum therapy was not felt to offer convincing benefit (5).

By the beginning of the 1940s, it was clear that the recently developed antibiotics (penicillin, streptomycin) and other antimicrobial agents (sulfonamides) were more effective and safer than serum in the treatment of bacterial infections. It is not surprising that a revolutionary new method for separating and concentrating gamma globulin from human plasma (6) developed by E. J. Cohn and co-workers at Harvard Medical School, was not widely appreciated for its therapeutic implications. This plasma-derived gamma globulin rich fraction was labeled immune serum globulin (ISG). While this antibody-rich material clearly offered advantages over the older serum preparations, there were limitations to its use as well (Table 3).

As noted in the early trials of serum therapy, the effectiveness of antibody therapy was dose-dependent. Unfortunately, it was found that ISG was poorly tolerated if given by intravenous infusion, presumably due to aggregation of IgG molecules and activation of the complement system (7). ISG must, therefore, be given by intramuscular injection. These injections are generally painful and the size of the dose is limited by the muscle mass (and pain threshold) of the recipient. In any event, rarely can more than 150 mg/kg of ISG be given in a single injection. Thus, while serum antibodies were concentrated several-fold by Cohn's fractionation procedure, the antibody dose that could be administered with ISG was still quite limited. In practice, this dose limitation for ISG has not precluded its usefulness for prophylaxis of infectious disease in immunodeficient patients, but has clearly limited its role in therapy of established infections.

Nevertheless, it was not long before investigators began to explore the important hypothesis that antibody therapy plus antibiotic therapy might result in additive or even synergistic efficacy in treating infections. Numerous animal models of infection were employed to demonstrate this effect (8). However, clinical trials of such combined therapy produced more modest results. For example, Waisbren treated 46 patients with infections (usually chronic) refractory to antibiotics alone by adding ISG to the drug regimen (9). Benefit resulting from the addition of ISG was observed in only six patients. Naturally, the dose of ISG was limited due to the intramuscular route of administration.

Directions for the Future

In recent years, there have been two major technological advances in the preparation of antibody-containing solutions which reestablish the viability of immu-

Table 3: Immune Serum Globulin.

Advantages	Disadvantages
"Pure" globulin	No IgM
Concentrated antibodies	Anaphylaxis (IV)
Easy to handle and store	

notherapy as a therapeutic modality in treating infections: the rendering of human gamma globulin safe for intravenous infusion, and the development of monoclonal antibodies. As early as 1962, Barandun and co-workers offered suggestions for procedures to modify immunoglobulin preparations to prevent aggregation and thus reduce adverse effects when given intravenously (7). Importantly, it was recognized that harsh chemical or enzymatic treatment of IgG may damage the molecule and reduce or abolish its natural function (7, 10). A number of methods have now been developed for preparing gamma globulin for intravenous infusion (Table 4) (11).

The maximal dosage of intravenous immunoglobulins (IGIV) is not limited by pain or other acute adverse reactions (with rare exception). Rather, dosage is limited by theoretical concerns, such as blockage of Fc receptors of phagocytic cells in septic patients, and practical issues, such as the high cost of IGIV. Currently, it is not recommended that dosages of IGIV exceed 500 mg/kg per infusion in the septic patient. In order to maximize the amount of antibody delivered per dosage, a number of hyperimmune IGIV preparations have recently been developed, and several of these are currently under investigation in clinical trials. Table 5 provides a list of such preparations known to the author to be in trial at this time. In all cases, the study designs are either open, in which all patients receive both an antimicrobial agent plus the IGIV, or controlled, in which patients are randomized to receive standard antimicrobial therapy alone versus in combination with IGIV.

The author has recently conducted experiments in a guinea pig model of acute *Pseudomonas aeruginosa* pneumonia which illustrate the rationale and application of hyperimmune IGIV in treatment of infection (12–14). These studies utilized a hyperimmune globulin enriched in antibodies against the most common serotypes of *Pseudomonas aeruginosa*. High-titered human plasma was identified by serologic screening of large numbers of plasma donors (15). For study, guinea pigs were infected by intratracheal instillation of lethal-sized bacterial inocula. Animals were treated two hours later by intravenous infusion of globulin (500 mg/kg). Initial experiments documented improved survival for globulin recipients (Figure 1). Subsequent experiments revealed superior efficacy of the hyperimmune globulin as compared to a conventional (non-hyperimmune) IGIV preparation (Figure 2). Importantly, the addition of

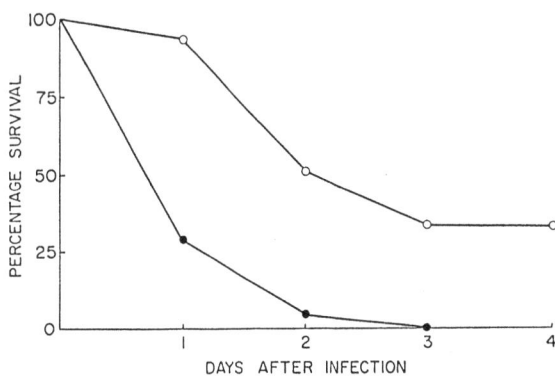

Figure 1: Survival from *Pseudomonas aeruginosa* pneumonia (strain 220, type 1) for guinea pigs treated 2 h after infection with a single dose of 5 % hyperimmune Pseudomonas immunoglobulin G (500 mg/kg) (n = 36) (○), or 5 % albumin (n = 33) (●). Cumulative survivals were greater among the globulin-treated group (P < .001).

Table 4: Methods to render immunoglobulin safe for intravenous infusion.

Reduction and alkylation
Enzyme treatment (pepsin)
Acidification (pH 4.25)
DEAE column chromatography

Table 5: Intravenous hyperimmune immunoglobulin preparations currently in clinical trials for infectious diseases.

Pseudomonas aeruginosa	Cytomegalovirus
Cutter	Cutter
Armour	Biotest
Sandoz	J5 Anti-endotoxin
Group B Streptococcus	Sandoz
Sandoz	Re Anti-endotoxin
Pneumococcal/*Haemophilus influenzae*	Hyland
Hyland	
Biotest	

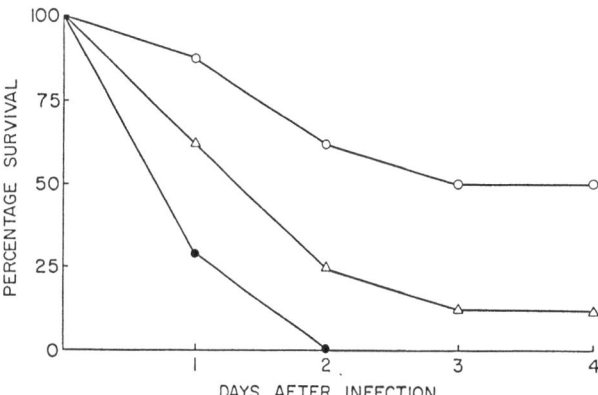

Figure 2: Survival from *Pseudomonas aeruginosa* pneumonia (strain 220) for guinea pigs treated 2 h after infection with hyperimmune Pseudomonas globulin (n = 16) (○), nonhyperimmune immunoglobulin (n = 16) (△), or albumin (n = 16) (●). Survivals were greater for treatment with hyperimmune globulin than with nonhyperimmune globulin (*P* = .06).

an antibiotic plus the antibody preparation offered increased therapeutic efficacy as compared to either agent alone (Figure 3). Early clinical trials with this preparation have confirmed these encouraging observations (16). Clearly, the development of hyperimmune IGIV preparations which can be given in high dosage offers an exciting new opportunity for treatment of serious infections.

While the development of high-titered polyclonal antibody preparations from human plasma may open a new era in immunotherapy of infection, these preparations clearly have limitations of their own (Table 6). One of the most important drawbacks in the use of plasma-derived polyclonal antibodies is the necessity to administer unneeded antibody protein along with the desired antibody. The net result is that rather large amounts of antibody protein must be administered in order to achieve therapeutic effects. Monoclonal antibodies may circumvent this dilemma.

Monoclonal antibodies are traditionally produced by fusing sensitized murine B lymphocytes with myeloma cells, thus resulting in a 'hybridoma' cell line. These hybridomas provide a continous source of a monoclonal antibody and clones can be selected by serologic and functional screening for those producing the most desirable antibody products (e.g. acceptable binding coefficient, opsonic or neutralizing activity, etc.). Experimental studies in animal models suggest that as long as one has selected an acceptably active antibody product, monoclonal antibodies can provide therapeutic efficacy in treating infections. Furthermore, since only the desired antibody is administered, therapeutic efficacy is achieved using protein dosages which are a fraction of those needed with polyclonal antibodies. The data displayed in Table 7 were obtained in the previously described guinea pig model of *Pseudomonas aeruginosa* pneumonia and clearly illustrate this phenomenon. Thus, it is likely that in the near future, clinical trials of immunotherapy of infection will be conducted using monoclonal rather than polyclonal antibodies.

Monoclonal antibodies are not without their own concern, however. For example, murine monoclonal antibodies obviously contain foreign protein and can sensitize human recipients. Development of human monoclonal antibodies with in vitro and in vivo activity against infectious agents has been described (R.F. Hector et al., 27th Interscience Conference on Antimicrobial Agents and Chemotherapy, New York, 1987, Abstract No. 547.) and may circumvent these problems with murine protein. However, Epstein-Barr viral transformation of human B lymphocyts is a commonly used technique in the production of

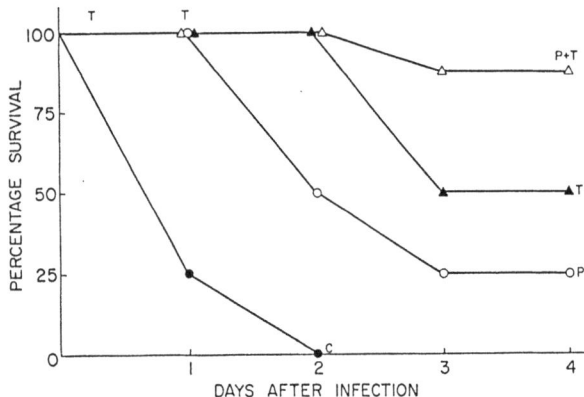

Figure 3: Survival from *Pseudomonas aeruginosa* pneumonia for guinea pigs treated 2 h after infection with albumin (n = 16) (C), hyperimmune Pseudomonas globulin alone (n = 16) (P), or treated 2 h and 24 h after infections with tobramycin, 1.7 mg/kg/injection (n = 16) (T), or with a combination of hyperimmune globulin plus tobramycin, as above (n = 16) (P + T). Survivals in P + T group greater than in P alone ($P = .01$) or T alone ($P = .06$) groups.

Table 6: Drawbacks of polyclonal immunoglobulin therapy.

1. High dosage required
2. Safety of plasma-derived product
3. Product standardization
4. Product availability

Table 7: Dose-dependent antibody-mediated protection from Type 1 *Pseudomonas aeruginosa* pneumonia.

Hyperimmune globulin			Monoclonal antibody (IT-1)		
Dose (mg/kg)	Serum concentration antibody (μg/ml)[a]	Survival[b] (%)	Dose (mg/kg)	Serum concentration antibody (μg/ml)[a]	Survival[c] (%)
100	< 1.3	0	1.0	1.77	0
250	1.38	0	2.5	4.65	50
500	2.69	33	5.0	6.15	75
–	–	–	20.0	14.60	100

[a] One hour after infusions (anti IT-1).
[b] 12 per group.
[c] 6 per group.

human monoclonal antibodies, and the presence of Epstein-Barr virus genome in these preparations must be considered. Furthermore, humans cannot be as readily immunized with the desired antigen as can mice.

Recent development of chimeric antibodies, produced by cell lines transfected with immunoglobulin genome from both murine and human sources, may alleviate some of these difficulties (17). In this technique, genome encoding for the variable region (Fab) of the immunoglobulin molecule is taken from mice immunized with the desired epitope. This genome is then combined with human genome encoding for the constant region (Fc) of the immunoglobulin molecule. The expression vector then produces an immunoglobulin molecule which is only partially murine, thus reducing the potential for sensitization to foreign protein. Yet another dilemma pertaining to monoclonal antibodies of any source is the potential for anti-idiotypic antibody formation. Anti-id antibodies may neutralize the activity of the monoclonal if used in a prolonged fashion.

At this point, the relative costs, safety and efficacy of polyclonal versus monoclonal antibody preparations for treatment of infection are not well defined. It is safe to say, however, that methods for rapid delivery of therapeutic amounts of human antibodies against a variety of infectious agents are now available.

Reference

1. Finland, M.: The serum treatment of lobar pneumonia. New England Journal of Medicine 1930, 202: 1244–1247.
2. Goodner, K., Miller, D. K.: The protective action of type I antipneumococcus serum in mice: II. The course of the infectious process. Journal of Experimental Medicine 1935, 62: 375–391.
3. Cross, A. S., Zollinger, W., Mandrell, R., Gemski, P., Sadoff, J.: Evaluation of immunotherapeutic approaches for the potential treatment of infections caused by K1-positive Escherichia coli. Journal of Infectious Diseases 1983, 147: 68–76.
4. Kurlander, R. J., Hall, J.: Comparison of intravenous gamma globulin and a monoclonal anti-Fc receptor antibody as inhibitors of immune clearance in vivo in mice. Journal of Clinical Investigation 1986, 77: 2010–2018.
5. Finland, M.: Adequate dosage in the specific serum treatment of pneumococcus type I pneumonia. American Journal of Medical Science 1936, 192: 849–864.
6. Cohn, E. J., Oncley, J. L., Strong, L. E., Hughes, W. L., Armstrong, S. H.: Chemical, clinical and immunological studies on the products of human plasma fractionation. I. The characterization of protein fractions of human plasma. Journal of Clinical Investigation 1944, 23: 417–432.
7. Barandun, S., Kistler, P., Jeunet, F.: Intravenous administration of human gammaglobulin, Vox Sanguinis 1962, 7: 157–174.
8. Fisher, M. W.: Synergism between human gamma globulin and chloramphenicol in the treatment of bacterial infections. Antibiotics & Chemotherapy 1957, 7: 315–320.
9. Waisbren, B. A.: The treatment of bacterial infections with the combination of antibiotics and gamma globulin. Antibiotics & Chemotherapy 1957, 7: 322–333.
10. Lundblad, J. L., Londeree, N., Mitra, G.: Characterization of various intravenous immunoglobulin preparations. Journal of Infection 1987, 15: Supplement 1, 3–12.
11. Alving, B. M., Finlayson, J.S.: Table of immunoglobulin preparations. In: Alving, B. M., Finlayson, J. S. (ed.): Immunoglobulins: characteristics and uses of intravenous preparations. U.S. Department of Health and Human Service, Food & Drug Administration, Washington D.C., DHHS Publication No. (FDA)-80-9005; 1980: 234.
12. Pennington, J. E., Pier, G. B., Small, G.J.: Efficacy of intravenous immune globulin for treatment of experimental Pseudomonas aeruginosa pneumonia. Journal of Critical Care 1986, 1: 4–10.
13. Pennington, J. E., Small, G. J., Lostrom, M. E., Pier, G. B.: Polyclonal and monoclonal antibody therapy for experimental Pseudomonas aeruginosa pneumonia. Infection and Immunity 1986, 54: 239–244.
14. Pennington, J. E., Small, G. J.: Passive immune therapy of experimental Pseudomonas aeruginosa pneumonia in the neutropenic host. Journal of Infectious Diseases 1987, 155: 973–978.
15. Collins, M. S., Roby, R. E.: Protective activity of an intravenous immune globulin (human) enriched in antibody against lipopolysaccharide antigens of Pseudomonas aeruginosa. American Journal of Medicine 1984, 76 (3A): 168–174.
16. Class, I., Junginger, W., Kloss, Th.: Einsatz von Pseudomonasimmunglobulin bei beatmeten patienten einer interdisziplinaren chirurgischen intensivstation. Infection 1987, Supplement 2, 15: S67–S70.
17. Morrison, S. L., Johnson, M. J., Herzenberg, L. A., Oi, V. T.: Chimeric human antibody molecules: Mouse antigen-binding domains with human constant region domains. Proceedings of the National Academy of Science USA 1984, 81: 6851–6855.

T-Cell Mediated Immunopathology in Viral Infections

R. M. Zinkernagel

> Virus-specific cytotoxic T cells are crucially involved in host recovery from primary infection. Due to the immunological destruction of infected host cells, immunopathological damage may determine the severity of disease caused by poorly cytopathic or non-cytopathic viruses. Some forms of virally induced hepatitis or of acquired immunodeficiency may be mediated by immunopathologically active virus-specific T cells.

Major transplantation antigens play a crucial role in lymphocyte interactions among themselves as well as with other somatic cells (1–4). Their biological function was first indicated by the finding that susceptibility to certain diseases is linked, albeit weakly, to the major transplantation antigens coded by the major histocompatibility gene complex (MHC; HLA in humans, H-2 in mice) (5).

The most significant (relative risk, > 5) degrees of susceptibility or resistance linked to certain HLA antigens have been found for such diseases as ankylosing spondylitis, Reiter's disease, narcolepsy, Yersinia arthritis, salmonella arthritis, psoriatic arthritis, acute anterior uveitis, psoriasis vulgaris, and dermatitis herpetiformis. Although this list is incomplete, most diseases have salient features regarded as characteristically autoimmune or autoaggressive, which may indicate that viral or other intracellular infections are often the instigators of diseases for which susceptibility is linked to the MHC.

In higher vertebrates, the function of the immune system is to maintain homeostasis. The two main branches of the system, cellular and humoral immunity, very efficiently defend the host against acute cytopathic infectious agents. The main targets of T cells are intracellular agents, while those of antibodies are primarily extracellular ones (6, 7). However, this immune defense is not equally efficient against all viruses and bacteria, and many other pathogens such as protozoa, metazoa, or tumor cells may escape immune attack since they are more or less out of the reach of efficient immune surveillance (6, 7).

T-cell immunity is most efficient against acute intracellular agents such as cytopathic viruses. T-cell activity is easily measurable in a classical ^{51}Cr-release cytotoxicity assay in vitro (4). T-cell mediated lysis of virus-infected target cells is virus specific, since only target cells infected with the proper virus are lysed, but, lysis of virus-infected cells depends additionally upon a match of the classical transplantation antigens between T cells and target cells (8, 4). Many experiments over the past 12 years have documented the following general rules governing lymphocyte-lymphocyte and lymphocyte-somatic cell interactions. T-cells recognize self-transplantation antigens together with foreign antigenic determinants exclusively on cell surfaces; T-cell specificity for self-transplantation antigens a) is specific for polymorphic determinants b) is targeted during differentiation in the thymus (9, 10); c) determines the effector function of T cells; cytotoxic T cells recognize class I, i.e. the classical transplantation antigens, whereas differentiation promoting T cells (helper or DTH T cells) are specific for class II (4); d) regulates T-cell responsiveness, i.e. the quality and quantity of cytotoxic T-cell response is regulated by class I, that of differentiation-promoting T cells by class II major histocompatibility gene products (11–13) e) reflects the binding capacity of MHC molecules (14) to antigenic fragments resulting from processing of antigen originating from within (via class I transplantation antigens) cells or from without (via phagocytosis in phagolysosomes and presentation by class II transplantation antigens) (15–19). The quality of the fragment binding capacity of MHC antigens directly determines immune responsiveness. Accordingly, vertebrate hosts with MHC-alleles that cannot bind particular antigenic fragments will not be able to respond to that antigen. It is probable that tolerance to self-peptides and T-cell receptor defects may also influence non-responsiveness, but the manner in which the T-cell receptor(s) recognize self-MHC products plus fragments or fragments alone is still unclear. It has recently become apparent that immunological tolerance to self antigens (i.e. absence of T-cell reactivity to normal self-antigens) is also MHC-restricted (20).

There are some consequences of practical medical importance derived from the fact that T cells recognize

Institut für Pathologie, Universitäts-Spital Zürich, Sternwartstraße 2, 8091 Zürich, Switzerland.

antigen fragments only on transplantation antigens. Cells not expressing transplantation antigens, irrespective of whether they are infected or modified (such as tumor cells), escape immune surveillance (21–24). MHC-disease associations may be explained by differential antigen binding to transplantation antigens (11, 12, 15, 17–19). MHC-polymorphism, i. e. the frequent variability of transplantation antigens between individual humans or mice, may guarantee that effective immune responses are optimally distributed in a species (12); as a side effect it causes the transplantation reaction. The evidence summarized suggests that both transplantation reactions and antiviral cytotoxic T-cell reactivity may reflect identical recognition mechanisms (12, 17).

Role of Cytotoxic T Cells

Virus-specific cytotoxic T cells dominate early cellular immune responses against viruses and seem to be potently protective (4, 25). The physiological role of cytolytic T cells (26, 27) may be questioned by asking why T cells lyse infected cells, and why they mediate cell and tissue destruction to combat intracellular infectious agents. There is evidence that cytotoxic T cells destroy virus-infected cells before viral progeny are assembled (25), thus eliminating the virus during the eclipse phase of virus replication. In the case of cytophatic viruses, virus elimination via immunological host cell destruction is an efficient way to prevent virus spread as well as the resulting more extensive virus-mediated cell and tissue damage. In the case of non-cytopathic viruses, however, this immunological defense mechansm becomes less efficient, because host cells are destroyed not by virus but only be the T-cell immune response; because T cells apparently cannot distinguish cytopathic from non-cytopathic viruses in infections caused by these viruses, immune-mediated cell and tissue damage results in immunopathology, (4, 6, 7, 28–31).

Damage Caused by T cell-Mediated Immunoprotection

Examples of infections with non-cytopathic viruses are lymphocytic choriomeningitis (LCM) in mice (29, 30) and hepatitis B in humans (32). Lymphocytic choriomeningitis disease in mice develops only in immunocompetent animals after intracerebral injection of LCM virus. Mice lacking T cells or those immunosuppressed by irradiation or cytostatic drugs do not develop inflammatory reactions or LCM disease, but they fail to eliminate the virus and as a result become LCMV-carriers (28–30). LCM disease has been carefully analyzed and has been clearly shown to be T cell-mediated (33). Lethal LCM disease apparently depends upon effector T cells being preferentially selected by the acutely infected leptomeninges or liver cells (31). The resulting LCMV-induced hepatitis in mice has been monitored histologically and by the determination of changes in serum levels of aminotranferases and alkaline phosphatase. The kinetics of histological disease manifestations, increases of liver enzyme levels in the serum, and cytotoxic T-cell activities in livers and spleens all correlated and were dependent upon several parameters such as the LCMV-isolate, the virus dose and route of infection, and the general genetic background of the murine host. Of the mouse strains tested, Swiss mice and A-strain mice were more susceptible than C57BL or CBA mice; BALB/c and DBA/2 mice were least susceptible. The degree of immunocompetence of the murine host is also important in that T-cell deficient nu/nu mice never developed hepatitis, whereas nu/+ or +/+ mice always did. In addition, local cytotoxic T cell activity played a role in mouse hepatitis; mononuclear cells isolated from livers during the period of overt hepatitis were two to five times more active than equal numbers of spleen cells.

Thus, LCMV-induced hepatitis in mice is an immunopathologically mediated disease caused by T-cell mediated destruction of infected liver cells. Overall, this disease parallels many aspects of acute viral hepatitis in humans, which is caused by hepatitis B virus.

In both LCMV hepatitis and hepatitis B, disease depends upon the balance between the rate of virus spread and the immune response. An efficient T-cell mediated immune response leads to rapid elimination of the virus, limited cell and tissue damage, and therefore limited disease. The absence of an immune response results in unchecked growth of virus, leading to a virus-carrier state. Slow and low immune responsiveness allows extensive spread of virus with chronic T-cell mediated tissue destruction, a classical situation of immunopathological conflict.

Since major transplantation antigens generally bind foreign antigen fragments accurately and thus determine whether a T-cell response is efficiently induced, they may drastically influence the balance between virus and immune mediated tissue damage. Among many other variables characteristic for either the virus or the host, severity of disease has been shown to be determined by major transplantation antigens in both hepatitis B virus infections in humans (5) and in LCMV infections in mice (34).

Virus-Triggerd Acquired Immune Suppression

It had been known for some time that LCMV causes immunosuppresion in mice (6, 29, 30). When re-evaluating this in various mouse strains using varying LCMV-isolates, we found that an LCMV infection in mice suppressed their capacity to mount an IgM or IgG response to vesicular stomatitis virus (VSV). It also rendered them considerably more susceptible to this virus, which does not measurably replicate in adult mice and is usually non-pathogenic for mice if infected subcutaneously or intravenously.

The extent of immune suppression by LCMV depended upon the following parameters: 1) Different virus isolates had different effects on immune response. LCMV-WE and some other LCMV isolates such as LCMV-AGG or LCMV-DOC caused immunosuppression, whereas LCMV-ARM did so only rarely. 2) Mouse strains differed considerably with respect to susceptibility to this immunosuppression; the MHC played some role, still poorly defined, but non-MHC genes also had a major influence. 3) The kinetics of induction of the described impairment of mice to respond to a subsequent virus infection with T-cell independent IgM and/or strictly T-cell dependent IgG paralleled that usually characteristic for the induction of an anti-LCMV T-cell response, starting on day 6 after LCMV infection and reaching maximum levels around day 8–10. (4) The inability to mount an IgM and/or IgG anti-VSV response after LCMV infection of mice was transient or of rather long duration (up to 4–5 months, the longest period measured to date), again dependent upon the LCMV-isolate and the inoculum used and on the mouse strain which was infected.

The following experimental results (35) suggest that the antiviral T-cell response, simular to the response to LCMV-hepatitis, is responsible for immunosuppression. When connataly infected LCMV-carrier mice were evaluated with respect to their immune responsiveness, they were found to mount anti-VSV IgM and IgG responses comparable to normal control mice. T-cell deprived nude mice infected with LCMV also had normal IgM responses. This indicates that LCMV alone is not immunosuppressive and that the observed immune suppression is not caused by the action of interferons on VSV. In contrast, LCMV-infected nude mice inoculated with LCMV immune cytotoxic T cells exhibited suppressed antibody responses. Also, while LCMV-infected mice failed to exhibit an antibody response, similarly infected mice treated with anti-CD8 antisera (anti-Lyt 2) some days before initiation of the VSV infection mounted normal IgM and IgG responses (35).

These results are compatible with the view that antiviral cytotoxic T cells are responsible for immune suppression in this model infection. Accordingly, LCMV may infect lymphocytes and antigen-bearing cells, which are involved in antibody responses; these infected cells are then in turn destroyed by anti-LCMV specific cytotoxic T cells.

Although LCMV infection in mice may differ from HIV-1 infections in humans with respect to the kinetics of induction of immunodeficiency, the tropisms of the virus, etc., it nevertheless exhibits many of the characteristics which make obvious a translation of these findings to AIDS in humans: for example, tropism for lymphohemopoietic cells, translation of these findings to AIDS in humans: for example, tropism for lymphohemopoietic cells, immunosuppression, difficulties in inducing appreciable in vivo protective neutralizing antibodies, the capacity to induce wasting disease in neonatal or adult mice, and the ability to induce a virus carrier state in immunoincompetent fetuses (by vertical transmission from the mother) or in newborns as well as in immunocompetent adults (29, 30). The antiviral T cell-response destroys part of the immune system because it is virus-infected, such a pathogenetic mechanism may also apply to HIV-1 infection in humans, causing such severe manifestations as AIDS. It is not the HIV-1 infection of T cells, antigen-bearing cells or macrophages that causes cell lysis, but rather the anti-HIV cytotoxic T cells which destroy infected host lymphocytes (36). The result is that the same cells which are essential for mounting an immune response are destroyed because they are infected. The consequences of this proposal may be that under carefully selected conditions, anti-CD8 antibodies or a possibly more selective treatment to eliminate anti-HIV specific cytotoxic T cells completely may be used to ameliorate AIDS.

Conclusion

The process of T-cell restriction and recognition is now nearly understood with regard to the structure of transplantation antigens and the T-cell receptor, with a few details of how the T-cell receptor recognizes antigen fragments in the context of transplantation antigens remaining to be defined. It has become apparent that immune protection by T cells and T-cell mediated immunopathology are two sides of the same medal – it is a question of balance between parasite and host factors that will determine the T-cell mediated pathophysiology of infectious disease. The reviewed evidence suggests that infectious agents may be responsible for many if not most HLA-associated and immunopathologically mediated diseases. Possibly, even arteriosclerosis, rheumatoid arthritis and other chronic diseases now considered to be degenerative diseases may also be triggered by infectious agents and maintained by an unbalanced immune response.

References

1. Davis, M. M., Chien, Y., Gascoigne, N. R. J., Hedrick, S. M.: A murine T cell receptor gene complex: isolation, structure and rearrangement. Immunological Review 1984, 81: 235–258.
2. Katz, D. H., Hamaoka, T., Dorf, M. E., Maurer, P. H., Benacerraf, B.: Cell interactions between histoincompatible T and B lymphocytes. IV. Involvement of the immune response (Ir) gene in the control of lymphocyte interactions in responses controlled by the gene. Journal of Experimental Medicine 1973. 138: 734–739.
3. Marrack, P., Kappler, J.: The T cell receptor. Science 1987, 238: 1073–1079.
4. Zinkernagel, R. M., Doherty, P. C.: MHC-restricted cytotoxic T cells: studies on the biological role of polymorphic major transplantation antigens determining T cell restriction-specificity, function and responsiveness. Advances in Immunolgy 1979, 27: 52–142.
5. Dausset, J., Svejgaard, A.: HLA and disease. Munksgaard, Copenhagen, 1977, p. 9–316.
6. Mims, C. A.: Pathogenesis of infectious disease. Academic Press, London, 1972, p. 1–160.
7. Zinkernagel, R. M., Hengartner, H., Stitz, L.: On the role of viruses in the evolution of immune responses. British Medicine Bulletin 1985, 41: 92–97.
8. Zinkernagel, R. M., Doherty, P. C.: Restriction of in vitro T cell mediated cytotoxicity in lymphocytic choriomeningitis within a syngeneic or semiallogeneic system. Nature 1974, 248: 701–702.
9. Bevan, M. J., Fink, P. J.: The influence of thymus H-2 antigens on the specificity of maturing killer and helper cells. Immunological Review 1978, 42: 4–19.
10. Zinkernagel, R. M., Callahan, G. N., Althage, A., Cooper, S., Streilein, J. W., Klein, J. J.: The lymphoreticular system in triggering virus-plus-self-specific cytotoxic T cells: evidence for T help. Journal of Experimental Medicine 1978, 147: 897–911.
11. Benacerraf, B., McDevitt, H. O.: Histocompatibility-linked immune response genes. Science 1972, 175: 273–279.
12. Doherty, P. C., Zinkernagel, R. M.: A biological role for the major histocompatibility antigens. Lancet 1975, 28: 1406–1409.
13. Zinkernagel, R. M., Althage, A., Cooper, S., Kreeb, G., Klein, P. A., Sefton, B., Flaherty, L., Stimpfling, J., Shreffler, D., Klein, J.: Ir genes in H-2 regulate generation of anti-viral cytotoxic T cells. mapping to K or D and dominance of unresponsiveness. Journal of Experimental Medicine 1978, 148: 592–606.
14. Bjorkman, P. J., Saper, M. A., Samraoui, B., Bennett, W. S., Strominger, J. L., Wiley, D. C.: The foreign antigen binding site and T cell recognition regions of class I histocompatibility antigens. Nature 1987, 329: 512–518.
15. Buus, S., Sette, A., Colon, S. M., Miles, C., Grey, H. M.: The relation between major histocompatibility complex (MHC) restriction and the capacity of Ia to bind immunogenic peptides. Science 1987, 235: 1353–1358.
16. Germain, R. N.: The ins and outs of antigen processing and presentation. Nature 1986, 322: 687–689.
17. Guillet, J. G., Lai, M.-Z., Briner, Th. J., Buus, S., Sette, A., Grey, H. M., Smith, J. A., Gefter, M. L.: Immunological self, nonself discrimination. Science 1987, 235: 865–870.
18. Kourilsky, P., Claverie, J.-M.: The peptidic self model: a hypothesis on the molecular nature of the immunological self. Annuals of the Institute Pasteur, Section C. Immunology 1986, 137D: 3–21.
19. Townsend, A. R. M., Rothbard, J., Gotch, F. M., Bahadur, G., Wraith, D., McMichael, A. J.: The epitopes of influenza nucleoprotein recognized by cytotoxic T lymphocytes can be defined with short synthetic peptides. Cell 1986, 44: 959–968.
20. Kappler. J. W., Staerz, U. D., White, J., Marrack, P.: Self tolerance eliminates T cells specific for Mls-modified products of the major histocompatibility complex. Nature 1988, 332: 35–40.
21. Bernards, R., Schrier, P. I., Houweling, A., Bos, J. L., van der Eb, A. J.: Tumorigenicity of cells transformed by adenovirus type 12 by evasion of T cell immunity. Nature 1983, 305: 776–781.
22. Burgert, H. G., Maryanski, J. L., Kvist, S.: E3/19K protein of adenovirus type 2 inhibits lysis of cytolytic T lymphocytes by blocking cell-surface expression of histocompatibility class I antigens. Proceedings of the National Academy of Sciences of the USA 1987, 84: 1356–1360.
23. Festenstein, H., Garrido, F.: MHC antigens and malignancy. Nature 1986, 322: 502–503.
24. Goodenow, R. S., Bogel, J. M., Linsk, R. L.: Histocompatibility antigens on murine tumors. Science 1985, 230: 777–783.
25. Zinkernagel, R. M., Althage, A.: Antiviral protection by virus-immune cytotoxic T cells: infected target cells are lysed before infectious virus progeny is assembled. Journal of Experimental Medicine 1977, 145: 644–651.
26. Cerottini, J. C., Brunner, K. T.: Cell-mediated cytotoxicity, allograft rejection and tumor immunity. Advances in Immunology 1974, 18: 67–132.
27. Podack, E. R., Lowrey, D. M., Lichtenhelf, M., Olsen, K. J., Aebischer, T., Binder, D., Rupp, F., Hengartner, H.: Structure, function and expression of murine and human Perforin 1 (P1). Immunological Reviews 1988, (in press).
28. Doherty, P. C., Zinkernagel, R. M.: T cell-mediated immunopathology in viral infection. Transplantation Reviews 1974, 19: 89–120.
29. Hotchin, J.: Persistent and slow virus infections. In: Monographs in virology. Karger, Basel, 1971, Volume 3, p. 1–211.
30. Lehmann-Grube, F.: Lymphocytic choriomeningitis virus. In: Virological monographs. Springer, Heidelberg, 1971, Volume 10, p. 1–173.
31. Zinkernagel, R. M., Haenseler, E., Leist, T. P., Cerny, A., Hengartner, H., Althage, A.: T cell mediated hepatitis in mice infected with lymphocytic choriomeningitis virus. Journal of Experimental Medicine 1986, 164: 1075–1092.
32. Eddleston, A. L. W. F., Williams, R.: HLA and liver disease. British Medicine Bulletin 1978, 34: 295–300.
33. Cole, G. A., Nathanson, N., Prendergast, R. A.: Requirement for theta-bearing cells in lymphocytic choriomeningitis virus-induced central nervous system disease. Nature 1972, 238: 335–337.
34. Zinkernagel, R. M., Pfau, C. J., Hengartner, H., Althage, A.: Susceptibility to murine lymphocytic choriomeningitis maps to class I MHC genes – a model for MHC/disease associations. Nature 1985, 316: 814–817.
35. Leist, T. P., Eppler, M., Rüedi, E., Zinkernagel, R. M.: Virus triggered AIDS in mice is a T cell mediated immunopathology caused by virus-specific cytotoxic T cells: prevention by tolerance or by treatment with anti-CD8 antibodies. Journal of Experimental Medicine 1988, 167: 1749–1754.
36. Walker, C. M., Moody, D. J., Stites, D. P., Levy, J. A.: $CD8^+$ lymphocytes can control HIV infection in vitro by suppressing virus replication. Science 1986, 234: 1563–1566.

New Diseases
and Disease Epidemiology

Adherence and Proliferation of Bacteria on Artificial Surfaces

G. Peters

Several bacteria are able to cause polymer-associated infections. Staphylococci, especially coagulase-negative staphylococci, are by far the predominant organisms involved. The pathogenesis of these infections is characterized by the ability of staphylococci to adhere to and grow on polymer surfaces. In the course of polymer colonization they produce an extracellular slime substance of presumably complex glycoconjugate nature. This substance obviously possesses several biological properties. It strongly interferes with several host response mechanisms, especially granulocyte function and opsonophagozytosis. Furthermore, it interferes with the action of antibiotics on the staphylococcal cell. Thus, the slime substance may protect the embedded staphylococci on the polymer surface against normal host defense and chemotherapy, resulting in the persistence of the infectious focus. Many of the clinical problems associated with polymer infections can be explained by these pathomechanisms. The future goal will be to modify polymers used in medicine to avoid adhesion or further growth on the polymer surface.

Bacterial adhesion to and growth on solid surfaces is a widely occurring phenomenon in nature. Many bacteria grow under conditions in which they are attached to natural surfaces (1–3). There is even evidence that their physiological behaviour is adapted to this mode of growth, which exhibits substantial differences from growth in a liquid environment. Many of these bacteria are also able to adhere to and grow on synthetic surfaces with undesirable consequences resulting. For example, marine bacteria growing on ship walls can cause fouling, and industrial polymers colonized by bacteria can undergo changes in their properties and may be degraded due to enzymatical attack by these microorganisms.

In medicine, bacterial adhesion to solid surfaces is involved in the development of dental plaque formation (3) and plays an important role in the development of implant or catheter-related infections (4). The majority of these biomaterials used in medicine is made out of synthetic polymers like polyvinylchloride, polyethylene, polyurethane or silicone. Besides thrombosis, infection is the most severe complication associated with the use of these materials. The number of patients involved is steadily increasing due to the progress of modern medicine. Therefore, the so-called "plastic surface infections" have to be accepted as a special type of opportunistic nosocomial or even iatrogenic infection. In addition to several bacteria belonging to the normal microflora of human skin and mucous membranes, such as staphylococci, streptococci and *Enterobacteriaceae*, other bacteria such as pseudomonads and *Acinetobacter* spp. as well as fungi like candida are able to cause these infections. However, staphylococci and especially coagulase-negative staphylococci are by far the predominant organisms involved. Therefore the following overview will especially focus on plastic surface infections caused by coagulase-negative staphylococci.

Clinical Aspects

Coagulase-negative staphylococci are the by far most frequently isolated organisms in infections of liquor shunt systems, intravascular catheters, catheters for continuous ambulant peritoneal dialysis, and heart valves. They are also predominantly responsible for late-onset infections of transvenous endocardial pacemaker electrodes and joint prostheses. They are further involved in infections of hemodialysis shunts, vascular prostheses, breast prostheses and artificial ocular lenses. The clinical manifestations of the disease depend on the kind of plastic device involved. For instance, intravascular catheter related infections or heart valve infections are associated with septicemia, while infections of breast and hip prostheses are associated with inflammation or pathological tissue reaction. Consequently, different clinical symptoms occur. Mild fever and chill episodes, as well as anemia and splenomegaly in more chronic cases, are associated with recurrent septicemia, whereas loosening of the prostheses or capsular fibrosis are signs of hip

---

Institute of Medical Microbiology and Hygiene, University of Cologne, Goldenfelsstr. 19–21, D-5000 Cologne 41, FRG.

prostheses or breast prostheses infection, respectively. A more common feature of all coagulase-negative staphylococcal plastic surface infections is the somewhat mild course of the disease. The onset of the disease is differentiated between early-onset and late-onset infection. In most cases the infection originates at the time of either surgery or catheter insertion. Hematogenous infections are considered to occur more rarely. A special clinical phenomenon of plastic surface infections caused by coagulase-negative staphylococci is that the host is generally not able to overcome the infection despite having a normal immune system and despite the low virulence of the bacteria. The same is true for chemotherapy that fails despite the use of substances with proven high in vitro activity.

Attachment to Polymer Surfaces

Several aspects of the pathogenesis of staphylococcal plastic foreign body infections have been elucidated in recent years. The first insights were obtained by scanning electron microscopy investigations of artificially or naturally infected intravenous catheters (5–10). According to these data coagulase-negative staphylococci are able to adhere to and grow on polymer surfaces and to produce an extracellular slime substance in the further course of colonization. The final result is a thick matrix composed of multiple staphylococcal cell layers and copious amounts of the extracellular slime substance. Host products such as fibronection may be additionally involved in in vivo infections. Similar observations have been made by investigating other polymer devices such as transvenous endocardial pacemaker leads (11). Figure 1 shows a representative example of the morphology described above. Thus coagulase-negative staphylococci adherent to polymer surfaces reveal a special type of growth which is very different from that in or on artificial media. This aspect is important pointing out the only relative value of in vitro tests like those for antibiotic susceptibility performed under such artificial conditions. It is furthermore hypothesized that the slime matrix may protect the embedded staphylococci against host defense mechanisms and antibiotics (7).

The attachment of staphylococci to polymer surfaces seems to be mediated by various complex mecha-

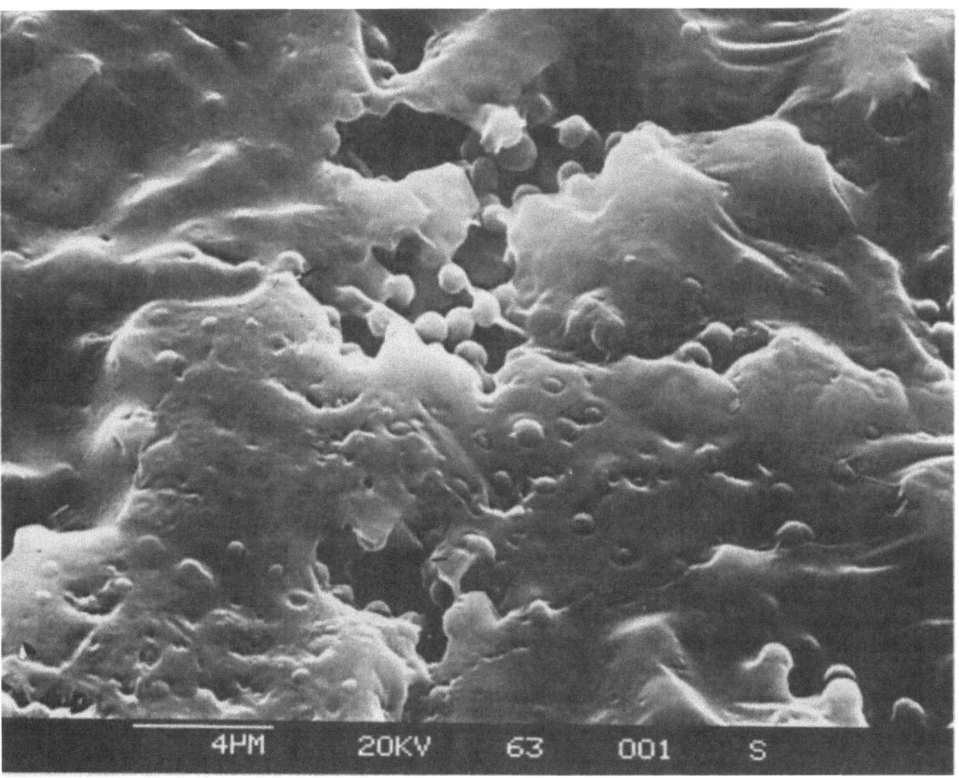

Figure 1: Adhering staphylococcal cells on a polyethylene surface partly covered by a matrix of extracellular slime substance (in vitro infection with *Staphylococcus epidermidis* KH11, scanning electron micrograph).

nisms. Hydrophobic interaction and electrostatic attraction have been shown to be unspecific mechanisms (12–13). These mechanisms depend on the surface characteristics of both the polymer and the staphylococcal cell. However, the in vivo situation is expected to be different and even more complex, since host factors are also involved (Figure 2). Shortly after implantation or insertion the polymer surface will become coated by serum or tissue substances (proteins). This may lead to a more specific interaction between receptor-like structures on the staphylococcal cell surface and the proteincoated polymer surface. These in vivo mechanisms of adhesion are still not fully understood and warrant further investigation.

Extracellular Slime Substance

It has been already mentioned that staphylococci adherent to the polymer surface produce enormous amounts of an extracellular slime substance (ESS). As known so far, most coagulase-negative staphylococci of the *Staphylococcus epidermidis*-group are able to produce ESS. However, the amount of slime produced as well as the still undiscovered chemical nature of the slime may be different in various strains. The substance adheres loosely to the staphylococcal cell surface and encloses many cells in a cell cluster. The ESS is water-soluble and can therefore be removed to great extent from the cells by washing, at least in vitro (14–15). These properties clearly separate the ESS from true capsules as defined for gram-positive cocci. The substance is probably identical or at least very similar to the mucoid substance described in association with the colonization of liquor shunts by *Staphylococcus* S II A (16). The ESS produced by most of the *Staphylococcus epidermidis* strains shows a strong reactivity with some mannose-specific lectins and poly-L-lysine, which can be used as a preliminary marker. There is some evidence, that the ESS may be a complex glycoconjugate (14–15). It seems proven that mannose, galactose and glucuronic acid are genuine constituents of the slime substance since these monosaccharides are not present in the peptidoglycan or teichoic acid of the cell wall of *Staphylococcus epidermidis*.

Interference with Host Defense Mechanisms

Data from in vitro and animal experiments accumulated so far suggest a high biological potency of the ESS (Table 1). These data strongly imply that the ESS can interfere with several host defense mechanisms. The blastogenic response of human peripheral mononuclear cells — mainly T-cells — to the stimulation with polyclonal stimulators is substantially altered (Figure 3). The degree of inhibition depends on the concentration of ESS and the time that ESS is present in the assay mixture (17). Furthermore, in surviving cells undergoing blastogenesis the surface structures associated with either helper/inducer- or cytotoxic/suppressor-cells are mostly not expressed (17). Surprisingly, cytotoxic cell activity is also inhibited as is the viability of myeloma cells (18). The underlying mechanisms and the clinical relevance of these phenomena are still unknown, especially with regard to the foreign body infection itself. The blastogenesis of B-cells stimulated with pokeweed mitogen

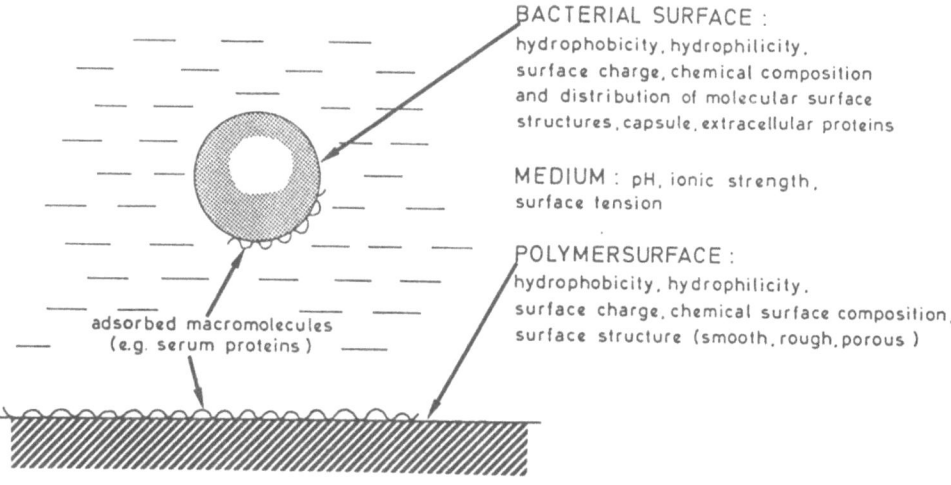

Figure 2: Hypothetical model: Factors influencing bacterial adhesion to polymers. Taken from B. Jansen et al. (see text).

Table 1: Biological properties of extracellular slime substance of *Staphylococcus epidermidis*.

1. Adhesion-like property
    adhesion to mammalian cells (?)
    attachment to polymer surfaces (?)
    intercell-adherence (cell-cluster-formation)
2. Interference with host defense mechanisms
    inhibition of T-cell blastogenesis
    inhibition of B-cell blastogenesis
    inhibition of immunoglobulin production
    enhancement of PMN adherence
    inhibition of PMN chemotaxis
    stimulation of PMN degranulation
    inhibition of bacterial opsonization
    inhibition of PMN chemiluminescence
    inhibition of *Staphylococcus epidermidis*-uptake by PMN
3. Enhancement of *Staphylococcus epidermidis* virulence in mice
4. Interference with the action of anti-staphylococcal antibiotics

is also inhibited in a dose-response manner (Figure 4), as is the subsequent immunoglobulin synthesis (18). These in vitro findings may be interpreted as evidence of a possible interference of ESS with the production of specific antibodies. However, these results have to be confirmed in further investigations.

The interference of ESS with several polymorphonuclear leukocyte) (PMN) functions could be of significant importance for the pathogenesis of staphylococcal foreign body infections. The substance is not cytotoxic to PMN, even in high concentrations as measured by trypan-blue exclusion and LDH-release.

On the contrary, ESS appears to be a strong chemotaxin. However, PMN pretreated with ESS revealed a decreased ability for directed migration in response to known chemotactic stimuli such as FMLP and zymosan-activated serum (ZAS), presumably C5a (19–20). Since this effect was especially pronounced with ZAS, interference with a possible C5a-receptor on the PMN membrane must be considered. Slime-pretreated PMN also showed increased degranulation, especially of specific granules (lactoferrin), possibly leading to a decreased ability for intracellular killing (19–20). Slime pretreatment has also been shown to inhibit PMN chemiluminescence in a dose-related manner (F. Schumacher-Perdreau et al., Third European Congress of Clinical Microbiology, The Hague, 1987, Abstract No. 61). These in vitro results regarding various PMN functions suggest the possibility of a substantial interference of staphylococcal ESS with PMN bacterial uptake and subsequent intracellular killing (opsonophagocytosis). Indeed, in investigations using the new model of surface phagocytosis (21), an assay more suitable to the in vivo situation of polymer infection, it was shown that the ESS interferes with staphylococcal uptake by PMN (19–20). Uptake by PMN of *Staphylococcus epidermidis* grown for 18 hours on a plastic surface was less than that of *Staphylococcus epidermidis* grown for only 2 hours. In contrast, for a *Staphlococcus aureus* strain used as control no difference in uptake after 2 and 18 hours incubation was found (Figure 5). In parallel scanning electron microscopy investigations *Staphylococcus aureus* revealed no slime production after 18 hours' growth on the plastic surface whereas *Staphy-*

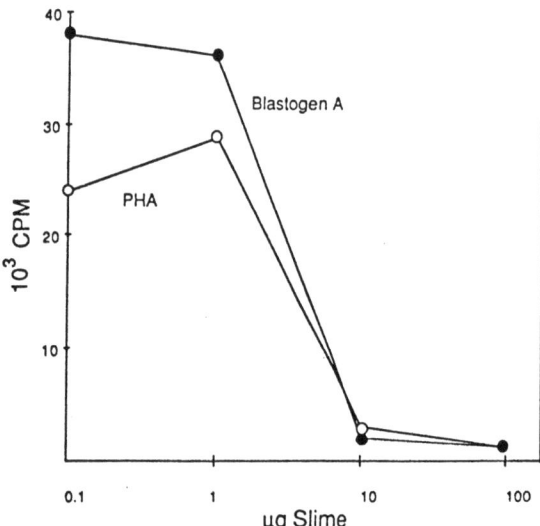

Figure 3: Inhibitory effect of extracellular slime substance on the blastogenic response of human peripheral mononuclear cells stimulated with phytohemagglutinin (PHA) or streptococcal blastogen A. Taken from Reference No. 18.

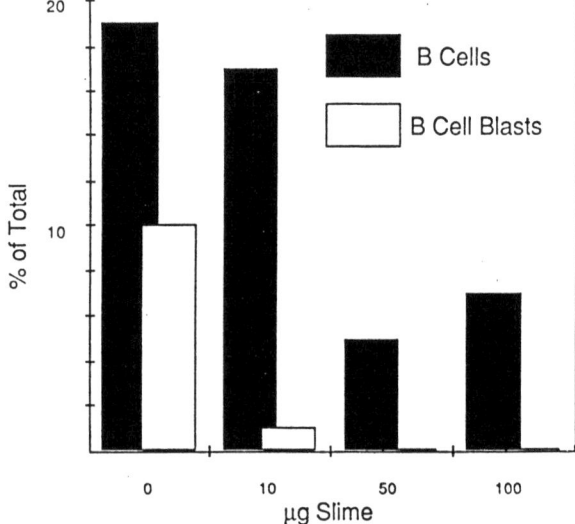

Figure 4: Inhibitory effect of extracellular slime substance on B-cell response to stimulation with pokeweed mitogen. Taken from Reference No. 18.

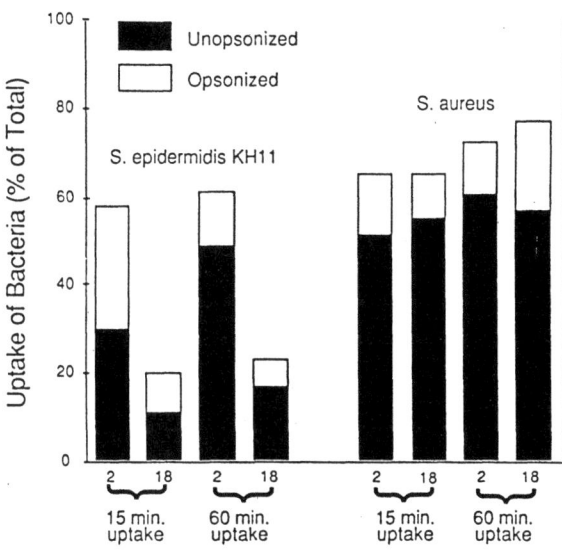

Figure 5: Surface phagocytosis of *Staphylococcus epidermidis* KH 11 and *Staphylococcus aureus* Cowan I (control) after different incubation times in plastic tissue culture plates. Uptake of bacteria by PMN expressed as percentage of total adherent bacteria in the wells. Taken from Reference No. 20.

Table 2: MICs of various antibiotics against *Staphylococcus epidermidis* V 2 in pmS 110-broth, a medium promoting ESS-production, and in Mueller-Hinton broth (standard MIC-medium, modified from Reference No. 15).

Antibiotic	MIC (mg/l)			
	Inoculum of 10^4 CFU		Inoculum of 10^7 CFU	
	Mueller-Hinton	pmS 110	Mueller-Hinton	pmS 110
Penicillin	0.19	0.39	0.19	3.12
Oxacillin	0.79	3.12	1.56	6.25
Vancomycin	12.5	50	6.25	> 100
Clindamycin	0.39	0.39	0.19	12.5
Ciprofloxacin	0.09	0.79	1.56	25
Gentamicin	0.19	1.56	0.79	> 100
Netilmicin	0.39	6.25	0.79	25

lococcus epidermidis was nearly encased in a slime matrix. Thus, there is strong evidence that the extracellular slime substance of *Staphylococcus epidermidis* — at least of certain strains — is antiphagocytic and can inhibit opsonophagocytosis of staphylococci embedded in slime on the surface of a foreign body in vivo. There are preliminary data from animals to support this hypothesis. Using a subcutaneous catheter infection model in mice it has been shown that the incidence of infection is significantly greater if strong slime-producing strains are used (22). In another mouse model the simultaneous intraperitoneal injection of extensively washed *Staphylococcus epidermidis* and slime isolated from the same strain resulted in high mortality whereas the injection of the bacteria without slime did not lead to death (15). All affected mice died within 48 hours after challenge due to septicemia (positive heart blood cultures) without any sign of an intraperitoneal abscess. Thus, the ESS seems to interfere with the function of peritoneal macrophages and invading PMN.

Protection against Antibiotics

It has also been postulated that ESS may be responsible for the protection of the embedded staphylococci against administered antibiotics. Matrices up to 140 μm thick observed by scanning electron microscopy in infected devices could act as a penetration barrier against antibiotics. This hypothesis is supported by the observation that the MIC of various antibiotics is significantly higher for *Staphylococcus epidermidis* adherent to a polymer surface or grown in a medium promoting slime production compared to the MIC in a standard medium (Table 2) (15, 23). Similar results have been obtained in bacterial killing experiments (15). Recently it was shown that the uptake of ^{3}H-labeled gentamicin is inhibited by ESS. The cell wall/cell membrane-associated radioactivity as well as the intracellular activity were significantly lower in cells grown in a medium promoting slime production than in those grown in the standard medium (Mueller-Hinton) (F. Schumacher-Perdreau et al., 88th Annual Meeting of the American Society for Microbiology, Miami Beach, 1988, Abstract No. B223). Thus, the ESS may interfere with the uptake of antibiotics into the staphylococcal cell wall and cytoplasma. This could explain the failure of antibiotic therapy despite the use of substances with proven in vitro activity.

Concluding Remarks and Future Aspects

The ability of coagulase-negative staphylococci, at least of most strains of human origin to adhere to and grow on surfaces and to produce extracellular slime may be a phylogenetically old property acquired during the evolution process. The production of ESS appears to be associated with the growth of staphylococci on surfaces, and it enables them to stick together in large cell clusters, allowing close contact and substance exchange. It may further enable the embedded staphylococci to stay in a somewhat dormant state, thereby permitting survival in below optimal environmental conditions. Thus the production of extracellular slime could be essential for the staphylococci to live on their natural surface, the skin and mucous membranes of humans or animals, without injuring the host. However, if a plastic foreign body is placed into the host, a new surface is presented to the staphylococci. Their natural mode of growth on this new surface may then result in infection of the tissue surrounding the device.

It is evident from the data presented on pathogenesis that prevention of bacterial adhesion or the rapid elimination of the bacteria shortly after adhesion would be the most appropriate strategy against polymer-related infections. The use of perioperative antibiotic prophylaxis is certainly one possibility. However, the amount of clinical data available is still inadequate to evaluate and propose a sufficient regimen. Another approach is to synthesize polymers with intrinsic anti-adhesive properties, or to coat polymers with or incorporate into the polymer substances which hinder adhesion or kill bacteria shortly after adherence. Preliminary investigations have shown that adhesion of *Staphylococcus epidermidis* to HEMA-grafted polyetherurethanes with high affinity for albumine is low compared with that to unmodified polyetherurethanes (24). Furthermore it seems possible to incorporate anti-staphylococcal antibiotics such as oxacillin, ciprofloxacin, clindamycin and vancomycin into the polyurethane matrix either by swelling agents or by solvent casting procedures (B. Jansen et al., 88th Annual Meeting of the American Society for Microbiology, Miami Beach, 1988, Abstract No. A105). The result is a delayed release of the antibiotic from the modified polyetherurethanes, leading to a rapid killing of adherent staphylococci. A much more elegant way of course would be to introduce chemical groups into the polymer surface with intrinsic bactericidal activity. For this purpose especially, glow discharge methods for the modification of polymers could be used. Further basic research is warranted to evaluate these possibilities for the prevention of plastic foreign body infections.

References

1. Fletcher, M., Loeb, G. L.: Influence of substratum characteristics on the attachment of a marine pseudomonad to solid surfaces. Applied and Environmental Microbiology 1979, 36: 67–72.
2. Cheng, K. J., Irvin, R. T., Costerton, J. W.: Autochthonous and pathogenic colonization of animal tissues by bacteria. Canadian Journal of Microbiology 1981, 27: 461–490.
3. Gibbons, R. J.: Adherent interactions which may affect microbial ecology in the mouth. Journal of Dental Research 1984, 63: 378–385.
4. Sugarman, B., Young, E. J.: Infections associated with prosthetic devices. CRC Press, Fla., Boca Raton, 1984.
5. Locci, R., Peters, G., Pulverer, G.: Microbial colonization of prosthetic devices. III. Adhesion of staphylococci to lumina of intravenous catheters perfused with bacterial suspensions. Zentralblatt für Bakteriologie, Parasitologie und Hygiene, I. Abteilung, Originale B, 1981, 173: 300–307.
6. Peters, G., Locci, R., Pulverer, G.: Microbial colonization of prosthetic devices. II. Scanning electron microscopy of naturally infected intravenous catheters. Zentralblatt für Bakteriologie, Parasitologie und Hygiene, I. Abteilung, Originale B, 1981, 173: 293–299.
7. Peters, G., Locci, R., Pulverer, G.: Adherence and growth of coagulase-negative staphylococci on surfaces of intravenous catheters. Journal of Infectious Diseases 1982, 146: 479–482.
8. Christensen, G. D., Simpson, W. A., Bisno, A. L., Beachey, E. H.: Adherence of slime-producing strains of *Staphylococcus epidermidis* to smooth surfaces. Infection and Immunity 1982, 37: 318–326.
9. Franson, T. R., Sheth, N. D., Rose, H. D., Sohnle, P. G.: Scanning electron microscopy of bacteria adherent to intravascular catheters. Journal of Clinical Microbiology 1984, 20: 500–505.
10. Marrie, T. J., Costerton, J. W.: Scanning and transmission electron microscopy of in situ bacterial colonization of intravenous and intraarterial catheters. Journal of Clinical Microbiology 1984, 19: 687–693.
11. Peters, G., Saborowski, F., Locci, R., Pulverer, G.: Investigations on staphylococcal infection of intravenous endocardial pacemaker electrodes. American Heart Journal 1984, 108: 359–364.
12. Hogt, A. H., Dankert, J., de Vries, J. A., Feijen, J.: Adhesion of coagulase-negative staphylococci to biomaterials. Journal of General Microbiology 1983, 129: 2959–2968.
13. Ludwicka, A., Jansen, B., Wadström, T., Switalski, L. M., Peters, G., Pulverer, G.: Attachment of staphylococci to various polymers. In: Shalaby, S. W., Hoffman, A. S., Ratner, B. D., Horbett, T. A. (ed.): Polymers as biomaterials. Plenum Publishing Corporation, New York, 1984, p. 241–255.
14. Ludwicka, A., Uhlenbruck, G., Peters, G., Seng, P. N., Gray, E. D., Jeljaszewicz, J., Pulverer, G.: Investigation on extracellular slime produced by *Staphylococcus epidermidis*. Zentralblatt für Bakteriologie, Mikrobiologie und Hygiene (A) 1984, 258: 256–267.
15. Peters, G., Schumacher-Perdreau, F., Jansen, B., Bey, M., Pulverer, G.: Biology of *Staphylococcus epidermidis* extracellular slime. In: Pulverer, G., Quie, P. G., Peters, G. (ed.): Pathogenicity and clinical significance of coagulase-negative staphylococci. G. Fischer Verlag, Stuttgart, 1987, p. 15–31.
16. Bayston, R., Penny, S. R.: Excessive production of mucoid substance in Staphylococcus S II A: a possible factor in colonization of Holter shunts. Developmental Medicine and Child Neurology 1972, 14, Supplement 27: 25–28.
17. Gray, E. D., Peters, G., Verstegen, M., Regelmann, W. E.: Effect of extracellular slime substance from *Staphylococcus epidermidis* on the human cellular immune response. Lancet 1984, i: 365–367.
18. Gray, E. D., Regelmann, W. E., Peters, G.: Staphylococcal slime and host defenses: effects on lymphocytes and immune function. In: Pulverer, G., Quie, P. G., Peters, G. (ed.): Pathogenicity and clinical significance of coagulase-negative staphylococci. G. Fischer Verlag, Stuttgart 1987, p. 45–54.

19. Johnson, G. M., Lee, D. A., Regelmann, W. E., Gray, E. D., Peters, G. Quie, P. G.: Interference with granulocyte function by *Staphylococcus epidermidis* slime. Infection and Immunity 1986, 54: 13–20.
20. Johnson, G. M., Regelmann, W. E., Gray, E. D., Peters, G., Quie, P. G.: Staphylococcal slime and host defenses: effects on polymorphonuclear granulocytes. In: Pulverer, G., Quie, P. G., Peters, G. (ed.): Clinical significance and pathogenicity of coagulase-negative staphylococci. G. Fischer Verlag, Stuttgart 1987, p. 33–44.
21. Lee, D. A., Hoidal, J. R., Clawson, C. C., Quie, P. G., Peterson, P. K.: Phagocytosis by polymorphonuclear leukocytes of *Staphylococcus aureus* and *Pseudomonas aeruginosa* adherent to plastic, agar, or glass. Journal of Immunological Methods 1983, 63: 103–114.
22. Christensen, G. D., Simpson, W. A., Bisno, A. L., Beachey, E. H.: Experimental foreign body infections in mice challenged with slime producing *Staphylococcus epidermidis*. Infection and Immunity 1983, 40: 407–410.
23. Sheth, N. D., Franson, T. R., Sohnle, P.G.: Influence of bacterial adherence to intravascular catheters on in-vitro antibiotic susceptibility. Lancet 1985, ii: 1266–1268.
24. Jansen, B., Schareina, S., Steinhauser, H., Peters, G., Schumacher-Perdreau, F., Pulverer, G.: Development of polymers with anti-infectious properties. Polymer Material Science and Engineering 1987, 57: 43–52.

Current Knowledge of *Chlamydia* TWAR, an Important Cause of Pneumonia and Other Acute Respiratory Diseases

J. T. Grayston[1,2]*, S. P. Wang[2], C. C. Kuo[2]

This article reviews the current knowledge of the TWAR strain, a newly recognized chlamydia organism that causes acute respiratory infection, especially atypical pneumonia. Information is presented under the following topics: introduction and history of the organism; microbiology and classification, including the proposal for a new chlamydia species, *Chlamydia pneumoniae*; laboratory diagnosis by isolation and serology; endemic TWAR disease and evidence for etiology, including studies in university students, in hospitalized pneumonia patients in three cities, and in a health maintenance organization from 1963 to 1974 and from 1985 to 1987; epidemic TWAR disease both country-wide in Denmark, Norway and Sweden 1981–1983, and localized in Finland and other countries; treatment including laboratory determination of antibiotic and sulfa drug sensitivity of the TWAR organism; population TWAR antibody prevalence; and studies by other investigators.

The term atypical pneumonia came into use to describe pneumonias that were different from typical pneumococcal pneumonia with lobar consolidation. In the antibiotic era, the atypical pneumonias have been recognized much more frequently and the understanding of the etiology of these pneumonias has been evolving continuously. Originally, most were thought to be due to viruses. Pneumonia due to the influenza viruses was recognized, and several other viruses (including respiratory syncytial virus, adenovirus and parainfluenza viruses) were shown to cause pneumonia, particularly in children but also in adults. Many bacteria, including *Streptococcus pneumoniae*, cause atypical pneumonia. Less common diseases (e.g. psittacosis, Q fever) cause numerous atypical pneumonias in certain circumstances. With the discovery of *Mycoplasma pneumoniae*, the major cause of atypical pneumonias was thought to have been found. However, in recent years, two new important causes of pneumonia have been identified: the legionella organisms, and the TWAR organisms.

TWAR is a strain designation, which was derived from the laboratory codes of the first two isolates TW-183 and AR-39 (1). TW-183 was isolated in 1965 from the conjunctiva of a control child in a trachoma vaccine study in Taiwan. It was the 183rd chick embryo egg yolk sac isolate of a *Chlamydia* organism from a series of studies of trachoma. The strain could not be typed as a trachoma strain by the mouse toxicity prevention test. Several years later when cell culture for *Chlamydia* was developed, it was found that the inclusions of TW-183 formed in cell culture were round and dense and unlike *Chlamydia trachomatis* strains. It was therefore assumed to be a *Chlamydia psittaci* strain. So far there has been no evidence that a syndrome of eye disease is caused by the TWAR organism. AR-39 was isolated from a throat swab of a University of Washington student with pharyngitis in 1983 (1). All subsequent isolates have come from throat swabs of patients with acute respiratory disease.

This review of the TWAR organism will aim at providing a survey of what is now known about the role of TWAR in human infection. We first undertook studies of TWAR in respiratory infection in 1983, and published the first report suggesting a role of this organism in respiratory disease in 1985 (2). It is possible to make some rather broad statements about the importance of TWAR infections because retrospective serological studies have been used to acquire knowledge of the epidemiology of TWAR.

---

[1]Department of Epidemiology, and [2]Department of Pathobiology, School of Public Health and Community Medicine SC-36, University of Washington, Seattle, Washington 98195, USA.

Microbiological Characterization

The order *Chlamydiales* has one family, *Chlamydiaceae*, and one genus, *Chlamydia*. There are now two recognized species, *Chlamydia trachomatis* and *Chlamydia psittaci* (3). *Chlamydia trachomatis* is the species that causes the eye disease trachoma and sexually transmitted disease with genital tract infections in both sexes, which have become well known only over the past decade. *Chlamydia trachomatis* is now recognized as the most common cause of sexually transmitted disease in the USA. *Chlamydia psittaci* is the species that cause psittacosis (also called ornithosis). The organisms are common in many animal and bird species and cause febrile respiratory tract disease and pneumonia in humans when transmitted from pet birds (and certain wild birds) or in turkey or duck processing plants.

Originally, we considered TWAR to be a strain of *Chlamydia psittaci* because it was clearly not *Chlamydia trachomatis* on the basis of its inclusion morphology and failure to react with *Chlamydia trachomatis* specific monoclonal antibody (1). Recent laboratory results suggest that TWAR does not belong to either recognized species. These results include immunological, fine structure and DNA analysis studies (4–7). All TWAR strains are identical to each other with respect to all the parameters studied.

The TWAR organism shares the *Chlamydia* genus specific antigen as demonstrated by immunofluorescence staining of inclusions using genus specific monoclonal antibodies. The TWAR strains show no crossreactions in the micro-immunofluorescence test with *Chlamydia trachomatis* or *Chlamydia psittaci* strains. So far, only a single TWAR serotype has been found. Monoclonal antibodies specific for the TWAR strain have been produced.

Ten TWAR strains, including TW-183, have been serially passaged in HeLa cell culture for characterization (4). TWAR organisms form intracytoplasmic inclusions in cultured cells which appear round and dense on Giemsa stain. The inclusions contain no glycogen (they are iodine stain negative). Electron microscopy has shown that the TWAR elementary bodies have a morphology and structure distinct from those of other chlamydial organisms (5). Figure 1 is an electron micrograph showing elementary bodies of TWAR and *Chlamydia trachomatis*. The TWAR elementary body is pleomorphic but typically pear shaped. The cytoplasmic mass is round and there is a large periplasmic space. The TWAR elementary bodies contrast with the round, dense elementary bodies of *Chlamydia trachomatis* and *Chlamydia psittaci* which have a narrow or barely discernible periplasmic space. The TWAR reticulate bodies are similar to those of the other *Chlamydia* species and undergo the same intracellular developmental cycle.

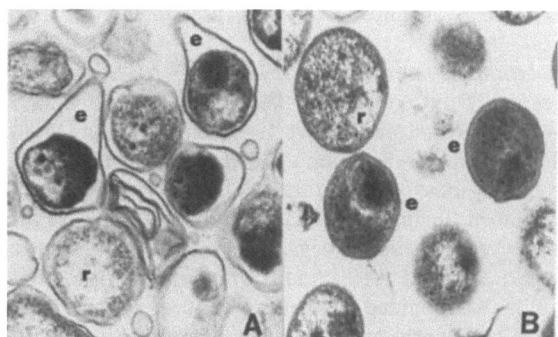

Figure 1: Electron micrograph of (A) *Chlamydia* TWAR (isolate AR-388) organisms and (B) *Chlamydia trachomatis* serovar H (UW-4) organisms (x 80,000). e: elementary body, r: reticulate body. Micrograph supplied through the courtesy of Dr. Emil Chi.

Unlike *Chlamydia trachomatis* and most *Chlamydia psittaci* strains, TWAR organisms contain no extrachromosomal DNA (plasmids) (6). TWAR is readily distinguished from *Chlamydia trachomatis* or *Chlamydia psittaci* by restriction endonuclease analysis, whereas identical or nearly identical restriction patterns have been observed among the TWAR isolates (6). The G + C content of TWAR DNA (40 mol %) was found to be intermediate between *Chlamydia trachomatis* and *Chlamydia psittaci* (7).

Table 1 shows that TWAR shares less than 10% relatedness (homology) in DNA sequence with *Chlamydia trachomatis* and *Chlamydia psittaci* (7). The TWAR strains tested showed 94% or more relatedness with each other. The *Chlamydia trachomatis* strains showed similar high relatedness with each other, but there was considerable heterogenicity among the *Chlamydia psittaci* strains.

Because of its unique DNA, morphology and immunological characteristics, we propose that the TWAR organism be designated a third species of *Chlamydia*, called *Chlamydia pneumoniae* (submitted to the International Journal of Systematic Bateriology). The TW-183 strain will be the prototype. The TWAR organism is the only strain (or serovar) recognized to date.

Table 1: Percentage of relatedness (homology) in DNA sequence in chlamydial strains. Three to five strains of each species were tested. From reference No. 7.

Unlabelled DNA	Labelled DNA		
	TWAR	*Chlamydia psittaci*	*Chlamydia trachomatis*
TWAR	94–100	≤5–8	≤5
Chlamydia psittaci	≤5–10	21–100	≤5–11
Chlamydia trachomatis	≤5–7	≤5–6	97–100

Laboratory Diagnosis of TWAR Infection

Isolation. Isolation and growth of TWAR strains has been difficult, otherwise they would probably have been identified earlier. We use techniques similar to those used for isolation of *Chlamydia trachomatis*, including both cell culture (HeLa 229) and the old-fashioned technique of culture in the yolk sac of embryonated chicken eggs. Both methods are equally sensitive but a larger amount of inoculum for further studies is obtained in the egg culture, and the presence of fewer organisms can be identified in the cell culture. McCoy cells are not as sensitive as HeLa 229 cells (4).

TWAR organisms are susceptible to temperature and to freezing and thawing (8). The organisms are rapidly inactivated at room temperature, only 1% remaining viable after storage for 24 h. At 4 °C, 70% of the organisms remain viable after storage for 24 h. Rapid freezing at −70 °C may inactivate 60% of the organisms. However, if the specimen is frozen more slowly by cooling it at 4 °C for up to 4 h before freezing to −70 °C, only 23% of the organisms are inactivated. Therefore, specimens should ideally be stored at refrigerator temperature and isolation done within 24 h, or specimens should be frozen at below −65 °C after 1–4 h of storage in a refrigerator (8). Chlamydia transport medium SPG or 2SP is used for storing specimens.

The real key to our success with isolation was the development of a TWAR monoclonal antibody which, conjugated to fluorescein, is used to identify inclusions in cell culture (1). A genus monoclonal antibody will also stain TWAR inclusions but does not identify the inclusion as TWAR. The fluorescent antibody stain is important because usually very few inclusions are seen.

Serological Tests. Two serological tests are used: the micro-immunofluorescence test with TWAR elementary body antigen is specific for TWAR (9), and the complement fixation test measures *Chlamydia* genus antibodies (10). Table 2 shows the serological reactions considered positive. The micro-immunofluorescence test distinguishes between antibodies in the IgM and IgG serum fractions. This has been helpful in determining whether infection is current or recent. The presence of IgG antibody indicating previous infection is used to determine population prevalence.

The usual way of determining the sensitivity of a serologic test for detection of infection with a microorganism is to measure the serologic results in persons from whom the organism is isolated. This is difficult to do with TWAR, because isolation has been accomplished from relatively few persons. However, in the data that are available, the micro-immunofluorescence serologic test has been shown to be highly sensitive, being positive in 24 of 25 patients from whom the organism was isolated. The one patient who did not show current infection by our definition of positivity in the serologic test had a titer of 128 in the IgG serum fraction, which fell to 64 two months later. No TWAR IgM antibody was detected. This patient demonstrated a four-fold fall in the chlamydia complement fixation titer from 16 to 4 over the two months, suggesting that there had been a recent infection.

The specificity of the test has best been demonstrated by the study of acute respiratory disease in students at the University of Washington. Since July 1984, when the TWAR monoclonal antibody became available, the organism has been isolated from 11 of 13 patients with positive serology. The opportunity to test persons serologically during several epidemics of TWAR infections has increased our confidence in the specificity of the micro-immunofluorescence test with TWAR antigen. A high percentage of epidemic sera showed TWAR antibodies indicating current infection compared to the rare occurrence of such antibodies in several population samples.

We have presented extensive data showing the absence of cross-reactions in our micro-immunofluorescence test between antibody against *Chlamydia trachomatis* and TWAR (9).

Serological Response in Primary Infection and Reinfection. Interpretation of patterns of serological responses is important in serological studies of patients and in seroepidemiology. We have identified two patterns of antibody response to TWAR infection (11). We believe that one is a response to primary or first TWAR infection and the other to reinfection. The primary response has been seen in most young persons, university students and military trainees infected with TWAR. The reinfection response has been most common in older adults. Table 3 shows that the first TWAR infection is accompanied by chlamydia complement fixing antibodies, and that the complement fixing antibodies usually appear first. One of the striking findings about the

Table 2: Serological tests used to study TWAR infections with definition of positive results.

Micro-immunofluorescence with TWAR elementary body antigen
    Current infection (acute phase):
        fourfold antibody titer rise
        IgM antibody titer ⩾ 16
        IgG antibody titer ⩾ 512
    Past infection:
        IgG antibody titer ⩾ 16 and ⩾ 512

Complement fixation with chlamydia antigen (not specific for TWAR)
        fourfold antibody titer rise
        antibody titer ⩾ 64

Table 3: Serological response pattern in primary TWAR infection and reinfection (most definitive examples).

	Antibody titers		
	TWAR Micro-immunofluorescence		Chlamydia complement fixation
	IgM	IgG	
First infection (primary)			
Acute serum	0	0	16
Convalescent serum (3 weeks)	128	0	128
Convalescent serum (8 weeks)	32	256	32
Reinfection (secondary)			
Acute serum	0	16	0
Convalescent serum (3 weeks)	0	1024	0

primary response is the relatively long time required for the development of TWAR antibody in the micro-immunofluorescence test. Antibody in the IgM fraction may not appear for three weeks after the onset of symptoms. Antibody in the IgG fraction may not reach diagnostic titer levels for six to eight weeks. In reinfection there is often no complement fixing antibody and no IgM antibody response. On the other hand, the IgG antibody response may appear within one to two weeks and often rises to a high titer ($\geqslant 512$). Not all infected individuals have such distinctive response patterns. As with all biological tests there are individual variations. Further, in reinfection disease, when IgG antibody is already present, there may be a low IgM antibody titer rise with or without a rise in the IgG antibody titer.

Both the timing of collection of the specimens and the response pattern are important in interpreting TWAR antibody results in paired serums. Convalescent serum obtained less than 21 days after onset may not contain TWAR antibody. Conversely, the absence of complement fixing and IgM antibody in reinfection may make it difficult to identify recent infection.

Clinical Laboratory Tests. Routine laboratory tests are generally not useful in diagnosing TWAR infection. White blood cell counts are either normal or slightly increased. Erythrocyte sedimentation rates are often elevated. As yet there has been no study of the presence of cold agglutinins in TWAR infection.

Endemic TWAR Disease and Evidence of TWAR Etiology

Acute Respiratory Disease in University of Washington Students. Our longest study of TWAR, now five years old, has been performed in University of Washington students. The original report of this study covered the first 2.5 years of the study (1). Table 4 shows the results of serologic and isolation tests for TWAR in 647 students. The frequency of TWAR infection in 1986 and 1987 was less than in the first three years of the study. The highest percentage of TWAR positive patients was in 1983. There were only three cases of illness associated with TWAR infection in 1986 and 1987, compared to 17 in the first three years. In 1988, there were two cases confirmed by isolation by the end of February which suggests there may be an upswing in the incidence of TWAR infection.

Twenty student patients were identified as having TWAR infection by isolation of the organism or by micro-immunofluorescence. The organism was isolated from 12, all but one of whom had positive serological tests. While in 1983 and the first half of 1984 the organism was isolated from only two of eight patients positive serologically, the frequency of isolation has been very high since July 1984. Including the two 1988 cases, 11 isolates have been obtained from 13 serologically positive cases. This is as good as could be expected with almost any microorganism. The isolation results strengthen the evidence of an etiologic association of the TWAR organism with acute respiratory tract disease.

Table 4: Occurrence of TWAR infections in University of Washington students with acute respiratory disease.

Diagnosis	Number with TWAR infection[a]/Number tested				
	1983	1984	1985	1986	1987
Pneumonia	5/28	3/28	4/30	2/33	0/21
Bronchitis	1/18	1/27	2/39	0/36	1/21
Other	1/38	0/115	0/118	0/30	0/68
Total no. with TWAR infection	7	4	6	2	1
No. of TWAR isolations	2	3	5	1	1

[a] Both serological (acute antibody) and isolation evidence of TWAR infection.

Table 4 also shows that there has been a strong tendency for TWAR to be associated with lower respiratory tract disease, either pneumonia or bronchitis. Over the five years of the study, 10% of the patients with pneumonia and 4% with bronchitis had TWAR infection. Although only one student with TWAR infection had pharyngitis without evidence of lower respiratory tract disease, pharyngitis and sinusitis frequently accompanied the lower respiratory tract diseases associated with TWAR infection. Sinusitis was identified in four, and severe sore throat, often with laryngitis, was present in 13 of the 19 TWAR pneumonia and bronchitis cases. In addition, a biphasic illness, in which severe sore throat was the first syndrome, was observed in seven of the patients. Sore throat, usually with hoarseness, often resulted in a clinic visit. When no pathogenic bacteria were found on culture, the patients were treated symptomatically, and improved. After two to three weeks their illness relapsed with symptoms that led to the diagnosis of pneumonia or bronchitis. In 12 of the 14 TWAR pneumonia patients chest radiographs were performed, and all demonstrated single pneumonic lesions, except one considered to demonstrate bronchopneumonia.

While the illness in the students was generally mild and none required hospitalization, they did require bedrest. Many of the patients failed to recover promptly from their infection and many had a persistent cough for one to two months. These symptoms often responded to a course of tetracycline after the TWAR infection had been identified.

Acute Respiratory Disease in the Group Health Cooperative of Puget Sound. We have carried out a similar study of acute respiratory infections in a wider age group in the Group Health Cooperative (HMO) in Seattle; in 1985 in a suburban primary health care clinic (Lynnwood) (11) and in 1986–87 in the emergency and off-hours clinic for the eastside of King County serving a population of 109,000. Table 5 shows that there was a decline in the frequency of TWAR infection after 1985 similar to that observed in the University students. Bronchitis was a much more common diagnosis than pneumonia in these patients, at least in part because the patients were often not available for study until after the acute stage of their illness. As with the University students, evidence of TWAR infection was found most frequently in lower respiratory infection. However, in these Group Health patients TWAR infections were found in three patients with primary sinusitis, two with pharyngitis, and one each with fever of undetermined origin and upper respiratory tract illness without fever or pharyngitis. One patient classified as having bronchitis had an equally prominent sinusitis. Three of the patients, one each with pharyngitis, sinusitis and fever of undetermined origin, had had repeated episodes of similar illness in the year preceding the diagnosis of TWAR infection. Also of interest was the finding that two of the patients with pneumonia had been diagnosed as having sarcoidosis, one during the current illness and one in the past.

Table 5: Results of studies of TWAR infection in patients of the Group Health Cooperative of Puget Sound with acute respiratory disease.

	Lynnwood 1985		Eastside 1986–1987	
	Number tested	Percent TWAR positive	Number tested	Percent TWAR positive
Pneumonia	7	14	63	5
Bronchitis	153	8	106	3
Sinusitis	12	8	45	4
Pharyngitis	76	1	91	1
Fever of undetermined origin	4	0	35	3
Other upper respiratory tract infection	26	0	129	1
	278	5	470	2

We isolated the organism from only two of the 26 seropositive patients. Most were seen later in the course of their illness than the University students, and many had received prior antibiotic therapy. Some of the cases classified as bronchitis could have had unrecognized pneumonitis earlier in their illness.

TWAR Infection in Hospitalized Patients with Pneumonia. In collaboration with Dr. Thomas Marrie, we carried out a retrospective serologic study of 301 consecutively seen patients with community-acquired pneumonia admitted to the Victoria General Hospital in Halifax, Nova Scotia, from November 1981 to August 1984 (12). The difficulty in interpretation of TWAR serologic results is especially great in older patients with reinfection, where complement fixing and micro-immunofluorescence IgM antibodies are usually not present. Despite this problem, it was possible to show that 18 (6%) of the pneumonia cases had evidence of current or recent TWAR infection. The mean age of the patients was 64 years. Sixteen were males and two females.

Pneumonia associated with the presence of acute phase TWAR antibody had no characteristic clinical or radiographic features when compared with pneumonia without acute phase chlamydia antibody. Six of the TWAR patients, all of whom had preexisting serious chronic disease, had severe illness, and two died. Both patients who died had a complicated hospital course and concomitant infections.

While determination of the primary cause of pneumonia is often not precise, and many cases are of unknown etiology, TWAR was the third most common etiologic agent identified as the cause of pneumonia in the study (Table 6). A number of established etiologic agents of respiratory infection were identified less often than TWAR.

We recently completed another retrospective serologic study in collaboration with Dr. Victor Yu and associates, in hospitalized pneumonia patients admitted to three Pittsburgh hospitals over a period of one year (1986–1987). Of 359 pneumonia cases, 8% had evidence of TWAR infection (several had other bacterial pathogens in addition). Again, *Streptococcus pneumoniae* and *Haemophilus influenzae* were most commonly associated with pneumonia followed by TWAR and *Legionella* species.

We also conducted another retrospective serological study of hospitalized patients with pneumonia, which was not always community-acquired. Serum specimens taken between October 1980 and April 1981 from 198 pneumonia patients in the Veterans Administration of Harborview hospitals in Seattle 1981 from 198 pneumonia patients in the Veterans Administration and Harborview hospitals in Seattle were tested for antibody against TWAR and some viruses and mycoplasma. Twenty (10%) had serologic evidence of recent TWAR infection. Fifteen of 142 (11%) had evidence of influenza A virus infection. Only four patients (3%) showed complement fixing antibody against *Mycoplasma pneumoniae* suggesting recent infection. No patient had evidence of infection with more than one of these organisms.

The hospital records of the patients with acute TWAR antibody and an equal number of matched controls were examined for clinical characteristics, laboratory test results, treatment and course during the hospital stay. The controls closely matched the cases for age (mean 52.5 versus 52.1 years), sex (both 16 M:4 F) and onset date (mean 2.11.81 versus 2.13.81). They were not matched for acquisition of pneumonia in the community or in hospital. We found that in 9 of the 20 pneumonia patients with TWAR antibody the onset of pneumonia was in hospital. However, 12 of the 20 control patients had apparently hospital-acquired pneumonias, suggesting that nosocomial pneumonia is common in these hospitals. Table 7 shows that the mean age of the community-acquired pneumonia patients with TWAR infection was 61 years compared to 43 years for the nosocomial pneumonia patients with TWAR infection. While the ages of the control patients were affected by the matching process, those with community-acquired pneumonia were older on average than those with nosocomial disease. While in five of these TWAR patients the onset of pneumonia was during the first week after hospital admission, in four the onset was in the period 18 to 247 days after admission. These nosocomial pneumonia cases were seen in both hospitals. There was no clustering of their onset dates which extended from December through April. Seven of the nine TWAR patients were admitted with multiple injuries as a result of trauma. The other two underwent major surgery. The mode of transmission in the hospital was not determined. All the patients with hospital-acquired pneumonia had been intubated and all had undergone some surgical procedure.

It was not possible clinically or radiographically to distinguish pneumonia associated with TWAR antibody from pneumonia in the controls. This was also true for the patients with influenza A infection. Most cases and controls had preexisting chronic diseases (Table 7).

TWAR Infection in Seattle 1963–1976. In another study from Seattle that presents more information on the endemic occurrence of TWAR infections, we investigated pneumonia in the Group Health Cooperative from the end of 1963 through 1976. Those studies primarily investigated the *Mycoplasma pneumoniae* etiology of pneumonia and involved mostly outpatients (13). They showed that 12 of 1000 mem-

Table 6: Etiologic agents found in hospitalized patients with community-acquired pneumonia in Halifax, Nova Scotia, November 1981 to August 1984.

Etiologic agent	Number of patients (%)
Streptococcus pneumonia	26 (9)
Haemophilus influenzae	19 (6)
TWAR	18 (6)
Influenza A	16 (5)
Legionella spp.	12 (4)
Mycoplasma pneumoniae	10 (3)

Table 7: Results of retrospective TWAR serological study in patients with pneumonia in Harborview and Veterans' Administration hospitals, Seattle, 1980–1981.

	Patients (n = 20) TWAR positive	Controls (n = 20) TWAR negative
Community-acquired pneumonia	11	10
Mean Age	61 years	59 years
Hospital-acquired pneumonia	9	10
Mean Age	43 years	45 years
Preexisting disease		
Alcohol abuse	6	8
COPD	5	4
Cardiac failure	4	3
Dementia	0	3

COPD = chronic obstructive pulmonary disease.

bers of the cooperative had pneumonia yearly (12 year average) and that 15 % of the pneumonia cases were due to Mycoplasma pneumoniae. The serum bank from this study has proved invaluable over the years, and we have recently tested over 1,000 paired sera, stratified by age, sex and time, for TWAR antibody. While evaluation of the findings in these antibody studies is still underway, it is now clear that TWAR infections in Seattle occurred as early as 1963, and continued through 1974. Of the sera studied from persons five years of age and older, 3–15 % in each year showed evidence of recent TWAR infection, with an overall average of 7 %. We suspect that this is an underestimation of the number of pneumonia cases associated with TWAR infection due to the timing of collection of the serum specimens. Some of the convalescent serum specimens were collected 10 to 14 days after the acute specimen.

There were no cases of TWAR infection in patients under the age of five. There was approximately equal frequency of TWAR infection in pneumonia patients in the age groups above five years, with no significant differences by age or by sex.

Including the studies in university students and hospitalized pneumonia patients, we have studied some Seattle sera from most years since 1963. There has been no evidence of epidemic occurrence of TWAR infection and no years without TWAR infection being diagnosed, although there was clearly a higher incidence in some years than in others. Overall, TWAR infection has occurred in 6–12 % of both outpatients and hospitalized patients with pneumonia in six different studies.

Epidemic TWAR Disease in Scandinavia

Country-wide TWAR epidemics in Denmark, Norway and Sweden 1981–1983. Studies of TWAR infection in Denmark suggest that a TWAR epidemic occurred there in the early 1980s (14). A publication from the Public Health Laboratory in Norway showed a large jump in the reported cases of ornithosis in 1981 (15). Table 8 shows the reported cases of ornithosis in Norway, Sweden and Denmark from 1980 to 1985. The occurrence of ornithosis closely correlated with chlamydia complement fixation test results. The number of reported cases increased in Norway in 1981, 1982 and 1983 before falling off closer to the original rate. A similar increased incidence, although not as sharp, was seen in Sweden with a slower fall-off. In Denmark the increase in reported cases did not occur until 1982.

Table 9 shows the results of testing sera from these three countries for TWAR antibody. In each case the sera had been submitted to the country's National Public Health Laboratory with the diagnosis of possible ornithosis. Our collaborators in this study included Carl Mordhorst, Anne-Lise Bruu and Sirkka Vene. The results shown are from sera in which chlamydia complement-fixing antibody was found.

The large increase in incidence of reported cases in 1981 was associated with acute phase TWAR antibody. The sera tested represented all areas of the countries. Even though the total number of cases in Denmark did not increase in 1981, the prevalence of TWAR antibody in the complement-fixation positive

Table 8: Notified cases of ornithosis by year in Scandinavia.

	1980	1981	1982	1983	1984	1985
Norway	55	404	585	333	54	75
Sweden	86	255	235	197	163	117
Denmark	70	83	434	309	86	86

Table 9: Results of TWAR immunofluorescence tests in sera submitted for ornithosis documentation which showed chlamydia complement-fixation antibody.

	Number tested	Percent with acute phase TWAR antibody					
		1980	1981	1982	1983	1984	1985
Norway	127	NT[a]	75	88	NT[a]	10	NT[a]
Sweden	147	13	67	65	34	20	19
Denmark	577	17	49	49	56	55/5[b]	11

[a] NT = not tested.
[b] To June 1984/after June 1984.

sera submitted for ornithosis documentation did increase sharply. While the high percentage of sera showing TWAR antibody fell off after 1982 in Norway and Sweden, it remained high in Denmark until June 1984, the latter half of 1984 showing a very low prevalence. Only a few sera were available for testing after 1982 in Norway.

Despite the fact that retrospective serological study for TWAR is dependent on the timing of collection of sera, a high frequency of TWAR antibody was found in all three countries during the epidemic years. The fact that 10–20 % of ornithosis sera had acute TWAR antibody in the nonepidemic periods suggests that TWAR infection is endemic as well as causing epidemics in Scandinavia.

Clinical information was available on some patients from the epidemic in Denmark who were tested for TWAR (11). Of 73 persons in whom acute TWAR antibody was demonstrated in 1982, 31 were diagnosed as having pneumonia. A number of these patients had severe illnesses; 16 were hospitalized. Although none died, two had life-threatening spreading pneumonitis involving all areas of the lung. Both of these patients required ventilatory assistance and intravenous antibiotics, and the outcome of their illness was in doubt for several days. Both were middle-aged males in good health. The patients without pneumonia were diagnosed as having bronchitis, sinusitis or pharyngitis. Several had influenza-like illnesses followed by periods of cough and feeling tired.

Localized TWAR Epidemics in Finland. Table 10 presents data on a series of localized pneumonia epidemics in Finland that were associated with the development of TWAR antibody. The epidemic in civilians in 1978 in Kajaani provided the first evidence that the TW-183 strain isolated in 1965 was associated with human disease (2). This was an unusual pneumonia epidemic in that it was not recognized clinically, but on the basis of a chest radiograph survey for tuberculosis carried out in April and May 1978. The radiologist reading the films found an unusual incidence of acute pneumonitis and a retrospective study was undertaken. Sera from the patients were found to have chlamydia complement fixation antibodies. It was shown by micro-immuno-fluorescence with chlamydia antigens that 32 of the 34 persons with pneumonitis had serologic evidence of recent TWAR infection. When questioned three weeks later, 28 of the patients reported they had had a recognised illness around the time of their X-rays and about half had been given an antibiotic by their physician, although the diagnosis of pneumonia was not made. Five patients were completely asymptomatic, one was not available for a case history, and all had been well enough on the day that their radiograph was obtained to attend school or to be present at another site for the survey.

One of the military epidemics was in a battalion stationed just outside Kajaani and occurred from February to June 1978, covering the time of occurrence of a nearby civilian outbreak. We do not know the length of the civilian epidemic because it was made into a "common source like", brief, high-incidence epidemic by the common diagnostic method, the chest radiograph survey, which was carried out over two weeks.

Systematic laboratory studies of etiology of acute respiratory tract infections in military conscripts in Finland began in 1970 (16). Between 1970 and 1976, 4,000 such tests were carried out, and only three

Table 10: Circumscribed TWAR epidemics in Finland, pneumonia case rates, and results of the chlamydia complement-fixation (CF) and TWAR micro-immunofluorescence (IF) tests.

Epidemic		Pneumonia cases		Chlamydia CF		TWAR Micro-IF	
		Number	Rate/1000	Number tested	Percent positive	Number tested	Percent positive
Civilian Kajaani[a]	April–May 1978	35	17	34	82	34	91
Military							
Oulu[b]	March–Oct 1977	211	84	86	43	15	73
Kajaani[b]	Feb–June 1978	103	69	24	71	15	73
Tammisaari[b]	Jan–June 1985	60	60	35	51	13	100
Sodankyla[c]	June–Dec 1985	85	71	59	51	55	62

[a] Only one Kajaani civilian epidemic patient was chlamydia CF positive and TWAR micro-IF negative. Two of 34 had neither CF or micro-IF antibody.
[b] All sera tested for TWAR from Oulu, Kajaani and Tammisaari were CF positive.
[c] Of the 27 paired sera from Sodankyla that were CF positive, all were TWAR micro-IF positive. Of 28 CF negative sera, 7 were positive for TWAR.

showed chlamydia complement-fixation antibody. In 1977 and 1978 clusters of complement-fixation positive pneumonia were found in one base each year. Between 1978 and 1983 there were only a few sporadic complement-fixation positive results. In 1984 there were a few more, but it was not until 1985 that additional clusters of complement-fixation positive cases were found. They were in one camp during the first half of the year and at another during the second half. The size of the military groups with clusters of complement-fixation positive pneumonia shown in Table 10 varied from 1,000 to 2,500, and the rate of pneumonia from 60 to 84 per 1,000 persons. The epidemics lasted five to seven months. For the small population size this suggests a very slow spread for a respiratory agent.

Table 10 shows that in the Tammisaari epidemic all 13 tested had TWAR antibody. In the first three military epidemics, all the pneumonia patients tested for TWAR antibody had chlamydia complement-fixation antibody. In the Sodankyla epidemic, 27 of the 55 paired sera tested for TWAR antibody had complement-fixation antibody and all 27 showed TWAR infection. Seven of 28 sera negative for chlamydia complement-fixation antibody had evidence of current TWAR infection (16).

There were three cases of recurrent pneumonia in the same individual during the same epidemic. In each case the second episode of pneumonia was demonstrated radiographically to be in a different area of the lung, and in each case the trainee had received penicillin or ampicillin treatment of his pneumonia during the first episode. One of the recurrent episodes of pneumonia, perhaps a relapse, occurred three weeks after the onset of the first episode, while the others were two and three months after the first episode. In each case the trainee was hospitalized both times for pneumonia. TWAR etiologic data was available only for the second pneumonia episodes, but in each case the serologic pattern suggested reinfection with a very high IgG antibody titer and no or a low IgM and complement-fixation antibody titer. On the basis of population antibody studies, we postulate that reinfection with TWAR is common. This actual demonstration of reinfection in the epidemic situation fits the hypothesis but is surprising in the short interval between infections, suggesting that TWAR infection does not produce good protective antibody. This is similar to other chlamydial infections.

In the first two military epidemics in 1977 and 1978, the presence of chlamydia complement-fixation positive serologic reactions in the pneumonia cases was not established until late in the epidemic periods, and most of the patients were treated with penicillin or penicillin-like drugs, rather than tetracycline or erythromycin. While a control study was not done, it was possible to compare the TWAR antibody response in patients receiving penicillin or ampicillin and those receiving tetracycline for treatment. Although this comparison was not a designed study, the differences were so great that they appear meaningful. Of the patients in the first two epidemics whose sera were tested with TWAR antigen, nine received treatment with penicillin or ampicillin or both, and six received treatment with tetracycline only. There was a striking difference in the micro-immunofluorescence IgG antibody response to TWAR in the two groups. Four of the patients receiving penicillin developed IgG antibody at a titer of ⩾ 1024. The others had IgG antibody titers ranging from 64 to 512. Only one of the patients receiving tetracycline developed an IgG antibody titer ⩾ 32 and that patient had a titer of 64. A similar depressive effect on IgM TWAR antibody was not seen, and diagnostic serologic IgM titers were demonstrated. This finding is not without precedence, since Karl Meyer observed many years ago that prompt tetracycline treatment of psittacosis infections depressed the complementfixation antibody response (17).

In the Tammisaari garrison a special serologic study was done of entire companies of conscripts during the TWAR pneumonia epidemic. The findings suggested that 20–25% of the recruits underwent TWAR infection during the epidemic period. This would mean that 25 cases of pneumonia were recognized in 250 infected men, indicating that there were many mild or asymptomatic TWAR infections during the epidemic period (16).

Since 1985 there has been a continuing TWAR outbreak in Finland. While Finland escaped the country wide TWAR epidemics as in Norway, Denmark and Sweden in 1981–1983, it appears to have had a similar TWAR outbreak in 1986–1987.

By monitoring serum specimens submitted from military garrisons, evidence was found of TWAR infections in the Kajaani garrison in 1987. Prospective studies were done by Drs. P. Saikku and M.-K. Ekman. The epidemic lasted five months and peaked in March–April 1987. Pharyngeal swab specimens and paired blood samples were obtained in 86 of the military trainees during the epidemic. Dr. Saikku brought these specimens to Seattle and ten TWAR strains were isolated in our laboratory. Forty-seven of the specimens were obtained from outpatients over four days during the peak of the epidemic in late March. Although most had symptoms of acute respiratory infection, their illnesses were not considered severe enough to warrant hospitalization or a chest radiograph. Of the 47 patients, 16 had serologic evidence of TWAR infection, the organism being isolated from six of those with positive serological tests and none of those with negative serological tests. The other four TWAR isolates were obtained from hospitalized patients. Of the ten trainees from whom the TWAR organism was isolated, five showed the serologic pattern of a first infection, and five the pattern of reinfection. Chlamydia complement-fixing and TWAR micro-immunofluorescence IgM antibody was present in each of those considered to have a first infection. IgM antibody was absent in the patients considered to have reinfection and complement-fixing antibody appeared only in one, a patient who developed pneumonia. The reinfection cases all had four-fold IgG antibody titer rises up to 1024. The one patient with a reinfection antibody pattern who had pneumonia was the only one of the group hospitalized, while three of those with first infections had pneumonia and four were hospitalized. With one exception, the men with a primary infection had a longer illness and required more antibiotic treatment (usually two courses) than those with reinfection, two of whom required no treatment. The exception was the patient with reinfection who had pneumonia and was hospitalized. This patient had a prolonged illness of at least 25 weeks. Despite ten days of doxycycline therapy (150 mg/day) in the first episode of pneumonia-like illness, the patient had recurrent illness with a continuing cough. He developed erythema nodosum and later a bilateral fan-shaped infiltrate extending from the hilum of the lung. His illness was diagnosed as sarcoidosis. The patient experienced gradual resolution of this radiographic chest abnormality in July and August during the last two months of his military service.

These findings suggest that reinfection with the TWAR organism can be milder or more severe than initial infection. The trainees with reinfection disease probably had their first infection a relatively short time prior to the reinfection. They may have been infected earlier in the epidemic or during the year prior to military training when TWAR infection was common in Finland. It is possible that the patient who developed sarcoidosis was exhibiting a manifestation of an immunopathological reaction to TWAR reinfection, similar to that which has been demonstrated with *Chlamydia trachomatis* reinfection, both in the eye with the development of chronic trachoma (18), and in the female genital tract with chronic scarring of the fallopian tubes (19), resulting in infertility and ectopic pregnancy.

Paired serum specimens were obtained from 86 men in a company of recruits at Kajaani in March and at the end of their training in October. The serological results suggested that 70–75% of those susceptible were infected with TWAR during the epidemic. Nine percent of those developing antibody had pneumonia. This confirms the earlier estimation of a 1:10 ratio between pneumonia and non-pneumonia cases in TWAR infections during epidemics in military trainees (16). Others had various upper respiratory tract symptoms, and a few were asymptomatic.

Other Localized TWAR Epidemics. Other epidemics have been identified by micro-immunofluorescence serological tests with TWAR antigen. Two such epidemics were identified in Denmark. One occurred in 1976 in a Nike anti-aircraft battalion stationed outside Copenhagen. The men had acute respiratory infections, including some cases of pneumonia. In 1979 there was an outbreak among inhabitants of the island of Als that lies just south of Jutland. The outbreak occurred over the first six months in 1979, and the major clinical manifestation was an influenza-like illness with fever (14). The island's physicians, who became quite aware of this outbreak, did not see any similar cases among workers who came to a factory on Als by bridge from the Jutland mainland.

In collaboration with Pether, we have shown that the TWAR organism caused an epidemic of acute respiratory disease in a British boy's school in 1980, which Pether had reported as being associated with chlamydia complement-fixation antibody, but with no certain avian source (20). In collaboration with Anne-Lise Bruu, we identified TWAR as the cause of an outbreak of pneumonia and other acute respiratory infections in the county of Hordaland, Norway (which includes Bergen) in the winter of 1987. We have also recently obtained serological evidence of a TWAR outbreak in a US Army camp in 1984.

There are many reports in the literature of outbreaks of pneumonia and acute respiratory tract infections in both military and civilian groups, in which chlamydia complement-fixing antibodies have been detected without a convincing avian source (21–27). It seems likely that many of these outbreaks were due to TWAR infection. One of the most intriguing was in association with a number of cases of perimyocarditis. Sutton and his colleagues reported an epidemic of "urban psittacosis" in Chicago from 1961–1967, most cases occurring in 1963 and 1964 (28, 29). They found 40 cases of myocarditis with complement-fixing antibody as evidence of chlamydial infection out of 319 cases of myocarditis seen during this time span. There were 245 cases of chlamydial infection similarly diagnosed without myocarditis, many with acute febrile illnesses and acute respiratory disease, including pneumonia. While some of their patients with myocarditis and other syndromes gave a history of contact with psittacine birds or other birds or animals, no direct evidence of *Chlamydia psittaci* infection in any of these possible hosts was demonstrated. By studying many controls they presented convincing evidence that chlamydia complement-fixation antibody in the myocarditis patients suggested an etiologic relationship with a chlamydia agent that they assumed to be *Chlamydia psittaci*. It seems entirely possible that these cases could have been caused by TWAR.

Susceptibility of TWAR to Antimicrobial Agents

We have recently obtained laboratory data on antibiotic and sulfa drug sensitivity of TWAR organisms that support clinical observations (30). Table 11 shows that tetracycline and erythromycin are the most effective drugs as with other chlamydia. Sulfa drugs are not effective against TWAR, which is different from *Chlamydia trachomatis* although similar to most *Chlamydia psittaci* strains.

While clinical experience has shown that tetracycline and erythromycin are effective against TWAR organisms, intensive prolonged therapy is recommended. Until the results of comparative clinical studies are available, our current recommendation for treatment is 2 g tetracycline or erythromycin daily for 10 to 14 days. An alternate therapy schedule could be 1–1.5 g daily for 21 days.

Population Antibody Prevalence

We have tested sera from adults in a number of countries around the world for TWAR antibody (9). These sera come from population samples and studies of various disease, but the test results showed a remarkable similarity. Table 12 shows that in each country the prevalence of antibody was high, in each area a higher rate being found in men than in women. The average prevalence ranged from 25% in Nova Scotia to over 50% in Taiwan with an overall average of 40% in the seven countries. These rates are much higher than those observed in the same sera for all *Chlamydia trachomatis* serovars. We found that about 4% of males and up to 10% of females have *Chlamydia trachomatis* antibody in both these adult populations and in other populations tested (9).

Since this early publication on population antibody prevalence (9), we have had considerable experience with serological tests in isolation-proven TWAR cases and in TWAR epidemics. The results have shown that TWAR antibody at a titer of 16 for the IgM and IgG serum fractions is significantly associated with TWAR infection. In our earlier publications, when we knew less about patterns of serologic response to TWAR infection, we used a conservative interpretation and considered an antibody titer of 32 to be positive and of 16 to be questionable. Using a titer of 16 as positive had the effect of changing the average adult prevalence of TWAR antibody from 40% (Table 12) to 50%.

Figure 2 shows antibody prevalence by age in Denmark. We had enough serum from all age groups in Denmark and Seattle to study prevalence by age. The only difference in the rates in Seattle and in Denmark is that the big jump in prevalence in teenagers occurred in the age group 15 to 19 years in Seattle and 10 to 14 years in Denmark (9). The antibody rates are very

Table 11: Minimum inhibitory concentrations of four antibiotics and one sulfa drug for eight TWAR strains in HeLa 220 cell culture.

	MIC values (μg or U/ml)	
	Viability	Infectivity
Tetracycline	0.05–0.1	0.05–0.1
Erythromycin	0.01–0.05	0.01–0.05
Penicillin	>100	0.1–0.2
Ampicillin	>100	0.8–1.6
Sulfisoxazole	>400	≥400

Table 12: Prevalence of TWAR antibody in adults from different areas of the world. IgG antibody was demonstrated at titers of 32 to 256 in the microimmunofluorescence test.

Country[a]	Number tested	Percent with TWAR antibody	
		Male	Female
Seattle, USA	1042	45	36
Taiwan	64	59	52
Denmark	555	48	41
Finland	271	47	36
Nova Scotia, Canada	200	35	18
Japan	196	45	–
Panama	934	–	40

[a] The sera from Nova Scotia and Panama were from mostly well persons. The sera from Seattle and Denmark were from both well persons and persons with respiratory illnesses. The sera from Finland and Japan were from sexually transmitted disease patients.

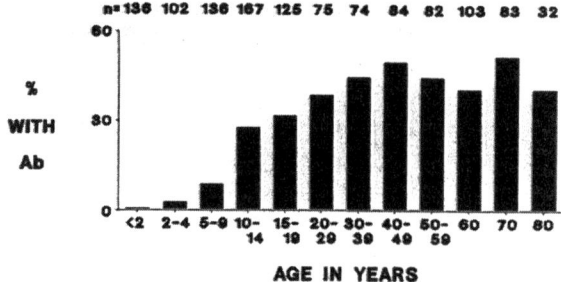

Figure 2: TWAR antibody by age group in Denmark in sera obtained 1977 to 1979. IgG antibody was demonstrated at a titer of 32 to 256 by the micro-immunofluorescence test.

low in young children in both countries; they begin to increase in teenagers, continue to increase until middle age and remain high into old age. The persistence of TWAR antibody into old age, a phenomenon not seen with *Chlamydia trachomatis* where antibody prevalence falls off sharply after the age of 40 to 50, suggests that reinfection with TWAR is common. In view of the expected decay of antibody after infection, the finding of TWAR antibody in nearly 50% of the adult population at one time suggests that most people are infected and reinfected during their life.

Age and sex infection rates in all our studies suggest that the age-sex TWAR antibody prevalence data is a good indication of infection rates. The infection is rare under five years of age, at least in the United States and Scandinavia, then the infection rate is rather similar throughout life into very old age. These age and sex rates suggest that transmission of TWAR may frequently occur outside the family, in schools, or in places of work or recreation.

We have found no evidence of a bird or animal host for TWAR. No avian source could be found for the Finnish epidemics. Our Seattle patients had no pet birds and few animals. Only a world-wide host with frequent human contact could produce the antibody prevalence rates observed. We have tested dogs and cats, and found no TWAR antibody. While the details of transmission of TWAR are not yet known, it is probably a pathogen spread entirely on a human-to-human basis.

TWAR Studies by Other Investigators

Investigators at the Institute of Ophthalmology in London have reported isolation of a *Chlamydia* agent from a specimen taken in 1967 from the eye of a child with trachoma in Iran that was similar immunologically to TW-183 in the micro-immunofluorescence test (31, 32). They have reported the results of serologic studies with their TWAR-like antigen in the micro-immunofluorescence test with sera from the UK and other countries. They found no evidence of association with eye disease, but did not study respiratory disease. They did find an increasing frequency of antibody in eye clinic patients in the UK from 1981 to 1984 (from 10% to 25%). While no interpretation was offered, we believe this provides evidence that Great Britain underwent a TWAR epidemic in the early 1980s similar to that observed in Scandinavia. Their antibody prevalence results closely parallel those discussed above, except that they show more variability in the frequency of antibody by country (32). At the Annual Meeting of the American Lung Association on May 9, 1988, C. M. Davis and colleagues presented a study of pneumonia patients in the Little Rock, Arkansas, Veterans Administration Hospital. They found serologic evidence of TWAR infection in 21, or 11%, of their patients.

Acknowledgement

These studies were supported in part by a Public Health Service grant No. AI-21885 from the National Institutes of Health, USA.

References

1. **Grayston, J. T., Kuo, C. C., Wang, S. P., Altman, J.:** A new *Chlamydia psittaci* strain called TWAR from acute respiratory tract infections. New England Journal of Medicine 1986, 315: 161–168.
2. **Saikku, P., Wang. S. P., Kleemola, M., Brander, E., Rusanen, E., Grayston, J. T.:** An epidemic of mild pneumonia due to an unusual *Chlamydia psittaci* strain. Journal of Infectious Diseases 1985, 151: 832–839.
3. **Moulder, J. W., Hatch, T. P., Kuo, C. C., Schachter, J., Storz, J.:** Genus 1. *Chlamydia* Jones, Rake and Stearns 1945, 55. In: Krieg, N. R. (ed.): Bergey's manual of systematic bacteriology. Volume 1. Williams and Wilkins, Baltimore, 1984, p. 729–739.
4. **Kuo, C. C., Chen, H. H., Wang, S. P., Grayston, J. T.:** Identification of a new group of *Chlamydia psittaci* strains called TWAR. Journal of Clinical Microbiology 1986, 24: 1034–1037.
5. **Chi, E. Y., Kuo, C. C., Grayston, J. T.:** Unique ultrastructure in the elementary body of *Chlamydia* species strain TWAR. Journal of Bacteriology 1987, 169: 3757–3763.
6. **Campbell, L. A., Kuo, C. C., Grayston, J. T.:** Characterization of the new *Chlamydia* agent, TWAR, as a unique organism by restriction endonuclease analysis and DNA: DNA hybridization. Journal of Clinical Microbiology 1987, 25: 1911–1916.
7. **Cox, R. L., Kuo, C. C., Grayston, J. T., Campbell, L. A.:** Deoxyribonucleic acid relatedness of *Chlamydia* species strain TWAR to *Chlamydia trachomatis* and *Chlamydia psittaci*. International Journal of Systematic Bacteriology 1988, 38: 265–268.
8. **Kuo, C. C., Grayston, J. T.:** Factors affecting the viability and the growth in HeLa 229 cells of the TWAR strain of *Chlamydia*. Journal of Clinical Microbiology 1988, 26: 812–815.
9. **Wang, S. P., Grayston, J. T.:** Micro-immunofluorescence serological studies with the TWAR organism. In: Oriel, J. D., Ridgway, G., Schachter, J., Taylor-Robinson, D., Ward, M. (ed.): Chlamydial infections. Cambridge University Press, Cambridge, 1986, p. 329–332.
10. **Meyer, K. F., Eddie, B., Schachter, J.:** Psittacosis-lymphogranuloma venereum agents. In: Lennette, E. H., Schmidt, N. J. (ed.): Diagnostic procedures for viral and rickettsial infections. American Public Health Association, New York, 1965, p. 869–903.
11. **Grayston, J. T., Kuo, C. C., Wang, S. P., Cooney, M. K., Altman, J., Marrie, T. J., Marshall, J. G., Mordhorst, C. H.:** Clinical findings in TWAR respiratory tract infections. In: Oriel, J. D., Ridgway, G., Schachter, J., Taylor-Robinson, D., Ward, M., (ed.): Chlamydial Infections. Cambridge University Press, Cambridge, 1986, p. 337–340.

12. Marrie, T. J., Grayston, J. T., Wang, S. P., Kuo, C. C.: Pneumonia associated with the TWAR strain of *Chlamydia*. Annals of Internal Medicine 1987, 106: 507–511.
13. Foy, H. M., Kenny, G. E., Cooney, M. K., Allan, I. D.: Long-term epidemiology of infections with *Mycoplasma pneumoniae*. Journal of Infectious Diseases 1979, 139: 681–687.
14. Mordhorst, C. H., Wang, S. P., Grayston, J. T.: Epidemic 'ornithosis' and TWAR infection, Denmark 1976–85. In: Oriel, J. D., Ridway, G., Schachter, J., Taylor-Robinson, D., Ward, M. (ed.): Chlamydial infections. Cambridge University Press, Cambridge, 1986, p. 325–328.
15. Bruu, A.-L., Aasen, S., Tjaland, S., Birkeland Flugsrud, L.: An outbreak of ornithosis in Norway in 1981. Scandinavian Journal of Infectious Diseases 1984, 16: 145–152.
16. Kleemola, M., Saikku, P., Visakorpi, R., Wang, S. P., Grayston, J. T.: Pneumonia epidemics in military trainees in Finland caused by TWAR, a new *Chlamydia* organism. Journal of Infectious Diseases 1988, 157: 230–236.
17. Meyer, K. F., Eddie, B.: The influence of tetracycline compounds on the development of antibodies in psittacosis. American Review of Tuberculosis and Pulmonary Diseases 1956, 74: 566–571.
18. Grayston, J. T., Wang, S. P., Yeh, L. J., Kuo, C. C.: The importance of reinfection in the pathogenesis of trachoma. Reviews of Infectious Diseases 1985, 7: 717–725.
19. Patton, D. L., Kuo, C. C., Wang, S. P., Halbert, S. A.: Distal tubal obstruction induced by repeated *Chlamydia trachomatis* salpingeal infections in pigtailed macques. Journal of Infectious Diseases 1987, 155: 1292–1299.
20. Pether, J. V. S., Noah, N. D., Lau, Y. K., Taylor, J. A., Bowie, J. C.: An outbreak of psittacosis in a boy's boarding school. Journal of Hygiene 1984, 92: 337–343.
21. Eng, J., Flottorp, A.: Para-ornithose. An epidemi av akutt luftveisinfeksjon med positiv lygranum-KBR. Tidsskrift for den Norske Laegeforening 1957, 77: 51–56.
22. Huseklepp, H., Oeding, P.: Ornithose. Nordisk Medicin 1957, 57: 370–373.
23. Orstavik, I., Loe, K. G., Davidsen, F. S.: Adenovirusinfeksjoner och ornithose blant militaere rekrutter. Nordisk Medicin 1969, 82: 1073–1077.
24. Andersson, E., Kjerulf-Jensen, K.: Ornithosis. Ugeskrift for Laeger 1957, 119: 1171–1174.
25. Löffler, H., Spengler, G. A., Riva, G., Stücki, P., Mangold, R.: Über gehäuftes Vorkommen von Lungeninfiltraten in Rekrutenschulen. Schweizerische Medizinische Wochenschrift 1956, 86: 967–975.
26. Fraser, P. K., Hatch, L. A., Shell, G. H., LeClerq, L. G. H., Pratt, D. W.: Minor respiratory illness caused by an agent of the psittacosis (lymphogranuloma-venereum group). Lancet, 1964, ii: 306–308.
27. Sundstrom, S., Bruu, A.-L., Jenum, P. A., Anestad, G.: Ornitoseepidemi. Garrisonen i Porsanger i 1982. Tidsskrift for den Norske Laegeforening 1986, 106: 820–823.
28. Sutton, G. C., Morrissey, R. A., Tobin, J. R., Anderson, T. O.: Pericardial and myocardial disease associated with serological evidence of infection by agents of the psittacosis-lymphogranuloma venereum group (*Chlamydiaceae*). Circulation 1967, 36: 830–838.
29. Sutton, G. C., Demakis, J. A., Anderson, T. O., Morrissey, R. A.: Serologic evidence of a sporadic outbreak in Illinois of infection by *Chlamydia* (psittacosis-LVG agent) in patients with primary myocardial disease and respiratory disease. American Heart Journal 1971, 81: 597–607.
30. Kuo, C. C., Grayston, J. T.: In vitro drug susceptibility of *Chlamydia* TWAR. Antimicrobial Agents and Chemotherapy 1988, 32: 257–258.
31. Dwyer, R. S. T. C., Treharne, J. D., Jones, B. R., Herring, J.: *Chlamydia* infection: results of microimmunofluorescence tests for the detection of type-specific antibody in certain chlamydial infections. British Journal of Venereal Diseases 1972, 48: 452–459.
32. Forsey, T., Darouger, S., Treharne, J. D.: Prevalence in human beings of antibodies to *Chlamydia* IOL-207, an atypical strain of *Chlamydia*. Journal of Infection 1986, 12: 145–152.

Current Status of Antiviral Chemotherapy for Genital Herpes Simplex Virus Infection: Its Impact on Disease Control

L. Corey

Acyclovir is an effective treatment for herpes simplex virus (HSV) infection. Its use produces improvement in symptoms and reduces the frequency of recurring disease. During chronic suppressive acyclovir therapy, breakthrough recurrences and asymptomatic viral shedding are common. Adverse reactions or signs of toxicity from acyclovir have been minimal. Early treatment does not prevent the estabilshment of latent HSV infection, the transmission of genital HSV infection, or asymptomatic viral shedding. Patient awareness of atypical lesions and modification of sexual activity are important aspects affecting transmission. Acyclovir resistance is being reported with increasing frequency, especially in patients infected with the human immunodeficiency virus. The development of additional antiviral agents would be beneficial in continuing the progress toward control of HSV infection.

The nucleotide analogue acyclovir has been shown to be an effective drug for the treatment of mucotaneous herpes simplex virus (HSV) infection (1, 2). Other antiviral agents have demonstrated clinical utility in selected patient populations with HSV infection (3–5). However, despite the advent of effective therapy for HSV infection, current evidence indicates that antiviral chemotherapy is having little impact in stopping the transmission and/or acquisition rates of genital HSV infection in the USA. This paper reviews current achievements in the chemotherapy of genital HSV infection and suggests new approaches to achieve clinical and epidemiological control of infection.

Current Status of Antiviral Chemotherapy for Treating Acute Episodes of Genital HSV Infection

HSV infection in immunologically normal individuals has a broad clinical spectrum that includes asymptomatic infection, recurrent, localized, oral-labial or genital lesions, severe frequently recurring disease, and episodes associated with systemic complications such as erythema multiforme, eczema herpeticum or recurrent aseptic meningitis (6). Primary genital HSV infection is characterized by widely spaced bilaterally distributed lesions, often complicated by fever, headache, malaise, myalgia and, in 10 % of the cases, aseptic meningitis. Untreated genital lesions last up to a month. In first-episode genital herpes, systemic rather than topical therapy is preferred because of the wide anatomic distribution of virus in the genitourinary tract. Acyclovir given by topical, oral and intravenous routes is effective in treating both primary and nonprimary genital HSV infections. Such treatment decreases the duration of lesions by 29, 35 and 57 %, the duration of viral shedding by 55, 80 and 85 %, and the duration of pain by 26, 44 and 57 %, respectively (7–14). It is recommended that all patients with painful and ulcerated first-episode genital lesions be treated with oral acyclovir in a dose of 200 mg five times daily for 7–10 days. Unfortunately, there is no evidence that treatment of first-episode genital HSV infection with acyclovir has any effect on reducing the frequency of subsequent recurrence rates (15).

In recurrent genital HSV infection in immunocompetent people, topical acyclovir shortens the duration of viral shedding but does not significantly effect the duration of pain or time to healing (16). Similarly, oral acyclovir does not reduce symptoms of recurrent genital HSV episodes but does decrease the duration of viral shedding and slightly reduces the time to healing (13, 17). Tables 1 and 2 summarize current recommendations for the use of acyclovir in treating genital herpes infections.

Suppressive Acyclovir Therapy

Rates of recurrent genital herpes vary with time of infection. Most patients who seek medical attention for symptomatic genital HSV infection report five to eight recurrences per year (6). In several studies, over

Departments of Laboratory Medicine, Medicine and Microbiology, University of Washington, Seattle, Washington 98195, USA.

Table 1: Current status of antiviral chemotherapy of mucocutaneous HSV infections with acyclovir.

Patient status and disease	Treatment and benefits
Immunosuppressed	
Acute symptomatic first or recurrent episodes	i.v. or oral relieves pain and speeds healing; topical for localized external lesions
Suppression of reactivation	i.v. or oral taken daily prevents recurrences during high risk periods (e.g. immediately after organ transplant)
Immunocompetent	
Symptomatic first episode	oral treatment is choice; i.v. may be used if severe disease or neurologic complications are present; topical in patients without cervical, urethral or first episode pharyngeal involvement
Symptomatic recurrent gential herpes	oral shortens course and viral excretion; not recommended for all episodes
Suppression of recurrent gential herpes	oral daily prevents reactivation of symptomatic recurrences; licensure limited to 6 months
First episodes of oral-labial HSV	oral not studied; possibly effective
Recurrent episodes	oral of minimal benefit
Suppression of recurrence (UV provoked)	oral offers possible prevention if started 24 h prior to exposure and continued
Herpetic whitlow	oral beneficial (anecdotal)
Proctitis	oral shortens course
Corneal ulcer	topical

Table 2: Dosage regimen of acyclovir treatment of HSV infections.

Immunocompetent patients	
CNS infection	i.v. 10 mg/kg every 8 h, 10 days; oral not recommended
First episode gential herpes	i.v. 5 mg/kg every 8 h, 5 days
	oral 200 mg 5 times/day, 10 days
Recurrent genital herpes	oral 200 mg 5 times/day, 5 days
Suppression of HSV infection	oral 200 mg t.i.d. or 400 mg b.i.d.
Immunosuppressed patients	
Acute lesions	i.v. 5 mg/kg every 8 h, 7–14 days
	oral 200–400 mg 5 times/day, 7–14 days
	topical 4–6 times/day, 7–10 days
Suppression of HSV infection	oral 400 mg t.i.d. (higher dosages can be used)

2.000 patients with frequently recurring genital HSV infection (4–12 episodes per year) were given acyclovir in doses of 200 mg two to five times daily for up to two years. With daily therapy, 65 to 85 % of the patients remained completely free of recurrences during treatment (18–21). Such suppressive therapy produces relief of symptoms and has been of major medical and psychosocial benefit to these patients. The issues in chronic suppressive therapy are the duration of therapy, the emergence of resistance in the patient populations for which this treatment regimen should be utilized, and the dosage form.

The dosage of acyclovir used for chronic suppressive therapy of genital herpes has varied among studies. Early observations suggested that 200 mg capsules taken two, three, four or five times daily were of similar efficacy (18–21). Cost and potential long-term toxicities require simple and convenient dosage regimens to achieve maximum compliance. The use of twice-daily 400 mg doses has been found to be an optimal initial regimen in immunocompetent patients. Recent preliminary data indicate that once-daily dosing with 800 mg may be effective in preventing recurrences and may result in enhanced compliance (22). After two to three months of therapy, it is often possible to reduce the dose to 200 mg three times daily or 400 mg once daily. On these regimens more than 90 % of persons with frequently recurrent genital herpes who are immunocompetent have a significant reduction in the number of clinical recurrences.

About 25 % of persons on suppressive therapy have a breakthrough recurrence during each three-month period. Thus, it is likely that most patients on chronic suppressive therapy will, at some time, experience a breakthrough recurrence. In long-term studies the frequency of breakthrough recurrences is not changed during the period that medication is given (23). Compared with untreated recurrences, breakthrough recurrences are associated with milder symptoms, shorter duration of viral shedding, and shorter duration of lesions (18, 21). Data are not available on the effect of chronic suppressive acyclovir on the frequency of asymptomatic genital tract excretion of HSV and how this may impact the subsequent risk of transmission of disease. Published reports and our own experience indicate that occasional cases of transmission may occur during therapy. The event usually occurs from sexual activity at the time of a mild breakthrough recurrence (24).

No data are available to suggest that short-term acyclovir is useful as a "morning-after pill" to protect seronegative individuals from primary infection after contact with a sexual partner who has active lesions. If acyclovir increased the frequency of asymptomatic primary infection, this strategy may even be harmful.

Toxicity of Suppressive Acyclovir

Many patients desire to take oral acyclovir for prolonged periods for which studies of potential toxicity are inadequate. Preclinical animal studies of acyclovir showed no drug-related carcinogenicity, effect on fertility, or abnormal fetal development (25). Acyclovir has been shown to be mutagenic in two of 11 in vitro systems. The implications of the results of chronic suppressive acyclovir therapy in humans, including its use during conception and pregnancy, are unknown. Until studies defining its role and safety in pregnancy are available, the use of oral acyclovir in pregnancy cannot be advocated. Chronic suppressive therapy in doses of 200 mg two to five times daily has had no effect on spermatogenesis (26). Side effects of daily suppressive oral acyclovir are uncommon. In a multicenter trial that included more than 1,000 patients taking suppressive therapy for one year, no significant clinical or laboratory toxicity was observed (23).

Clinical Indications for the Use of Acyclovir for Recurrent Genital HSV Infection

The most common criterion on which to base a decision about the use of intermittent versus chronic suppressive acyclovir therapy is the number and severity of the recurrences (27). Patients with frequently recurring genital herpes who have considerable physical discomfort, emotional upset and increased potential for transmission of infection to sexual partners are candidates in persons with six or more recurrences per year ($1.50–2.00 per day for medication). Fewer recurrences are probably best managed with intermittent oral therapy. People with frequent recurrences who are minimally symptomatic and not at risk of transmitting infection to an uninfected partner also may be best served by intermittent therapy. Studies indicate that it takes from five to seven days of therapy before clinical effects can be seen (18, 21). Intermittent use, for example weekend therapy, has been associated with subsequent clinical recurrences and transmission, indicating that acyclovir must be administered on a daily basis (28, 29).

Acyclovir Therapy During Pregnancy

First-episode primary genital herpes at or near term can cause high morbidity in the mother and infant. In this setting intravenous acyclovir may be useful (30, 31). Recurrent genital herpes late in the third trimester of pregnancy is a theoretical indication for short-term suppressive acyclovir therapy to prevent an episode of disease near the time of delivery and thus avoid the need for cesarean section. The incidence of HSV infection in neonates born to women with HSV-2 antibody is low (about one in 2,000 births). Routine use of acyclovir in seropositive women to prevent neonatal HSV infection is not indicated. Among women with frequently recurring genital HSV infection, which necessitates a high rate (50 %) of cesarean section deliveries, effective prophylaxis would be desirable. However, no studies are available showing the safety or utility of suppressive oral acyclovir in pregnancy, especially its effect on asymptomatic viral shedding.

Emergence of Resistance

In vitro resistance to acyclovir can result from thymidine kinase (TK)-deficient, TK-altered, or DNA polymerase-resistant strains of HSV (32, 33). Thymidine kinase deficiency is the most common mechanismen of resistance of HSV to acyclovir (34–36). Animal studies have suggested that TK-deficient mutants are less virulent and less able to establish neural latency (37), although some strains can do so (38).

Acyclovir-resistant strains of HSV have been recovered from patients who have never been treated with acyclovir (39). The clinical significance of acyclovir resistance is further confounded by isolation of TK-deficient mutants from lesions in patients who have responded to treatment with acyclovir (40); no clear relationship has been established between response to prophylactic therapy and in vitro testing of specific clinical isolates (41). Similarly, the relationship between in vitro resistance to acyclovir and the subsequent development of breakthrough recurrences during suppressive therapy is unclear. In some studies breakthrough isolates with resistance to acyclovir in vitro have found, whereas in others HSV isolates were susceptible (21, 41).

Most resistant isolates have been recovered from immunocompromised patients undergoing multiple courses of therapy for established infection. Increasing acyclovir resistance has recently been seen in patients infected with human immunodeficiency virus (HIV) who have received intermittent and/or suppressive acyclovir therapy for long periods. Resistance has been associated with persistent cutaneous lesions, which can be cleared by the use of alternative antiviral chemotherapy, especially intravenous foscarnate. The observations indicate that acyclovir-resistant mutants can cause severe disease. Thus, continued surveillance of HSV strains associated with breakthrough recurrences and/or persistent mucotaneous HSV infection is needed. Routine in vitro testing of HSV isolates for acyclovir sensitivity is not recommended. Isolates from patients who report persistent HSV infections while on therapy, especially those from patients who have HIV infection, should be tested for acyclovir resistance. If the recent increase in acyclovir resistance in HIV-infected patients continues, alternative antiviral chemotherapy may be required.

Current Epidemiology of Genital HSV Infection in the USA

HSV infections continue to be widespread in the USA. Between 1969 and 1984, visits to practitioners for genital herpes increased tenfold (42, 43). At the Sexually Transmitted Diseases (STD) Clinic of the King County Hospital in Seattle, Washington, genital HSV infections accounted for 8.2 % of all new patient visits between 1980 and 1984, and 7.6 % from 1985 through 1987. Neonatal HSV infection increased from four cases per 100,000 live births in the years 1970–1973 to 15.8 cases per 100,000 live births in the years 1982–1984 (44).

Recent surveys show that the seroprevalence of HSV-2 infection is much more widely distributed and more frequent than clinical illness. Of the women attending the King County STD Clinic between 1984 and 1986, 46 % possessed HSV-2 antibodies. Similar rates of infection have been found in men and women attending other clinics (A. Nahmias, personal communication). Seroprevalence of HSV-2 infection in the general U.S. population varies between 20 and 50 %, depending on race, socioeconomic status, demographics and history of past sexual behavior (45). These data indicate the widespread difference between the seroprevalence of HSV-2 and its frequency of diagnosis, even in STD clinics, and suggest that many genital HSV-2 infections are either asymptomatic, underdiagnosed or both.

Inapparent and Asymptomatic HSV Infection: Its Importance in Disease Acquisition and Transmission

Several questions remain unanswered concerning the pathogenesis and clinical spectrum of genital HSV infection. For example, it is not known whether all persons with HSV antibody are latently infected with virus, and whether all intermittently reactivate. The titer of virus shed from asymptomatic episodes is lower than that from symptomatic episodes, but it is unknown whether infected carriers transmit infection. Recent studies using in situ hybridization show latent HSV in trigeminal nerve root ganglia and/or recurrences of lesions after primary inoculation in nearly all seropositive persons or animals (46, 47). On this basis it must be assumed that people who are HSV-2 seropositive have latent ganglionic infection.

The importance of asymptomatic carriers in disease transmission has been illustrated in several studies. Two have shown that source partners with unrecognized lesions account for at least half of the cases of transmission of first-episode genital herpes (48, 49). Many of these seropositive persons have mild genital lesions which are undiagnosed. Obtaining an accurate medical history of genital herpes is difficult. It has been shown that when an anamnestic history revealed no genital herpes, prospective evaluation and repeat questioning often indicated atypical genital ulcerations that had not been recognized as genital HSV infection by either the patient or the physician (49). This suggests that seropositive persons who claim they are asymptomatic may in fact have atypical mildly symptomatic lesions that are recognized only when the patient is educated about the clinical manifestations of the disease. Antiviral chemotherapy and counseling of these patients might be a means of interrupting disease transmission.

While unidentified lesions are important in the transmission of infection, asymptomatic carriers also transmit genital herpes (24). Recently, genital HSV infection was shown to have occurred from HSV in semen given by insemination from a donor with asymptomatic primary genital HSV-2 infection (50).

A Perspective

Much progress has been made in the therapy of HSV infection in the past decade, but the diversity of clinical lesions, the wide anatomic distribution of HSV in the genitourinary tract and the unavailability of modern diagnostic methods in many clinical settings result in underdiagnosis of HSV infections. The advent of effective antiviral chemotherapy does not appear to have changed the epidemiology of genital HSV infection because of the high rate of unrecognized infection by both patients and practitioners. In the last decade research has concentrated on identification of the symptomatic carrier with typical disease and/or frequent recurrences. The role of persons with mild or ignored symptoms and the asymptomatic carrier needs to be addressed. This will require the continued development and use of accurate diagnostic assays and virologic studies for discriminating episodes of HIV-1 and -2 infection. Chronic latency with periodic shedding of virus poses a major challenge to effective antiinfective therapy.

Acknowledgement

This work was supported by NIH Grant AI-20381.

References

1. Elion, G.: Selectivity of action of an antiherpetic agent 9-(2-hydroxyethoxymethyl) guanine. Proceedings of the National Academy of Sciences of the USA 1977, 74: 5716.
2. Dorsky, D. I., Crumpacker, C. S.: Drugs 5 years later. Annals of Internal Medicine 1987, 207 (Supplement 6): 859–874.
3. Pazin, G. H., Harger, J. H., Armstrong, J. A.: Leukocyte interferon for treating first episodes of genital herpes in women. Journal of Infectious Diseases 1987, 156: 891–898.
4. Mindel, A., Kinghorn, G., Allison, J. E.: Treatment of first attack genital herpes, acyclovir versus Inosine Pranobex. Lancet 1987, i: 1171–1173.
5. Sacks, S. L., Portnoy, J., Loweed, D.: Clinical course of recurrent genital herpes and treatment with foscarnate: results of a Canadian multicenter trial. Journal of Infectious Diseases 1987, 155: 178–186.
6. Corey, L., Adams, H. G., Brown, Z. A., Holmes, K. K.: Genital herpes simplex virus infection: clinical manifestations, course and complications. Annals of Internal Medicine 1983, 98: 958–972.
7. Bryson, Y. J., Dillon, M., Lovett, M., Acuma, G., Taylor, S., Cherry, J. D., Johnson, B. L., Wiesmeier, E., Growdon, W., Creagh-Kirk, T., Keeney, R.: Treatment of first episodes of genital herpes simplex virus infection with oral acyclovir; a randomized double blind controlled trial in normal subjects. New England Journal of Medicine 1983, 308: 916–921.
8. Corey, L., Benedetti, J., Critchlow, C., Mertz, C., Douglas, J., Fife, K., Fahnlander, A., Remington, M. L., Winter, C., Dragavon, J.: Treatment of primary first-episode genital herpes simplex virus infections with acyclovir: results of topical, intravenous, and oral therapy. Journal of Antimicrobial Chemotherapy 1983, 12 (Supplement B): 79–88.
9. Corey, L., Fife, K. H., Benedetti, J. K., Winter, C. A., Fahnlander, A., Conner, J. D., Hintz, M. A., Holmes, K. K.: Intravenous acyclovir for the treatment of primary genital herpes. Annals of Internal Medicine 1983, 98: 914–921.
10. Fiddian, A. P., Kinghorn, G. R., Goldmeier, D., Reese, E., Rodin, P., Thin, R. N. T., deKonig, G. A. J.: Topical acyclovir in the treatment of genital herpes: a comparison with systemic therapy. Journal of Antimicrobial Chemotherapy 1983, 12 (Supplement B): 67–77.
11. Mertz, G. J., Critchlow, C. W., Benedetti, J., Reichman, R. C., Dolin, R., Connor, J., Redfield, D. C., Savoia, M. C., Richman, D. D., Tyrell, D. L., Miedzinski, L., Portnoy, J., Keeney, R. E.: Double blind placebo controlled trial of oral acyclovir in first-episode genital herpes simplex virus infection. Journal of the American Medical Association 1984, 252: 1147–1151.
12. Mindel, A., Adler, M. W., Sutherland, S., Fiddian, A. P.: Intravenous acyclovir treatment for primary genital herpes. Lancet 1982, i: 697–700.
13. Nilsen, A. E., Aasen, T., Halsos, A. M., Kinge, B. R., Tjotta, E. A. L., Wilkstrom, K., Fiddian, A. P.: Efficacy of oral acyclovir in treatment of initial and recurrent genital herpes. Lancet 1982, ii: 572–573.
14. Thin, R. N., Nabarro, J. M., Parker, J. D., Fiddian, A. P.: Topical acyclovir in the treatment of initial genital herpes. British Journal of Venereal Disease 1983, 59: 116–119.
15. Mindel, A., Weller, I. V. D., Faherty, A., Sutherland, S., Fiddian, A. P., Adler, M. W.: Acyclovir in first attacks of genital herpes and prevention of recurrences. Genitourinary Medicine 1986, 62: 28–32.
16. Corey, L., Benedetti, J. K., Critchlow, C. W., Remington, M. L., Winter, C. A., Fahnlander, A. L., Smith, K., Salter, D., Keeney, R. E., Davis, L. G., Hintz, M. A., Conner, J. D., Holmes, K. K.: Double blind controlled trial of topical acyclovir in genital herpes simplex virus infections. American Journal of Medicine 1982, 73 (Supplement 1A): 326–334.
17. Reichman, R. C., Badger, G. J., Mertz, G. J., Corey, L., Richman, D. D., Connor, J. D., Redfield, D., Savoia, M. C., Oxman, M. N., Bryson, Y., Tyrrell, D. L., Portnoy, J., Creigh-Kirk, T., Keeney, R. E., Ashikaga, T., Dolin, R.: Treatment of recurrent genital herpes simplex infections with oral acyclovir: a controlled trial. Journal of the American Medical Association 1984, 251: 2103–2107.
18. Douglas, J. M., Critchlow, C., Benedetti, J., Mertz, G. J., Conner, J. D., Hintz, M. A., Fahnlander, A., Remington, M., Winter, C., Corey, L.: A double-blind study of oral acyclovir for suppression of recurrences of genital herpes simplex virus infection. New England Journal of Medicine 1984, 310: 1551–1556.
19. Halsos, A. M., Salo, O. P., Lassus, A., Tjotta, E. A. L., Havi, T., Gabrielsen, B., Fiddian, A. P.: Oral acyclovir suppression of recurrent genital herpes: a double-blind, placebo-controlled crossover study. Acta Dermato-Venereologica 1985, 65: 59–63.
20. Mindel, A., Faherty, A., Hindley, D., Adler, M. W., Weller, I. V. D., Sutherland, S., Fiddian, A. P.: Prophylactic oral acyclovir in recurrent genital herpes. Lancet 1986, ii: 57–59.
21. Straus, S. E., Takiff, H. E., Mindell, S., Seidlin, M., Bachrach, S., Lininger, L., DiGiovanna, J. J., Western, K. A., Smith, H. A., Nusinoff-Lehrman, S., Creagh-Kirk, T., Alling, D. W.: Suppression of frequently recurring genital herpes; a placebo controlled double blind trial of oral acyclovir. New England Journal of Medicine 1984, 310: 1545–1550.
22. Mindel, A., Faherty, A., Carney, O., Patou, G., Freris, M., Williams, P.: Long term suppressive acyclovir therapy – dosage and safety in patients with recurrent genital herpes. Lancet 1988, i: 926–928.
23. Mertz, G., Jones, C., Mills, J., Fife, K. H., Lemon, S., Stapleton, J. T., Hill, E. L., Davis, L. G., and the Acyclovir Study Group: Long term acyclovir suppression of frequently recurring genital herpes simplex virus infection: a multicenter double blind trial. Journal of the American Medical Association 1988, 260 (Supplement 2): 201–206.
24. Rooney, J. F., Felser, J. M., Ostrove, J. M., Strause, S. E.: Acquisition of genital herpes from an asymptomatic sexual partner. New England Journal of Medicine 1986, 34: 1561–1564.
25. Tucker, W. E.: Preclinical toxicology of acyclovir: an overview. American Journal of Medicine, Acyclovir Symposium, 1982, p. 27–30.
26. Douglas, J. M., Davis, L. G., Remington, M. L., Paulsen, C. A., Perrin, E. B., Goodman, P., Conner, J. D., King, D., Corey, L.: A double-blind placebo-controlled trial of the effect of chronic oral acyclovir on sperm production in men with frequently recurrent genital herpes. Journal of Infectious Diseases 1988, 157: 588–593.
27. Gold, D., Corey, L.: Acyclovir prophylaxis for herpes simplex virus infection. Antimicrobial Agents and Chemotherapy, 1987, 361–367.
28. Straus, S. E., Seidlin, M., Takiff, H. E., Rooney, J. F., Nusinoff-Lehrman, S., Bachrach, S., Felser, J. M., Giovanna, J. J., Grimes, G. J., Krakauer, H., Hallanan, C., Alling, D.: Double blind comparison of weekend and daily regimens of oral acyclovir for suppression of recurrent genital herpes. Antiviral Research 1986, 6: 151–159.

29. Shepp, D. H., Dandliker, P. S., Flournoy, N., Meyers, J. D.: Once-daily intravenous acyclovir for prophylaxis of herpes simplex virus reactivation after marrow transplantation. Journal of Antimicrobial Chemotherapy 1985, 16: 389–395.
30. Brown, Z. A., Vontver, L. A., Benedetti, J., Critchlow, C. W., Sells, C. J., Berry, S., Corey, L.: Effects on the infants of first episode genital herpes during pregnancy. New England Journal of Medicine 1987, 317: 1247–1251.
31. Lagrew, D. C., Furlow, T. G., Hager, D., Yarrish, D. L.: Dissemianted herpes simplex virus infection in pregnancy: succesful treatment with acyclovir. Journal of the American Medical Association 1984, 252: 2038–2039.
32. Coen, D. M., Schaffer, P. A.: Two distinct loci confer resistance to acycloguanosine in herpes simplex virus type 1. Proceedings of the National Academy of Sciences of the USA 1980, 77: 2265–2269.
33. Crumpacker, C. S., Schnipper, L. E., Marlowe, S. I., Kowalsky, P. N., Hershey, B. J., Levin, M. J.: Resistance to antiviral drugs of herpes simplex virus isolated from a patient treated with acyclovir. New England Journal of Medicine 1982, 306: 343–346.
34. Barry, D. W., Lehrman, S. N., Ellis, M. N.: Clinical and laboratory experience with acyclovir-resistant herpesviruses. Journal of Antimicrobial Chemotherapy 1986, 18 (Supplement B): 75–84.
35. Dekker, C., Ellis, M. N., McLaren, C., Hunter, G., Rogers, J., Barry, D. W.: Virus resistance in clinical practice. Journal of Antimicrobial Chemotherapy 1983, 12 (Supplement B): 137–152.
36. Burns, W. H., Santos, G. W., Leitman, P. S., Saral, R., Laskin, O. L., McLaren, C., Barry, D. W.: Isolation and characterization of resistant herpes simplex virus after acylcovir therapy. Lancet 1982, i: 421–423.
37. Field, H. J., Darby, G.: Pathogenicity in mice of strains of herpes simplex virus which are resistant to acyclovir in vitro and in vivo. Antimicrobial Agents and Chemotherapy 1980, 17: 209–216.
38. Parris, D. S., Harrington, J. E.: Herpes simplex virus variants resistant to high concentrations of acyclovir exist in clinical isolates. Antimicrobial Agents and Chemotherapy 1982, 22: 71–77.
39. McLaren, C., Corey, L., Dekker, C., Barry, D. W.: In vitro sensitivity to acyclovir in genital herpes simplex viruses from acyclovir treated patients. Journal of Infectious Diseases 1983, 148: 868–875.
40. Meyers, J. D.: Treatment of herpesvirus infections in the immunocompromised host. Scandinavian Journal of Infectious Disease 1985, Supplement 47: 128–136.
41. Nusinoff-Lehrman, S., Douglas, J. M., Corey, L., Barry, D. W.: Recurrent genital herpes and suppressive oral acyclovir therapy: relationship between clinical outcome and in vitro drug sensitivity. Annals of Internal Medicine 1986, 104: 786–790.
42. Division of Sexually Transmitted Diseases, Center for Prevention Services, Centers for Disease Control: Genital herpes infection – United States, 1966–1984. Morbidity and Mortality Weekly Report 1986, 35: 402–404.
43. Chuang, T.-Y., Su, W. P. D., Perry, H. O., Ilstrup, D. M., Kurland, L. T.: Incidence and trend of herpes progenitalis: a 15 year population study. Mayo Clinic Proceedings 1983, 58: 436–441.
44. Sullivan-Bolyai, J., Hull, H. F., Wilson, C., Corey, L.: Neonatal herpes simplex virus infections in King County, Washington, Journal of the American Medical Association 1983, 250: 3059–3062.
45. Corey, L., Spear, P. G.: Infections with herpes simplex viruses. Parts I and II. New England Journal of Medicine 1986, 314: 686–691, 749–757.
46. Stevens, J. G., Wagner, E. K., Rao, G. B., Cook, M. L., Feldman, L. T.: RNA complementary to a herpes virus alpha gene mRNA is prominent in latently infected neurons. Science 1987, 235: 1056–1059.
47. Croen, K. D., Ostrove, J. M., Dragovic, L. J., Smialek, J. E., Straus, S. E.: Latent herpes simplex virus in human trigeminal gnaglia: detection of an immediate early gene "anti-sense" transcript by in situ hybridization. New England Journal of Medicine 1987, 317: 1427–1432.
48. Mertz, G. J., Schmidt, O., Jourden, J. L., Guinan, M. E., Remington, M. L., Fahnlander, A., Winter, C., Holmes, K. K., Corey, L.: Frequency of acquisition of first episode genital infection with herpes simplex virus from symptomatic and asymptomatic source contacts. Sexually Transmitted Diseases 1985, 12: 33–39.
49. Mertz, G. J., Coombs, R. W., Ashley, R., Jourden, J., Remington, M., Winter, C., Fahnlander, A., Guinan, M., Ducey, H., Corey, L.: Transmission of genital herpes in couples with one symptomatic and one asymptomatic partner: a prospective study. Journal of Infectious Diseases 1988, 157: 1169–1177.
50. Moore, D. E., Zarutskie, P. W., Soules, M. R., Ashley, R., Dragavon, J., Remington, M., Corey, L.: Transmission of genital herpes by artificial insemination with a donor experiencing asymptomatic primary HSV-2 infection. Journal of the American Medical Association (in press).

Induction and Maintenance Therapy for Opportunistic Infections in Patients with AIDS

M. A. Sande

The acquired immunodeficiency syndrome (AIDS) has clearly illustrated the vital role of an effective cellular immune system in the successful chemotherapy of many infections. Most drugs used to treat fungal, protozoan, viral, and some bacterial infections are capable of inhibiting growth of the pathogen (static), but do not kill or destroy it. These static agents require an effective cellular immune (monocyte-macrophage) system to ensure that the infecting organism(s) is eradicated and relapse prevented. The cellular immune system is severely impaired in patients with advanced human immunodeficiency virus (HIV) infection (AIDS). Thus, a more aggressive approach to therapy of infections complicating HIV disease is emerging. This approach, which includes an initial induction phase followed by a chronic suppressive or maintenance phase, comprises a strategy that mimics the approach of the oncologist to chemotherapy of malignancies.

Justification for Two-Stage (Induction-Maintenance) Antimicrobial Strategy

Many of the clinical infections that complicate advanced HIV infection or AIDS are due to the reactivation of latent infections acquired earlier in life but held "in check" by an intact cellular immune response. As the HIV destroys this system by, among other things, relentlessly destroying the T4 (helper) lymphocytes, these organisms are activated and begin to proliferate, ultimately producing clinical disease. Since reconstitution of this immune system generally does not occur, control of infection is nearly completely dependent on antimicrobial chemotherapy. It is therefore not surprising that most of these infections are incurable, and that most, while characterized by an initial clinical and microbiological response to treatment, will progress once drugs are discontinued. Gradually over the past seven years a strategy has emerged by trial and error that utilizes a two-phase approach to chemotherapy.

Initially, an induction phase using conventional-dose antimicrobial therapy is used to control the acute infection, to ameliorate symptoms, and to reduce organism titers. This strategy is based on the assumption that higher-dose therapy will rapidly lower the titer of organisms. Since residual viable organisms apparently persist, it is usually necessary to follow the induction phase of treatment with chronic suppressive or maintenance chemotherapy after allowing for a therapeutic interval that typically ensures cure in the non-AIDS patient. This has been approached by using the same drug that was used in the induction phase (but in a lower dose or with less frequent administration), another less toxic drug, or one that can be administered orally. The following are some of the infections that have been managed in this manner.

Pneumocystic Pneumonia

Pneumocystis carinii pneumonia (PCP) is an illness that occurs in more than 80% of AIDS patients. Historically, PCP occurring as a complication of corticosteroid therapy or in patients with hematological malignancies could be cured with a two- to three-week course of parenteral pentamidine or high-dose trimethoprim-sulfamethoxazole. While this approach is successful in controlling infection in over 80% of AIDS patients, up to 50% of them will relapse in the six- to nine-month period following discontinuation of therapy (1). If maintenance therapy is employed, however, relapse rates can be reduced to less than 5% in that time period (2). It is interesting that most of the maintenance regimens that have been tested appear to be effective, including therapy with orally administered trimethoprim-sulfamethoxazole, Fansidar®, inhaled aerosolized pentamidine at various doses administered every 14 days, and parenteral pentamidine given every two to four weeks. Numerous studies are currently in progress to identifiy the least toxic, most practical, and most effective regimen.

Toxoplasmosis

Patients with advancing HIV infection also become susceptible to activation of *Toxoplasma gondii*, a common protozoan parasite latently present in nearly 50% of the American population. While the acute infection in the normal host is either asymptomatic or present as a "mononucleosis-like syndrome", reactivation in the AIDS patient, who has a falling T4 lymphocyte count, usually presents as focal lesion(s) in the brain. Patients with this infection respond remarkably well to oral therapy with sulfadiazine and pyrimethamine. The mass lesion will usually improve or disappear completely (as judged by computed tomographic scanning) after several weeks of therapy, but reappearance of the lesion or relapse will occur in most patients if therapy is discontinued. Therefore, maintenance therapy is employed by most physicians caring for AIDS patients (3).

Fungal Infections

HIV-infected patients are also susceptible to infection with pathogenic fungi. Cryptococcal meningitis is a common infection in the AIDS patient population, occurring in up to 10% of the patients; more than 150 cases of this infection have been treated at San Francisco General Hospital since 1981 (S. L. Chuck and M. A. Sande, unpublished observation). Whether these cases represent reactivation or newly acquired infections is not clear. Amphotericin B (0.5–0.8 mg/kg/day i.v.) is highly effective in ameliorating symptoms, producing a drop in cryptococcal antigen titers and usually eliminating cryptococci from the cerebrospinal fluid. 5-flucytosine is often added in the initial phase of therapy, but its value in the AIDS patient has yet to be determined, and it appears to add significantly to bone marrow toxicity. If therapy is discontinued after a six- to ten-week course (which is adequate to cure the vast majority of cryptococcal infections in non-AIDS patients), relapse will occur in most patients (4). Various maintenance regimens, including amphotericin (1 mg/kg i.v. once a week, a regimen that appears to be quite effective, although published data are sparse) and orally administered ketoconazole, have been employed. Although relapses have been observed with both regimens, patients at San Francisco General Hospital who received maintenance therapy had a longer median survival (S. L. Chuck and M. A. Sande, unpublished observation). It is hoped that fluconazole, a new imidazole derivative with excellent activity against cryptococci and improved penetration into the cerebrospinal fluid, will prove even more useful in this setting.

Another fungal infection that may be reactivated when the cellular immune system is destroyed by the HIV is caused by *Histoplasma capsulatum*. Reactivation of histoplasmal infection leads to widespread hematogenous dissemination of the organism to the lungs, liver, spleen, lymph nodes, and bone marrow. Response to conventional (induction-phase) doses of amphotericin is often good, with resolution of clinical symptoms and clearing of the fungemia, but relapse is common after therapy is discontinued (5). Ketoconazole appears to constitute effective maintenance therapy for preventing relapses. We have observed patients who, because they "felt so good", discontinued maintenance therapy after a year and subsequently relapsed within three weeks.

Bacterial Infections

Certain bacterial infections that are primarily controlled by the cellular immune system under normal conditions follow the same pattern of response to antimicrobial therapy in patients with advanced HIV infection. For example, these patients seem to be particularly susceptible to persistent bacteremia caused by non-typhoidal strains of the genus *Salmonella* (6). Although the salmonellal bacteremia is cleared rapidly by therapy with ampicillin, trimethoprim-sulfamethoxazole, chloramphenicol, or ceftriaxone, bacteremia will usually recur when therapy is discontinued. We have successfully used orally administered ciprofloxacin, up to 750 mg b.i.d., as maintenance or suppressive therapy to control salmonellal infections in patients with AIDS (S. M. Hahn, J. L. Gerberding and M. A. Sande, unpublished observation). In two cases in which ciprofloxacin was discontinued after several months, relapse occurred within three weeks.

Viral Infections

Latent cytomegalovirus infection can be documented by antibody studies in approximately 50% of the American population. When activated in the patient with advanced HIV infection, cytomegalovirus most commonly produces a progressive retinitis that may lead to blindness. Ganciclovir (DHPG) administered intravenously is effective in most cases in stopping the progression of retinal destruction, and in some cases leads to the regression of concomitant edema and visual impairment (7). However, if therapy with ganciclovir is discontinued after a two-week induction period, the progressive retinitis resumes, but again can usually be controlled with maintenance therapy consisting of periodic ganciclovir administration (7).

Conclusion

The need for studies to determine the most effective, least toxic, and most practical regimens for both inductive and suppressive phases is urgent, and pharmaceutical firms should be urged to continue the search for new agents to fill this need. Although this two-phase approach can minimize relapses and, it is hoped, maximize quality of life by reducing the suffering from active infection, it at best remains a temporizing measure until control of the underlying HIV infection is achieved and measures to reconstitute the cellular immune system are developed.

Thus, AIDS has taught us a valuable lesson about the critical interaction between antimicrobial chemotherapy and the cellular immune system, an interaction that is necessary for the successful treatment of many infectious diseases. Moreover, experience with this patient population has clearly demonstrated the need for a new approach to chemotherapy of AIDS-associated opportunistic infections, an approach that utilizes an induction phase followed by maintenance or suppressive therapy.

M. A. Sande

Department of Medicine, University of California, San Francisco School of Medicine and the Medical Service, San Francisco General Hospital, 1001 Potrero Avenue, Room 5H22, San Franciso, California 94110, USA.

References

1. Kovacs, J. A., Masur, H.: *Pneumocystis carinii* pneumonia: therapy and prophylaxis. Journal of Infectious Diseases 1988, 158: 254–259.
2. Fischl, M. A., Dickinson, G. M., La Voie, L.: Safety and efficacy of sulfamethoxazole and trimethoprim chemoprophylaxis for *Pneumocystis carinii* pneumonia in AIDS. Journal of the American Medical Association 1988, 259: 1185–1189.
3. Luft, B. J., Remington, J. S.: Toxoplasmic encephalitis. Journal of Infectious Diseases 1988, 157: 1–6.
4. Dismukes, W. E.: Cryptococcal meningitis in patients with AIDS. Journal of Infectious Diseases 1988, 157: 624–628.
5. Graybill, J. R.: Histoplasmosis and AIDS. Journal of Infectious Diseases 1988, 158: 623–626.
6. Celum, C. L., Chaisson, R. E., Rutherford, G. W., Barnhart, J. L., Echenberg, D. F.: Incidence of salmonellosis in patients with AIDS. Journal of Infectious Diseases 1987, 156: 998–1002.
7. Drew, W. L.: Cytomegalovirus infection in patients with AIDS. Journal of Infectious Diseases 1988, 158: 449–456.

New Technology and Drug Design

Nucleic Acid Hybridization: A Rapid Method for the Diagnosis of Infectious Diseases

N. Dattagupta[1], E. Huguenel[1], P. Rae[1], D. Crothers[2]*

A new method is described for the rapid identification of microorganisms in clinical samples by DNA-DNA hybridization. In this procedure, nucleic acids are labelled nonradioisotopically in the sample, which is then incubated with a panel of immobilized unlabelled DNAs from different organisms as probes. The sample labelling is a photochemical reaction between the nucleic acids in cell lysates and an isopsoralen derivative covalently linked to a biotin moiety for detection. Results are given of the application of the procedure to the identification of pathogens in clinical specimens of urine and cerebrospinal fluid.

Nucleic acid hybridization is a technique that has been widely used in research laboratories in studies of gene structure and function, and it is now being adapted to the identification of specific microbes and viruses according to the presence of particular DNA or RNA sequences in a clinical sample. The base pairing of a DNA or RNA probe to sample nucleic acids is a highly specific process guided by conditions of temperature and solvent composition. Alteration of these conditions allows variation in the rate, the extent or the precision of hybridization, and this manipulability makes nucleic acid hybridization a potentially more powerful diagnostic or identification technique than conventional immunoassay. A small number of nucleic acid probe assays have been approved recently by the U.S. Food and Drug Administration for clinical use (1). Although the technology has been advanced enough for application to the diagnosis of some infectious diseases, it still suffers from the disadvantages of low sensitivity, difficulty of operation, and the absence of a unified format that is appropriate to the great variety of laboratory conditions under which diagnostic tests are run.

This article describes how the identification of a microorganism in an unknown sample can be achieved in a new and simple way by a single hybridization of DNA in the sample with a panel of immobilized DNA probes. For an identification by conventional hybridization procedures, aliquots of the nucleic acids from the sample are immobilized onto solid supports, then each is hybridized individually with an excess of a labelled probe. The multiple hybridizations required by this method for the detection of an unknown organism cannot be avoided unless a mixture of probes could be used in a way that each probe is somehow differentially labelled so that it can be distinguished from the others during the detection of hybrids. Currently, however, diagnoses of infectious diseases by nucleic acid hybridization are done simply by probing samples for the presence or absence of one candidate causative organism at a time.

While studying the processes of photochemical labelling of DNA, we found that some furocoumarin derivatives can very effectively label unpurified nucleic acids, even in crude cell lysates. It was already well known that psoralens can complex with DNA in living cells and cause mutations by crosslinking the DNA under conditions of ultraviolet irradiation (2). It was also known that isopsoralen derivatives such as angelicin (3) can only form monoadducts with double-stranded DNA and thus cannot crosslink. Hence, a derivative of isopsoralen is an ideal choice for a photolinker through which one can label nucleic acids with a reporter moiety such as biotin, which in turn can be detected in a number of conventional ways. We therefore had synthesized compounds in which a biotin residue is attached to an angelicin via a polyethylene oxide linker, and showed that one such compound, biotin-polyethylene glycol-angelicin (BPA), can label DNA in a cell lysate with a detectable biotin. The structure of biotin-PEG-angelicin is shown below:

---

[1] Molecular Diagnostics, Inc., Miles Research Center, West Haven, Connecticut 06516, USA.
[2] Department of Chemistry, Yale University, New Haven, Connecticut 06511, USA.

Since DNA can be labelled directly in a clinical specimen such as a sample of urine or cerebrospinal fluid, as we show below, a single hybridization with a panel of immobilized probes will identify microbe(s) in the test sample that may be responsible for clinical presentation. This makes the process much simpler in diagnostic and clinical laboratories than the conventional hybridization method. The technique we have developed has been used with cloned and whole genomic DNAs as immobilized probes, with the latter being sufficient to identify microorganisms at the genus level.

Materials and Methods

Hybridization of a Radiolabelled Probe DNA to Other DNAs. A dot matrix of immobilized denatured DNAs of several microorganisms plus human DNA was prepared in the amounts indicated in Figure 1 on a sheet of nitrocellulose. The filter was prehybridized in 50 % formamide, 5 × SSPE and 5 × Denhardt's solution at 42 °C for 4 h, and then hybridization was under the same conditions overnight at a probe concentration of about 10 ng/ml. The ^{32}P-labelled probe was nick-translated *Escherichia coli* DNA. Post-hybridization treatment of the filter included three 5 min washes at room temperature in 1 × SSC (1 × SSC is 0.15 M NaCl plus 0.015 M sodium citrate), 0.1 % SDS, and then two 15 min washes in 0.1 × SSC, 0.1 % SDS at 65 °C.

Photolabelling DNA in Clinical Samples. A known volume of clinical sample was adjusted to 1.2 N NaOH and boiled for 5 min. After this lysis step, sufficient solid boric acid was added to each sample to adjust the pH to neutrality. Nucleic acid in the sample was then photolabelled by adding biotin-PEG-angelicin to the sample and irradiating the mixture for 60 min with a UV Transilluminator (TL-33, UV Products, San Gabriel, California, USA) at a distance of about 10 cm. The photolabelled samples were then added directly to hybridization solution as indicated below.

Hybridization of Sample DNA to Unlabelled DNA Probe Panels. Dot matrices of immobilized, denatured probe DNAs were prepared on 5 × 2 cm sheets of nitrocellulose by spotting 0.5 µg amounts of DNA from the organisms indicated in Figures 2 and 3, wetting the sheets for 5 min on paper saturated with 0.5 N NaOH to denature the DNA in situ, rinsing the sheets in 1.5 M NaCl, 0.5 M Tris-HCl, pH 7.5, and then baking the sheets at 80 °C under vacuum to affix the DNA. Prehybridization of the sheets was for 30 min at 68 °C in 3 × SSC, 0.02 M Na pyrophosphate, 5 % nonfat dry milk and 10 % polyethylene glycol. Hybridization of the labelled sample was accomplished by adding 300 µl of the labelled sample to 1.1 ml of a solution of the components of the prehybridization mix plus 1 mg/ml herring sperm DNA, prewarmed to 68 °C, and then incubating the mixture with a filter sheet at 68 °C for 2 h. After hybridization, the sheets were washed in 0.1 × SSC, 0.1 % SDS and then in 0.1 × SSC alone for 30 min each at 68 °C.

Detection of Hybrids. This was accomplished either by using anti-biotin colloidal gold conjugate as described by Tomlinson et al. (4), or by enhanced chemiluminescence (unpublished data). Chemiluminescence detection involved reacting biotinylated DNA hybrids with anti-biotin-linked horseradish peroxidase, and assaying for peroxidase using isoluminol and H_2O_2, with iodophenol added as an enhancer. Emitted light was detected photographically using Polaroid films.

Results

Whole Genomic DNAs as Probes for the Identification of Microorganisms

In conventional hybridizations, synthetic oligonucleotides or cloned specific segments of a genome are

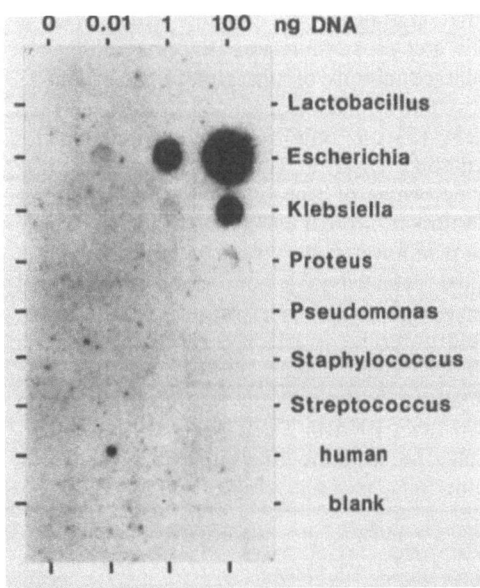

Figure 1: Cross reactivity among whole genomic DNAs of bacteria commonly involved in urinary tract infections. A dot matrix of immobilized denatured DNAs of several microorganisms plus human DNA was prepared in the amounts indicated on a sheet of nitrocellulose. The filter was then hybridized with ^{32}P-labelled *Escherichia coli* genomic DNA as described in the text.

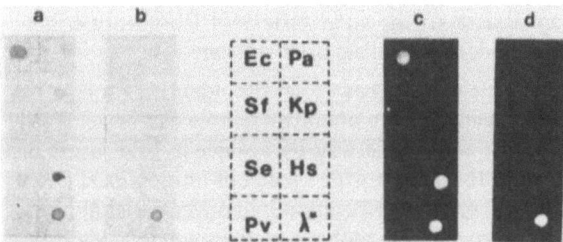

Figure 2: Reverse hybridization of photolabelled clinical urine samples to panels of unlabelled probe DNAs from bacteria commonly involved in urinary tract infection. Biotin in photolabelled DNA hybrids was detected either by colloidal gold (panels a and b) or by enhanced chemiluminescence (panels c and d). Abbreviations in the center key panel: Ec, *Escherichia coli;* Sf, *Streptococcus faecalis;* Se, *Staphylococcus epidermidis,* Pv, *Proteus vulgaris;* Pa, *Pseudomonas aeruginosa,* Kp, *Klebsiella pneumoniae;* Hs, *Homo sapiens;* λ*, immobilized biotinylated phage lambda DNA.

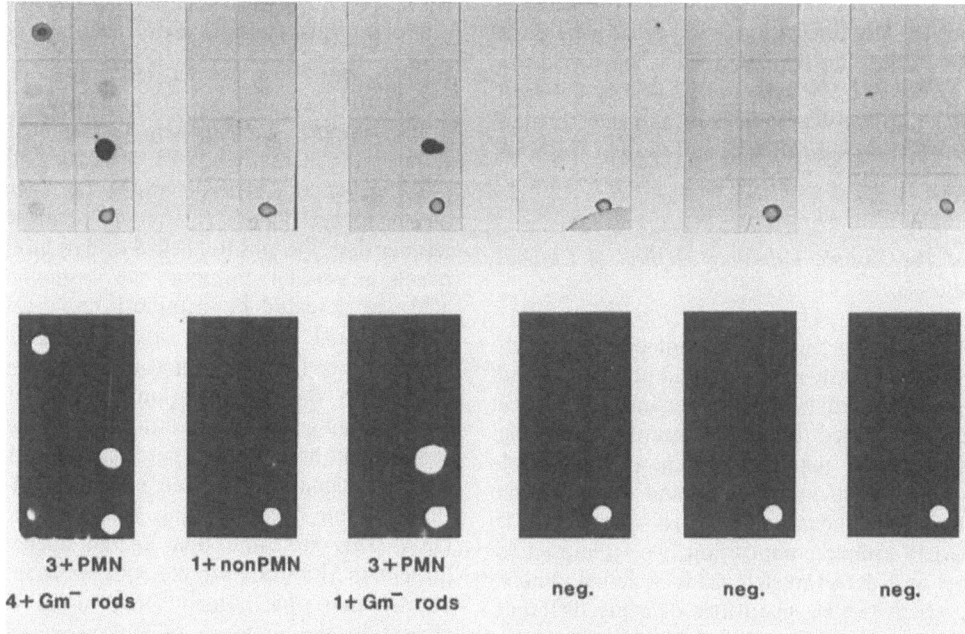

Figure 3: Reverse hybridization of photolabelled clinical spinal fluid samples to panels of unlabelled probe DNAs from bacteria commonly involved in meningitis. The designations below each pair of panels indicate the results of microscopic analysis of each fluid. Quantities of bacteria and polymorphonuclear leukocytes (PMNs) are estimated on a scale of 1+ to 4+, which correlate quantitatively as follows: 1+ represents 1–10 cells per high power microscopic field, or 10,000 cells/ml; 2+ represents 20–30 cells per high power microscopic field, or 50,000 cells/ml; 3+ represents > 30 cells per high power microscopic field, or 100,000 cells/ml; 4+ represents > 50 cells per high power microscopic field, or > 100,000 cells/ml. Spinal fluid panels were prepared by immobilizing probe DNAs as follows, beginning with the upper left sector and following in a clockwise fashion: *Haemophilus influenzae;* blank; *Escherichia coli; Homo sapiens;* biotinylated phage lambda DNA; *Klebsiella pneumoniae; Streptococcus faecalis; Neisseria meningitidis* or *Neisseria gonorrhoeae.*

used as probes. We found that by adjusting the conditions of hybridization, it is possible to use whole genomic DNAs as probes for the identification of a microorganism to the genus level. This affords some advantages over the standard use of cloned segments of a genome or of oligonucleotides. The much greater extent of sequence homology between a whole genomic DNA probe and a homologous genome, where potentially all sequences can hybridize, gives a stronger signal than does a hybridization involving homology between only a portion of a genome and a cloned segment as probe, so that the efficiency of the whole process is greater. Rapid signal detection is also facilitated by base pairing among overlapping complementary strands of the labelled DNA, which produces networks of hybridized nucleic acids at the appropriate target sites on a solid support. This is particularly helpful for enhancing the sensitivity of nonisotopic detection methods. The supply of probe DNA depends only on the growth of cells and a simple purification of the DNA from cell lysates; no recombinant DNA procedures are required, and quality control of probes involves only standard microbiological identification of bacteria and simple physical characterization of the DNA.

To show that our conditions of DNA hybridization allow discrimination among urinary tract pathogens, we prepared a panel of spots of immobilized denatured DNA of five genera of bacteria commonly involved in urinary tract infections, and then challenged the panel with ^{32}P-labelled whole genomic DNA of *Escherichia coli* as a probe. The panel comprised DNA from *Escherichia coli, Klebsiella pneumoniae, Proteus mirabilis, Staphylococcus epidermidis* and *Streptococcus faecalis*, as well as from *Lactobacillus acidophilus,* which is a common contaminant of improperly collected urine, and from *Pseudomonas aeruginosa*, which is an agent commonly responsible for hospital-acquired infections. Figure 1 shows the results of such a hybridization. As expected, the probe hybridized proportionately with the 100, 1 and 0.01 ng spots of homologous DNA in the second row from the top of the matrix. There is also hybridization to the *Klebsiella* DNA spots to the extent of about 1% that of homologous DNA hybridization, and the 100 ng *Proteus* DNA spot shows a signal comparable in strength to that of the 0.01 ng *Escherichia coli* spot. This cross-reactivity between *Escherichia coli* DNA and the DNAs of *Klebsiella* spp. and *Proteus* spp. is actually less than that predicted from the published extent of relatedness among the three microorganisms (5). Earlier DNA hybridization studies that were done under conditions less stringent than ours had indicated 10–20 % DNA sequence homology between *Escherichia* spp. and *Klebsiella* spp., and an estimated 1–2 % between *Escherichia* spp. and *Proteus* spp. (5).

Utility of the Sample Labelling Method in Clinical Assays

The finding that nucleic acid present in a crude cell lysate prepared directly in urine could be biotinylated by our photochemical method was encouraging, since this obviated the need for time consuming and often complicated sample preparation steps prior to labelling. To verify that our labelling and hybridization techniques were robust enough to tolerate wide differences in sample composition, we attempted to photolabel and detect nucleic acids in actual clinical samples, where varying quantities of many different substances may be present along with leukocytes, other cell types and drugs, all of which have the potential for inhibiting or interfering with the assay. The two kinds of samples we examined were clinical urine samples and clinical cerebrospinal fluid samples. These fluids are compositionally different and also exhibit a somewhat different spectrum of infecting organisms. The most common pathogen causing urinary tract infections is *Escherichia coli*, accounting for 60 to 90 % of all cases. A number of other gram-negative enteric organisms also cause the disease, among them *Klebsiella pneumoniae*, *Proteus mirabilis*, *Proteus vulgaris* and *Pseudomonas aeruginosa*. In addition, gram-positive organisms such as *Streptococcus faecalis* and *Staphylococcus epidermidis* and also yeast (*Candida* spp.) contribute to a small percentage of infections (6). In the case of meningitis, the most common pathogens vary according to the population, with *Escherichia coli*, group B streptococci and *Listeria monocytogenes* most common in neonates, *Haemophilus influenzae*, *Streptococcus pneumoniae* and *Neisseria meningitidis* most common in younger children, and *Streptococcus pneumoniae* and *Neisseria meningiditis* most common in older children and adults (7). In both kinds of samples, it can be seen that a variety of organisms are capable of causing the disease, and any technique employed for diagnostic purposes must be able to accommodate and discriminate a wide variety of pathogens.

Our initial clinical testing was done with clinical urine samples obtained from the Microbiology Department at Bridgeport (Connecticut) Hospital, and with clinical cerebrospinal fluid samples obtained from the Microbiology Department of Primary Children's Hospital, Salt Lake City, Utah. In both cases, the photolabelling and hybridization were performed and our own results obtained without prior knowledge of the hospital identification results obtained by standard microbiological analysis in the hospital laboratory.

Figure 2 shows a set of hybridization panels representative of the results obtained with clinical urine samples. In between the clinical panels is shown a schematic panel indicating the relative positions of the genomic probe DNAs immobilized on the panel. Panels (a) and (c) represent a urine sample that was photolabelled and hybridized to two panels in parallel. For one, the biotinylated nucleic acid was detected by anti-biotin colloidal gold conjugate (Panel a) and the other by enhanced chemiluminescence (Panel c). In both cases a positive signal located on the hybridization panel in the position corresponding to the location of *Escherichia coli* genomic probe DNA can be clearly seen. In addition, a strong signal is observed in Panels (a) and (c) at the location corresponding to immobilized human DNA. This indicated that human nucleic acid was present in the urine sample, and we have found (see below) that the human DNA signal corresponds closely to the presence of leukocytes in the urine. The signal in the lower right corner of each panel corresponds to the position of biotinylated, immobilized phage lambda DNA used as a positive control for the biotin detection reactions. Panels (b) and (d) represent the results obtained for a different urine sample; in this case there was no detectable signal coming from any of the probe DNA positions on the panel, indicating that this particular urine sample was not infected with any of the organisms represented by our probe panel. The hospital clinical diagnoses of these two particular urine samples corresponded exactly with our diagnoses made by DNA hybridization, namely that the first sample had a clinically significant level of *Escherichia coli* in it and that the second sample was not infected.

We have performed our photolabelling and hybridization method on a number of clinical urine samples obtained over a period of several months, and the results of this initial clinical analysis are summarized in Tables 1 and 2. We found a very good correlation between the hospital laboratory diagnosis and the bacterial DNA hybridization diagnosis for the 74 samples examined (Table 1). Most of the discordant results arose from our failing to detect bacteria in some of the samples which, by hospital diagnosis, were clearly infected. This probably reflects the fact that our assay method has a present sensitivity level of 50,000–100,000 bacteria. Significantly, out of 29 infected samples for which there was a detectable hybridization signal, only one was misdiagnosed, which illustrates the high degree of specificity of the hybridization reaction. Two other urines, indicated in Table 1, were reported initally by the hospital as positive, using a rapid screen method that relies on the binding of safranin dye to bacterial

Table 1: Correlation of conventional culture and hybridization diagnoses for 74 urine samples.

		Culture negative	Conventional culture diagnosis					
			ESC	KLE	PRO	PSE	STR	STA
Hybridization diagnosis	NEG	31	8	1	–	1	1	1
	ESC	2[a]	19	–	–	–	–	–
	KLE	–	1	1	–	–	–	–
	PRO	–	–	–	5	–	–	–
	PSE	–	–	–	–	–	–	–
	STR	–	–	–	–	–	–	–
	STA	–	–	–	–	–	–	3

[a] Screen (+), culture (−)
NEG negative; ESC = *Escherichia coli;* KLE = *Klebsiella pneumoniae;* PRO = *Proteus vulgaris;*
PSE = *Pseudomonas aeruginosa;* STR = *Streptococcus faecalis;* STA = *Staphylococcus epidermidis*

cells in urine. Upon culture, however, these two urines were found to be negative ($< 10^4$ CFU/ml). It is possible that our positive hybridization results on these samples are due to high levels of non-viable bacteria which would give positive screen and hybridization results but negative culture results.

These same clinical urine samples were scored for the presence of human DNA by hybridization and were also analyzed for the presence of human leukocytes using a simple leukocyte esterase assay which is often used as a rapid urine screen for pyuria, an accepted clinical sign of urine infection (8). The results (Table 2) indicated a correlation between the leukocyte esterase assay result and the DNA hybridization result, with 88 % of the esterase-positive urines scored as human DNA-positive. Out of 16 esterase-negative urines, ten were scored as positive by DNA hybridization. One likely reason for this significant discordance is that many urine metabolites known to interfere with the esterase assay and thus give false-negative results would not necessarily interfere with the photolabelling and hybridization reactions.

In a similar fashion, we examined the utility of our assay in the diagnosis of bacteria in cerebrospinal fluid. A representative set of hybridization panels is shown in Figure 3. In this experiment, six different spinal fluid samples were subjected to our labelling and hybridization method, the hybridized nucleic acid being detected by either chemiluminescence (top panels) or immunogold (bottom panels). The hospital's microscopic analysis of these fluids is shown below each pair of panels. In the single case where a high level of gram-negative rods (designated as 4+) was observed in the sample, which was confirmed as *Haemophilus influenzae* by subsequent culture diagnosis, we observed a hybridization signal corresponding in location on the panel to the *Haemophilus influenzae* probe DNA. Two other samples contained low levels of gram-negative rods (1+); these bacteria were not detected by our hybridization method. Two of the samples contained high levels of white cells − 3+ PMN (polymorphonuclear leukocytes) − and both of these samples showed strong hybridization signals on the panel corresponding to the human probe DNA position. The other samples were negative by hybridization, and these results were confirmed by hospital diagnosis.

A summary of our clinical testing of spinal fluids is shown in Tables 3 and 4. Of 94 samples examined,

Table 2: Correlation of leukocyte esterase assay and DNA hybridization assay for the detection of human cells in 78 urine samples.

		Leukocyte esterase assay	
		Human positive	Human negative
Hybridization diagnosis	Human positive	55	10
	Human negative	7	6

Table 3: Correlation of conventional culture and hybridization diagnoses for 94 cerebrospinal fluid samples.

		Conventional culture		
		Negative	Haemophilus influenzae	Neisseria meningitidis
DNA	Negative	86	2[a]	1
	Haemophilus influenzae	–	5	–
	Neisseria meningitidis	–	–	–

[a] One of these had 1+ gram-negative rods, and sample volume was 1/5 of usual.

Table 4: Correlation of microscopic analysis and DNA hybridization diagnoses of 94 cerebrospinal fluid samples.

		Microscopic analysis	
		Negative PMNs	Positive PMNs
DNA	Negative	50	13[a]
	Human DNA	5	26

[a] Microscopic analysis indicated 1+ PMNs, which corresponds to fewer than 10^4 PMNs per ml of fluid.

86 were judged negative for bacteria by DNA hybridization (Table 3), and these were confirmed as negative) by the hospital laboratory. Of the seven fluids diagnosed as containing Haemophilus influenzae by the hospital laboratory, we were able to detect Haemophilus influenzae in five of them. The other two Haemophilus influenzae-containing fluids and one Neisseria meningitidis-containing fluid were not diagnosed correctly by the hybridization method, probably due to problems in sample handling prior to labelling. These 94 samples were also examined microscopically by the hospital for the presence of PMNs, which indicates spinal fluid infection or inflammation. We found good agreement between the microscopic analysis and DNA hybridization results (Table 4), with 13 of the discordant results explainable by the finding of very low (less than 10^4/ml) levels of PMNs in these samples.

Discussion

We have shown that the photolabelling compound biotin-PEG-angelicin can label nucleic acids present in a cell lysate that has been prepared directly in complex body fluids such as urine and cerebrospinal fluid. Furthermore, these labelled nucleic acids are hybridizable and we have shown that hybridization can take place without first purifying the labelled nucleic acid away from the cell lysate. The hybridization format we have developed, in which a single, labelled nucleic acid sample is hybridized to a panel of different immobilized probe DNAs, allows us to discriminate with a single hybridization reaction among a wide variety of microorganisms present in clinical materials. The lack of requirements for purification of the sample nucleic acid prior to sample labelling or hybridization are distinct advantages of the assay method.

Other important features of the method are the use of unfractionated genomic DNAs as probes and their immobilization on a solid support such as nitrocellulose paper. In conventional hybridization techniques where an unknown sample is immobilized on a solid support and challenged with multiple labelled probe DNAs, whole chromosomal DNAs have been used as probes for the identification of bacteria involved in periodontal disease (9) and for the detection of mycobacteria in cultured clinical isolates (10). The advantage of our format is that the identification of an organism in a clinical sample can be achieved by a single hybridization reaction, since the probe DNAs are immobilized. Another advantage is that the probe panel can easily be enlarged to accomodate additional probe DNAs, and individual panels can be tailored to meet particular diagnostic needs. Furthermore, our method is not restricted to the use of genomic DNAs as probes, since we have correctly identified the gender of human cell samples by labelling the nucleic acids in the cell lysates and hybridizing with an immobilized cloned human Y chromosome-specific DNA probe.

At present, the sensitivity of our method using nonisotopic detection methods is 50,000–100,000 bacterial cells, which can be insufficient for some clinical applications where high sensitivity is critical. By coupling our sample labelling technique with a sample amplification method that we are developing, we will have a highly sensitive method of DNA hybridization with wide applications in clinical and research laboratories.

Acknowledgements

We thank E. Carlson, H. Chabot, E. Hall, A. Lyga, J. Shapiro, S. Tomlinson and S. Wayne for their technical contributions to this work and Dr. W.-D. Busse for encouragement and comments.

References

1. Young, F. A.: DNA probes: fruits of the new biotechnology. Journal of the American Medical Association 1987, 258: 2404–2406.
2. Song, P.-S., Tapley, Jr., K. J.: Photochemistry and photobiology of psoralens. Photochemistry and Photobiology 1979, 29: 1177–1197.
3. Brodin, F., Carlassare, F., Baccichietti, F., Guiotto, A., Rodrighiero, P., Vedaldi, D., Dall'Acqua, F.: 4,5'-Dimethylangelicin: a new DNA-photobinding monofunctional agent. Photochemistry and Photobiology 1979, 29: 1063–1070.
4. Tomlinson, S., Lyga, A., Huguenel, E., Dattagupta, N.: Detection of biotinylated nucleic acid hybrids by antibody-coated gold colloid. Analytical Biochemistry 1988, 171: 217–222.
5. Brenner, D. J.: Facultatively anaerobic gram-negative rods, family I. Enterobacteriaceae. In: Krieg, N. R. (ed.): Bergey's manual of systematic bacteriology. Volume I. Williams and Wilkins, Baltimore, 1984, p. 408–420.

6. Clarridge, J. E., Pezzlo, M. T., Vosti, K. L.: Laboratory diagnosis of urinary tract infections. In: McCarthy, L. R. (ed.): Cumitech 2A. American Society for Microbiology, Washington, DC, 1987.
7. Ray, C. G., Wasilauskas, B. L., Zabransky, R.: Laboratory diagnosis of central nervous system infections. In: McCarthy, L. R. (ed.): Cumitech 14. American Society for Microbiology, Washington, DC, 1982.
8. Stansfield, J. M.: The measurement and meaning of pyuria. Archives of the Diseases of Childhood 1982, 37: 257–262.
9. French, C. K., Savitt, E. D., Simon, S. L., Eklund, S. M., Chen, M. C., Klotz, L. C., Caccaro, K. K.: DNA probe detection of periodontal pathogens. Oral Microbiology and Immunology 1986, 1: 58–62.
10. Roberts, M. C., McMillan, C., Coyle, M. B.: Whole chromosomal DNA probes for rapid identification of *Mycobacterium tuberculosis* and *Mycobacterium avium* complex. Journal of Clinical Microbiology 1987, 25: 1239–1243.

New Technology and Immunospecific Reactions in Helminthic Diseases

B. Gottstein

> The success which has been and will be achieved in immunological control and prevention of helminthic diseases is closely related to technological developments in molecular biology and molecular and cellular immunology. The primary need for identification, isolation and characterization of relevant parasite epitopes is emphasized. T- and B-cell epitope mapping has provided parasite molecules suitable for investigation in various host-parasite interactions. The molecular cloning of the respective gene fragments, using various expression vectors, makes it possible to synthesize the parasite molecules in carrier host cells that have been adapted to specific problems. Described as an example is the use of live attenuated *Salmonellae* vaccine strains for the expression of *Echinococcus multilocularis* genes which are subsequently used in investigations regarding the induction of protective cellular and humoral immunity.

The increased interest in the search for a detailed understanding of parasitism due to infectious worms, i.e. helminths, has resulted in the study of a wider range of parasites. The investigation of host-parasite relationships has moved beyond the more direct consideration of pathology toward biochemical, physiological, immunological, ecological, epidemiological and molecular biological problems. Early work on the biochemistry of helminths has greatly influenced parasite chemotherapy. Biochemical knowledge has served to explain the action of curative agents and has also indicated differences between hosts and parasites which may be exploited in the search for selective toxicity. In recent decades special attention has been paid to the immunology of helminth infections. Helminths generally induce antibody responses that are useful for immunodiagnosis. Parasites are seldom eliminated by the hosts' natural immune response; rather they are involved in producing chronically persistent infections. For this reason a major area of interest has been the elucidation of the nature of the hosts's response and how parasites avoid it, and, within these mechanisms, the possible role of external active (immunomodulation, immunotherapy, vaccination) and passive (genetic control of protective immunity) immunological interferences. Especially in the area of vaccination, the current surge of interest has been kindled by the spectacular success of recombinant DNA technology and by major advances in our understanding of the host effector mechanisms, which are or might be responsible for protection. In the same respect, from the advanced knowledge of basic immunology it could be concluded that the induction and maintenance of cell-mediated immune response is of major importance in helminth immunology. The analysis of the immunochemical configuration of antigenic determinants and their immunological functions has become a crucial matter of investigation. It has become clear that the ability of antigenic determinants to stimulate appropriate responses in hosts is variable and may be dependent on the genetic background and immune status of the host, as well as on adjuvants, carrier molecules and an acceptable way of administration regarding vaccines (1). Novel presentation routes utilizing evolved recombinant DNA technology to incorporate the antigenic helminth protein as a surface or internal component in not only live attenuated enteric but also tissue-invading bacteria or virus may offer an attractive alternative to any traditional routes. Furthermore, anti-idiotypic antibodies, which carry the internal image of a parasite antigen, may represent an effective alternative tool for use as a vaccine, based on the ability of anti-idiotypes to mimic foreign antigen-structures.

Scientists involved in diagnosis, control and treatment of parasitoses are all confronted by the complexity of the life-cycle of most helminths. Consequently, this offers a great challenge for researchers to work in close collaboration at multiple levels within various disciplines. New technology applied to helminths and their hosts provides new tools of fundamental importance to the control of parasitoses. In this respect, molecular biology will play a vital role in developing these new tools not only for molecular biologists, but also for immunologists, clinicians, entomologists, epidemiologists, taxonomists, environmental

---

Institute of Parasitology, University of Zürich, Winterthurerstraße 266a, CH-8057 Zürich, Switzerland.

hygienists and all other scientists involved in the fascinating multidisciplinary field of helminthology.

Host-Parasite Interactions

As metazoan parasites, helminths have a complicated level of organization compared to other pathogenic organisms. The mostly chronic form of the diseases caused by helminths and the long persistance of organisms from one or more stages of the parasite require the development of highly sophisticated immune evasion, immune tolerance or immune suppression mechanisms. Trematodes, such as schistosomes, have bodies that are covered by a potentially vulnerable, plasma membrane-bounded surface. They release a wide variety of metabolic molecules which are involved in humoral and cellular immune reactions. Some, such as a recently described 28 K schistosomula surface polypeptide, might be relevant in the stimulation of protective immunity (2). Others have a functional property in interfering with host immunity. It has been shown, for instance, that schistosomes may be covered by host immunoglobulins bound to their surface by Fc receptors (3). The IgG is partially cleaved by a secreted parasite protease, and the peptides released by this reaction inhibit macrophage activation and depress macrophage-mediated cytotoxicity for schistosomula. Nematodes, on the other hand, have a tough outer tegument that, to a certain degree, confers protection against immune attack. Nevertheless, a constant antigen turnover and release invokes a strong humoral and cellular immune reaction, which seems to be more important with tissue-dwelling nematodes than with intestinal worms. In several diseases caused by infection with nematodes, the pathology associated with infections is caused not by the direct activities of the parasite but by the immunological and inflammatory responses of the host. The larvae (metacestodes) of taeniid cestodes, which are important in human and veterinary medicine, develop in tissue or internal organs of infected intermediate hosts, and a strong humoral and cellular immune response is usually induced (4). The propagation of these cestodes depends on the survival of the metacestodes for the remaining life of the host. Thus the ability of the parasite to evade host immune reactions during these stages is an essential requirement for the successful transmission of infection. Immune mechanisms which affect these established metacestodes are therefore of major interest for research of the protective role of immunity. Consideration of immune responses to these stages is also important because cellular reactions around degenerating metacestodes may be responsible for the pathogenic effects of infection (e.g. *Taenia solium*) and for the lesions which cause economic loss in domestic animals (e.g. *Taenia ovis*). In certain intermediate hosts of *Echinococcus multilocularis* (e.g. humans, various mice strains) the unrestrained proliferation of larvae is not affected despite a marked lymphoproliferative activity in the B-cell areas of lymphoid tissues. The progressive growth of the metacestode mass results in or from depression of the cytotoxic cellular response involving macrophages, eosinophils and neutrophils, but the humoral mechanism remains functional (5). This idea is supported by the observation that T-cell suppressed mice fail to limit the metastasis formation and growth of *Echinococcus multilocularis* (6).

Helminth Antigens

The identification and analysis of helminth molecules has become a major area of research in helminthology. Mostly, identification of parasite molecules consists solely of the biochemical or immunological analysis of proteins, glycoproteins, or glycoconjugates resolved on polyacrylamide gels. Assignment of functional roles to most of the identified molecules has not yet been achieved, but it is becoming clear that research in purification of mainly hydrophobic membrane-associated and hydrophilic excreted-secreted molecules and their structure-function analysis will be of primary importance for molecular parasitologists. Cooperation between the disciplines of molecular biology, parasitology, immunology and biochemistry will ensure progress in future research on helminth antigens. In this report, some current, arbitrarily selected antigenic polypeptides from *Echinococcus multilocularis* and other helminth species serve as examples to illustrate recent advances made in this area as well as some problems remaining to be solved.

Echinococcus multilocularis: Parasite and Immunodiagnostic Antigens

The life-cycle of *Echinococcus multilocularis*, a small tape-worm, involves two mammalian hosts. The main definitive hosts are foxes, in whose intestines the adult stage of the worm occurs. Intermediate hosts are herbivorous and omnivorous species in which development of the metacestode (larva) takes place. Human and animal intermediate hosts become infected by ingesting eggs passed in the feces of infected definitive hosts. The infection with metacestodes in intermediate hosts follows a progressive course and is severely harmful to the host. Dysfunction is caused by local, massive, proliferative extension of the parasite in the liver and the formation of metastatic lesions in other organs. The infection usually results in death of the host: lethality has been reported to be about 90 % in certain endemic areas (7). *Echinococcus multilocularis* is restricted to the

Northern Hemisphere, and cases of alveolar echinococcosis in humans are diagnosed relatively frequently in central Europe, the Soviet Union, some areas of Asia (China, Japan) and western Alaska. In Switzerland, for instance, 145 new cases of alveolar echinococcosis were diagnosed between 1970 and 1983 (8). An understanding of the biological events which occur during infection is necessary to visualize the diversity of interactions to which host and parasite are subjected. When *Echinococcus* eggs are ingested by a suitable intermediate host, the oncospheres hatch and become activated in the small intestine. Lytic secretions of the oncosphere then facilitate its passage into the intestinal mucosa and the host's circulatory system, through which they usually reach the target organ for post-oncospheral development. This process involves the formation of primary vesicles followed by exogeneous budding and proliferation, resulting in the formation of a solid cellular parasite tumour which infiltrates the surrounding tissue. The proliferative mode of *Echinococcus multilocularis* causes constant and direct contact between parasite and host tissue. The result is early recognition by and continuous humoral and cellular immune stimulation of the host.

The need for the identification of antigens specific to *Echinococcus multilocularis* is based on the aim of early presurgical detection of patients with alveolar echinococcosis, and discrimination of these patients from those with cystic echinococcosis in regions where both *Echinococcus* species (*multilocularis* and *granulosus*) occur sympatrically. Recent work has resulted in the identification, purification and characterization of an antigenic polypeptide from the *Echinococcus multilocularis* metacestode which showed several promising characteristics (9, 10, 11). Comparison of patients' antibody reactivity to the Em2-antigen and an antigen fraction (Em1) containing antigenic components shared by *Echinococcus granulosus* and *Echinococcus multilocularis* permitted a serologic differentiation in 95% of human *Echinococcus granulosus* and *Echinococcus multilocularis* infections. The use of Em2-antigen in sero-epidemiological studies performed in several areas endemic for *Echinococcus multilocularis* resulted in the detection of several cases of asymptomatic but active alveolar echinococcosis. Due to early detection most of the patients could be successfully treated by radical surgical resection of the parasite lesion. Antibodies to the Em2-antigen were detected in symptomatic and asymptomatic clinical cases of alveolar echinococcosis, cases of inactive echinococcosis (12) and cases of seroconversion after highly probable egg infection without detectable alveolar echinococcosis (11). The operating characteristics of the Em2-antigen resulted in positive and negative predictive values both of $> 99\%$ (11). Furthermore, antibody-detection to Em2-antigen was also suggested to be useful for monitoring *Echinococcus multilocularis*-infected patients following treatment (13).

The Em2-antigen was characterized by SDS-PAGE, isoelectric focusing, immunoprecipitation and protein immunoblotting. The antigenic polypeptide was shown to have a relative molecular mass of 54,000 and an isoelectric point at pH 4.8. Antigen is required in large amounts for large-scale sero-epidemiological studies; therefore, its production by new methods such as recombinant DNA techniques is anticipated to be of practical interest.

Recombinant DNA Technology

The adaptation of molecular biological techniques for investigations in helminthology represents a break-through in the study of immunospecific reactions to helminth antigens, although this was achieved relatively late compared to the use of such methods in virology, bacteriology or protozoology. This delay is mainly attributable to the complexity of helminths, which more closely resemble humans than bacteria. The genome size of helminths is estimated to be approximately 10^8 base pairs, while that of bacteria is approximately 10^6, that of protozoa approximately 10^7, and that of humans approximately 10^9. Cloning and expressing helminth genes (obtained from complementary DNA [cDNA] or genomic DNA) in *Escherichia coli*, for example, can circumvent many of the problems encountered when using classical immunochemical methods, such as those associated with unstable or low-amount proteins. Expression of helminth antigens has been achieved in *Escherichia coli* and other bacteria using both plasmid and bacteriophage vectors. Plasmid expression vectors (circular DNA molecules) have an origin of replication, a selective (drug resistance) marker and a promoter/operator linked to a DNA sequence into which a helminth DNA or cDNA insert can be cloned. The DNA sequence is usually a part of a structural bacterial gene. The recombinant proteins may then be expressed as a fusion of two proteins. A disadvantage of plasmids as vectors is that they usually do not grow well if the size of helminth DNA is too large (> 10 kb). For larger DNA fragments the insertion into bacteriophages is considered to be more suitable.

Bacteriophage lambda has been modified to become an excellent expression vector in the form of λgt11. The bacteriophage is temperature-sensitive lysogenic and possesses the *Escherichia coli* β-galactosidase gene with one Eco R1 cloning site at a point corresponding to the C-terminal region. Helminth polypeptides expressed in this vector are fused to the C-terminal end of β-galactosidase. Eukaryotic genes such as those from helminths lack promoter and ribosomal binding sites recognized by *Escherichia coli*. It is therefore necessary to rely on the transcriptional and translational regulatory signals from the bacterium. Good expression vectors have strong promoters and are under the negative control of a repressor, which is inactivated either by a temperature change or by a classical inducer. The repression is needed to prevent the expression of fusion proteins, which may be toxic to Escherichia coli, during multiplication of bacteria until synthesis of the proteins is needed for immunological screening.

The identification of recombinant proteins, expressed from DNA sequences coding for helminth antigens, is performed immunologically using either hyperimmune polyclonal or monoclonal antibodies. Problems encountered due to background reactivities of antibodies with contaminating Escherichia coli-antigens or with β-galactosidase can be surmounted by immunosorption with these antigenic components in solid-phase. A more efficient approach is to subclone helminth gene fragments using modified gene expression vector systems such as pKK-233-MTTL, where the expressed helminth gene products are only fused to four amino acids originating from the plasmid genome. Overexpression in such a system may also result in recombinant antigens directly applicable to immunodiagnosis, as no bacterial polypeptide is present which may interfere immunologically. A very efficient way to obtain pure recombinant polypeptides free of contaminating bacterial fragments has been developed by Norbert Müller and coworkers (personal communication), who established a new plasmid cloning system, pVB1, by which antigen-coding helminth DNA sequences could be expressed at a very high level. The pVB1 plasmid carries an ampicillin resistance marker and the gene (mgl B) of the galactose binding-protein. Galactose binding-protein is an abundant protein of Escherichia coli, Salmonella and some other bacteria, and is exported actively into the hydrophilic space (periplasm) between the inner (cytoplasmic) and outer membrane of the bacterial cell. In this way, Müller and coworkers cloned Echinococcus multilocularis cDNA into the Eco R1 restriction site of pVB1, which is located at the C-terminal end of mgl B. The recombinant fusion proteins were exported, like the galactose binding wild-type protein, into the periplasm. Subsequently they could easily be isolated from bacterial cultures by osmotic shock procedures (14) without lysis of the bacterial cells, finally isolating the fusion protein from culture supernatant.

Recombinant Helminth Antigens

Echinococcus multilocularis. A cDNA expression library derived from mRNA of metacestodes from Echinococcus multilocularis was constructed in the Escherichia coli expression vector λgt11 and screened with parasite-specific sera of human patients (15). Various recombinant proteins were shown to bind only antibodies from patients with alveolar echinococcosis. One isolated clone synthesized a fusion protein which was rapidly degraded. The intracellular degradation process provided two distinct polypeptides with M_r of 31,000 and 33,000, respectively (II/3-antigen). The immunodiagnostic value of the II/3-antigen was evaluated by high-resolution mini-Western-blot with sera from patients with homologous and various heterologous helminth infections, indicating a diagnostic sensitivity of 98 % and an overall specificity of 96 %. The recombinant II/3-antigen may be useful for immunodiagnosis of human alveolar echinococcosis and for further studies in specific immunoprophylaxis.

Schistosomes. An excellent review on the chemical nature, immunological protectivity and gene cloning of defined antigens of Schistosoma has been recently published (16). About 40 different Schistosoma gene libraries have now been established in different laboratories. In one of them, a gene encoding for a 28 K antigen has been cloned and fully sequenced (2). Immunization of rats, hamsters and monkeys has been achieved with this recombinant antigen, and protection against a natural challenge infection with live cercariae in rats and hamsters (67 % and 52 % protection, respectively) has been reported (2).

Filariidae. Brugia malayi is a filarial nematode which infects humans and various animal species. A genomic DNA expression library has been established and screening with antibodies generated against the infective third-stage larvae has resulted in the identification of genus- and species-specific recombinant clones. The recombinant antigens may be candidates for further studies in immunoprophylaxis and diagnosis of Brugia malayi infection.

New Trends in Vaccination

Immunogen Selection and Epitope Mapping

To effectively plan a new generation of vaccines it is generally accepted that one must consider that the potential response of the host is regulated by the interaction of stimulating and suppressing epitopes, resulting in dominance of certain molecule sites over others. It has become clear that both B- and T-cell cooperation is not random but is guided by preferential pairing of sites within a single molecule (17). Cell-mediated immunity is especially important in helminth infections (18). Stimulation by helminth-specific antigens can induce clonal expansion of parasite-specific T-cells which may act by direct cytotoxicity or by indirect effect on other cells such as natural killer cells, or, as mentioned above, on antibody-synthesizing B-cells. In this way, analysis of proliferative and cytotoxic activities of subcloned cultures of T-cells, or, more efficiently, of cloned T-cell cultures stimulated with helminth antigens, can provide relevant information about the importance of cell-mediated immunity. One major challenge for molecular immunologists in helminthology is to identify T-cell epitopes on vaccine candidate antigens. Factors influencing the property of immunodominant T-cell sites, such as self-tolerance, idiotype networks, suppression phenomenon and other regulatory mechanisms within the host's immune response, are either intrinsic to the structure of the antigen or extrinsic to the antigen. Some biochemical characteristics can be used for predicting the presence of T-cell epitopes. For example, the presence of amphipatic α-helices in macromolecules is considered to be important for T-cell recognition. A computer algorithm has been designed to search proteins for amino acid sequences resulting in the conformational formation of amphipatic α-helices (19). For a helix to be amphipatic, the hydrophobicity of the amino acids in the sequence must oscillate with a period like that of the helix, in order to place hydrophilic residues on one side and hydrophobic ones on the other (20). Some characteristics are provided by the absence of coil propensity or the presence of lysine at the -COOH terminus. Among other points which remain largely unresolved are antigen polymorphism and the placement of T(helper)-cell epitopes for induction of protective antibody formation or antibody-independent cell-cytotoxicity.

Mode of Vaccine Delivery

An appealing approach for making recombinant products into better vaccines is the use of recombinant virus (e. g. vaccinia virus) and bacteria (e. g. attenuated *Salmonella*) as a delivery system for helminth antigens. The vaccination potency should be increased markedly by incorporating helminth gene fragments encoding B-cell and T-cell epitopes, preferably on the same molecule.

Salmonella. *Salmonella* species such as tissue-invading *Salmonella typhi* or *Salmonella typhimurium* can be rendered avirulent by mutation without impairing their immunogenicity (21). Attenuation can be obtained by introducing genetically defined, non-reverting mutations into specific genes of the *Salmonella* chromosome. Mutations such as in the *gal* E or *aro* A genes prohibit the growth of bacteria in vivo. Genetic determinants encoding for potentially protective helminth epitopes can be readily introduced into these attenuated *Salmonella* strains. For instance, the recombinant plasmid pVB1 mentioned previously has been introduced into *Salmonella thyphimurium* LT 2 M1C. The fusion protein was expressed and constituted up to 30% of the total cell protein (N. Müller, personal communication). The *Echinococcus multilocularis* derived gene fragment used was relatively short, and some observations with different clones indicated a limitation in length with regard to transportation of the gene products into the periplasm. Of great significance was the observation by another group which showed that mice vaccinated in a similar way developed a cellular immune response to β-galactosidase, using pXY411 as expression vector system (22). If humoral and cellular immunity to a recombinant helminth antigen can be stimulated, then a number of interesting immunological questions might be answered using recombinant *Salmonella* vaccines. For example, it may be possible to determine whether a local immune response in the lung, the urogenital tract, or in the gut of humans or animals can be stimulated using appropriate attenuated *Salmonella* species. One objection to the use of *Salmonella typhi* or *Salmonella typhimurium* has been the possibility of an existing immunity in a given community against a bacterium species. If this is the case then an attenuated variant of another species might be used to deliver antigens, as, unlike vaccinia, hundreds of serologically distinct species of *Salmonella* are known.

Vaccinia. Foreign genes can be inserted into a non-essential region of the vaccinia virus genome without impairing its infectivity. One major advantage of this mode of delivery is that protein products of these genes may be glycosylated and processed for secretion or membrane insertion. Such recombinant clones are known to induce both B- and T-cell response in vivo and the persistence of antigen-encoding gene expression by vaccinia virus-infected cells can be expected to provide a strong stimulation of the immune system with the possibility that certain cell-surface presented recombinant antigens will be more immunogenic than the in vitro isolated products (23). Vaccinia has the potential to be an extremely valuable vector because it can incorporate up to 25 kb pairs of foreign DNA.

Anti-Idiotypes

The part of lymphocytic receptors and antibody molecules which recognizes and binds an antigenic epitope is termed a paratope. This antigen binding site is in its physical structure complementary to the antigen against which the lymphocytic receptor or the antibody has been raised. When antibodies are developed against a paratope they are in a similar way complementary in shape to the paratope and thus, they mimic the structure of the original antigen of that paratope. Such antibodies are termed "anti-idiotype antibodies". Anti-idiotype antibodies play a major role in immunoregulation (24). Due to the ability of anti-idiotype antibodies to mimic foreign antigens, their use as idiotype vaccines has been envisaged. This was suggested to be of special interest if the antigen is of a non-peptide nature, which means that it cannot be synthesized by recombinant DNA techniques. In this way, rat monoclonal anti-idiotype antibodies were used to immunize LOU rats against a *Schistosoma mansoni* 38K glycoprotein antigen. The glycanic nature of one of the major epitopes of that antigen had limited its molecular biological production. In the rat model, the anti-idiotype vaccination has been shown to be at least as effective as when using conventional (antigen of parasite origin) vaccination procedures (25).

Conclusion

Investigations at the molecular level occupies a crucial position in all areas of research in helmintic diseases. The understanding of host-parasite interactions and their subsequent alterations aimed at therapy and prophylaxis in the host is rapidly progressing as such interactions are studied increasingly at the level of gene structure. Genes or gene fragments can be specifically identified by direct screening with nucleotide probes, or by screening gene expression with adequate antibodies. Such genes can be engineered basically in any direction, opening a tremendous spectrum of possibilities for future investigations regarding diagnosis, treatment, prophylaxis and control of helminthic diseases. From the clinical and epidemiological standpoints, the future of research in helminthic diseases requires not only the development of highly sophisticated technology and the acquisition of basic knowledge in helminthology, but also a solid link to all other disciplines of work in non-molecular domains, and a bilateral flow of information to fieldworkers and scientists working in other fields of infectious disease.

References

1. **Kaye, P. M.**: Antigen presentation and the responses to parasite infection. Parasitology Today 1987, 3: 293–299.
2. **Balloul, J. M., Sondermeyer, P., Dreyer, D., Capron, M., Grzych, J. M., Pierce, R. J., Carvallo, D., Lecocq, J. P., Capron, A.**: Molecular cloning of a protective antigen of schistosomes. Nature 1986, 362: 149–153.
3. **Capron, A.**: Mechanisms of evasion of host immune response in *Schistosoma* infections. Fortschritte der Zoologie 1982, 27: 259–264.
4. **Rickard, M. D., Williams, J. F.**: Hydatidosis/cysticercosis: immune mechanisms and immunization against infection. Advances in Parasitology 1982, 21: 229–296.
5. **Heath, D. D.**: Immunobiology of *Echinococcus* infections. In: Thompson, R. C. A. (ed.): The Biology of *Echinococcus* and Hydatid Diseases. George Allen & Unwin, London, 1986, p. 164–188.
6. **Baron, R. W., Tanner, C. E.**: The effect of immunosuppression on secondary *Echinococcus multilocularis* infections in mice. International Journal of Parasitology 1976, 6: 31–42.
7. **Schantz, P. M., Gottstein, B.**: Echinococcosis (Hydatidosis). In: Walls, K. W., Schantz, P. M. (ed.): Immunodiagnosis of Parasitic Diseases. Volume 1. Academic Press, Orlando, Fla., 1986, p. 69–107.
8. **Gloor, B.**: Echinokokkose beim Menschen in der Schweiz, 1970–1983. Thesis of Medicine, University of Zürich, Switzerland, 1987.
9. **Gottstein, B., Fey, H., Eckert, J.**: Serological differentiation between *Echinococcus granulosus* and *Echinococcus multilocularis* infections in man. Parasitology Research 1983, 69: 347–356.
10. **Gottstein, B.**: Purification and characterization of a specific antigen from *Echinococcus multilocularis*. Parasite Immunology 1985, 7: 201–212.
11. **Gottstein, B., Lengeler, C., Bachmann, P., Hagemann, P., Kocher, P., Brossard, M., Witassek, F., Eckert, J.**: Sero-epidemiological survey for alveolar echinococcosis (by Em2-ELISA) of blood donors in an endemic area of Switzerland. Transactions of the Royal Society of Tropical Medicine and Hygiene 1987, 81: 960–964.
12. **Rausch, R. L., Wilson, J. F., Schantz, P. M., McMahon, B. J.**: Spontaneous death of *Echinococcus multilocularis*: cases diagnosed serologically (by Em2-ELISA) and clinical significance. American Journal of Tropical Medicine and Hygiene 1987, 36: 576–585.
13. **Lanier, A. P., Trujillo, D. E., Schantz, P. M., Wilson, J. F., Gottstein, B., McMahon, B. J.**: Comparison of serologic tests for the diagnosis and follow-up of alveolar hydatid disease. American Journal of Tropical Medicine and Hygiene 1987, 37: 609–615.
14. **Neu, H., Heppel, L.**: The release of enzymes from *Escherichia coli* by osmotic shock and during the formation of spheroblasts. Journal of Biological Chemistry 1965, 240: 3685–3692.
15. **Vogel, M., Gottstein, B., Müller, N., Seebeck, T.**: Production of a recombinant antigen of *Echinococcus multilocularis* with high immunodiagnostic sensitivity and specificity. Molecular and Biochemical Parasitology 1988, (in press).
16. **Simpson, A. J. G., Cioli, D.**: Progress towards a defined vaccine for schistosomiasis. Parasitology Today 1987, 3: 26–28.
17. **Celada, F., Sercaz, E. D.**: Preferential pairing of T-B specificities in the same antigen: the concept of directional help. Vaccine 1988, 6: 94–98.
18. **Baldwin, C. L., Goggeeris, B. M., Morris, W. I.**: T-cell clones in immunoparasitology. Parasitology Today 1988, 4: 40–45.
19. **Margalit, H., Spouge, J. L., Cornette, J. L., Cease, K. B., DeLisi, C., Berzofsky, J. A.**: Prediction of immunodominant helper T-cell antigenic sites from the primary sequences. Journal of Immunology 1987, 138: 2213–2229.
20. **Berzofsky, J. A.**: Features of T-cell recognition and antigen structure useful in the design of vaccines to elicit T-cell immunity. Vaccine 1988, 6: 89–93.
21. **Germanier, R.**: Immunity in experimental Salmonellosis. I. Protection induced by rough mutants of *Salmonella typhimurium*. Infection and Immunity 1970, 2: 309–315.

22. Brown, A., Hormaeche, C. D., Dermaco de Hormaeche, R. Winther, M. D., Dougan, G., Maskell, D. J., Stocker, B. A. D.: An attenuated *aro* A *Salmonella typhimurium* vaccine elicits humoral and cellular immunity to cloned beta-galactosidase in mice. Journal of Infectious Diseases 1987, 155: 86–92.
23. Langford, C. J., Edwards, S. J., Smith, G. L., Mitchell, G. F., Moss, B., Kemp, D. J., Anders, R. F.: Anchoring a secreted plasmodial antigen on the surface of recombinant vaccinia infected cells increases its immunogenicity. Molecular Cell Biology 1986, 6: 3191–3199.
24. Jerne, N. K.: Towards a network theory of the immune system. Annals of Immunology 1974, 125: 373–389.
25. Grzych, J. M., Capron, M., Lambert, P. H., Dissous, C., Torres, S., Capron, A.: An anti-idiotype vaccine against experimental schistosomiasis. Nature 1985, 316: 74–76.

Molecular Targets of Chemotherapeutic Agents Against the Human Immunodeficiency Virus

E. De Clercq

> There are a multitude of virus-specific proteins and steps in the replicative cycle of the human immunodeficiency virus (HIV) that could act as targets for potential drugs against the acquired immune deficiency syndrome (AIDS). The reverse transcriptase has proven to be the principal if not the sole target for the anti-HIV activity of 2′,3′-dideoxynucleoside analogues [i.e. 3′-azido-2′,3′-dideoxythymidine (AZT), 2′,3′-dideoxycytidine (DDC) and 2′,3′-didehydro-2′,3′-dideoxythymidine (D4T)], following intracellular phosphorylation of these nucleoside analogues to their 5′-triphosphates. Sulfated polysaccharides such as heparin, dextran sulfate and pentosan polysulfate block virus adsorption to the outer cell membrane, which implies that these compounds do not have to be taken up by the cells to achieve their anti-HIV activity. Several other viral processes (i.e. uncoating, integration, transcription and assembly) and viral proteins (i.e. protease, *tat* protein, *rev* protein and RNase H) have been identified as attractive targets for antiviral chemotherapy, and an intensive search for specific inhibitors of these functions continues.

The replicative cycle of any virus can, quite schematically, be divided in ten major steps: (i) virus adsorption to the cell membrane, (ii) virus penetration into the cell, (iii) uncoating or release of the viral genome, (iv) transcription of the viral genome to either RNA or DNA, (v) translation of the viral mRNA to "early" proteins (primarily RNA or DNA polymerases), a process that is replaced by integration of the viral DNA genome into the cellular genome when it concerns oncogenic RNA or DNA viruses, (vi) replication of the viral genome (whether integrated or not), (vii) transcription of the viral genome to mRNA, (viii) translation of the viral mRNA to "late" proteins (primarily capsid proteins), (ix) assembly of the viral nucleic acid and proteins, and (x) release of the virus particles (referred to as "budding" for some viruses, e.g. retroviruses) by the cell.

In its replicative cycle (Figure 1), human immunodeficiency virus type 1 (HIV-1), the causative agent of the acquired immune deficiency syndrome (AIDS), follows a pattern similar to that of the conventional viruses: adsorption, penetration, uncoating, and reverse transcription of the viral RNA genome to double-stranded DNA, which is first circularized before being integrated as proviral DNA into the cellular genome. As the proviral DNA is an integral part of the chromosome, its replication occurs concomitantly with the replication of cellular DNA, and hence this stage in the retrovirus replicative cycle cannot be considered specific for the virus. The expression of the viral proteins follows the classical flow of transcription, translation and post-translational processing. Additionally, as a major peculiarity, the virion proteins of human retroviruses

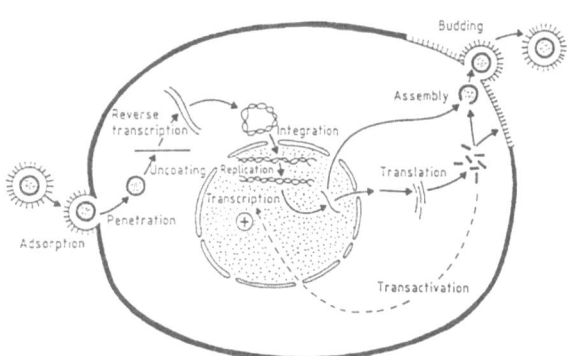

Figure 1: Major steps in the replicative cycle of HIV-1. These major steps can further be resolved in different events: adsorption of virus to cell receptor is followed by fusion between virus and cell; reverse transcription not only pertains to transcription of viral RNA to DNA but also implies degradation of the residual RNA by the "hybrid" ribonuclease (RNase H), duplication of the minus strand DNA to double-stranded DNA, and circularization of the latter; processing of viral proteins requires several post-translational modifications such as myristylation, glycosylation and proteolytic cleavage; and transactivation can be effected by both *tat* and *rev* proteins, and, in addition to *tat* and *rev*, other virus-encoded proteins play a regulatory role in the replication and infectivity of HIV-1.

Rega Institute for Medical Research, Katholieke Universiteit Leuven, Minderbroedersstraat 10, B-3000 Leuven, Belgium.

have the possibility of orchestrating their own expression via both positive and negative regulatory proteins (transactivation). Once the HIV-1 particles have been assembled they are released, as retroviruses normally are, through "budding" (Figure 1). Hence the replicative cycle of HIV-1 offers a wealth of targets that could be exploited in the design of chemotherapeutic agents for the treatment of AIDS (1, 2).

Viral mRNA transcribed from the minus strand of the HIV-1 proviral DNA contains three open reading frames (ORFs) that encode the viral capsid (*gag*) proteins, polymerase (*pol*) proteins, envelope (*env*) glycoproteins, and five additional proteins not commonly found in other retroviruses: *tat, rev, vif, vpr* and *nef* (3) (Figure 2). In addition, the DNA plus strand of HIV-1 contains an open reading frame that may ultimately encode a protein that has yet to be identified (4). The genomic organization of HIV-2 is very similar to that of HIV-1. However, HIV-2 contains an open reading frame designated *vpx* (previously called X-ORF) that is not found in HIV-1. It is located in the central region of the genome between the *pol* open reading frame and the *env* open reading frame (5). The *vpx* gene encodes a protein (p14) that may function as a specific RNA binding protein. Due to the presence of this unique protein, HIV-2 may respond differently from HIV-1 in its susceptibility to some anti-HIV agents.

The proteins specified by the viral genome are directly involved in crucial steps of the virus replicative cycle (Figure 3): *env* gp120 is involved in the binding of the virions to the cell membrane, reverse transcriptase and RNase H in the reverse transcription of the viral RNA genome to proviral DNA, *end* in the integration of proviral DNA in cellular DNA, *tat* and *rev* in the transcription of proviral DNA to mRNa, and *pro* in the cleavage of the *gag-pol* precursor protein to its final products. As all these proteins seem innately associated with the replicative cycle of HIV-1, they may serve as adequate target molecules for the design of inhibitors that would specifically interfere with their function. In addition to the viral proteins depicted in Figure 3, *vif* and *nef* may also be considered appropriate targets. As *nef* is a negative regulator of virus expression, measures to enhance rather than block its function should be envisaged.

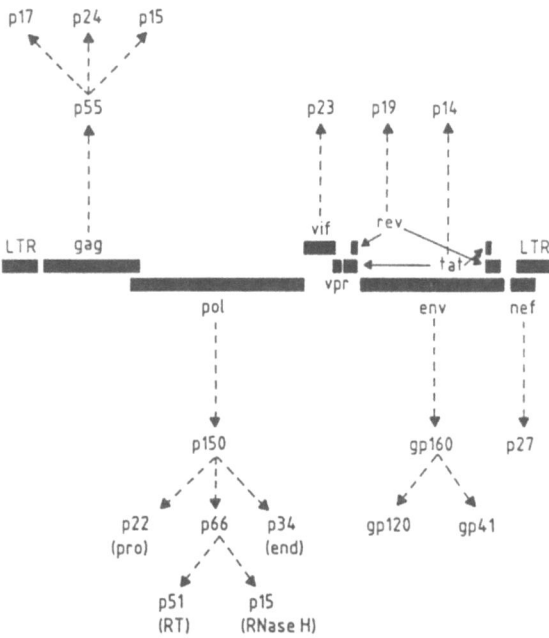

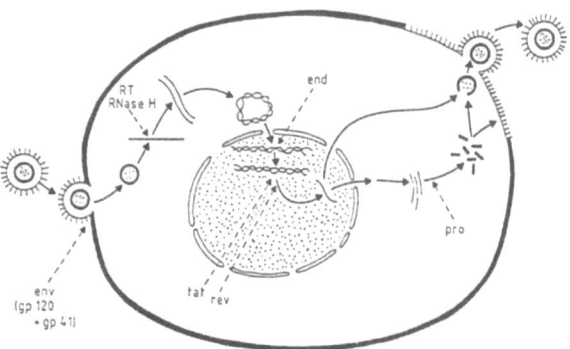

Figure 2: Genomic organization of HIV-1 and proteins encoded by the HIV-1 genome: *LTR*, long terminal repeats located at the 5'- and 3'-ends; *gag*, group-specific antigens; *pol*, polymerase [encompasses *pro* (protease), *RT* (reverse transcriptase), *RNase* H (ribonuclease H), and *end* (endonuclease, also referred to as *int* for integrase)]; *vif*, virion infectivity factor (previously referred to as *sor* for short open reading frame); *vpr*, viral protein R (a protein of unknown size and function); *tat*, trans-acting transcriptional activator; *rev*, regulator of expression of virion proteins (previously referred to as *art* for anti-repression transactivator or *trs* for trans-acting regulator of splicing); *env*, envelope glycoproteins; *nef*, negative factor (previously referred to as 3'*orf* for 3' open reading frame). The genomic organization of HIV-2 is very similar to that of HIV-1. However, HIV-2 contains an open reading frame (ORF) designated *vpx* (previously called X-ORF) that is not found in HIV-1.

Figure 3: Role of viral proteins in the replicative cycle of HIV-1: glycoprotein gp120 is involved in the virus adsorption process; the RT (p51) + RNase H (p15) complex is required for the reverse transcription reaction; *end* (p34) effects the integration of the proviral DNA in the cellular genome; the expression of the viral proteins is positively regulated by *tat* (p14) and *rev* (p19), predominantly at the transcription level; and *pro* (p22), which is itself formed autocatalytically, cleaves the *gag-pol* precursor protein to its products p17, p24, p15, p22 (*pro*), p66 [p51 (RT) + p15 (RNase H)] and p34 (*end*). In addition to *tat* and *rev*, *vif* (p23) and *nef* (p27) also act as regulatory genes that orchestrate virus expression: *vif* as a positive regulator and *nef* as a negative regulator. Exactly where they interfere in the virus replicative cycle has not been rigorously determined.

Virus Adsorption

The initial event in the infection of target cells by HIV-1 (and HIV-2) is the attachment of the HIV-1 envelope glycoprotein gp120 to its cellular receptor, CD4. The HIV-binding site has been mapped to residues 37–53 of the CD4 protein (6), opening the way to the design of peptide analogs that may interfere with the HIV-receptor interaction. Peptide T, an octapeptide composed of Ala-Ser-Thr-Thr-Thr-Asn-Tyr-Thr, may be regarded as a first step toward designing antagonists of the HIV-cell binding event. Although peptide T has been claimed to inhibit HIV infectivity for T4 lymphocytes by preventing its interaction with the CD4 receptor (7, 8), these findings have not gained wide acceptance (9).

Alternatively, binding of HIV-1 to $CD4^+$ lymphocytes, and thus infectivity of HIV-1 for these cells, can be blocked by soluble forms of CD4 (10), and these results have been widely confirmed (11–14). Whether CD4, given its antigenic nature, represents a viable modality is another matter, however, and this problem will have to be addressed before CD4 or fragments thereof can be used in a clinical setting.

HIV adsorption to its target T lymphocytes can also be blocked by less sophisticated substances such as heparin, dextran sulfate and other sulfated polysaccharides (15–17). These polyanionic substances had been known for more than two decades before they were suggested as potential anti-HIV agents (1) because of their putative effect on the virus adsorption process (18). In fact, heparin and dextran sulfate were found to be very efficient and highly selective inhibitors of HIV-1 replication (19, 20). Although these anionic polysaccharides suppress the binding of HIV to $CD4^+$ cells (15–17), this inhibitory effect should not be viewed as the consequence of a specific interaction of dextran sulfate or its congeners with the CD4 receptor; dextran sulfate does not interfere with the binding of monoclonal antibody (OKT4) to CD4 (D. Schols, M. Baba, R. Pauwels, J. Desmyter and E. De Clercq, unpublished data). Furthermore, dextran sulfate and other sulfated polysaccharides are also inhibitory to the replication of various enveloped viruses other than HIV, i.e. herpes simplex virus, cytomegalovirus, vesicular stomatitis virus and Sindbis virus, which do not require the CD4 receptor for invading the cells (unpublished data).

Sulfated polysaccharides are not indiscriminately active against HIV-1. Certain structural requirements have to be met. Ideally, there should be two (or three) sulfate groups per monosaccharide unit, as is the case with dextran sulfate and pentosan polysulfate (Figure 4). Chondroitin sulfate and dermatan sulfate, which contain only one sulfate group per disaccharide unit, have little if any activity against HIV-1 (Table 1), and dextran that has been stripped of its sulfate groups has no anti-HIV activity at all.

The importance of the sulfate group is attested by the fact that unsulfated polysaccharides such as curdlan and lentinan become active against HIV following sulfation (21). Furthermore, following "supersulfation" (sulfation of the remaining free hydroxyl groups) dermatan sulfate and chondroitin sulfate become equally active as dextran sulfate and pentosan polysulfate. The molecular size of the sulfated polysaccharides is another important structural parameter. For dextran sulfate to impart optimal anti-HIV-1 activity, the molecular weight should be 5,000–10,000, but even with dextran sulfate samples of an average molecular weight of 1,000, appreciable anti-HIV-1 activity has been noted (unpublished data).

From Table 1 it is clear that heparin, dextran sulfate, pentosan polysulfate, λ-carrageenan and mannan sulfate are extremely selective in their anti-HIV-1 activity: with a selectivity index of about 10,000, dextran sulfate and pentosan polysulfate rank among the most selective anti-HIV-1 agents which have ever been described. Of particular concern is the anticoagulant activity of sulfated polysaccharides, which is, in fact, the major indication for the clinical use of heparin. From Table 1 (last column) it is clear,

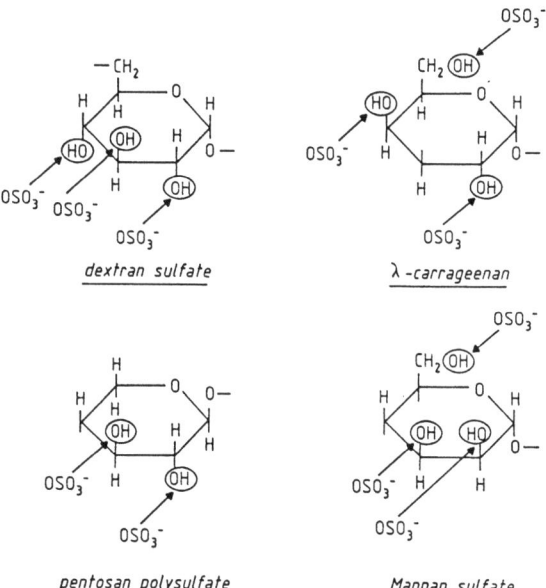

Figure 4: Repeating monosaccharide units (with their putative linkages) in dextran sulfate, pentosan polysulfate, λ-carrageenan and mannan sulfate: α-D-glucose, xylopyranose, α-D-galactose and α-D-mannose, respectively. Shown are the hydroxyl groups which are prone to sulfation. Thus, maximally three sulfate groups can be accommodated per hexose unit (only two for pentosan polysulfate). The molecular weights (MW) of the sulfated polysaccharides examined were as follows: dextran sulfate (MW = 1000–500000), pentosan polysulfate (MW = 3100), λ-carrageenan (MW = not determined) and mannan sulfate (MW = 30000).

Table 1: Potency and selectivity of sulfated polysaccharides as inhibitors of HIV-1 in MT-4 cells. All data taken from Reference No. 17, except for mannan sulfate (unpublished data).

Compound[a]	Anti-HIV-1 activity			Anticoagulant activity (U/mg)	Anti-HIV-1 activity ED50[e] (U/ml)
	ED50[b] (µg/ml)	CD50[c] (µg/ml)	SI[d]		
Heparin	0.58	> 2500	> 4300	177	0.103
Dextran sulfate	0.3	> 2500	> 8300	14.7	0.0044
Pentosan polysulfate	0.19	> 2500	> 13150	14.4	0.0027
λ-carrageenan	0.54	> 625	> 1150	4.2	0.0023
Mannan sulfate	1.2	> 2500	> 2000	20	0.024
Chondroitin sulfate	230	> 2500	> 10	0.5	0.115
Dermatan sulfate	> 625	> 2500	–	< 0.01	–

[a] Compounds added immediately after virus infection.
[b] 50 % effective dose, or compound concentration required to protect 50 % of the virus-infected cells against the cytopathic effect of HIV-1.
[c] 50 % cytotoxic dose, or compound concentration required to reduce the viability of mock-infected cells by 50 %.
[d] Selectivity index, or ratio of CD50 to ED50.
[e] Same as in footnote b but now expressed in anticoagulant units.

however, that all sulfated polysaccharides exert their inhibitory effect on HIV-1 replication at doses which are well below the anticoagulant threshold.

Virus Penetration (Virus-Cell Fusion)

Following binding of the HIV envelop glycoprotein to the CD4 receptor, the viral lipid bilayer fuses with the lipid bilayer of the cell. This fusion would be mediated by a specific domain located at the N-terminus of gp41. This fusogenic domain would become active only after the precursor gp160 has been cleaved (by a trypsinlike endopeptidase) (22) to the gp120-gp41 heterodimer. The N-terminal fusogenic domain of gp41 may itself mediate fusion between the viral lipid bilayer and that of the cell, as well as mediate syncytium formation between infected and uninfected cells. HIV may operate according to the same protocol by which myxo- and paramyxoviruses effect fusion and syncytium formation. In the latter case, virus infectivity and syncytium formation can be abrogated by carbobenzoxy di- and tripeptides (23–25) and longer peptides with amino acid sequences that resemble those of the N-terminal regions of the glycoproteins generated following proteolytic cleavage (26, 27). Extrapolating from the experience with myxo- and paramyxoviruses, the interaction of the N-terminal sequence of gp41 with the cell surface may be considered an attractive target. Likewise, the use of oligopeptides homologous to the gp41 N-termini may be an attractive approach to specifically inhibit the infectious cycle of HIV.

Virus Uncoating

Virus uncoating has been recognized as the target for the antiviral action of several entero- and rhinovirus inhibitors, i.e. arildone (28), dichloroflavan (BW 683C) (29), 4′-ethoxy-2′-hydroxy-4,6′-dimethoxychalcone (Ro 09-0410) (30), 5-[7-[4-(4,5-dihydro-2-oxazolyl)phenoxy]heptyl]-3-methylisoxazole (WIN 51711) (31) and 2-[(1,5,10,10a-tetrahydro-3H-thiazolo[3,4-b]isoquinolin-3-ylidine)amino-4-thiazole acetic acid (44081 R.P.) (32). The specific anti-influenza A action of amantadine, which directly interacts with the viral matrix (M_2) protein (33), could also be interpreted as resulting from the inhibition of virus uncoating, provided at least that the M_2 protein is involved in the uncoating process.

The interaction of WIN 51711 and of the structurally related WIN 52084 with human rhinovirus has been resolved at the atomic level (34). The 3-methylisoxazole group of these compounds inserts itself into the hydrophobic interior of the β-barrel of the structural viral protein VP1, and the oxazoline group covers the access to an ion channel leading from the surface to the interior of the virion (Figure 5). By filling the "holes" in VP1, the WIN compounds make the viral capsid structure more rigid and thus prevent its disassembly. The holes in VP1 confer sufficient flexibility to the viral capsid to allow its disassembly, and, as such holes are likely to be conserved among various viruses, the HIV-1 p24 capsid protein may be expected to contain similar hydrophobic pockets (35). If so, it may be possible to design compounds that can enter and fit snugly into the hydrophobic pocket of the p24 capsid protein, and these compounds may thus act as uncoating inhibitors.

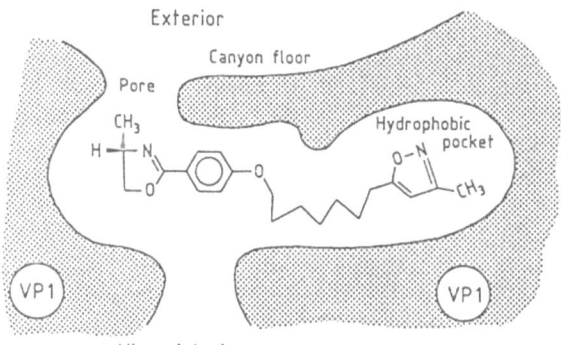

Figure 5: Diagrammatic representation of "docking" of the virus uncoating inhibitor WIN 52084 into the "hole" formed by the structural viral protein VP1 of human rhinovirus 14 (adapted from Reference No. 34). The 3-methylisoxazole group and the seven-membered aliphatic chain are inserted into the hydrophobic interior of the VP1 β-barrel, whereas the oxazoline group covers the entrance to an ion channel (pore) in the floor of the canyon on the viral surface. Viral disassembly may be inhibited by preventing collapse of the VP1 hydrophobic pocket or by blocking the flow of ions from the exterior into the virus interior.

Reverse Transcription

In view of its unique role in the replicative cycle of retroviruses, the reverse transcriptase associated with HIV has been envisaged as the most obvious chemotherapeutic target. Site-directed mutations, i.e. Asp → His at residue 185, have been found to completely destroy reverse transcriptase activity, and such mutations are also expected to deter virus growth (36).

Suramin was the first compound shown to protect T4 cells against the infectivity and cytopathic effects of HIV-1 (37). Suramin was evaluated for this purpose because it had been found previously to be a potent inhibitor of reverse transcriptase (RT) of several murine and avian retroviruses (38), and hence its anti-HIV-1 activity could be ascribed to an inhibitory effect on the HIV-1-associated reverse transcriptase (which by no means excludes additional targets for the antiviral action of suramin). Following investigations with suramin, several other reverse transcriptase inhibitors were found to selectively inhibit the replication of HIV-1 in vitro: Evans Blue (39), aurintricarboxylic acid (40) and phosphonoformate (41). Meanwhile, azidothymidine (AzddThd) (42) and dideoxycytidine (ddCyd) (43) had appeared as effective inhibitors of HIV-1 replication, and it became immediately clear that the 2',3'-dideoxynucleoside analogues were significantly more selective in their anti-HIV-1 action than suramin or phosphonoformate and their congeners.

By now, various nucleoside analogues have been identified as potent and selective anti-HIV agents, and from a structural viewpoint they fall into several classes: 2',3'-dideoxynucleosides, 2',3'-dideoxy-2',3'-didehydronucleosides, 3'-azido- or 3'-fluoro-or 2'-fluoro(ara)-substituted derivatives of 2',3'-dideoxynucleosides, carbocyclic derivatives of 2',3'-dideoxy-2',3'-didehydronucleosides, acyclic nucleosides (4-hydroxy-1,2-butadienyl derivatives) and acyclic nucleotides (2-phosphonylmethoxyethyl derivatives) (Figure 6). From a comparative examination of the potency and selectivity of the 2',3'-dideoxynucleoside analogues (Table 2), it appears that most of the compounds inhibit HIV-1 replication at a concentration of $\leq 1 \mu M$ (FddThd even at a concentration of 0.001 μM), and that their selectivity index generally exceeds two orders of magnitude.

Other nucleoside analogues, i.e. carbovir, FaraddAdo (51), phosphonylmethoxyethyladenine (PMEA) (52), adenallene and cytallene (53), were not included in Table 2 because they have not been evaluated in the

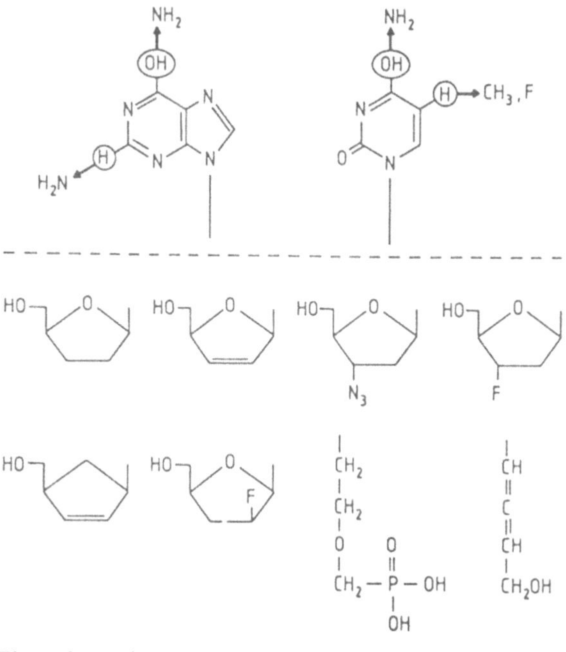

Figure 6: Unifying scheme for nucleoside analogues which have been found active as anti-HIV agents: 2',3'-dideoxynucleosides — ddAdo, ddGuo, ddIno, ddDAPR, ddCyd, ddThd, ddFCyd; 2',3'-dideoxy-2',3'-didehydronucleosides — ddeCyd (D4C), ddeThd (D4T); 3'-azido-2',3'-dideoxynucleosides — AzddAdo, AzddGuo, AzddDAPR, AzddThd, AzddUrd; 3'-fluoro-2',3'-dideoxynucleosides — FddGuo, FddDAPR, FddThd, FddUrd, FddCyd; carbocyclic 2',3'-dideoxy-2',3'didehydroguanosine (carbovir); 2'-fluoro-ara-2',3'-dideoxynucleosides — FaraddAdo, FaraddIno; 9-(2-phosphonylmethoxyethyl)adenine (PMEA) and derivatives (PMEDAP, PMEMAP); 9-(4-hydroxyl-1,2-butadienyl)adenine (adenallene) and 1-(4-hydroxy-1,2-butadienyl)cytosine (cytallene).

Table 2: Potency and selectivity of 2′,3′-dideoxynucleoside analogues as inhibitors of HIV-1 in MT-4 cells. Data taken from References No. 44–50.

Compound[a]	ED50[b] (µg/ml)	CD50[c] (µg/ml)	SI[d]
AzddThd (AZT)	0.006	3.5	583
ddCyd (DDC)	0.06	37	616
ddThd	0.2	>125	>625
ddeCyd (D4C)	0.13	7.9	61
ddeThd (D4T)	0.01	1.2	120
FddThd	0.001	0.197	197
AzddUrd	0.36	244	677
FddUrd	0.04	16	400
ddAdo (DDA)	6.4	890	139
ddGuo	7.6	486	64
AzddGuo	1.4	190	136
FddGuo	2.4	231	96
ddDAPR	3.6	404	112
AzddDAPR	0.3	44	147
FddDAPR	4.5	360	80

[a] Compounds added after a 2-hour virus adsorption period.
[b] 50 % effective dose, or compound concentration required to protect 50 % of the virus-infected cells against the cytopathic effect of HIV-1.
[c] 50 % cytotoxic dose, or compound concentration required to reduce the viability of mock-infected cells by 50 %.
[d] Selectivity index or ratio of CD50 to ED50.

same assay system in parallel with the 2′,3′-dideoxynucleoside analogues. However, in the assay systems in which they were examined they gave selectivity indexes of about two orders of magnitude, comparable to those of azidothymidine, dideoxycytidine and dideoxyadenosine.

In the reverse transcriptase reaction, suramin is assumed to act as a template analogue, phosphonoformate as a product analogue, and the nucleoside analogues as substrate analogues. Suramin inhibits reverse transcriptase activity competitively with respect to the template [poly(A)], suggesting that the drug interacts with the template-binding site of the enzyme (38). Various structural analogues of suramin (54) may act in a similar fashion. Whereas suramin and phosphonoformate do not require any metabolic conversion, the nucleoside analogues must first be converted to their triphosphate form before they can interact with the reverse transcriptase. This requires three phosphorylation steps for all nucleoside analogues, except for the phosphonylmethoxyethyl derivatives, which only require two phosphorylation steps to be converted to their putatively active forms.

As has been directly demonstrated with the triphosphate of azidothymidine (AzddThd) (55, 56), all 2′,3′-dideoxynucleoside triphosphates may inhibit the reverse transcriptase reaction competitively with respect to the natural substrates, but, in addition, they may also serve as alternate substrates for the reaction. The resulting incorporation of the 2′,3′-dideoxynucleoside monophosphate into DNA would obviously lead to chain termination, as the 3′-hydroxyl group needed for further chain elongation is missing in the 2′,3′-dideoxynucleosides. For a selected number of 2′,3′-dideoxynucleoside 5′-triphosphates, i.e. AzddTTP, ddTTP, FddTTP and ddeTTP, K_i values have been determined, not only with HIV-1 reverse transcriptase but also with the cellular DNA polymerases α, β and γ (56–61). Where the affinities of the thymidine triphosphate analogues for the different DNA polymerases were compared, their K_i values for HIV-1 reverse transcriptase were invariably lower (by several orders of magnitude) than for DNA polymerases α, β, γ, indicating their selective affinity for the reverse transcriptase.

Selective inhibition of reverse transcriptase has been proven for only a few nucleoside analogues (AzddThd, ddThd, FddThd and ddeThd). For the other 2′,3′-dideoxynucleoside analogues depicted in Figure 6, it can only be surmised that they are specifically targeted at the reverse transcriptase step. For the carbocyclic (carbovir) and acyclic (PMEA, PMEDAP, PMEMAP, adenallene, cytallene) compounds, a targeted action at reverse transcriptase implies that these unusual nucleoside analogues are previously phosphorylated to their active triphosphate forms. Whether these compounds are actually phosphorylated and which enzymes are responsible for this phosphorylation remain issues for further investigation.

Conversion of the nucleoside analogues to their triphosphate form is a *conditio sine qua non* for their action at the reverse transcriptase level (62, 63), and the rate and extent by which the nucleoside analogues are phosphorylated intracellularly to their triphosphates may vary enormously depending on the sort of compounds (64) and the nature of the cells (65). Thus, not only the affinity for the reverse transcriptase but also the ease by which the compounds are phosphorylated to their triphosphates will determine how efficiently they ultimately block virus replication. The successive phosphorylation steps in the metabolic activation of the compounds also provide the opportunity for the intervention of either positive or negative regulating factors. Examples of such regulators are thymidine, which stimulates the phosphorylation of ddCyd to ddCTP (66), and ribavirin, which inhibits the phosphorylation of AzddThd to AzddTTP (67). The former enhances the inhibitory effect of ddCyd on HIV replication, the later antagonizes the inhibitory effect of AzddThd on HIV replication (66–68).

Proviral DNA Integration

Closely associated with the reverse transcriptase is ribonuclease H, which is responsible for the degradation of the viral mRNA template after it has been transcribed to DNA. RNase H may be detached from reverse transcriptase by proteolytic cleavage, and it still retains activity after detachment. Its role as a target for chemotherapeutic intervention has not yet been assessed. Following the initial transcription of the genomic RNA to DNA, the latter must be duplicated and circularized before it can be integrated as proviral DNA into the cellular genome. As this integration requires the help of a virus-specified endonuclease, it should in principle serve as a plausible target, but, again, no compounds have so far been identified that would specifically interfere with this event.

Viral DNA Replication and Expression

To specifically block the replication of viral DNA or its transcription to RNA, or the splicing of the latter and its translation to protein, the use of oligodeoxynucleotides of well-defined length that are complementary to part of the viral genome could be envisaged. These complementary oligonucleotides may be expected to hybridize to their target sequence in the viral DNA (or RNA) and thus suppress the viral replication, transcription or translation machinery. This approach was originally called "hybridization competition" and has more recently been termed the "antisense" approach (Figure 7). Oligodeoxynucleotides, complementary to the viral genome, have indeed been shown to inhibit the replication of Rous sarcoma virus (69), and, more recently, of HIV-1 as well (70). However, antisense oligonucleotides suffer from a number of problems, e.g. poor uptake by the cells, premature degradation by nucleases and lack of stability of the hybrid formed with the target DNA or RNA sequence.

To overcome these difficulties, several strategies have been followed: conjugation with poly(L-lysine) to increase cellular uptake of the oligonucleotides (71); substitution of the phosphodiester groups by thiophosphates to protect the oligonucleotides against degradation by nucleases (72); replacement of the negatively charged phosphodiester groups by the neutral methylphosphonates, which enables the molecules to both penetrate the cells and resist degradation by nucleases (73–75); conversion of the (natural) β-configuration of the N-glycosidic bond to the α-configuration (76) to allow formation of a more stable duplex with the target DNA (or RNA); and covalent coupling of an intercalating agent to the oligonucleotide, also aimed at stabilizing the ensuing duplex with the target DNA or RNA

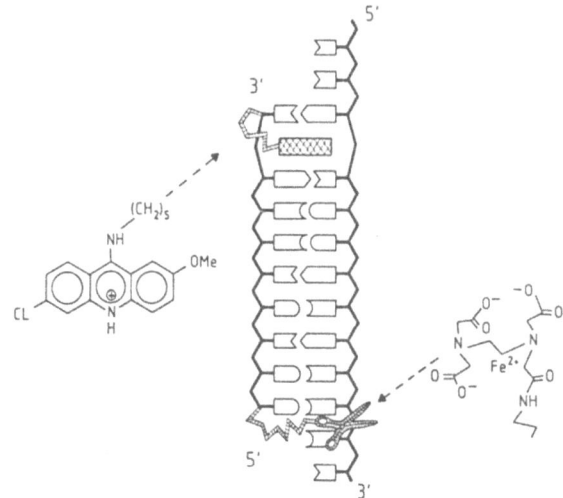

Figure 7: The "antisense" approach. Schematic representation of an oligonucleotide (left) that, because of its complementary base sequence, hybridizes to its target DNA or RNA (right) (adapted from C. Hélène's Figure 6 in Reference No. 78). At its 3′ end, the oligonucleotide is covalently linked to an intercalating agent (acridine), which is intended to stabilize the hybrid. At its 5′ end, it is covalently linked to EDTA-Fe^{2+}, which acts as a nucleic acid-cleaving reagent. The length of the oligonucleotide has been arbitrarily chosen: it may be extended to 14 or 16 bases to enhance the specificity of binding. Resistance of the oligonucleotide to premature degradation by nucleases may be conferred by substitution of methylphosphonates or phosphorothioates for the usual phosphate linkages.

(77). Some of these modifications, which have all been tried separately, will probably have to be combined in the same molecule in order to create the ideal antisense drug. Also, the optimal chain length of the oligonucleotides will have to be defined, so as to impart the greatest specificity. For the oligonucleotide methylphosphonates, a chain length of 14 or 16 has been estimated as sufficient (75).

The different possibilities offered by oligonucleotides as inhibitors of gene expression have been recently reviewed (78). If the oligonucleotide is equipped with a nucleic acid-cleaving device such as EDTA-Fe^{2+}, which in the presence of molecular oxygen is capable of generating hydroxyl radicals that can cleave the target DNA strand ("affinity cleaving") (Figure 7), such an approach may be successful in obtaining deletions of part of the viral genome. If so, it may be reasonable to envision the possibility that virus-infected cells may eventually be cleared from the viral genome, even during the latent stage of the infection.

Transcription of Viral RNA

The transcription of viral mRNA is positively controlled by virus-specified proteins, i.e. *tat* and *rev*, and thus these proteins appear to be suitable targets for chemotherapeutic attack. The *tat* protein may achieve transactivation by several means, in particular by increasing the rate of transcription from the long terminal repeat (LTR) promotor. The *tat* protein would bind to a region of 50–100 base pairs (called the TAR site) near the 3'end of the LTR. According to recent evidence (79), *tat* protein would form a dimeric structure (Figure 8), with the dimers held together by metal (e.g. Cd^{2+}) bridges between the cysteine residues of the monomer interfaces. In addition to Cd^{2+}, Zn^{2+} and Cu^{2+} may also be considered candidate metals that bind to *tat* in vivo. If indeed the dimeric structure and the metals are necessary for *tat* to bind to TAR and to transactivate the transcription of viral mRNA, any chemotherapeutic attempt at removing the metal ions or preventing dimerization may be worth pursuing. Thus, metal chelators should be investigated as possible anti-HIV agents, as should cysteine analogues and/or specific peptide analogues that mask the dimerization site. The study of cysteine analogue D-penicillamine may be a step in this direction. According to some reports (80, 81), which have not yet been confirmed, D-pencillamine may have a selective inhibitory effect on the replication of HIV-1.

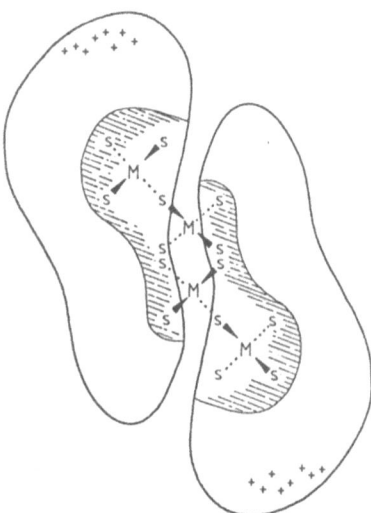

Figure 8: Schematic presentation of the *tat* dimer (adapted from Reference No. 79), with four metal ions (M) coordinated in tetrahedral geometry by 14 cysteine residues (S). Each monomer would contribute seven cysteine residues. The positive charges (+) represent the basic region of the protein that may participate in the binding of *tat* to its specific binding site (TAR) on the 5' long terminal repeat (LTR) of the proviral DNA genome.

Translation of Viral RNA

It may be possible to specifically suppress the translation of viral mRNA using complementary (antisense) oligonucleotides that hybridze with the target mRNA in the region of the initiation codon (AUG). As discussed above, some problems would have to be overcome before the antisense oligonucleotides could reach their target, but, provided they are delivered intact at their destination, they may be expected to markedly inhibit the functioning of the sense strand mRNA and shut off its translation to protein.

As the mature retroviral *gag* and *pol* proteins are derived from a (*gag-pol*) polyprotein precursor by post-translational cleavage, and as this cleavage is catalyzed by an HIV gene product (*pro*), this HIV protease represents another attractive chemotherapeutic target. The HIV protease belongs to the aspartyl proteases (82–84). It contains the sequence Asp-Thr-Gly, which is conserved in the active site of the aspartyl proteases. In the HIV protease this sequence occurs at positions 25–27. If Asp-25 is replaced by an asparagine residue, proteolytic activity of the enzyme is abolished, HIV *gag* p55 is no longer cleaved to *gag* p17, p24 and p15, and the mutant virions synthesized under these conditions are unable to infect other cells (84). Thus, a single mutation that blocks the activity of the HIV protease may also block the infectivity of the virus, and hence, specific inhibitors of the HIV protease may be expected to render the virus noninfectious. A strongly conserved pattern, X-Y-Pro-Z (where X is generally small and hydrophobic, Y is aromatic or large and hydrophobic, and Z is small and hydrophobic) has been found for the cleavage site of retroviral proteases (85), and this can be instructive in designing specific inhibitors of HIV protease. So far, however, no such specific inhibitors have been reported.

Another post-translational event that appears to be an attractive target for anti-HIV drugs is the glycosylation process. The viral envelope glycoprotein gp120, involved in the binding of HIV-1 to the CD4 receptor, is extremely heavily glycosylated (31–36 N-linked glycanes per gp120 molecule). It may be anticipated, therefore, that HIV virions formed in the presence of the glycosylation inhibitors would have a reduced ability to adsorb to the cell membrane and induce virus-cell fusion and would thus show impaired infectivity.

The first glycosylation inhibitor shown to inhibit infectivity of HIV-1 was 2-deoxy-D-glucose (86) (Figure 9). More recently, 1-deoxynojirimycin and castanospermine (a plant alkaloid isolated from the seeds of the Australian chestnut tree, Castanospermum australe) were also shown to interfere with HIV-induced syncytium formation and viral infectivity (87–89). Deoxymannojirimycin did not show any anti-retrovirus activity (87, 90). Castanospermine and 1-deoxynojirimycin are structurally related to D-glucose, as is 2-deoxy-D-glucose (Figure 9); deoxymannojirimycin (Figure 9) is in fact a mannose derivative (Figure 4). The mechanism of action of deoxymannojirimycin is quite different from that of castanospermine and 1-deoxynojirimycin. The latter inhibit the glucosidases, whereas the former inhibits the mannosidases that are involved in the trimming of N-linked oligosaccharides. During this trimming process the terminal glucose moieties of the oligosaccharides are removed by glucosidases I and II, after which the terminal mannose moieties are split off by mannosidases IA and IB. Only after this trimming has taken place can the oligosaccharide develop into its mature form, which requires the successive addition of N-acetylglucosamine, galactose and N-acetylneuraminic acid (NANA). From the observation that castanospermine and 1-deoxynojirimycin, but not deoxymannojirimycin, affect the infectivity of HIV-1, it may be inferred that limited trimming of the viral glycoproteins, involving only the outermost glucose and not the mannose residues, is required for virion maturation.

Although the glycosylation process may be regarded as an attractive target for anti-HIV chemotherapy, it should be recognized that glycosylation inhibitors have to be used at relatively high concentrations ($>$ 1 mM) (87, 89) to achieve their inhibitory effects on HIV-1 replication. Also, the doses at which castanospermine and its congeners were found to inhibit HIV-induced cytopathogenicity in MT-4 cells (Table 3) are much higher than the doses at which sulfated polysaccharides (Table 1) and 2',3'-dideoxynucleoside analogues (Table 2) inhibit viral cytopathogenicity in MT-4 cells. It is doubtful, therefore, that the dose required for castanospermine to inhibit HIV-1 replication is therapeutically attainable. Yet the glycosylation of the viral glycoproteins should be envisaged as a valuable target for the design of anti-HIV agents, and perhaps newly designed inhibitors should be aimed at one of the final steps in the maturation of the glycoproteins, e.g. the addition of NANA, as this may be the site where the greatest specificity could be accomplished.

Virus Assembly and Release (Budding)

Virus assembly per se has not been identified as the sole target for the action of any antiviral compound. Yet on theoretical grounds, virus assembly may just be as good a target for prospective inhibitors as virus disassembly has proven to be for the virus uncoating inhibitors (see above). Whereas uncoating inhibitors must reduce the flexibility of the viral capsid structure so as to prevent disassembly (35), virus assembly inhibitors should work the other way around and thus enhance capsid flexibility.

Budding of retrovirus particles has long been recognized as one of the sites where interferon acts, and indeed, human interferon alpha (HuIFN-α) and beta (HuIFN-β) but not gamma (HuIFN-γ) have been found to suppress HIV replication in vitro (91–93). The anti-HIV activity of interferon inducers such as the mismatched double-stranded RNA poly(I).poly(C_{12},U) (ampligen) (94, 95) may at least in part be mediated by the induction of interferon. Poly(I).poly(C_{12},U) is apparently more effective against HIV infection than could be accounted for by the amounts of interferon it induces (95). Since double-stranded RNA not only induces interferon bio-

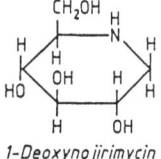

Figure 9: Glycosylation inhibitors: 2-deoxy-D-glucose, castanospermine, 1-deoxynojirimycin and 1-deoxymannojirimycin.

Table 3: Potency and selectivity of glycosylation inhibitors against HIV-1 in MT-4 cells (unpublished data).

Compound[a]	ED50[b] (µg/ml)	CD50[c] (µg/ml)	SI[d]
2-Deoxy-D-glucose	> 500	> 500	—
Castanospermine	200	> 500	> 2.5
1-Deoxynojirimycin	> 250	> 250	—
1 Deoxymannojirimycin	> 250	> 250	—

[a] Compounds added after a 2-hour virus adsorption period.
[b] 50 % effective dose, or compound concentration required to protect 50 % of the virus-infected cells against the cytopathic effect of HIV-1.
[c] 50 % cytotoxic dose, or compound concentration required to reduce the viability of mock-infected cells by 50 %.
[d] Selectivity index, or ratio of CD50 to ED50.

synthesis but also activates certain enzymes induced by interferon, the greater efficacy of the double-stranded RNA over interferon in protecting the cells against HIV infection may result from the activation of such enzymes. The most obvious candidate is the $2'$-$5'$ oligoadenylate synthetase, which, when switched on, synthesizes $2'$-$5'$ oligoadenylate, which in turn functions to activate a latent ribonuclease specific for single-stranded RNA. It would seem worth exploring to what extent this pathway contributes to the anti-HIV effects observed with interferon and double-stranded RNAs.

Conclusion

Several events in the HIV replicative cycle have been identified as targets for chemotherapeutic intervention: virus adsorption to the cell, virus-cell fusion, virus uncoating, reverse transcription of the viral RNA to proviral DNA, integration of the proviral DNA into the cellular genome, replication of the viral DNA and its expression (transcription, translation), transactivation by regulatory proteins such as the *tat* protein, processing of the viral precursor proteins (proteolytic cleavage, glycosylation), and finally, virus assembly and release (budding). For some of these targets, potent and selective inhibitors that achieve a marked activity against HIV have been found: sulfated polysaccharides (such as heparin, dextran sulfate, pentosan polysulfate, λ-carrageenan and mannan sulfate), which block virus adsorption to the cell, and $2',3'$-dideoxynucleoside analogues (such as $2',3'$-dideoxycytidine and -thymidine, $2',3'$-dideoxy-$2',3'$-didehydrocytidine and -thymidine, and $3'$-azido- and $3'$-fluoro-$2',3'$-dideoxythymidine and -uridine), which operate at the reverse transcriptase level (following intracellular conversion to their $5'$-triphosphates). For other, ostensibly attractive targets such as HIV uncoating, proviral DNA integration, proteolytic cleavage of viral precursor proteins, and virion assembly, no specific inhibitors have been reported so far. Yet the specificity of these events is such that it would seem quite feasible to design specific inhibitors. For a number of compounds active against HIV, e.g. glycyrrhizin (96), amphotericin (97) and oxetanocin (98), the target has not been revealed. For other compounds (e.g. suramin), which have been found to interact with one particular target (e.g. reverse transcriptase), other targets (e.g. virus adsorption) cannot necessarily be excluded. As our insight into the various steps of the HIV replicative cycle continues to grow, an increasing number of potential targets (e.g. the phosphorylation of the CD4 receptor) (99), may become apparent. Consequently, the further search for effective anti-HIV agents will profit from the multitude of targets available for chemotherapeutic attack of the virus.

Acknowledgements

The original investigations of the author are supported in part by the AIDS Basic Research Programme of the European Community and by grants from the Belgian Fonds voor Geneeskundig Wetenschappelijk Onderzoek (projects No. 3.0040.83 and 3.0097.87), the Belgian Geconcerteerde Onderzoeksacties (project No. 85/90-79), and Janssen Pharmaceutica. I thank Christiane Callebaut for her dedicated editorial help.

References

1. De Clercq, E.: Chemotherapeutic approaches to the treatment of the acquired immune deficiency syndrome (AIDS). Journal of Medicinal Chemistry 1986, 29: 1561–1569.
2. De Clercq, E.: Perspectives for the chemotherapy of AIDS. Anticancer Research 1987, 7: 1023–1038.
3. Gallo, R., Wong-Staal, F., Montagnier, L., Haseltine, W. A., Yoshida, M.: HIV/HTLV gene nomenclature. Nature 1988, 333: 504.
4. Miller, R. H.: Human immunodeficiency virus may encode a novel protein on the genomic DNA plus strand. Science 1988, 239: 1420–1422.
5. Henderson, L. E., Sowder, R. C., Copeland, T. D., Benveniste, R. E., Oroszlan, S.: Isolation and characterization of a novel protein (X-ORF product) from SIV and HIV-2. Science 1988, 241: 199–201.
6. Jameson, B. A., Rao, P. E., Kong, L. I., Hahn, B. H., Shaw, G. M., Hood, L. E., Kent, S. B. H.: Location and chemical synthesis of a binding site for HIV-1 on the CD4 protein. Science 1988, 240: 1335–1339.
7. Pert, C. B., Hill, J. M., Ruff, M. R., Berman, R. M., Robey, W. G., Arthur, L. O., Ruscetti, F. W., Farrar, W. L.: Octapeptides deduced from the neuropeptide receptor-like pattern of antigen T4 in brain potently inhibit human immunodeficiency virus receptor binding and T-cell infectivity. Proceedings of the National Academy of Sciences of the USA 1986, 83: 9254–9258.
8. Ruff, M. R., Martin, B. M., Ginns, E. I., Farrar, W. L., Pert, C. B.: CD4 receptor binding peptides that block HIV infectivity cause human monocyte chemotaxis. FEBS Letters 1987, 211: 17–22.
9. Barnes, D. M.: Debate over potential AIDS drug. Science 1987, 237: 128–130.
10. Smith, D. H., Byrn, R. A., Marsters, S. A., Gregory, T., Groopman, J. E., Capon, D. J.: Blocking of HIV-1 infectivity by a soluble, secreted form of the CD4 antigen. Science 1987, 238: 1704–1707.
11. Fisher, R. A., Bertonis, J. M., Meier, W., Johnson, V. A., Costopoulos, D. S., Liu, T., Tizard, R., Walker, B. D., Hirsch, M. S., Schooley, R. T., Flavell, R. A.: HIV infection is blocked in vitro by recombinant soluble CD4. Nature 1988, 331: 76–78.
12. Hussey, R. E., Richardson, N. E., Kowalski, M., Brown, N. R., Chang, H.-C., Siliciano, R. F., Dorfman, T., Walker, B., Sodroski, J., Reinherz, E. L.: A soluble CD4 protein selectively inhibits HIV replication and syncytium formation. Nature 1988, 331: 78–81.
13. Deen, K. C., McDougal, J. S., Inacker, R., Folena-Waserman, G., Arthos, J., Rosenberg, J., Maddon, P. J., Axel, R., Sweet, R. W.: A soluble form of CD4 (T4) protein inhibits AIDS virus infection. Nature 1988, 331: 82–84.

14. Traunecker, A., Lüke, W., Karjalainen, K.: Soluble CD4 molecules neutralize human immunodeficiency virus type 1. Nature 1988, 331: 84–86.
15. Baba, M., Pauwels, R., Balzarini, J., Arnout, J., Desmyter, J., De Clercq, E.: Mechanism of inhibitory effect of dextran sulfate and heparin on replication of human immunodeficiency virus in vitro. Proceedings of the National Academy of Sciences of the USA 1988, 85: 6132–6136.
16. Mitsuya, H., Looney, D. J., Kuno, S., Ueno, R., Wong-Staal, F., Broder, S.: Dextran sulfate suppression of viruses in the HIV family: inhibition of virion binding to $CD4^+$ cells. Science 1988, 240: 646–649.
17. Baba, M., Nakajima, M., Schols, D., Pauwels, R., Balzarini, J., De Clercq, E.: Pentosan polysulfate, a sulfated oligosaccharide, is a potent and selective anti-HIV agent in vitro. Antiviral Research 1988: (in press).
18. De Somer, P., De Clercq, E., Billiau, A., Schonne, E., Claesen, M.: Antiviral activity of polyacrylic and polymethacrylic acids. I. Mode of action in vitro. Journal of Virology 1968, 2: 878–885.
19. Ito, M., Baba, M., Sato, A., Pauwels, R., De Clercq, E., Shigeta, S.: Inhibitory effect of dextran sulfate and heparin on the replication of human immunodeficiency virus (HIV) in vitro. Antiviral Research 1987, 7: 361–367.
20. Ueno, R., Kuno, S.: Dextran sulphate, a potent anti-HIV agent in vitro having synergism with zidovudine. Lancet 1987, i: 1379.
21. Yoshida, O., Nakashima, H., Yoshida, T., Kaneko, Y., Yamamoto, I., Matsuzaki, K., Uryu, T., Yamamoto, N.: Sulfation of the immunomodulating polysaccharide lentinan: a novel strategy for antivirals to human immunodeficiency virus (HIV). Biochemical Pharmacology 1988, 37: 2887–2891.
22. McCune, J. M., Rabin, L. B., Feinberg, M. B., Lieberman, M., Kosek, J. C., Reyes, G. R., Weissman, I. L.: Endoproteolytic cleavage of gp160 is required for the activation of human immunodeficiency virus. Cell 1988, 53: 55–67.
23. Nicolaides, E., DeWald, H., Westland, R., Lipnik, M., Posler, J.: Potential antiviral agents. Carbobenzoxy di- and tripeptides active against measles and herpes viruses. Journal of Medicinal Chemistry 1968, 1: 74–79.
24. Miller, F. A., Dixon, G. J., Arnett, G., Dice, J. R., Rightsel, W. A., Schabel, F. M., Jr., McLean, I. W., Jr.: Antiviral activity of carbobenzoxy di- and tripeptides on measles virus. Applied Microbiology 1968, 16: 1489–1496.
25. Norrby, E.: The effect of a carbobenzoxy tripeptide on the biological activities of measles virus. Virology 1971, 44: 599–608.
26. Richardson, C. D., Scheid, A., Choppin, P. W.: Specific inhibition of paramyxovirus and myxovirus replication by oligopeptides with amino acid sequences similar to those at the N-termini of the F_1 or HA_2 viral polypeptides. Virology 1980, 105: 205–222.
27. Richardson, C. D., Choppin, P. W.: Oligopeptides that specifically inhibit membrane fusion by paramyxoviruses: studies on the site of action. Virology 1983, 131: 518–532.
28. McSharry, J. J., Caliguiri, L. A., Eggers, H. J.: Inhibition of uncoating of poliovirus by arildone, a new antiviral drug. Virology 1979, 97: 307–315.
29. Tisdale, M., Selway, J. W.: Inhibition of an early stage of rhinovirus replication by dichloroflavan (BW683C). Journal of General Virology 1983, 64: 795–803.
30. Ninomiya, Y., Ohsawa, C., Aoyama, M., Umeda, I., Suhara, Y., Ishitsuka, H.: Antivirus agent, Ro 09-0410, binds to rhinovirus specifically and stabilizes the virus conformation. Virology 1984, 134: 269–276.
31. Fox, M. P., Otto, M. J., McKinlay, M. A.: Prevention of rhinovirus and poliovirus uncoating by WIN 51711, a new antiviral drug. Antimicrobial Agents and Chemotherapy 1986, 30: 110–116.
32. Alarcon, B., Zerial, A., Dupiol, C., Carrasco, L.: Antirhinovirus compound 44 081 R.P. inhibits virus uncoating. Antimicrobial Agents and Chemotherapy 1986, 30: 31–34.
33. Hay, A. J., Wolstenholme, A. J., Skehel, J. J., Smith, M. H.: The molecular basis of the specific anti-influenza action of amantadine. EMBO Journal 1985, 4: 3021–3024.
34. Smith, T. J., Kremer, M. J., Luo, M., Vriend, G., Arnold, E., Kamer, G., Rossmann, M. G., McKinlay, M. A., Diana, G. D., Otto, M. J.: The site of attachment in human rhinovirus 14 for antiviral agents that inhibit uncoating. Science 1986, 233: 1286–1293.
35. Rossmann, M. G.: Antiviral agents targeted to interact with viral capsid proteins and a possible application to human immunodeficiency virus. Proceedings of the National Academy of Sciences of the USA 1988, 85: 4625–4627.
36. Larder, B. A., Purifoy, D. J. M., Powell, K. L., Darby, G.: Site-specific mutagenesis of AIDS virus reverse transcriptase. Nature 1987, 327: 716–717.
37. Mitsuya, H., Popovic, M., Yarchoan, R., Matsushita, S., Gallo, R. C., Broder, S.: Suramin protection of T cells in vitro against infectivity and cytopathic effect of HTLV-III. Science 1984, 226: 172–174.
38. De Clercq, E.: Suramin: a potent inhibitor of the reverse transcriptase of RNA tumor viruses. Cancer Letters 1979, 8: 9–22.
39. Balzarini, J., Mitsuya, H., De Clercq, E., Broder, S.: Comparative inhibitory effects of suramin and other selected compounds on the infectivity and replication of human T-cell lymphotropic virus (HTLV-III)/ lymphadenopathy-associated virus (LAV). International Journal of Cancer 1986, 37: 451–457.
40. Balzarini, J., Mitsuya, H., De Clercq, E., Broder, S.: Aurin-tricarboxylic acid and Evans blue represent two different classes of anionic compounds which selectively inhibit the cytopathogenicity of human T-cell lymphotropic virus type III/lymphadenopathy-associated virus. Biochemical and Biophysical Research Communications 1986, 136: 64–71.
41. Vrang, L., Öberg, B.: PP_i analogs as inhibitors of human T-lymphotropic virus type III reverse transcriptase. Antimicrobial Agents and Chemotherapy 1986, 29: 867–872.
42. Mitsuya, H., Weinhold, K. J., Furman, P. A., St. Clair, M. H., Nusinoff Lehrman, S., Gallo, R. C., Bolognesi, D., Barry, D. W., Broder, S.: 3'-Azido-3'-deoxythymidine (BW A509U): an antiviral agent that inhibits the infectivity and cytopathic effect of human T-lymphotropic virus type III/lymphadenopathy-associated virus in vitro. Proceedings of the National Academy of Sciences of the USA 1985, 82: 7096–7100.
43. Mitsuya, H., Broder, S.: Inhibition of the in vitro infectivity and cytopathic effect of human T-lymphotropic virus type III/lymphadenopathy-associated virus (HTLV-III/LAV) by 2',3'-dideoxynucleosides. Proceedings of the National Academy of Sciences of the USA 1986, 83: 1911–1915.
44. Pauwels, R., De Clercq, E., Desmyter, J., Balzarini, J., Goubau, P., Herdewijn, P., Vanderhaeghe, H., Vandeputte, M.: Sensitive and rapid assay on MT-4 cells for detection of antiviral compounds against the AIDS virus. Journal of Virological Methods 1987, 16: 171–185.
45. Baba, M., Pauwels, R., Herdewijn, P., De Clercq, E., Desmyter, J., Vandeputte, M.: Both 2',3'-dideoxy-

thymidine and its 2′,3′-unsaturated derivative (2′,3′-dideoxythymidinene) are potent and selective inhibitors of human immunodeficiency virus replication in vitro. Biochemical and Biophysical Research Communications 1987, 142: 128–134.
46. Baba, M., Pauwels, R., Balzarini, J., Herdewijn, P., De Clercq, E.: Selective inhibition of human immunodeficiency virus (HIV) by 3′-azido-2′,3′-dideoxyguanosine in vitro. Biochemical and Biophysical Research Communications 1987, 145: 1080–1086.
47. Herdewijn, P., Pauwels, P., Baba, M., Balzarini, J., De Clercq, E.: Synthesis and anti-HIV activity of various 2′- and 3′substituted 2′,3′-dideoxyadenosines: a structure-activity analysis. Journal of Medicinal Chemistry 1987, 30:2131–2137.
48. Balzarini, J., Pauwels, R., Baba, M., Robins, M. J., Zou, R., Herdewijn, P., De Clercq, E.: The 2′,3′-dideoxyriboside of 2,6-diaminopurine selectively inhibits human immunodeficiency virus (HIV) replication in vitro. Biochemical and Biophysical Research Communications 1987, 145: 269–276.
49. Balzarini, J., Baba, M., Pauwels, R., Herdewijn, P., Wood, S. G., Robins, M. J., De Clercq, E.: Potent and selective activity of 3′-azido-2,6-diaminopurine-2′,3′-dideoxyriboside, 3′-fluoro-2,6-diaminopurine-2′,3′-dideoxyriboside, and 3′-fluoro-2′,3′-dideoxyguanosine against human immunodeficiency virus. Molecular Pharmacology 1987, 33, 243–249.
50. Balzarini, J., Baba, M., Pauwels, R., Herdewijn, P., De Clercq, E.: Anti-retrovirus activity of 3′-fluoro- and 3′-azido-substituted pyrimidine 2′,3′-dideoxynucleoside analogues Biochemical Pharmacology 1988, 37: 2847–2856.
51. Marquez, V. E., Tseng, C. K.-H., Kelley, J. A., Mitsuya, H., Broder, S., Roth, J. S., Driscoll, J. S.: 2′,3′-Dideoxy-2′-fluoro-ara-A. An acid-stable purine nucleoside active against human immunodeficiency virus (HIV). Biochemical Pharmacology 1987, 36: 2719–2722.
52. Pauwels, R., Balzarini, J., Schols, D., Baba, M., Desmyter, J., Rosenberg, I., Holy, A., De Clercq, E.: Phosphonylmethoxyethyl purine derivatives, a new class of anti-human immunodeficiency virus agents. Antimicrobial Agents and Chemotherapy 1988, 32: 1025–1030.
53. Hayashi, S., Phadtare, S., Zemlicka, J., Matsukura, M., Mitsuya, H., Broder, S.: Adenallene and cytallene: acyclic nucleoside analogues that inhibit replication and cytopathic effect of human immunodeficiency virus (HIV) in vitro. Proceedings of the National Academy of Sciences of the USA 1988, 85: 6127–6131.
54. Jentsch, K. D., Hunsmann, G., Hartmann, H., Nickel, P.: Inhibition of human immunodeficiency virus type 1 reverse transcriptase by suramin-related compounds. Journal of General Virology 1987, 68: 2183–2192.
55. Furman, P. A., Fyfe, J. A., St. Clair, M. H., Weinhold, K., Rideout, J. L., Freeman, G. A., Nusinoff-Lehrman, S., Bolognesi, D. P., Broder, S., Mitsuya, H., Barry, D. W.: Phosphorylation of 3′-azido-3′-deoxythymidine and selective interaction of the 5′-triphosphate with human immunodeficiency virus reverse transcriptase. Proceedings of the National Academy of Sciences of the USA 1986, 83: 8333–8337.
56. St. Clair, M. H., Richards, C. A., Spector, T., Weinhold, K. J., Miller, W. H., Langlois, A. J., Furman, P. A.: 3′-Azido-3′-deoxythymidine triphosphate as an inhibitor and substrate of purified human immunodeficiency virus reverse transcriptase. Antimicrobial Agents and Chemotherapy 1987, 31: 1972–1977.
57. Ono, K., Ogasawara, M., Iwata, Y., Nakane, H., Fujii, T., Sawai, K., Saneyoshi, M.: Inhibition of reverse transcriptase activity by 2′,3′-dideoxythymidine 5′-triphosphate and its derivatives modified on the 3′ position. Biochemical and Biophysical Research Communications 1986, 140: 498–507.
58. Vrang, L., Bazin, H., Remaud, G., Chattopadhyaya, J., Öberg, B.: Inhibition of the reverse transcriptase from HIV by 3′-azido-3′-deoxythymidine triphosphate and its threo analogue. Antiviral Research 1987, 7: 139–149.
59. Chen, M. S., Oshana, S. C.: Inhibition of HIV reverse transcriptase by 2′,3′-dideoxynucleoside triphosphates. Biochemical Pharmacology 1987, 36: 4361–4362.
60. Matthes, E., Lehmann, Ch., Scholz, D., von Janta-Lipinski, M., Gaertner, K., Rosenthal, H. A., Langen, P.: Inhibition of HIV-associated reverse transcriptase by sugar-modified derivatives of thymidine 5′-triphosphate in comparison to cellular DNA polymerases α and β. Biochemical and Biophysical Research Communications 1987, 148: 78–85.
61. Cheng, Y.-c., Dutschman, G. E., Bastow, K. F., Sarngadharan, M. G., Ting, R. Y. C.: Human immunodeficiency virus reverse transcriptase. Journal of Biological Chemistry 1987, 262: 2187–2189.
62. Balzarini, J., Kang, G.-J., Dalal, M., Herdewijn, P., De Clercq, E., Broder, S., Johns, D. G.: The anti-HTLV-III (anti-HIV) and cytotoxic activity of 2′,3′-didehydro-2′,3′-dideoxyribonucleosides: a comparison with their parental 2′,3′-dideoxyribonucleosides. Molecular Pharmacology 1987, 32: 162–167.
63. Starnes, M. C., Cheng, Y.-c.: Cellular metabolism of 2′,3′-dideoxycytidine, a compound active against human immunodeficiency virus in vitro. Journal of Biological Chemistry 1987, 262: 988–991.
64. Haertle, T., Carrera, C. J., Wasson, D. B., Sowers, L. C., Richman, D. D., Carson, D. A.: Metabolism and anti-human immunodeficiency virus-1 activity of 2-halo-2′,3′-dideoxyadenosine derivatives. Journal of Biological Chemistry 1988, 263: 5870–5875.
65. Balzarini, J., Pauwels, R., Baba, M., Herdewijn, P., De Clercq, E., Broder, S., Johns, D. G.: The in vitro and in vivo anti-retrovirus activity, and intracellular metabolism of 3′-azido-2′,3′-dideoxythymidine and 2′,3′-dideoxycytidine are highly dependent on the cell species. Biochemical Pharmacology 1988, 37: 897–903.
66. Balzarini, J., Cooney, D. A., Dalal, M., Kang, G.-J., Cupp, J. E., De Clercq, E., Broder, S., Johns, D. G.: 2′,3′-Dideoxycytidine: regulation of its metabolism and anti-retroviral potency by natural pyrimidine nucleosides and by inhibitors of pyrimidine nucleotide synthesis. Molecular Pharmacology 1987, 32: 798–806.
67. Vogt, M. W., Hartshorn, K. L., Furman, P. A., Chou, T.-C., Fyfe, J. A., Coleman, L. A., Crumpacker, C., Schooley, R. T., Hirsch, M. S.: Ribavirin antagonizes the effect of azidothymidine on HIV replication. Science 1987, 235: 1376–1379.
68. Baba, M., Pauwels, R., Balzarini, J., Herdewijn, P., De Clercq, E., Desmyter, J.: Ribavirin antagonizes inhibitory effects of pyrimidine 2′,3′-dideoxynucleosides but enhances inhibitory effects of purine 2′,3′-dideoxynucleosides on replication of human immunodeficiency virus in vitro. Antimicrobial Agents and Chemotherapy 1987, 31: 1613–1617.
69. Zamecnik, P. C., Stephenson, M. L.: Inhibition of Rous sarcoma virus replication and cell transformation by a specific oligodeoxynucleotide. Proceedings of the National Academy of Sciences of the USA 1978, 75: 280–284.
70. Zamecnik, P. C., Goodchild, J., Taguchi, Y., Sarin, P. S.: Inhibition of replication and expression of human T-cell lymphotropic virus type III in cultured cells by exogenous synthetic oligonucleotides complementary

to viral RNA. Proceedings of the National Academy of Sciences of the USA 1986, 83: 4143–4146.
71. Lemaitre, M., Bayard, B., Lebleu, B.: Specific antiviral activity of a poly(L-lysine)-conjugated oligodeoxyribonucleotide sequence complementary to vesicular stomatitis virus N protein mRNA initiation site. Proceedings of the National Academy of Sciences of the USA 1987, 84: 648–652.
72. Matsukura, M., Shinozuka, K., Zon, G., Mitsuya, H., Reitz, M., Cohen, J. S., Broder, S.: Phosphorothioate analogs of oligodeoxynucleotides: inhibitors of replication and cytopathic effects of human immunodeficiency virus. Proceedings of the National Academy of Sciences of the USA 1987, 84: 7706–7710.
73. Agris, C. H., Blake, K. R., Miller, P. S., Reddy, M. P., Ts'o, P. O. P.: Inhibition of vesicular stomatitis virus protein synthesis and infection by sequence-specific oligodeoxyribonucleoside methylphosphonates. Biochemistry 1986, 25: 6268–6275.
74. Smith, C. C., Aurelian, L., Reddy, M. P., Miller, P. S., Ts'o, P. O. P.: Antiviral effect of an oligo(nucleoside methylphosphonate) complementary to the splice junction of herpes simplex virus type 1 immediate early pre-mRNAs 4 and 5. Proceedings of the National Academy of Sciences of the USA 1986, 83: 2787–2791.
75. Ts'o, P. O. P., Miller, P. S., Aurelian, L., Murakami, A., Agris, C., Blake, K. R., Lin, S.-B., Lee, B. L., Smith, C. C.: An approach to chemotherapy based on base sequence information and nucleic acid chemistry. Annals of the New York Academy of Sciences 1987, 507: 220–241.
76. Morvan, F., Rayner, B., Leonetti, J.-P., Imbach, J.-L.: α-DNA VII. Solid phase synthesis of α-anomeric oligodeoxyribonucleotides. Nucleic Acids Research 1988, 16: 833–847.
77. Toulmé, J. J., Krisch, H. M., Loreau, N., Thuong, N. T., Hélène, C.: Specific inhibition of mRNA translation by complementary oligonucleotides covalently linked to intercalating agents. Proceedings of the National Academy of Sciences of the USA 1986, 83: 1227–1231.
78. Stein, C. A., Cohen, J. S.: Oligodeoxynucleotides as inhibitors of gene expression: a review. Cancer Research 1988, 48: 2659–2668.
79. Frankel, A. D., Bredt, D. S., Pabo, C. O.: Tat protein from human immunodeficiency virus from a metal-linked dimer. Science 1988, 240: 70–73.
80. Chandra, P., Sarin, P. S.: Selective inhibition of replication of the AIDS-associated virus HTLV-III/LAV by synthetic D-penicillamine. Arzneimittel-Forschung/Drug Research 1986, 36: 184–186.
81. Schulof, R. S., Scheib, R. G., Parenti, D. M., Simon, G. L., Di-Gioia, R. A., Paxton, H. M., Sztein, M. B., Chandra, P., Courtless, J. W., Taguchi, Y. T., Sun, D. K., Goldstein, A. L., Sarin, P. S.: Treatment of HTLV-III/LAV-infected patients with D-penicillamine. Arzneimittel-Forschung/Drug Research 1986, 36: 1531–1534.
82. Pearl, L. H., Taylor, W. R.: A structural model for the retroviral proteases. Nature 1987, 329: 351–354.
83. Katoh, I., Yasunaga, T., Ikawa, Y., Yoshinaka, Y.: Inhibition of retroviral protease activity by an aspartyl proteinase inhibitor. Nature 1987, 329: 654–656.
84. Kohl, N. E., Emini, E. A., Schleif, W. A., Davis, L. J., Heimbach, J. C., Dixon, R. A. F., Scolnick, E. M., Sigal, I. S.: Active human immunodeficiency virus protease is required for viral infectivity. Proceedings of the National Academy of Sciences of the USA 1988, 85: 4686–4690.
85. Pearl, L. H., Taylor, W. R.: Sequence specificity of retroviral proteases. Nature 1987, 328: 482.
86. Blough, H. A., Pauwels, R., De Clercq, E., Cogniaux, J., Sprecher-Goldberger, S., Thiry, L.: Glycosylation inhibitors block the expression of LAV/HTLV-III (HIV) glycoproteins. Biochemical and Biophysical Research Communications 1986, 141: 33–38.
87. Gruters, R. A., Neefjes, J. J., Tersmette, M., de Goede, R. E. Y., Tulp, A., Huisman, H. G., Miedema, F., Ploegh, H. L.: Interference with HIV-induced syncytium formation and viral infectivity by inhibitors of trimming glucosidase. Nature 1987, 330: 74–77.
88. Walker, B. D., Kowalski, M., Goh, W. C., Kozarsky, K., Krieger, M., Rosen, C., Rohrschneider, L., Haseltine, W. A., Sodroski, J.: Inhibition of human immunodeficiency virus syncytium formation and virus replication by castanospermine. Proceedings of the National Academy of Sciences of the USA 1987, 84: 8120–8124.
89. Tyms, A. S., Berrie, E. M., Ryder, T. A., Nash, R. J., Hegarty, M. P., Taylor, D. L., Mobberley, M. A., Davis, J. M., Bell, E. A., Jeffries, D. J., Taylor-Robinson, D., Fellows, L. E.: Castanospermine and other plant alkaloid inhibitors of glucosidase activity block the growth of HIV. Lancet 1987, ii: 1025–1026.
90. Sunkara, P. S., Bowlin, T. L., Liu, P. S., Sjoerdsma, A.: Antiretroviral activity of castanospermine and deoxynojirimycin, specific inhibitors of glycoprotein processing. Biochemical and Biophysical Research Communications 1987, 148: 206–210.
91. Ho, D. D., Hartshorn, K. L., Rota, T. R., Andrews, C. A., Kaplan, J. C., Schooley, R. T., Hirsch, M. S.: Recombinant human interferon alfa-a suppresses HTLV-III replication in vitro. Lancet 1985, i: 602–604.
92. Yamamoto, J. K., Barré-Sinoussi, F., Bolton, V., Pedersen, N. C., Gardner, M. B.: Human alpha- and beta-interferon but not gamma- suppress the in vitro replication of LAV, HTLV-III, and ARV-2. Journal of Interferon Research 1986, 6: 143–152.
93. Hartshorn, K. L., Neumeyer, D., Vogt, M. W., Schooley, R. T., Hirsch, M. S.: Activity of interferons alpha, beta, and gamma against human immunodeficiency virus replication in vitro. AIDS Research and Human Retroviruses 1987, 3: 125–133.
94. Mitchell, W. M., Montefiori, D. C., Robinson, W. E., Jr., Strayer, D. R., Carter, W. A.: Mismatched double-stranded RNA (ampligen) reduces concentration of zidovudine (azidothymidine) required for in vitro inhibition of human immunodeficiency virus. Lancet 1987, i: 890–892.
95. Montefiori, D. C., Mitchell, W. M.: Antiviral activity of mismatched double-stranded RNA against human immunodeficiency virus in vitro. Proceedings of the National Academy of Sciences of the USA 1987, 84: 2985–2989.
96. Ito, M., Nakashima, H., Baba, M., Pauwels, R., De Clercq, E., Shigeta, S., Yamamoto, N.: Inhibitory effect of glycyrrhizin on the in vitro infectivity and cytopathic activity of the human immunodeficiency virus [HIV (HTLV-III/LAV)]. Antiviral Research 1987, 7: 127–137.
97. Schaffner, C. P., Plescia, O. J., Pontani, D., Sun, D., Thornton, A., Pandey, R. C., Sarin, P. S.: Anti-viral activity of amphotericin B methyl ester: inhibition of HTLV-III replication in cell culture. Biochemical Pharmacology 1986, 35: 4110–4113.
98. Hoshino, H., Shimizu, N., Shimada, N., Takita, T., Takeuchi, T.: Inhibition of infectivity of human immunodeficiency virus by oxetanocin. Journal of Antibiotics 1987, 15: 1077–1078.
99. Fields, A. P., Bednarik, D. P., Hess, A., May, W. S.: Human immunodeficiency virus induces phosphorylation of its cell surface receptor. Nature 1988, 333: 278–280.

Modern Strategies in the Design of Antimicrobial Agents

J. K. Seydel

Several statistical and graphical methods and systems have been developed during recent decades to assist in a more rational approach to drug design. Together with an increased knowledge of molecular biology and the development of simple, suitable in vitro test systems, a better understanding of the various steps in drug action and their structural dependence has been achieved. The newly developed computerized techniques are especially helpful for the systematic development of new antibacterial agents. Three major applications of these techniques are reviewed: (1) Lead generation by computer graphics, molecular modelling and three-dimensional design; (2) Rationalization in the optimization procedure of lead compounds by quantitative structure-activity relationship (QSAR) techniques; and (3) Comparison of various biological activity data derived from test systems by multivariate data analysis to avoid unnecessary testing and to separate pharmacodynamic and pharmacokinetic effects.

Fortuitous findings have played an essential role in drug research and development, due to the enormous complexity of the biological systems. Indeed, most of the drugs used today have been discovered by a combination of serendipity and creativity. In most cases, when these circumstances result in the detection of an active compound, the mode of action, i.e. the properties of the specific receptor and the location of interaction with the drug, is unknown. Therefore the action of many drugs is not highly specific and side effects independent of the therapeutic effect may arise. There is no doubt that numerous potent drugs have been detected by mass screening and empirical guidelines. Nevertheless it has always been the aim of scientists involved in the development of new drugs to find a more rational approach to drug design. Potent drugs with a large therapeutic index against a great number and variety of diseases are still lacking. Progress in this respect is therefore not merely an academic interest but a practical, clinical, and, because of enormous screening costs, an economic challenge as well.

The development of suitable in vitro test systems, the increased knowledge of molecular biology, the application of modern quantitative structure-activity relationships, and the progress made in X-ray and nuclear magnetic resonance (NMR) techniques have enabled researchers to construct a more rational strategy of drug development. These improved conditions are especially favorable for the rational design of antiparasitic drugs, because of the possibility to study separately the structural requirements and the dependency relationships for the various steps involved in drug action. This is illustrated in Figure 1. After its administration the drug is absorbed from the intestinal tract, transferred into the bloodstream and distributed to the various tissues. Simultaneously the drug is eliminated unchanged and metabolized from the central blood compartment via bile and the kidneys. These pharmacokinetic processes determine the concentration of drug available in the tissues surrounding the parasites. Additionally, two other preconditions for drug action are a sufficient permeation of the cell wall of the microorganism and a significant affinity for certain enzymes or other targets essential for parasite growth.

These three aspects of drug action can possess widely differing structural requirements, the knowledge of which is of great importance for optimization drug. The pharmacokinetic properties and those properties responsible for permeation into bacterial cells are to a large extent determined by the sum of the lipophilic-hydrophilic properties of the molecule. In contrast, the affinity for the target (the specific receptor) requires high structural specificity, i.e. suitable conformation and charge distribution, and specifically localized lipophilic and hydrophilic areas. Therefore it seems reasonable to first optimize the structure for interaction with the specific receptor in an isolated simple test system, as optimization of the other steps is less structural specificity demanding. The understanding and interpretation of isolated steps is a necessary precondition for deriving causal connections between structure and biological effect. This can then lead to prediction of activity of drugs not yet synthesized, improvement of our under-

---

Borstel Research Institute, D-2061 Borstel, FRG.

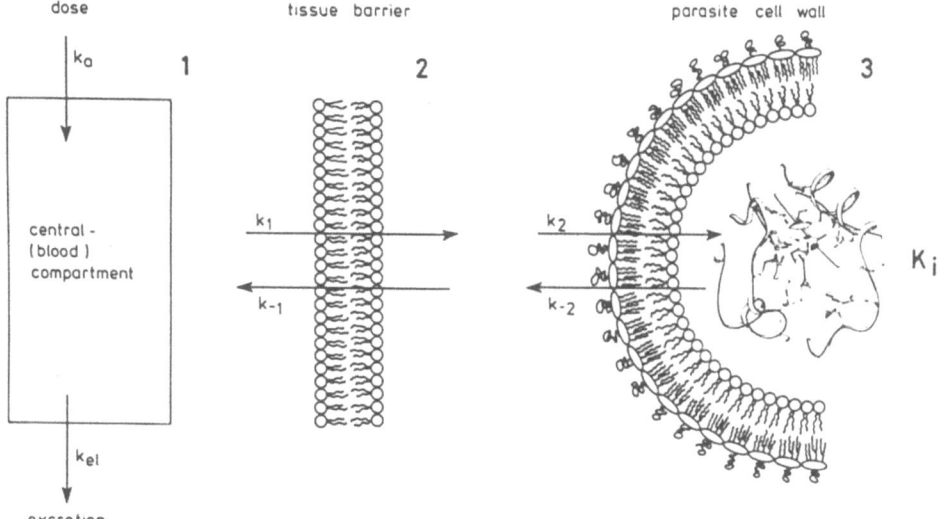

Figure 1: Factors possibly limiting the antiparasitic action of drugs:
1. Pharmacokinetic properties.
2. Properties responsible for the permeation of parasitic cell wall.
3. Affinity to the receptor (enzyme).

standing of drug action mechanisms on a molecular level, and development of highly specific compounds. Admittedly, the integration of information obtained in separate isolated test systems into the whole setting of drug action is still problematic because of nonlinearities involved.

Several mathematical, statistical, and graphical methods and systems are available to assist current efforts to derive quantitative structure-activity relationships, to prove working hypotheses, to find exceptions, to construct three-dimensional models of drug- and receptor molecules, and to calculate interaction energies even for molecules not yet synthesized (1–6). Depending on the level of information available, one method or a combination of these tools can be used in finding new leads or in guiding the optimization process. Thus there is not one but several new strategies in modern drug design. It is impossible to present a complete survey in this contribution rather, an admittedly subjective selection of special tools is presented.

1. Stepwise Approach in Development of a New Dihydrofolate Reductase Inhibitor
Using Computer Graphics (Receptor Structure Known)

The first crystal structure of a receptor complexed with an inhibitor molecule to be analyzed by X-ray studies was the *Escherichia coli*-derived dihydrofolate reductase (DHFR) and its complex with methotrexate

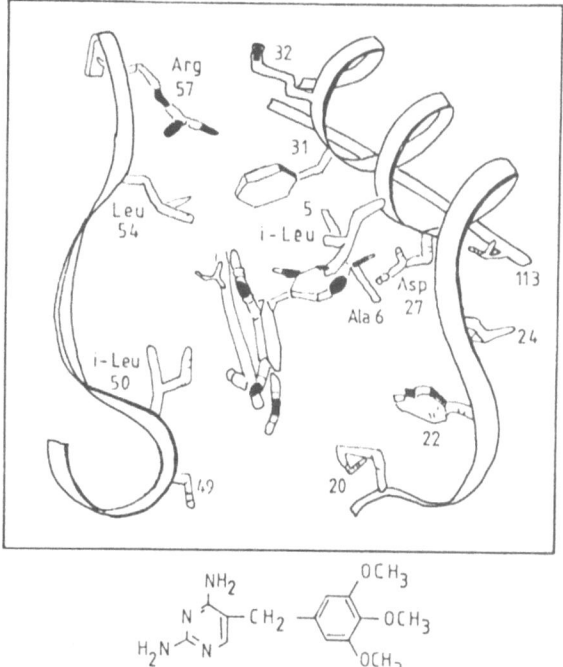

Figure 2: Schematic drawing of the binding site for trimethoprim in *Escherichia coli* DHFR (Taken from Reference No. 8).

(7). Later, similar studies were performed with DHFR from other bacterial and mammalian sources as well as with a DHFR/trimethoprim (TMP) complex. Trimethoprim specifically inhibits bacterial DHFR (8) (Figure 2). During investigations to devel-

Table 1: Cell-free (I_{50}) and whole cell (MIC) inhibitory activities (μmol/l) and lipophilic properties (log k'_r) of benzylpyrimidines.

			Escherichia coli (ATCC)			Mycobacterium lufu			
			I_{50}	MIC	MIC/I_{50}	I_{50}	MIC	MIC/I_{50}	log k'_r
R_3	R_4	R_5							
OCH_3	$OC_2H_4OCH_3$	OCH_3	0.0093	8.28	890	0.957	>128	> 133	−0.59
OCH_3	OCH_3 [b]	OCH_3	0.0045	1.50	333	0.325	>110	> 338	−0.36
OCH_3	Br	OCH_3	0.0017	1	588	0.152	26.5	174	0.82
OCH_3	_c	OCH_3	0.00039	56	143590	0.034	1.03	30.3	1.28

[a] Basic chemical structures

[structure of benzylpyrimidine with H_2N, N, H_2N, CH_3, CH_2, R_3, R_4, R_5 groups]

[b] TMP

[c] $O(CH_2)_3-NH-\langle\rangle-SO_2-\langle\rangle-NH_2$ (K-130)

op an inhibitor of mycobacterial DHFR, trimethoprim, which is inactive in whole cell systems of mycobacteria, was found to also exert inhibitory activity toward the isolated target enzyme, the activity against *Escherichia coli*-devired DHFR being about 50 times greater (Table 1) (8). This indicates the possibility that problems of permeation into the bacterial cell are responsible for the observed inactivity of trimethoprim toward whole cell mycobacteria (MIC > 128 μM). Unlike gram-negative bacteria, which possess a hydrophilic polysaccharide core, mycobacterial membranes consist of mycolic acids. Therefore the overall lipophilicity should be increased by adding suitable substituents. Furthermore, considering the three-dimensional structure of DHFR, it may be possible to increase the affinity for the target enzyme. Derivatives of trimethoprim were synthesized in such a way that a polarized SO_2-group could be localized in the vicinity of the Arg 57, similarly as described by Kuyper and coworkers (9) with a carboxylic acid group and as found for methotrexate. Using computer graphics the interaction of the energy-minimized form of model molecules was simulated. An interaction of the SO_2-group with Arg 57 of DHFR was possible for a few derivatives. The best fit was obtained for compound K-130 (Figure 3) with a spacer of three methylen groups between the aromatic sulfone and the benzyl moiety of trimethoprim.

The synthesized compound was tested against cell-free enzyme extracts derived from *Escherichia coli* and *Mycobacterium lufu* (10, 11). The latter is an atypical mycobacterial strain which shows significant similarities to *Mycobacterium leprae* in its drug sensitivity pattern (12). The new derivative was highly active with a similar increase in activity as described

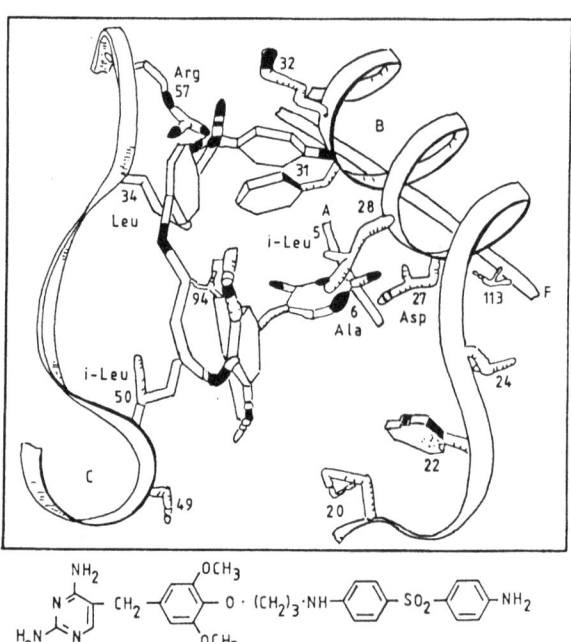

Figure 3: Schematic drawing of the binding site for K-130 in *Escherichia coli* DFHR (Reference No. 10)

by Kuyper for his carboxylic acid derivatives (9) (Table 1). As expected the new compound inhibited not only the isolated DHFR but was also highly active against whole cell mycobacteria. This was due to the increased lipophilicity (log k') (Table 1) of this molecule, which enabled the permeation of the lipid-rich cell wall of mycobacteria. This high inhibitor activity of K-130 versus mycobacteria was

Table 2: Effect of K-130 on multiplication of *Mycobacterium leprae* in mouse foot pads. Inoculation was performed 5 June 1985, drug treatment was started 5 June 1985, and drug treatment was terminated 20 March 1986.

Control	x 10^6 *Mycobacterium leprae*/foot pad					
	Harvest 1 (5 Oct 1985)	Harvest 2 (Dec 1985)	Harvest 3 (Jan 1986)	Harvest 4 (20 Mar 1986)	Harvest 5 (June 1986)	Harvest 6 (12 Dec 1986)
	0.826 ± 0.089	1.69 ± 0.10	2.47 ± 0.169	3.41 ± 0.113	3.64	4.29
DDS[a] 0.0001 %	0.78 ± 0.083	1.45 ± 0.10	1.85 ± 0.193	2.35 ± 0.08	2.91	3.90
K-130 0.03 %	0.47 ± 0.063	0.41 ± 0.043	0.13 ± 0.025	0.0	0.0	0.0
K-130 0.03 % + DDS[a] 0.0001 %	0.40 ± 0.069	0.30 ± 0.095	0.07 ± 0.023	0.0	0.0	0.0

[a]DDS = 4,4'-diaminodiphenylsulfon.

also shown in the mouse foot pad model (13) with *Mycobacterium leprae* infected mice. A dose of 0.03 % K-130 in the diet led to complete elimination of the bacteria from the foot pads. No regrowth occurred even nine months after stopping the treatment (Table 2) (14). The inhibitory activity of K-130 against gram-negative *Escherichia coli* is, however, lower when compared to trimethoprim, despite the increase in inhibitory activity toward the isolated DHFR derived from *Escherichia coli*.

As already discussed, gram-negative bacteria possess a lipopolysaccharide core, i. e. a hydrophilic surface. This consideration is supported by results of experiments using *Escherichia coli* with different degrees of cell wall damage (unpublished results). Bacterial growth kinetic techniques were used to follow the degree of inhibition of growth rate for several strains of *Escherichia coli* of the smooth, rough and deep rough types. K-130 was added to all cultures (5 µM). This concentration had only a small effect on the "normal" strain, but the inhibitory effect increased with the increase in cell wall damage, resulting in total inhibition of growth for the deep rough mutant (Figure 4). The assumption of a rate-limiting step in cell wall permeation was further confirmed by the results of NMR-binding measurements. A strong interaction between isolated bacterial polysaccharides (LPS) and K-130 was observed. No interaction occurred when the molecule was split into a 3,4,5-trimethoxybenzylpyrimidine and 4-amino-4'-propylaminodiphenylsulfone, indicating a specific interaction occurs, probably between the negatively charged LPS and the positively charged K-130. The rough mutants of *Escherichia coli* possess considerably smaller amounts of LPS as cell wall constituents, so that smaller amounts of K-130 are inactivated by being bound to cell wall constituents.

Following the propagated stepwise approach, the structural dependency of pharmacokinetic properties of benzylpyrimidines, especially of their biological half-life, was studied. This class of drugs can be

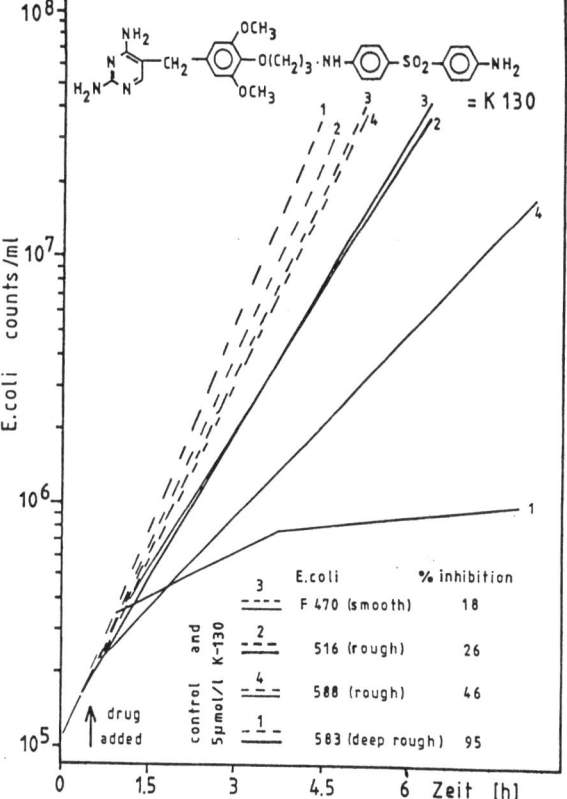

Figure 4: Bacterial growth kinetics of various *Escherichia coli* strains [smooth (3) to deep rough (1) mutants] in the absence and presence of 5 µM K-130.

favourably used in combination with sulfones and sulfonamides because of their synergistic effects (15). Therefore it would be desirable to influence the elimination rate of the benzylpyrimidine in such a way that it is similar to that of the sulfone or sulfonamide selected for combination. At the same time, this modification should not significantly decrease the antibacterial potency. This can only be done on a rational basis if the structural dependency has been quantitatively analyzed for the separate steps. The rate of elimination for benzylpyrimidines of the trimethoprim type showed a statistically significant dependence on the total lipophilicity of the derivatives (16). The lipophilicity is expressed by log P, the partition coefficient in the octanol/water system. The quantitative dependency of the rate constant of elimination (k_{el}), determined in rats, and the lipophilicity (log P) of eight derivatives is given in the following regression equation:

(Equation 1)
$$\log k_{el} = -0.328(0.11) \log P - 0.60 (0.1)$$
$$n = 8 \quad r = 0.96 \quad s = 0.09 \quad F = 57$$

The rate constant of elimination decreases with increasing lipophilicity, i.e. the biological half-life increases with increasing lipophilicity. In contrast the variation in the MIC for the same set of derivatives cannot be described by the change in their lipophilic properties. The regression equation is not statistically significant.

(Equation 2)
$$\log 1/\text{MIC } \textit{Escherichia coli} = 0.41(0.81)$$
$$\log P - 1.13(0.74)$$
$$n = 8 \quad r = 0.46 \quad s = 0.73 \quad F = 1.6$$

As stated above the interaction with the target receptor requires high structure-specificity and normally cannot be sufficiently described by measuring the global lipophilicity of the molecule. These properties can, however, describe transport phenomena. This first example documents the usefulness of a stepwise approach in the rational development of antibacterial agents using the various techniques of structure-activity relationship analysis.

Another aspect which should be considered in a rational design of chemotherapeutic agents is the possible administration of drug combinations, not necessarily in a fixed dosage form. The increase in knowledge of biochemical pathways in cell metabolism could be used for planning combined action of a synergistic type and thus decrease the risk of development of resistance. In addition the dosage for the single drug could be reduced, thus decreasing the risk of side effects. Checkerboard titration experiments have shown high synergism for a combination of K-130 with diaminodiphenylsulfone and, in addition, with a new inhibitor of ribonucleoside diphosphate reductase. This highly synergistic action could be expected on the basis of the enzymatic pathway.

2. Lead Generation, Three-Dimensional Design (Structure of Receptor Unknown)

The identification or construction of new parent structures is normally not accomplished by the standard QSAR-method. Generally, classical QSAR derives relationships between biological effects and physicochemical properties of substituents (see example No. 3). This then allows the estimation of biological effects of unsynthesized derivatives within a known class of compounds. New possibilities are opened up by the so-called 3D-design.

Since there is normally a lack of information concerning the molecular structure of the receptor, the assumption is made that there is a commonness among the molecules exerting a certain effect. The basic tenet is the existence of a receptor, which interacts with all molecules by means of a common type of interaction. This dates back to the "lock and key" concept of Paul Ehrlich. The three-dimensional arrangement of certain chemical groups, the so-called pharmacophore groups, is considered to be responsible for recognition by the receptor and its subsequent activation. This concept underlines the importance of the 3D-stereochemical features and offers a means of new lead generation with or without knowledge of the "construction" of the receptor. Although X-ray crystallography is the most direct approach for obtaining information on structural geometry, it should be kept in mind that molecules in the solid state may not correctly represent the geometry in solution or complexed with the receptor. Nuclear magnetic resonance studies in solution and theoretical simulations are therefore additional tools worthy of consideration. The new computerized techniques of molecular modelling permit not only the visualization of 3D-structures but also the comparison and superposition of 3D-structures of various active and inactive molecules for the recognition of common stereochemical features. The usefulness of this method has been demonstrated for various classes of compounds and has been reviewed in the literature (6, 17). It is the comparison of bioactive structures of β-lactam antibiotics which allows the investigation of biological receptors and enzyme binding sites. The comparison may involve an examination of the multiple conformations that are possible for a single molecule.

The β-lactam antibiotics exert a bactericidal effect by inhibition of the glycopeptide transferase, an enzyme which catalyzes the last step in cell wall biosynthesis. From the data available it appears that β-lactam antibiotics mimic the D-Ala-D-Ala portion of the enzyme substrate and bind very effectively to the substrate binding site. A comparison of penicillin or cephalosporin structures with D-Ala-D-Ala is given in Figure 5. Using computer graphics these structures can be superimposed and the similarity becomes even more evident. On the basis of this observation Cohen (17) tried to classify active and inactive β-lactam derivatives using the relationship between the β-lactam bond and the conformational position of the carboxylic acid group. The structures

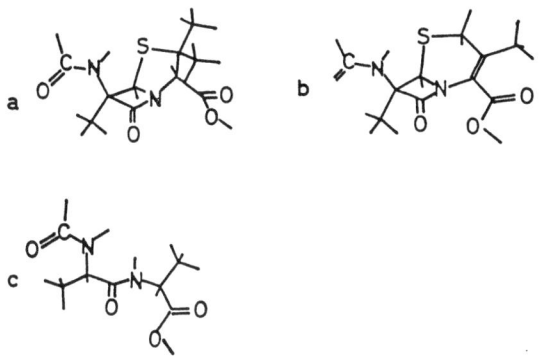

Figure 5: Comparison of (a) a 6-methyl substituted penicillin, (b) a 7-methyl substituted cephalosporins, and (c) the D-Ala-D-Ala fragment (Taken from Reference No. 6).

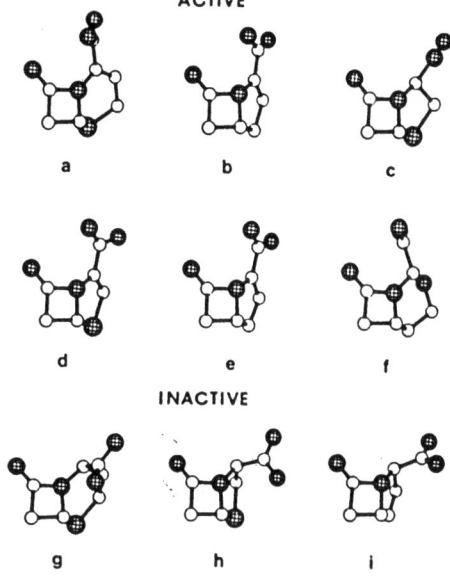

Figure 7: Three-dimensional features of the nine structures listed in Figure 6 (Taken from Reference No. 17).

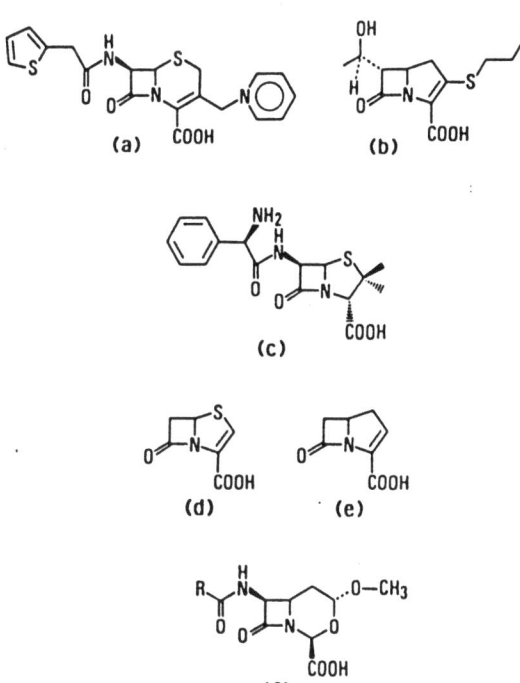

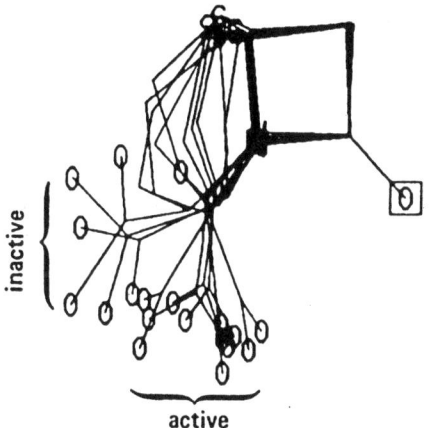

Figure 8: Geometrical separation between active and inactive structures (Taken from Reference No. 17).

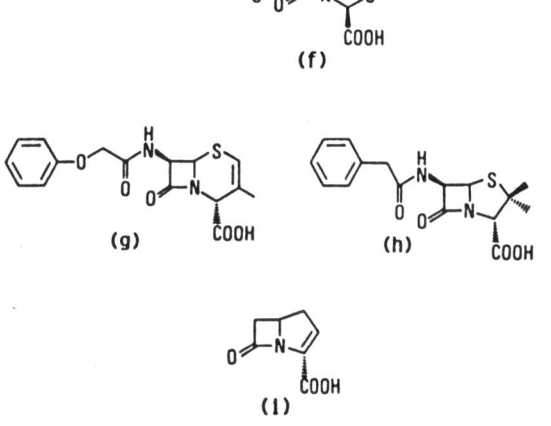

Figure 6: Representative molecules chosen for 3D-comparison (Taken from Reference No. 17).

used in that study are given in Figure 6. The conformational structure of the fused ring systems with the side chains ignored are given in Figure 7. Finally, the β-lactam portions of nine derivatives have been matched and it can be seen that the carboxylic acid groups are occupying two areas of conformational space which correspond to active and inactive derivatives (Figure 8). This is of course not a complete analysis of the structural requirements for the glycopeptide transpeptidase binding site. However, it can serve as a starting point to develop a map of the binding site which could be useful in the design of new inhibitors.

3. Use of the Classical LFE-Approach in Drug Optimization

The first step in drug development is to find a lead structure which can be used as a starting point for the following optimization process. This process can be directed toward different aims (Table 3). Normally in this situation the specific target is not known, nor is anything known about its structure. In this case the LFE-approach can be very helpful to guide the optimization process. This is done by a planned challenge of the unknown receptor site. Again, because of the complexity of biological systems, the stepwise approach is advocated starting with isolated test systems of low complexity. A training set of derivatives is synthesized by substituting the parent lead structure in such a way that a large range of changes in lipophilic, electronic, and steric properties, or others considered to be of importance, is achieved. One or a combination of these properties is considered to be responsible for the change in degree of interaction. By multiregression analysis those physicochemical properties which could explain the observed changes in biological response are detected and quantified. Using the derived regression equation it can be decided which derivative with estimated higher activity should be synthesized next.

This will be discussed in the example of the optimization process of inhibitors of dihydropteroic acid synthase derived from plasmodia. Sulfonamides and diaminodiphenylsulfones have been used in the therapy of malaria; use of the latter has been restricted because of side effects leading to methemoglobin formation. A QSAR analysis has been performed (18) on a series of sulfone derivatives using cell-free extracts of synthase derived from *Plasmodium berghei*. Guided by the results of QSAR analysis with a training set of nine derivatives, the inhibitory activity could be increased significantly and with only a limited number of derivatives synthesized. The results of QSAR analysis for the training set is summarized in the following equation:

(Equation 3)
$$\log 1/I_{50} = -6.20 \, \Delta \text{ ppm } 2/6H - 1.88$$
$n = 9 \quad r = 0.93 \quad s = 0.13$

Δ ppm is the NMR chemical shift observed for the protons in the 2/6 position compared to the 4'-unsubstituted derivative. This shift is used as an indicator of the electronic properties of the substituents. Changes in lipophilic effects did not contribute to the observed variation in inhibitory power.

To further increase the polarization of the SO_2-group measured by the chemical shift of the adjacent

Table 3: Possible aims for optimizations of drugs.

Optimization of pharmacological properties
1. Increase in activity
2. Increase in spectrum of activity
3. Increase in specificity
4. Decrease in toxicity

Optimization of pharmacokinetic properties
1. Bioavailability
2. Distribution
3. Metabolism
4. Elimination

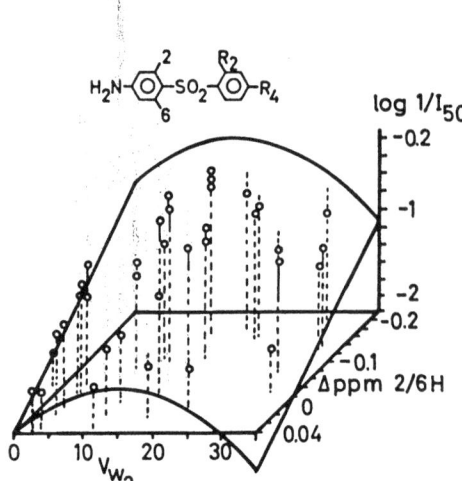

Figure 9: Activity surface of 2'4'-substituted 4-aminodiphenylsulfones (log $1/I_{50}$ versus dihydropteroate synthase of P. berghei, cell free system) as a function of Δ ppm (chemical shift of the 2/6 protons and V_{w2} of the substituents R_2.

protons, some disubstituted derivatives have been synthesized. The result shows that the achieved increase in biological activity is no longer solely dependent on the electronic properties of the substituent. The regression equation shows a decrease in statistical significance.

(Equation 4)
$$\log 1/I_{50} = -6.22 \, \Delta \text{ ppm } 2/6H - 1.76$$
$n = 14 \quad r = 0.825 \quad s = 0.36$

If the volume (V_w) or polarizability (MR) of the substituents in 2'-position are introduced, an increase in statistical significance is observed.

(Equation 5)
$$\log 1/I_{50} = -5.58 \, \Delta \text{ ppm } 2/6H + 0.032 \, V_{w2'} - 1.85$$
$n = 14 \quad r = 0.954 \quad s = 0.138 \quad F = 55.5$

This means there is a positive contribution of the volume of substituents in 2'-position. Additional derivatives were synthesized guided by Equation 5. The final results are summarized in both Figure 9 and the following equation:

(Equation 6)
log $1/I_{50}$ = $-5.9 \, \Delta$ ppm 2/6H + 0.093 $V_{w2'}$ $-$ 0.0029 $V_{w2'}^2$ $-$ 2.08
n = 41   r = 0.918   s = 0.20   F = 66.0

The results documented in Equation 6 indicate that no more potent analogues within this series can be found because substituents with stronger electron-releasing properties are not available and the positive influence of substituent volume in 2'-position passes through a maximum. The optimal activity has been reached by synthesizing a relatively small number of derivatives. These derivatives exceed the activity of 4-sulfa-5,6-dimethoxypyrimidine (Fanasil®) considerably. Later, the free space intramolecular conformational entropy (S) of these sulfones was calculated by Hopfinger (19) and correlated with the inhibitory activity (log $1/I_{50}$) against *Mycobacterium lufu*.

(Equation 7)
log $1/I_{50}$ = $-$ 0.0072 S + 6.24
n = 53   r = 0.918   s = 0.167   F = 173.6

This entropy value correlates with the physicochemical descriptors used in QSAR analysis to describe the effect on plasmodial synthase (see above) and on mycobacterial derived synthase.

S = 678.9 Δ ppm 2/6H $-$ 1.79 $V_{w2'}$ $-$ 60

This was the first time that a correlation of physicochemical property descriptors and theoretical values derived from conformational analysis was shown.

The consecutively performed structure-activity relationship analysis to explain observed variation in pharmacokinetic parameters revealed the major dependence of these parameters on lipophilic properties of the sulfone derivatives. The variation in total clearance (Cl_{tot}) using rats as test animals and the partition coefficient, D, into red blood cells for this series of sulfones can again nicely be described as a function of differences in their lipophilic properties (log k' or R_m).

(Equation 9)
log Cl_{tot} = $-$ 0.21 log k' + 0.18
n = 6   r = 0.93   s = 0.12

(Equation 10)
log D = 0.308 R_m + 0.133
n = 15   r = 0.91   s = 0.069

4. Multivariate Data Analysis in Drug Design

One of the major problems in drug research is to handle and analyze large amounts of information stemming from pharmacological screening data obtained in various test systems, for example from various bacterial strains and/or from pharmacokinetic studies. This is leading to a multidimensional parameter space, and inherent possible multiple intercorrelations are not easily detected. In such a situation the various methods of multivariate data analysis, as for example principal component (PC) analysis, are powerful tools. The aim of PC-analysis is to extract a reduced number of hypothetical new variables, the so-called principal components (PCs), from a set of intercorrelated variables (20). Similar information contained in different variables (tests) is extracted and combined in a reduced number of new variables. The number of original variables is reduced and concentrated in a smaller number of orthogonal PC-vectors. It becomes obvious which of the original parameters (tests) possess similar information content.

The first example explains the application of PC-analysis to a set of sulfones tested as inhibitors of dihydropteroic acid synthase derived from various bacterial strains either sensitive or resistant to sulfones (I_{50}), and against whole cell bacteria (MIC, I_{25} from bacterial growth kinetic studies with *Escherichia coli*) (21). This creates a data matrix of nine variables. From these nine original variables two significant new principal components have been extracted. The first principal component, PC1, contains 71.9% of the original information, and the second, PC2, contains 21.3%, i.e. 93.2% of the total variance of the original data set is contained in only two PCs. The loadings (contributions) of the original scaled activity variables on principal components after varimax rotation are given in Table 4 and the corresponding vector representation is shown in Figure 10. Inspection of the loadings show that PC1 is extracted from the activity data (I_{50}) obtained in the cell-free systems which are highly co-linear. This indicates that the structural preconditions for fit of the molecules to the target enzyme are essentially the same for the four different bacterial species, and in addition, also for the resistant and sensitive strain derived enzymes. This information is most valuable and excludes the possibility that resistance is due to changes in the conformation or amino acid sequence of the target enzyme. The second PC, PC2, is formed by linear

Table 4: Loadings of original, scaled activity variables on principal components (PC) after Varimax rotation (VR).

		PC1VR	PC2VR
I	log $1/I_{50}$ *M. lufu*, DDS-res.	0.962	0.194
II	log $1/I_{50}$ *M. lufu*, DDS-sens.	0.962	0.120
III	log $1/I_{50}$ *M. smegmatis*, DDS-res.	0.975	0.103
IV	log $1/I_{50}$ *M. smegmatis*, DDS-sens.	0.980	0.106
V	log $1/I_{50}$ *M. Leprae*, DDS-res.	0.954	0.265
VI	log $1/I_{50}$ *M. Leprae*, DDS-sens.	0.957	0.284
VII	log $1/I_{50}$ *E. coli*, DDS-sens.	0.879	0.209
VIII	log $1/I_{25}$ *E. coli*, DDS-sens.	0.038	0.951
IX	log 1/MIC *M. smegmatis*, DDS-sens.	0.333	0.862

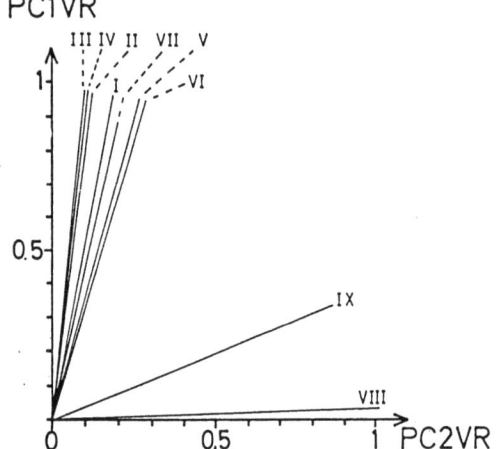

Figure 10: Activity vectors drawn according to the loadings given in Table 4.

combination of whole cell data (MIC, *Mycobacterium smegmatis*; I_{25}, *Escherichia coli*), indicating an additional influence of bacterial cell wall properties on the antibacterial effect. The PC scores, which are the contribution of the individual objects (derivatives) to the PC-vectors, can again be subjected to QSAR-analysis and the following significant relationship can be derived:

(Equation 11)
PC1 = -7.02Δ ppm $NH_2 + 1.813 f_i - 0.929$
n = 17   r = 0.969   s = 0.26   F = 108

Δ ppm NH_2 is the NMR chemical shift of the primary amino group protons in 4-position relative to those of the 4'-position unsubstituted derivative, and f_i indicates the degree of ionization of substituents in 4'-position. The activities derived in the cell-free system which are extracted in one new PC depend only on electronic features.

PC2 scores corresponding mainly to whole cell activites are best described by the high-pressure liquid chromatography (HPLC) lipophilicity parameter log k'. They show a bilinear dependence on log k' with a maximum at log k' = 0.83. Possibly, PC1 and PC2 reflect intrinsic activities at the active site of the enzyme and transport phenomena at the cell membrane, respectively.

The second example (22) describes an attempt to separate pharmacokinetic from pharmacodynamic influences by PC-analysis. The analysis is applied to a set of antibacterial sulfonamides. The pharmacokinetic parameters are derived in rats. The original data matrix consists of eight variables which are given in Table 5. They have been determined for 19 sulfapyridines. Three PCs containing 94.9 % of the original information could be extracted from the eight original variables (Table 6). It can be shown that the pharmacokinetic information is mainly extracted in PC1, whereas the antibacterial activity expressed as MIC and the calculated necessary maintenance dose (log 1/D) for therapy is extracted into PC2 (Table 7). PC3 is almost exclusively loaded by the volume of distribution, V_d. QSAR-analysis of PC scores show, in agreement with previous results (22, 23) that pharmacokinetic parameters as rate constant of elimination ($k_{elim.}$), as clearance (Cl_{tot}), as affinity constant for protein binding or as percent bound to serum albumin depend mainly on lipophilicity (log k')

Table 5: List of pharmacokinetic (rats) and pharmacodynamic parameters of 2-sulfapyridines subjected to PC-analysis.

$H_2N-\langle O \rangle-SO_2NH-\langle O \rangle-R$

1. log $k_{elim.}$ [h^{-1}]
2. log Cl_{total} [ml/min]   } Obtained after i.v. injection to rats; 1-compartment open model.
3. log V_d [ml]
4. log K_{ass} (rat serum protein)
5. logit (% bd.) (rat serum protein)
6. log 1/MIC (*Escherichia coli*-1 in vitro)
7. log 1/D^a
8. log 1/D$_\infty^b$

^{a}D = initial dose in mmol/l to give [SA^{free}] ≥ MIC. τ = 2h.
^{b}D$_\infty$ = maintenance dose to give [SA^{free}] ≥ MIC. τ = 4, 6, 8 h.
n = 19: (1) H (2) 5-Me (3) 6-Me (4) 4-Me (5) 5, 6-Me$_2$ (6) 5-Cl (7) 5-Br (8) 5-NO$_2$ (9) 5-Me$_2$N; o-substituted: (10) 3-Me (11) 3-Cl (12) 3-CN (13) 3-MeO (14) 3-EtO (15) 3-Me-5-Br (16) 3-Me-5-Cl (17) 3,5-Cl$_2$ (18) 3,5-Br$_2$ (19) 3-CN-5-Me.

Table 6: PC-analysis of 2-sulfapyridines.

PC$_i$	λ_i	Variance (%)	Cumulative (%)
1.	5.06	63.2	63.2
2.	1.69	21.1	84.3
3.	0.85	10.6	94.9
4.	0.23	2.9	97.8

Table 7: Loadings of original, scaled variables (from Table 5) on principal components (PC) after Varimax rotation.

	PC1	PC2	PC3
log $k_{elim.}$	0.75	−0.59	−0.12
log Cl_{tot}	0.73	−0.62	0.16
log V_d	−0.10	−0.11	0.98
log K_{Ass}	−0.80	0.35	0.34
logit (% bd)	−0.97	0	0.03
log 1/MIC	−0.40	0.88	0.13
log 1/D	0.05	0.94	−0.23
log 1/D$_\infty$	−0.40	0.91	−0.03

(Equation 12), whereas the antibacterial effect is determined by electronic properties (pKa) of the substituents (Equation 13).

(Equation 12)
$$PC1 = -1.17 \log k'_{pH\ 4.5} + 0.74\ I_0 + 0.376$$
$$n = 19 \quad r = 0.90 \quad s = 0.47$$

I_0 is an indicator variable indicating the presence (1) or absence (0) of a substituent in o-position.

(Equation 13)
$$PC2 = -0.603\ pKa + 4.53$$
$$n = 19 \quad r = 0.85 \quad s = 0.56$$

Conclusion

These methods and tools for a more rational drug design by no means replace the creativity required for drug research. Natural products, intelligent screening, identification of novel receptors and biochemical pathways will remain essential sources for new classes of bioactive compounds. In the various aspects of drug optimization, QSAR and multivariate data analysis have proven to be powerful tools. Together with computer graphics, visualization of three-dimensional structures and interaction of substrate molecules with receptors, and nuclear magnetic resonance and X-ray structure analysis, these methods will increasingly contribute to our understanding of drug action, stimulate our creativity and force us to design meaningful test systems. Three-dimensional modelling will also allow us to derive valid pharmacophore models even in the absence of knowledge about the construction of the receptor.

References

1. Seydel, J. K., Schaper, K.-J.: Chemische Struktur und biologische Aktivität von Wirkstoffen. Verlag Chemie, Weinheim, 1979.
2. Franke, R.: Optimierungsmethoden in der Wirkstoff-Forschung, Quantitative Struktur-Wirkungs-Analyse. Akademie-Verlag, Berlin, 1980.
3. Topliss, J. G. (ed.): Quantitative structure-activity relationships of drugs. Academic Press, New York, 1983.
4. Seydel, J. K.: Wirkstoffentwicklung – drug design. In: Kleemann, A., Lindner, E., Engel, E. (ed.): Arzneimittel-Fortschritte 1972–1985. VCH, Weinheim, 1987, p. 3–51.
5. Kier, L. B., Hall, L. H.: Molecular connectivity in structure-activity analysis. Wiley, Letchford, 1986.
6. Cohen, N. C.: Drug design in three dimensions. Advances in Drug Research 1985, 14: 41–145.
7. Matthews, D. A., Alden, R. A., Bolin, J. T., Freer, S. T., Hamlin, R., Xuong, N., Kraut, J., Peo, M., Williams, M., Hoogsteen, K.: Dihydrofolate reductase: X-ray structure of the binary complex with methotrexate. Science 1977, 197: 452–455.
8. Baker, D. J., Beddell, C. R., Champness, J. N., Goodford, P. J., Norrington, F. E. A., Smith, D. R., Stammers, D. K.: The binding of trimethoprim to bacterial dihydrofolate reductase. FEBS Letters 1981, 126: 49–52.
9. Kuyper, L. F., Roth, B., Baccanari, D. P., Ferone, R., Beddell, C. R., Champness, J. N., Stammers, D. K., Dann, J. G., Norrington, F. E. A., Baker, D. J., Goodford, P. J.: Receptor-based design of dihydrofolate reductase inhibitors: comparison of crystallographically determined enzyme binding with enzyme affinity in a series of carboxy-substituted trimethoprim analogues. Journal of Medicinal Chemistry 1982, 25: 1120–1123.
10. Czaplinsky, K.-H., Kansy, M., Seydel, J. K., Haller, R.: Design of a new substituted 2,4-diamino-5-benzylpyrimidine as inhibitor of bacterial dihydrofolate reductase assisted by molecular graphics. Quantitative Structure-Activity Relationships 1987, 6: 70–72.
11. Kansy, M.: Hemmstoffe der Folatbiosynthese: Entwicklung neuer Chemotherapeutika gegen *Mycobacterium leprae*. Thesis, Kiel University, Germany, 1986.
12. Seydel, J. K., Wempe, E.: Bacterial growth kinetics of *Mycobacterium lufu* in the presence and absence of various drugs alone and in combination. A model for the development of combined chemotherapy against *Mycobacterium leprae*. International Journal of Leprosy 1981, 50: 20–30.
13. Shepard, C. C.: The experimental disease that follows the injection of human leprosy bacilli into foot pads of mice. Journal of Experimental Medicine 1960, 112: 445–454.
14. Seydel, J. K., Rosenfeld, M., Sathish, M., Wiese, M., Schaper, K.-J., Hachtel, G., Haller, R., Kansy, M., Dhople, A. M.: Strategies in the development of new drugs and drug combinations against leprosy, demonstrated on the example of folate and gyrase inhibitors. Leprosy Research 1986, Supplement 3, 57: 235–253.
15. Hitchings, G. H. (ed.): Inhibition of folate metabolism in chemotherapy. Springer Verlag, Berlin, 1983.
16. Seydel, J. K.: Strategies in drug design. In: Mutschler, E., Winterfeld, E., (ed.): Trends in medicinal chemistry. VCH, Weinheim, 1987, p. 83–103.
17. Cohen, N. C.: β-lactam antibiotics: geometrical requirements for antibacterial activities. Journal of Medicinal Chemistry 1983, 26: 259–264.
18. Wiese, M., Seydel, J. K., Krüger, G., Pieper, H., Noll, K. R., Keck, J.: Multiple regression analysis of antimalarial activities of sulfones and sulfonamides in cell-free systems and principal component analysis to compare with antibacterial activities. Quantitative Structure-Activity Relationships 1987, 6: 164–172.
19. Hopfinger, A. J., Lopez de Compadre, R. L., Koehler, M. G., Emery, S., Seydel, J. K.: Quantitative Structure-Activity Relationships 1987, 6: 111–117.
20. Wold, S. in Massart, D. K. (ed.): Evaluation and optimizations of laboratory methods and analytical procedures. Elsevier, Amsterdam, 1978.
21. Coats, E. A., Cordes, H. P., Kulkarni, V. M., Richter, M., Schaper, K.-J., Wiese, M., Seydel, J. K.: Quantitative Structure-Activity Relationships 1985, 4: 99–109.
22. Schaper, K.-J., Seydel, J. K.: Multivariate methods in quantitative structure-pharmacokinetic relationship analysis. In: Seydel, J. K. (ed.): QSAR and strategies in the design of bioactive compounds. VCH, Weinheim, 1985, p. 173–189.
23. Seydel, J. K., Trettin, D., Cordes, H. P., Wassermann, O., Malyusz, M.: Quantitative structure-pharmacokinetic relationships derived on antibacterial sulfonamides in rats and their comparison to quantitative structure-activity relationships. Journal of Medicinal Chemistry 1980, 23: 607–613.

**Future Development and
Use of Anti-Infective Chemotherapy**

The Future Challenge of Infectious Disease

F. E. Young

Commissioner of Food and Drugs, U. S. Food and Drug Administration

The Challenge We Face Today

The infectious disease community can point to many successes in the past. In the late 1970s some felt we had the right to be complacent, as we believed we had virtually eliminated such dreaded diseases as smallpox, reduced the burden of schistosomiasis and malaria, and had begun to attack some venereal diseases. Indeed, we could be proud of the accomplishments and satisfied with the state of scientific knowledge that led to them, but nothing remains static. New infectious diseases are appearing as are more highly resistant strains of known diseases. Fortunately, at the same time, we find ourselves in the midst of an exciting technological revolution. Although new technologies require new ways of doing business, I am confident that the infectious disease community is capable of meeting the challenge.

Today we have new tools available to help us. In order to utilize these tools most effectively — to bring new products to the patients who most desperately need them — we must work together.

Promising New Tools

The new biotechnology promises an amazingly effective array of techniques in the fight against infectious diseases. First, biotechnology promises to alter secondary metabolites such as cephalosporin by introducing genes from other organisms. In this way, we will be able to obtain a greater variety of products that can achieve dramatic results. Many secondary metabolites have antibiotic activity for which they have been widely exploited clinically. While it has been said that the "Golden Age" of antimicrobial chemotherapy began in the 1950s, the advent of rDNA technology is introducing a new level of rationality and precision into the discovery and creation of new molecules. For example, advances in the knowledge of microbiological genetics and physiology have made possible manipulations that can produce new antibiotic molecules. Our capacity for altering metabolic pathways — and for moving them among species with rDNA techniques — is virtually unlimited. The number of possible permutations of chemical structures for new potential antimicrobial molecules is thus infinite. Already these promise to produce a new generation of cephalosporins and related antibiotics.

Secondly, biotechnology will help us to substantially augment the design of new therapies as well as to understand the underlying genetic basis of drug resistance. Already, we have been able to unveil the complete antigenic sequence of HIV and gain some idea of the functional roles of the proteins involved in the AIDS infection process. It is now possible to design and select chemotherapeutic agents that might inhibit unique portions of the HIV viral function. Two such agents currently under investigation are CD4 and dextran sulfate. Biotechnology has also enabled us to understand the antigenic structure of viruses. This information has been critically important in our attempts to develop vaccines, such as the recombinant hepatitis B vaccine. Work is presently underway to determine if this route will lead to a successful vaccine against AIDS.

Antibiotic resistance is an area in which biotechnology will certainly play a key role. We must continue to develop new derivatives of existing drugs because many infectious organisms use antibiotic resistance or antigenic modulation to protect themselves from the new therapeutic agents that are developed. It is clear that biotechnology can play a unique role in the development of new drugs, especially for desperately ill patients. However, it is not the only tool at our disposal.

Food & Drug Administration, Office of Health Affairs, Rockville, Maryland 28832, USA.

Antiviral Drugs and Antiparasitic Drugs

For years, we have been challenged by a number of viral and parasitic diseases that we could not control. This situation is changing. Even the proverbial common cold may have to yield to treatments we are presently investigating. To expedite the review of antivirals, the U.S. Food and Drug Administration (FDA) created in February 1988 in the Center for Drug Research and Review a division of anti-viral drug products, which focuses primarily on drugs indicated for the treatment of AIDS and AIDS-related disorders. The division also covers all other antivirals as well as drugs to treat tuberculosis, fungal infections and mycobacterial infections. Some of the antivirals presently being investigated include AL-721, dideooxyadenosine, dideoxycytidine, dextran sulfate and ansamycin. The division is also reviewing a number of anti-infective drugs, such as fluconazole for cryptococcal meningitis and candidiasis, and pentamidine isethionate for *Pneumocystis carinii* pneumonia (PCP).

The area of antiparasitic therapy has also entered a period of rapid growth and development. The FDA currently has several active Investigational New Drugs (INDs) and New Drug Applications (NDAs) for antiparasitic drugs. Antiparasitic drugs such as ivermectin have an unusually broad spectrum of activity against parasitic nematodes, such as the agent that causes onchocerciasis, also known as river blindness. This drug is effective at low concentrations and with minimal toxicity. There is no current approved therapy for neurocysticercosis, with its resultant neurological dysfunction; however, some promise has been shown by praziquantel, a drug currently approved for the treatment of all forms of schistosomiasis.

The antimalarials are also important. In the past few years the incidence of *Plasmodium falciparum* resistance to chloroquine has increased, posing a serious threat to life. A new drug currently under review offers much promise against this disease.

New Role of Immunomodulators

Another tool that will become more prominent in the near future is in the form of the immunomodulators, which are being made available through the new biotechnological techniques. These drugs are revolutionizing our approaches to therapy. Immunomodulators and the use of drugs in combination with them are being used more often, especially in the treatment of cancer and opportunistic infections associated with AIDS. Most likely, we will continue to see much more emphasis on combining immunomodulators with chemotherapeutic drugs. Many of these combinations are currently undergoing clinical investigation.

New Research Division Established

The FDA has recently announced the formal establishment of a new research division within the Center for Biologics Evaluation and Research, the Division of Cytokine Biology. Under Dr. K. Zoon as acting director, the division will be primarily responsible for conducting regulatory review and research on biological agents that affect cellular growth and development. These include interleukins, interferons, growth factors and immunomodulators. Many of these agents, like interleukin 2, various interferons, and CD4 soluble protein, have been developed through recombinant DNA technology. We believe this new division will expedite the development and review of therapies for AIDS, cancer and other serious diseases.

Development of New Therapies

The FDA review process forms the bridge by which new products enter the marketplace. Moreover, those who understand the process know that cooperation between government and industry is essential if the system is to function at its best. Recently, the FDA made some changes to streamline the process and to make sure that promising experimental treatments for life-threatening and serious diseases reach the patients who need them. The terrible disease AIDS has focused attention on these issues as never before.

The prime responsibility for ensuring the safety and efficacy of new drugs belongs to the manufacturers. The drug development process begins with the basic science that defines the compounds to be tested and suggests how it will be used. Once laboratory testing with animals shows the drug is safe enough, tests begin in progressive phases, with larger and larger groups of human subjects, to test safety and effectiveness. It is the FDA's job to review manufacturers' test method and results.

AIDS

The disease AIDS serves as the foremost example of why we must work together. Fighting a war requires a united front against the enemy. Any drug or biologic compound that will be a potential weapon against AIDS is given the highest priority in our review system. That would include, in most cases, drugs for opportunistic infections, the antivirals, the antineoplastics and the immunomodulators. We have a special designation for these drugs, called "1 AA", which means we have promised the American people to give every AIDS drug the shortest possible evaluation.

We know we have a hard battle ahead to conquer AIDS when we consider the difficulties in developing antivirals. Only seven antiviral agents have been licensed in the history of the FDA, in contrast to hundreds of antimicrobial agents. The approval of aztreonam (AZT) in record time required around-the-clock work from FDA staff, but even then such a rapid approval would not have been possible without close teamwork between the FDA and the drug sponsor. Early consultations between the FDA and the sponsor led to "gold-plated" clinical studies that produced unequivocal evidence of efficacy. The efficacy data enabled us to approve the drug, despite known toxicity, because it resulted in a favorable ratio of benefit-to-risk. The AZT example illustrates the importance of well-controlled clinical trials. These have proved by far to be the best means of developing safe and effective drugs quickly. If we work together throughout the drug review process, everyone will benefit – most importantly, the American public.

Guidelines

The FDA must do its part as well. As has been indicated, we are available for early consultation to help sponsors in the design of clinical trials. We are also working with experts in the field to develop guidelines for the clinical evaluation of anti-infective drugs, which will cover testing of drugs for systemic infections of adults and children. For clarification in this vitally important area, the FDA has issued a contract to the Infectious Diseases Society of America to review and update these guidelines. This close professional cooperation will benefit both the FDA and the sponsors of investigational new drugs – and ultimately the public as well. It will provide a splendid example of working together to facilitate the transfer of innovative therapies from the laboratory to the marketplace.

Treatment Investigational New Drugs (INDs)

The FDA is doing everything possible to help patients who are deperately ill to have access to promising investigational drugs. Hope is a precious commodity. It is imperative that we provide a streamlined way for patients to obtain such drugs once a reasonable body of safety and efficacy data exists. With AZT, we developed a model for accomplishing this. As soon as the FDA had evidence that AZT extended lives, we made the drug available to over 4,000 patients through a treatment protocol, before the final review for marketing was complete. We concluded that a formal provision should be written into FDA's regulations permitting expanded use of experimental drugs, and this was done last year.

These new regulations will help us to provide the very best possible care for patients. However, our need to help patients must be reconciled with our equally important need to study drugs thoroughly and carefully and base drug approval decisions first and foremost on good science. Our decisions will always be affected by the nature of the disease and the existence of available alternatives. The more serious and less treatable the disease, the greater the risk we – and the patients – are willing to accept. As I have testified to the U.S. Congress, I am very frustrated by the lack of treatment INDs the FDA has received to date. While six treatment INDs have been approved, only one is for AIDS. I have actively encouraged the pharmaceutical industry and others to pursue treatment INDs since, as I emphasised before, innovation is a product of teamwork.

The Future

The challenges that face us in the infectious disease community are great. If the public is to take full advantage of the scientific discoveries that are now taking place in the field of anti-infectives, we must work together to make sure that we sharpen our scientific expertise to keep pace with constant technological change. At the FDA, I am working hard to enhance our scientific environment to improve the drug review process. None of us can afford to be complacent and stand still when public health is at stake. We have worked hard to develop a system that stimulates research and development by being as predictable, consistent and efficient as possible, but that is only one side of the equation. We also need a partnership with the scientific community, as has been already pointed out.

We are at the threshold of an explosion in new therapeutic agents that can significantly prevent and reduce the burden of disease for mankind. As a former researcher myself, it gives me enormous pride and satisfaction to be the FDA Commissioner at a time when so many revolutionary technologies are being transferred successfully to the marketplace. These exciting endeavors hold real promise to conquer the infectious diseases that challenge us.

Acknowledgement

The Commissioner acknowledges the assistance of FDA staff member Wayne Matthews in preparing his remarks.

Barriers to Effective Anti-Infective Therapy: The Perspective of a Clinical Pharmacologist

The most fundamental barrier to optimal anti-infective therapy is the non-availability of safe and effective remedies. Medicines that have not cleared the regulatory approval process cannot be prescribed, nor can the sick benefit from them. Anti-infective therapy is perhaps the most dramatic component of the pharmaceutical revolution that has occurred worldwide over the last half-century. The health benefits of antibiotic research and development have been little short of miraculous, and society owes an enormous debt of gratitude to the responsible figures in academia, industry and government who have cooperated in the battle to prevent or cure infectious diseases.

The system in place has clearly served us well in the past — the question is whether it will do so in the future. For the pharmaceutical industry, pride in providing new remedies to the public cannot by itself justify the enormous expenditures required to bring such medicines to the marketplace; there must also be profits to maintain the vitality of the industry. The return on capital investment in pharmaceuticals depends on a number of factors, including the ability to charge a reasonable price for medicines, market exclusivity whenever possible, a significant market life for new products, and a cost of development that is not disproportionate to the expected return on investment.

Regulatory Barriers

The regulatory process for reviewing new drug applications has been lengthening in many countries, although anti-infectives (at least in the U.S.) seem to fare better in this regard then do other therapeutic categories. Even when approved, a new antibiotic is introduced into different countries at different times, so that a "drug lag" invariably exists, during which time a country lagging behind is deprived of the benefits of the drug and the manufacturer is denied profits from drug sales (1). In some countries, foreign clinical trial data are often considered insufficient basis for regulatory approval, thus prolonging the approval process and increasing its cost (2). Lengthy regulatory review tends to decrease the period of market exclusivity, since the patent clock is ticking away inexorably between the time of issuance of the patent and the time of marketing. In the USA and UK, recognition of this fact has prompted moves on the part of government to restore some of the lost patent life (3). On the other hand, the tendency to encourage and facilitate generic product substitution is eroding the de facto patent term extension that exists beyond the life of the patent in the absence of effective generic competition.

Threats of Litigation and Drug Withdrawal

In countries where society is increasingly litigious, legal costs and claims settlements represent another type of disincentive. In the USA, for example, there has been an exodus of firms from vaccine research, development, manufacture, and sales, related in large measure to fears about the unquantifiable risks of future litigation (4). The situation is paradoxical in view of the extraordinary benefits to society of past vaccine development programs directed against smallpox, poliomyelitis, measles, rubella, mumps, tetanus, diphtheria, and pertussis, as well as the acknowledged need for new vaccines for both the civilian and military populations. But the disincentives to vaccine research are formidable. Vaccine production is complex and expensive, with a lengthy production pipeline and consequent inventory and cash flow problems. The return on capital investment is low. The target populations, once vaccinated, often need no further vaccination; this situation with vaccines thus presents an impressive contrast to that with prescription drugs. As a disease is gradually eradicated by successful vaccine programs, the need for widespread vaccination diminishes. All these factors, added to a potential legal liability that is perceived as excessively onerous by manufacturers, have in essence driven most U.S. companies out of the vaccine business. Even if a successful anti-infective is developed, return of investment may be jeopardized if adverse reactions to the product are exaggerated or if a flurry of adverse events leads to media attention and political pressure to withdraw the drug from the market. Such pressures may be impossible to resist unless convincing pharmacoepidemiologic evidence can be quickly marshalled to indicate that the product's risk-benefit ratio is indeed acceptable when considered either independently or against the track record of competing products.

Impact of Cost Containment

While calculation of the costs of new drug development today need recalculation to update the older estimates of Hansen (5), there seems little doubt that the cost of drug development continues to escalate at the same time as pressures to contain drug costs are increasing with each passing year in every corner of the globe. Pharmaceuticals are generally acknowledged to be the most cost-effective component of health care, and they constitute only a small part of the health care budget in developed countries, but drug costs are a visible and easy target for those seeking to contain health care expenditures and whose decisions are usually guided by short-term savings rather than by long-term costs that might result from excessive restriction of prescribing.

The rising health care bill in most countries has predictably led to cost-containment efforts of various kinds. The rise in the cost of health care is related to such factors as an increasingly elderly population and the success of science in developing new diagnostic techniques, new medical devices, new surgical procedures, and, of course, new drugs. Many of these represent true advances in medical practice, but their availability usually, at least for the short term, means an increase in health care costs. A few years ago, an article appeared describing the risks and costs of two aminoglycoside antibiotics (6). One — the less expensive of the two — was also more nephrotoxic. The authors concluded, however, that on balance this more nephrotoxic drug represented the more attractive choice, because the increased nephrotoxicity, even if it occasionally might require renal dialysis, was not of sufficient magnitude in the target population to offset the lesser costs of the medicine. From the patient's standpoint, the safer drug is preferred in such a situation, needless to say. Quality of care suffers whenever a less expensive therapy is chosen and that therapy is not the best available in terms of therapeutic impact.

The advent of therapeutic substitution — the right of the pharmacist to dispense to a patient not the prescribed drug, but a completely different one that is in general capable of producing a similar therapeutic outcome — can be expected to have significant attraction for institutions seeking to contain health care costs, because it will confer on them negotiating advantage in the purchase of products for which there is market exclusivity and no generic subsitute available. If this practice becomes widespread, manufacturers of expensive new products may find it difficult, if not impossible, to establish a product's track record for safety and efficacy, since such a record requires substantial experience within a population for a proper assessment.

Criticism of "Me-Too" Products

Industry is often accused of "me-too" research, and the marketing of medicines that are "clones" of one another. Such criticism ignores the fact that exciting research areas are not secrets in world science, and hence it is to be expected that many scientists in the industry will be digging for therapeutic gold in the same scientific territory. This fact, coupled with the long time needed to develop research discoveries into marketed products, explains, at least in part, the "me-too" phenomenon. Nevertheless, it is of interest that half the drugs appearing on the WHO Essential Drugs List, which represents the most important drugs for a developing country to consider in devising a national formulary, are not the original compounds in their respective therapeutic classes, but the result of molecular modification or other research strategies designed to discover better or cheaper successors to the breakthrough innovation.

Academia-Industry Collaboration

Another type of barrier to the development of new anti-infectives is the suboptimal cooperation of academic and industrial scientists in the search for practical applications of basic research. Collaboration between these sectors has always existed to some degree, to be sure, and it would be fatuous to look on academia as the only place where basic research is performed, and industry as the only place where applied research occurs. Nevertheless, the substantial creative brain power residing in universities has, in the past, often not been effectively enlisted in the search for new medicines, commercial development often being scorned by academics as an inferior intellectual pursuit. Shrinking government support of research has changed this snobbish attitude to a considerable extent, and in the area of biotechnology, there has been an academic exodus into the industrial ranks, and strong consulting links exist between the two sectors.

Federal Support of Research

Notwithstanding the need for greater cooperation between academia and industry, federal support of research remains an important subsidy to commercial development of new medicines, and to the extent that budgetary belt-tightening cuts back on research support, some of the eventual fruits of such support, i.e., biomedical discoveries to help the sick, will not be harvested, or at least the harvest will be delayed. An exception, at the moment, to federal research cutbacks is the AIDS epidemic, where the grim downhill course of the disease and the absence of truly curative or preventive approaches have spawned massive government investment in research, as well as substantial academic and industrial commitment. AIDS represents our most dramatic infectious disease challenge for many reasons, not the least being the formidable obstacles to be overcome in the search for effective vaccines or treatments.

The Barrier of Ignorance

A large and heterogeneous set of barriers to optimal anti-infective therapy might be classified under the rubric of "ignorance", examples of which follow.

Misdiagnosis. An erroneously diagnosed infection can only be properly treated by accident. New entities like Legionnaires disease or Lyme disease are especially likely to be missed, but classic and well-known infections are missed every day.

Noncompliance. The frequency with which patients fail to follow prescribing directions is appalling (7). Sometimes such failure might be called "intelligent noncompliance", if the medicine is not needed or is not working properly, but often such is not the case. The efficacy of the best antibiotic will decrease if dosing is inadequate either in amount or duration.

Poor Prescribing Practices. After many years during which academia scorned most forms of perioperative antibiotic prophylaxis, it is now generally agreed that in certain surgical conditions, such prophylaxis can decrease morbidity. Yet while antibiotic experts stress that only a day or two of perioperative prophylaxis is required, surgical practice in many cases deviates from this advice, with some patients receiving no antibiotic, but many more being treated for needlessly long periods of time postoperatively (8). The result is wasted resources, needless drug toxicity, and the encouragement of superinfection or bacterial resistance.

Academic Obsession with Diagnostic Certitude. Many academics stress, to a ridiculous degree, the need to establish unequivocally the identity of the pathogenic microorganism before starting therapy, despite the fact that diagnostic tests are often impractical or not cost-effective because of expense, delay in return of reports, and misleading or misinterpreted data. While one cannot condone the prescribing of antibiotics that are unnecessary or unlikely to be effective, it is interesting that the decline of acute rheumatic fever and rheumatic heart disease in the USA seems most reasonably attributed to the substantial "promiscuous" use of penicillin and other antibiotics since 1946 (9).

Undeserved Worship of Antibiotics. In developed countries, there is a certain amount of patient pressure for antibiotic prescribing in infectious situations where medical opinion would disagree with such practice, but in Third World countries there is often a pathetic faith on the part of many patients in the ability of a few doses of antibiotic – often barely affordable – to cure almost anything from which the sick suffer.

Inadequate Attention to Baseline Variables Related to Outcome. Drugs tend to be approved for registration on the basis of their performance in population groups, while the proper practice of medicine involves the adaptation of treatment to the needs of individuals (10). Whenever possible, predictors of therapeutic or adverse response to medicines need to be measured so that choices or modifications of therapy can be made in advance rather than on a trial-and-error basis. Reliable prognosticators are to be preferred to clichés. The elderly, for example, are often said to require reduction in dosage, or increase in dosage interval, of certain antibiotics eliminated primarily by the kidney, because it is said kidney function decreases inexorably with advancing years. While this is statistically true on average, the elderly are by no means a homogeneous population (11). Some old people certainly have severe renal impairment, but others have little impairment, and some have kidney function indistinguishable from that of the healthiest young adult. To treat all elderly with reduced dosage of renally excreted medicines is to undertreat many patients. If renal function is an important factor in selecting dosage regimens, the focus should be on the elucidation of that function in all patients, regardless of age, rather than on the factor of age, which is only indirectly and imperfectly related to kidney function.

Inadequacies in Measurement of Drug Concentrations in Biological Fluids. Until several years ago, it was rare to measure drug levels in biological fluids except for forensic purposes or to diagnose the cause of an intoxication. Today it is possible to measure almost any drug in such fluids. But "to measure" is not synonymous with "to use intelligently". Drug concentrations are useless if they are not correctly interpreted. The question may be asked whether it is the parent compound or one or more metabolites, that determines therapeutic or toxic effect. It may also be asked whether more or less constant therapeutic levels are necessary for success (as with sulfonamides), or whether discontinuous therapy is effective (as with streptomycin in the treatment of tuberculosis or penicillin in the treatment of pneumococcal pneumonia). The importance of drug binding to proteins in blood or tissues must be determined. If "instant blood level monitoring" were technically possible, it is questionable whether would we know how to make use of such data for a given antibiotic.

The aminoglycoside antibiotics are a specific example. Appropriate assays are available for these drugs. We know that there is significant interindividual variation in their distribution in the body and in their elimination, and often no clear relationship between pharmacologic effect and plasma drug concentration. It is not known with certainty whether higher peak or trough plasma concentrations are associated with more toxicity, or whether the key factor is total dose or total duration of treatment. There are no well-defined therapeutic or toxic plasma level ranges for aminoglycoside antibiotics. It is not surprising, therefore, that aminoglycoside assays have not been dramatically effective in improving therapeutic outcome or decreasing the incidence of nephrotoxicity (12). Here, then, is a sad example of our technology outstripping our wisdom. In theory, measuring the levels of aminoglycosides in blood should be very useful, since undertreatment and overtreatment of serious gram-negative bacterial infections are equally unacceptable, but the reality seems far from the theory.

Conclusion

In conclusion, it is obvious that while we are in many ways remarkably well off with our current anti-infective armamentarium, we desperately need new and better drugs for many diseases such as malaria, Chagas' disease, trypanosomiasis, leishmaniasis, opportunistic fungal infections, and infections caused by *Mycobacterium avium-intracellulare* and resistant enterococci and staphylococci, to name a few. The ideal antibiotic does not as yet exist (13), and even for the most effective antibiotics, there is the nagging worry of microorganismal resistance.

Infectious diseases remain among the leading causes for patients' consulting of physicians, and still constitute a major cause of mortality as well as morbidity. The past half-century has witnessed remarkable progress in our ability to prevent or treat infection. The next half-century can be just as exciting if we recognize the barriers to optimal anti-infective therapy and work effectively to remove them.

L. Lasagna

Center for the Study of Drug Development, Tufts University, Boston, Massachusetts 02111, USA.

References

1. Wardell, W. M.: The drug lag revisited: comparison by therapeutic areas of patterns of drugs marketed in the United States and Great Britain from 1972 through 1976. Clinical Pharmacology and Therapeutics 1978, 24: 499–524.
2. Lasagna, L.: On reducing waste in foreign clinical trials and post-regulation experience. Clinical Pharmacology and Therapeutics 1986, 40: 369–372.
3. Kaitin, K. I., Trimble, A. G.: Implementation of the Drug Price Competition and Patent Term Restoration Act of 1984: a progress report. Journal of Clinical Research and Drug Development 1987, 1: 263–275.
4. Lasagna, L.: Impediments to vaccine research. Report based on conference sponsored by Medicine in the Public Interest, January 9–10, 1984. MIPI, Boston, 1984.
5. Hansen, R. W.: The pharmaceutical development process: estimates of development cost and times and the effects of proposed regulatory changes. In: Chien, R. (Ed.): Issues in pharmaceutical economics. DC Heath, Lexington, Massachusetts, 1979, p. 151–181.
6. Holloway, J. J., Smith, C. R., Moore, R. D., Feroli, E. R. Jr., Lietman, P. S.: Comparative cost effectiveness of gentamicin and tobramycin. Annals of Internal Medicine 1984, 101: 764–769.
7. Lasagna, L.: Patient compliance. In: McMahon, F. G. (ed.): Principles and techniques of human research and therapeutics, Volume X. Futura Publishing, Mount Kisco, New York, 1976.
8. Madan, M., Mehta, G., Weintraub, M., Lasagna, L., Liang, R.: Perioperative prophylaxis with cephalosporins. Clinical Pharmacology and Therapeutics 1984, 36: 712–715.
9. Massell, B. F., Chute, C. G., Walker, A. M., Kurland, G. S.: Penicillin and the marked decrease in morbidity and mortality from rheumatic fever in the United States. New England Journal of Medicine 1988, 318: 280–286.
10. Lasagna, L.: On assuring pharmacotherapeutic progress in the 21st century. British Journal of Clinical Pharmacology 1987, 23: 659–665.
11. Appley, M. H., Lasagna, L.: Who are the "elderly"? Report of a conference held June 23, 1986 on the definition of aging. Center for the Study of Drug Development, Boston, 1986.
12. Spector, R., Park, G. D., Johnson, G. F., Vesell, E. S.: Therapeutic drug monitoring. Clinical Pharmacology and Therapeutics 1988, 43: 345–353.
13. Lasagna, L.: Maximizing the benefits of antibiotics. Report based on conference sponsored by Medicine in the Public Interest, Tufts University, November 1985. MIPI, Boston, 1986.

Optimal Use of Antimicrobial Agents

The word "optimal" can have a number of different meanings. It clearly would indicate the best, but to define the best use of antimicrobial drugs is far from simple. What is optimal today may be passé tomorrow. That which is optimal for the moment may be shown to be toxic at some future date. To understand the optimal use of antimicrobial agents, it is necessary to review the indications for which antimicrobial drugs are used (1). Basically there are three forms of antimicrobial drug use. The first is in defined infections in which the pathogenic microorganism has been established by culture or other means of identification such as an unequivocal Gram stain. These infections actually are infrequent. In most situations, antimicrobial use is empiric; that is, the best possible diagnosis of the etiologic pathogens has been made on the basis of clinical and laboratory information available to the physician. There is empiric use of antimicrobial agents in patients with normal defenses, that is, in individuals with normal white cell counts, adequate immunoglobulin, and functioning complement, and there is empiric use in the immunocompromised patient. The latter patients may be immunocompromised either by disease or by treatment. The final use of antimicrobial agents is for the prevention of infection that would result from a surgical procedure or from exposure to an infectious agent in a situation in which a high probability of colonization and subsequent infection exists.

There are a variety of different infections that can be considered for a discussion of optimal therapy with antimicrobial agents. These infections range from those that are infrequent in the population to those that are common. Infrequent infections include meningitis, endocarditis, gram-negative pneumonia, peritonitis, osteomyelitis (hematogenous) and deep-seated fungal infections. Common infections are those such as sinusitis, pharyngitis, bronchitis, community-acquired penumonia, diarrhea, osteomyelitis (diabetes), (PID), viral infections of many sites, infection of the urinary tract or skin structure, and parasitic and cutaneous fungal infections. In many of these infections, it is extremely difficult to determine the optimal form of therapy, either with agents already available or with those agents that are currently under study or still being used only in in vitro experiments.

It is reasonable to consider both uncommon and common infections in attempting to determine the optimal therapy of different infections. Several uncommon infections will be analyzed here, and the current status of infections which are extremely common and prevalent in both developed and undeveloped nations will also be reviewed.

Meningitis

A large number of comparative studies have evaluated the effect of the combination of ampicillin plus chloramphenicol, the accepted therapy of unknown meningitis, versus the use of a single third generation cephalosporin such as cefotaxime or ceftriaxone (2). These studies have demonstrated that both antimicrobial drug programs are effective, but have failed to demonstrate unequivocably a superiority of the latter cephalosporin program. Nonetheless, many infectious disease experts would consider a third generation cephalosporin to be an optimal therapy at the present time for meningitis of unkown etiology. To analyze further the therapy of meningitis, it is important to realize that in many developing countries, the cost of the third generation cephalosporins in comparison to a drug such as chloramphenicol, which can be administered orally and which adequately penetrates the cerebrospinal fluid, may make it difficult if not impossible to achieve worldwide what probably is optimal therapy. Furthermore, since in an infection such as meningitis the optimal antimicrobial therapy must result in the rapid eradication of microorganisms that unchecked will result in a morbidity which makes survival of minor value, it is questionable whether even more active antimicrobial agents will significantly alter the morbidity of this disease (3). Antimicrobial drugs have probably gone as far as they can go in reducing both morbidity and mortality of the common causes of meningitis such as those due to *Haemophilus influenzae, Streptococcus pneumoniae* and *Neisseria meningitidis*. Further advances may be made in the therapy of meningitis due to organisms such as *Pseudomonas aeruginosa* or *Acinetobacter calcoaceticus*, but these infections are extremely uncommon, even on a worldwide basis, and it may be impossible even in cooperative studies to have sufficient numbers of patients to determine the optimal therapy in these less common central nervous system illnesses.

Currently available agents inhibit and rapidly kill most bacteria that cause meningitis as well as those pathogens that produce brain abscesses, such as staphylococci, microaerophilic streptococci and *Bacteroides* spp. However, optimal therapy for fungal, parasitic and viral nervous system infections is not available. The type of patients who develop these latter infections usually are those in whom therapy will only be adequate, and indeed it may never be possible to achieve an optimal therapy for a number of these uncommon central nervous system illnesses.

Further advances are needed in the therapy of central nervous system diseases such as *Herpes simplex* encephalitis, if one considers the morbidity associated with the infection. However, analysis of the data of studies with acyclovir suggests that much of the problem is related to a failure to rapidly recognize the disease and to institute therapy promptly. This is a problem common to the infrequent infections of a life-threatening nature.

Bronchitis

Bronchitis is an extremely common illness seen in both developed and developing nations, and many papers have been written about its therapy in the last several decades. Many acute exacerbations of bronchitis are related to air pollution, viral infections, and/or allergic reactions such as those that occur when pollens are in the air. It is not possible by physical examination, X-ray studies, or laboratory tests to establish unequivocably when a bronchial infection is of bacterial etiology. Thus it is extremely difficult to determine the optimal therapy (4). No single agent(s) has been unequivocably shown to be optimal. In fact, the proper length of therapy for this extremely common illness — 7, 10 or 14 days — is still unknown. In spite of extensive research, it is also unknown whether the concentration of antibiotic in sputum or in bronchial mucosa or the precise degree of activity against the common pathogens *Streptococcus pneumoniae*, *Haemophilus influenzae* and *Branhamella catarrhalis* is critical to the rapid resolution of this infection.

Gram-Negative Pneumonia

Another extremely important albeit rather uncommon infection is that of pneumonia due to aerobic gram-negative bacilli (5). Extended-spectrum penicillins such as mezlocillin, ticarcillin and piperacillin; third generation cephalosporins such as cefotaxime, ceftizoxime and ceftazidime; combinations of former beta-lactam agents with aminoglycosides; monobactams such as aztreonam; and the carbapenem imipenem have all achieved excellent therapeutic outcomes in many pulmonary infections due to aerobic gram-negative bacilli. Recently the quinolones such as ciprofloxacin have proved to have activity comparable to many of the parenterally administered agents, but whether optimal therapy should always be parenteral is still disputed. It may be asked whether it is possible to treat a patient in an intensive care unit with an antimicrobial agent without the selection of organisms resistant to the agent. If the patient's pulmonary function fails to improve, if intubation remains necessary, and/or if cardiac function remains suboptimal, the necessity to continue therapy with antimicrobial agents will result in the selection of a resistant bacterial or fungal flora, resulting in the failure of what appears to be the optimal drug to treat an aerobic gram-negative pulmonary infection. Thus the optimal therapy has not been achieved, even with the development of highly active drugs.

Endocarditis

Endocarditis is an uncommon disease in spite of the large numbers of patients with underlying valvular abnormalities. A number of excellent agents are available to treat the most common causative organisms such as streptococci and staphylococci, and in recent years the availability of extended-spectrum cephalosporins has made it possible to readily treat infections due to species such as *Haemophilus parainfluenzae*, *Haemophilus aphrophilus* and other related fastidious gram-negative species. At present, the optimal shortest course of therapy in order to decrease costs and secondary complications is not yet defined, and attempts are underway to shorten the duration of treatment, particularly the time required for hospitalization (6). However, delay in diagnosis and the complications of emboli and heart failure are intrinsic to the disease and will not respond to better antimicrobial agents. As more is learned about the pathophysiology of endocarditis, it has become increasingly apparent that other modalities such as surgery may be critical for the survival of patients with this infection, and the optimal program may ultimately be less important than the recognition of the optimal time to proceed to cardiac intervention (7). This has become particularly true as more is learned about fungal endocarditis and the rare endocarditis due to aerobic gram-negative bacteria.

Osteomyelitis

Osteomyelitis is an infection that requires long-term hospitalization and has been associated with frequent relapses. Hematogenous osteomyelitis is primarily a disease of children; patients should increasingly be treated with oral medications at home following a brief course of intravenous therapy within the hospital (8). A number of studies have demonstrated that oral therapy with beta-lactam antibiotics is just as advantageous as parenteral therapy, provided one takes into consideration the length of time the disease has been untreated and in particular the ability of some bacteria to survive in osteoclastic cells. Another important form of osteomyelitis is that which follows trauma or surgery. The advent of the oral quinolones may make it possible to replace long-term parenteral hospital therapy with oral therapy that can be continued for extended periods of time, allowing eradication of those small numbers of bacteria which persist within the osteoclastic and osteoblastic focci.

Intraabdominal Infections

It is interesting that the optimal therapy of intraabdominal infections is unknown in spite of extensive study. For the past two decades a variety of programs have been advocated to treat intraabdominal infections. Most authorities agree that anaerobic organisms are important, but the optimal anti-infective drug or combination of drugs has not been found (9). Studies have analyzed the value of single agents such as the beta-lactamase stable cephalosporins, the beta-lactamase inhibitors combined with extended-spectrum penicillins, and combinations of aminoglycosides with anti-anaerobic agents such as imidazoles or clindamycin. Significant differences in outcome illustrating that one agent is unequivocably superior to all other agents have not been achieved.

Urinary Tract Infections and Sexually Transmitted Diseases

Much of the discussion of optimal therapy has in recent years centered around considerations of the cost of therapy and the frequency of dosing rather than the ultimate outcome of the therapy, since success has been similar in many of the different programs (10). An example of disease in which optimal clinical use of antimicrobial agents should be readily achieved is urinary tract infections. It should be possible to develop a number of different optimal agents for single-dose therapy of acute lower urinary tract disease (11). Prophylactic programs to treat recurrent urinary infection have been established and validated with careful clinical trials, and self-administration of antibiotics for the woman with recurrent urinary tract infections may in many situations be optimal from a clinical and a cost point of view. The therapy of upper tract disease remains somewhat controversial, particularly when there is underlying structural abnormalities of the kidney. Nonetheless, optimal therapy for two weeks followed by urine cultures with subsequent longer therapy if bacteruria is detected should provide appropriate if not optimal therapy for these infections (12). Unfortunately, a disease such as bacterial prostatitis, when chronic, does not have an optimal form of therapy. Many antimicrobial agents have been tried with varying degrees of success. Even the new quinolone agents such as ciprofloxacin, norfloxacin, and ofloxacin have failed to achieve complete cures in this particular type of infection when it is due to certain pathogens.

It is possible to develop optimal clinical programs for the treatment of certain sexually transmitted diseases (13). First and foremost of these would be a disease such as syphilis, in which the development of resistance has not been a problem. Guidelines can be established for the optimal therapy of each stage of disease with penicillin, but alternative programs for the patient allergic to penicillin have not been established. This illustrates the difficulty of developing therapeutic programs in a disease in which the long-term consequences are of greatest concern. Even syphilis in the AIDS era may prove to be an infection in which optimal therapy is unknown. The question remains whether HIV-positive patients with syphilis should receive lifetime therapy rather than the usual short course. Therapy for gonorrhea and for chancroid can be made optimal by understanding the epidemiological factors of resistance in a particular community. Although gonorrhea has characteristically been a difficult disease for which to achieve optimal therapy, and the development resistance has resulted in a change in accepted programs practically every three to four years, as our understanding of most sexually transmitted diseases evolves, it should be possible to select therapeutic programs that will be optimal for the majority of the population.

Obstacles to Selecting Optimal Therapy

There are a number of situations in which achieving an optimal antimicrobial drug program for the future will remain a problem. There are illnesses in which the change of the organism characteristics will make it increasingly difficult to know which program is optimal at a particular time in a particular part of the world. Consider otitis media or pneumococcal pneumonia in a country such as Spain. There has been an increasing isolation of *Streptococcus pneumoniae* strains that are relatively resistant to penicillin. Thus selection of the optimal agent for therapy of otitis media is difficult, knowing this changing bacterial ecology. Pathogens that cause urinary tract infections have also been undergoing an evolutionary change; although *Escherichia coli* continues to be the most common organism causing acute lower tract infections, widespread use of antimicrobial agents such as the aminopenicillins and trimethoprim has resulted in *Escherichia coli* strains resistant to these first-line drugs. Skin structure infections such as chronic ulcers also are infections in which multiply resistant species such as the coagulase-negative staphylococci, methicillin-resistant *Staphylococcus aureus*, and cephalosporin-resistant species such as *Enterobacter cloacae*, *Pseudomonas aeruginosa* and *Citrobacter freundii* are isolated. Thus it is difficult to develop a program that is optimal in all clinical settings.

Another area of difficulty in selecting the optimal agent to use occurs in those situations in which there have been changes in the infecting pathogens. For example, we know that in otitis media, *Branhamella catarrhalis* is now considered the third most common pathogen, far surpassing *Streptococcus pyogenes*. Similarly, in pneumonia developing within the hospital, organisms such as *Acinetobacter* spp. may cause outbreaks. This organism is resistant to many of the available antimicrobial agents as are species such as *Pseudomonas maltophilia* and *Pseudomonas cepacia*, which have appeared following the introduction of some of the extended-spectrum cephalosporins and the carbapenem, imipenem. Hospital-acquired urinary tract infections are increasingly due to multi-resistant organisms that have developed in patients receiving agents directed at infections in other parts of the body, and even organisms resistant to the broad-spectrum quinolones have appeared when the quinolones have been inappropriately used continuously in patients with indwelling urethral catheters.

Another disease in which there is a major potential for problems in trying to develop an optimal clinical use of antibiotics is infectious diarrhea (14). The exact etiology is frequently difficult to rapidly determine, and there is a great potential for misuse of an agent with the selection of resistant organisms. To date this has not been noted with quinolone antibiotics, but ampicillin-, chloramphenicol-, and trimethoprim-resistant *Salmonella* and *Shigella* species have appeared in the Orient and in Latin American countries.

Certainly the chronic use of antimicrobial agents in aged patients with decubitus ulcers provides a substantial potential for the development of resistance and the selection of resistant bacteria that can easily be distributed in the environment of a chronic care facility. It is difficult if not impossible to define the optimal agent to utilize in such infections without causing an overgrowth of resistant bacteria or a fungal superinfection.

Therapy with Antifungal Agents

The optimal clinical therapy with antifungal agents poses a number of problems inherent to fungal infections that preclude easy identification of any optimal therapy (15). Currently it is difficult to document the presence of fungal infections before the fungi are deep-seated. The inability to rapidly recognize and identify the infection limits the ability of many agents to eradicate such infections. There have been adverse reactions associated with the use of antifungal agents, and a poor understanding of the pharmacology of antifungal agents has further impaired proper use, making an optimal clinical therapeutic program unclear. Controversy remains for example in the therapy of fungemia due to *Candida* spp. regarding duration of therapy with a drug such as amphotericin B (16). There is no agreement on the dose of amphotericin B to use after a fungemia has been detected. Optimal therapy of cryptococcal meningitis is still controversial in spite of large cooperative studies addressing this issue; it is unclear whether it is best to use amphotericin B plus flucytosine or higher dose amphotericin B alone. Finally, the patients who develop fungal infections are a small segment of the population, and unfortunately those that develop deep-seated infections are rarely cured; thus the selection of an optimal drug for long-term suppression of infection is extremely difficult. At present, studies are underway to determine whether some of the oral triazoles are as effective as amphotericin B administered twice weekly. Prophylaxis of fungal infection is an area in which no optimal program has been established (17). It is not known whether oral, nasal or aerosol use of amphotericin B will prevent colonization with fungi and subsequent infection. Orally administered antifungal agents do not eradicate fungi from the intestine, and the best agent has not been determined. The question of which patients would benefit most from antifungal prophylaxis also remains to be answered.

Therapy with Antiviral Agents

The optimal clinical use of antiviral agents is difficult to establish. Furthermore, it is difficult to persuade physicians to use an optimal program. Amantadine will prevent influenza A if administered before infection, but whether many physicians do this during an outbreak is questionable. There is a major potential for inappropriate use with the selection of resistant mutants if the drugs are widely used. The increasing use of acyclovir to prevent reactivation of herpes or the use of acyclovir in the treatment of herpes or zoster infections in AIDS patients may lead to the selection of more thymidine kinase resistant mutants. It is rare to test the susceptibility of isolates, and clinical failure in the AIDS patient frequently is attributed to the underlying disease rather than the selection of a resistant mutant. Thus these organisms may be disseminated in a hospital. Optimal therapy of the viral infection is also made difficult by the inability to rapidly provide a precise diagnosis (18). As antigen tests are used, it may be seen that early institution of therapy is truly beneficial.

Therapy with Antiparasitic Agents

The optimal use of antiparasitic drugs is far from established due to the lack of drugs available for a number of difficult parasitic infections. Anti-malarial agents, for example, should be used in a manner to decrease the potential of early resistance development. Combination drug programs should be further explored to achieve an optimal program, and prophylactic use by travellers to the developing nations should not predispose to rapid loss of activity of drugs through resistance development. The latter is an extremely important point as new drugs are developed. An ideal prophylactic program is not available for the prevention of *Plasmodium falciparum* infection or treatment of infection by this species when it is multidrug resistant. For some parasitic infections there are optimal drugs available such as praziquantel for schistosomiasis and ivermectin for river blindness due to *Onchocerra volvulus*.

In many ways the development of optimal agents for the therapy of parasitic infections is a goal achievable only for developed nations. Unless major improvements in sanitation and food delivery are achieved in developing nations, there will continue to be millions of individuals infected by parasites. Although such individuals can be treated optimally, infection will rapidly recur due to the poor sanitary conditions.

Important Factors in Preventing Failure of Therapy

There are a number of situations in which it is extremely easy to cause the destruction of effective antimicrobial agents through failure to use optimal programs of therapy. For example, the therapy of urinary tract infections in individuals with indwelling urethral catheters has been shown to be a way in which it is possible to select for resistant organisms (19). Thus it is important that practicing physicians understand the pathophysiology of the infection so that they learn how to administer optimal therapy. Another example of a situation in which optimal therapy may not be achieved is in that in which there is an inadequate dose of an antimicrobial agent in infections with high numbers of bacteria, since the large population of bacteria contains clones resistant to even the most effective agents, as has been shown by experience over the last 20 years. Finally, the extensive use of antimicrobial agents in chronic care facilities is a mechanism for the selection of resistant microorganisms and an illustration of a failure to understand the principles of optimal anti-infective therapy in a chronically aged population.

Extremely important in the selection of antimicrobial agents is the understanding of the optimal use of anti-infective agents as prophylaxis (20). Brief use of an agent for the prevention of infection due to specific microorganisms is the optimal form of prophylactic use. Although this is preached by infectious disease experts, it is performed infrequently in the community at large. The delivery of the agent so that the compound reaches the site of potential infection at the time the infection would be characteristically initiated is another goal. Yet antimicrobial agents are administered at improper times in relation to surgical procedures. Finally, greater flexibility in prophylactic programs is necessary to meet the demands of different situations that lie outside the circumstances for which the programs for "the masses" are developed. In selected situations, the approved or established prophylactic program is inappropriate due to the changing ecology of the bacterial environment.

Discussion

The question of who should decide which anti-infective therapy is optimal still remains. For many diseases, programs could be initiated by the Centers for Disease Control, as already has been established for the therapy of sexually transmitted diseases. Or, perhaps the Infectious Disease Society of America, the British Chemotherapy Society, or the Paul Erlich Society should develop programs of therapy for common and uncommon infections with alternative programs as well. It should be ascertained whether the determination of optimal anti-infective therapy is the goal of the FDA or the other regulatory organizations, or whether the current diagnosis-related groupings of disease for an infection should influence which therapy is optimal because of cost considerations.

Each physician wishes to have the optimal therapy for his/her patient. The unfortunate fact is that many physicians do not know which anti-infective therapy is optimal in terms of dose, route, or duration of administration (21). This results in inappropriate therapy in many situations. The newest agent may not be the best compound, nor may an older therapy still have value in light of what has been learned from careful studies in major medical centers. If anti-infective therapy is to be optimal, it will become the duty of the infectious disease specialist to direct how antimicrobial drugs are used as well as to educate those who must administer them. As oral antimicrobial agents of extended spectrum such as the quinolones or third-generation oral cephalosporins become available, guidelines must be developed, particularly with regard to dosage, duration of administration, and route of therapy (22).

There are other, much more complex questions that arise concerning the optimal use of antimicrobial drugs. For example, it must be determined whether the use of the most effective, most active agents to treat common infections by all physicians and surgeons will result in the loss of activity of the drug. This has been seen with antibiotics in the past and was first noted with penicillin used for *Staphylococcus aureus* infections. It must also be determined whether the prophylactic use of optimal therapeutic agents will cause the agents to be ineffective as therapeutic agents for bacterial, fungal, parasitic, or viral infections. Most physicians would probably treat his/her family prophylactically with the "best" agent if they were in a situation in which exposure to a serious pathogen has occurred.

Another question remaining to be answered is whether an agent should be used as the optimal therapy for a disease based on the in vitro or animal test results, particularly when clinical studies have failed to demonstrate a significant improvement in clinical or bacteriological outcome, despite in vitro studies showing the agent to be the most active compound. Furthermore, if an agent in a class clearly surpasses all other agents of the class microbiologically, it may be asked whether the other agents should even be used. Another question raised is whether the concept of "me too" should be one that results in the rejection of drugs that fail to show a statistically significant improvement over older therapy. For optimal clinical use of anti-infective drugs, the following factors must be considered: the optimal dosage and duration of therapy, and the appropriate agent administered by the appropriate route. It is important to cure the illness rapidly and effectively. It is necessary to avoid adverse reactions and, since physicians are dealing with an increasingly aged population taking many other drugs, to treat in a manner that does not cause interaction with the other drugs required by these patients. It is further necessary to protect the environment from the selection of resistant microorganisms or the selection in a patient of a fungus, and at the same time to administer drugs in a manner that is not economically destructive. The optimal clinical use of anti-infective drugs means that one should use them in adequate amounts, by the correct route, and for the proper length of time.

In many ways optimal antimicrobial therapy is an illusion. The concept of optimal therapy for every infectious disease is a dream-like elusion like that which believes anti-arrhythmic drugs, anti-cholesterol agents, or some of the new anti-cancer drugs will banish death. As John Donne said, "death be not proud, mighty and dreadful for thou art not so, those whom thou kills die not poor death." It should be our goal to achieve a proper, safe, effective therapy of the majority of infectious diseases. Voltaire noted that there was no best of all possible worlds. Candide never found it. Indeed as another writer, Lewis Carroll, noted, many times we are in a red queen's race. The goal of optimal therapy is one to be desired. However, it is necessary to place this goal in the perspective of what can be achieved given the economic and social constraints of our time.

H. C. Neu

College of Physicians & Surgeons, Columbia University, 630 West 168th Street, New York, New York 10032, USA.

References

1. **Neu, H. C.:** New antibiotics: Areas of appropriate use. Journal of Infectious Diseases 1987, 3: 403–417.
2. **Neu, H. C.:** Cephalosporins in the treatment of meningitis. Drugs 1987, 34 (Supplement 2): 135–153.
3. **Scheld, W. M.:** Pathogenesis and pathophysiology of pneumococcal meningitis. In: Sande, M. A., Smith, A. L., Root, R. K. (ed.): Bacterial meningitis. Churchill Livingstone, New York, 1985, p. 37–70.
4. **Chodosh, S.:** Acute bacterial exacerbations in bronchitis and asthma. American Journal of Medicine 1987, 82 (Supplement 4A): 154–163.
5. **Neu, H. C.:** Antimicrobial therapy of gram-negative bacillary pneumonia. In: Respiratory infections. Sande, M. A., Hudson, L. D., Root, R. K. (ed.): Churchill Livingstone, New York, 1986, p. 235–252.
6. **Wilson, W. R., Geraci, J. S.:** Treatment of streptococcal infective endocarditis. American Journal of Medicine 1985, 78 (Supplement 6B): 128–137.
7. **Neu, H. C.:** Infective endocarditis. In: Cheng, T. O. (ed.): The international textbook of cardiology. Pergamon Press, New York, 1986, p. 788–810.
8. **Gentry, L. O.:** Home management of osteomyelitis. Bulletin of the New York Academy of Medicine 1988, 64: 565–569.
9. **Nichols, R. L., Smith, J. W., Klein, D. B.:** Risk of infection after penetrating abdominal trauma. New England Journal of Medicine 1984, 311: 1065–1070.
10. **Quintiliani, R., Cooper, B. W., Briceland, L. L., Nightingale, C. H.:** Economic impact of streamlining antibiotic administration. American Journal of Medicine 1987, 82 (Supplement 4A): 391–394.
11. **Tolkoff-Rubin, N., Rubin, K. H.:** New approaches to the treatment of urinary tract infections. American Journal of Medicine 1987, 82 (Supplement 4A): 270–277.
12. **Andriole, V. T.:** Changing treatment patterns in urinary infections. Bulletin of the New York Academy of Medicine 1987, 63: 433–440.
13. **Stamm, W. E.:** Problems in the treatment of bacterial sexually transmitted diseases. American Journal of Medicine 1987, 82 (Supplement 4A): 307–310.
14. **Donowitz, M., Wicks, J., Sharp, G. W. G.:** Drug therapy for diarrheal disease: a look ahead. Reviews of Infectious Diseases 1986, 8 (Supplement 2): S188–201.
15. **Bennett, J. E.:** Rapid diagnosis of candidiasis and aspergillosis. Reviews of Infectious Diseases 1987, 9: 398–402.
16. **Medoff, G.:** Controversial areas in antifungal chemotherapy: short course and combination therapy with amphotericin B. Reviews of Infectious Diseases 1987, 7: 403–407.

17. **Meunier, F.:** Prevention of mycoses in immunocompromised patients. Reviews of Infectious Diseases 1987, 9: 408–416.
18. **Orga, P. L., Volovitz, B.:** Diagnosis and treatment of viral infections. Bulletin of the New York Academy of Medicine 1987, 63: 475–483.
19. **Kunin, C. M.:** Genitourinary tract infections in the patient at risk: extrinsic risk factors. American Journal of Medicine 1984, 76 (Supplement 5A): 131–140.
20. **Neu, H. C.:** Chemotherapy of infections. In: Braunwald, E., Isselbacher, K. J., Petersdorf, R. G., Wilson, J. D., Martin, J. B., Fauci, A. S. (ed.): Harrison's principles of internal medicine. McGraw-Hill, New York, 1987, p. 485–502.
21. **Neu, H. C.:** Antimicrobial activity, bacterial resistance, and antimicrobial pharmacology. American Journal of Medicine 1985, 78 (Supplement 6B): 17–22.
22. **Kunin, C. M., Lipton, H. L., Tupsai, T., Sacks, T., Scheckler, W. E., Jivani, A., Goic, A., Martin, R. R., Guerrant, R. L., Thanlikitkul, V.:** Social, behavioral, and practical factors affecting antibiotic use worldwide. Reviews of Infectious Diseases. 1987, 9 (Supplement 3): 270–285.

Views of Future Anti-Infective Therapy

W. Goebel, E. R. Moxon, L. S. Young

> In formal scientific literature it is sometimes difficult to capture the intuitive views and perceptions of scientists engaged in a particular aspect of investigation that affects the outcome of a major activity such as anti-infective therapy. In the setting of the symposium the reflections of three such research scientists were elicited in three areas that impinge on future developments, success and failures in anti-infective therapy: the management of microbial evolution, the application of understanding microbial pathogenesis and the management of altered host states.

I. Managing Microbial Evolution

W. Goebel

Genetic Flexibility

When we design, develop and finally apply antimicrobial drugs or vaccines directed against a microbial pathogen, we face in the beginning an apparently fixed genetic background in the microorganism. If this genetic background were to remain permanently fixed we would have solved the problem; the pathogen would be defeated by the successful drug or vaccine. In most cases, however, this is unfortunately not the case. The reason for therapy or vaccine failure lies in the flexibility of the DNA, which permanently leads to microevolutionary changes. The pressure put on the microorganism by the drug or by the host's defense mechanism will finally select those variants in the microbial population that have changed their response to the drug or have altered an antigenic determinant without significantly altering their virulence. The following discussion will deal only with those genetic mechanisms that have been shown to affect bacterial virulence.

Extrachromosomal Genes

The simplest and probably best known mechanism of aquiring new genetic information is the transfer of extrachromosomal elements (plasmids) by conjugation, transduction or transformation. A few examples include enterotoxin production in *Escherichia coli*, hemolysin synthesis in some *Escherichia coli* stains, adhesin production (e.g. K88, K99, CFAI/II), Vir-plasmids in *Salmonella, Shigella* and *Yersinia* spp. and tetanus toxin synthesis in *Clostridium tetani*. Clearly, the loss or the acquisition of these plasmids will infuence the virulence properties of the host.

Phage conversion of a bacterial host leads to toxin production and hence highly virulent variants of *Corynebacterium diphtheriae,* pyogenic type A streptococci, *Clostridium botulinum* types C and D and hemorrhagic *Escherichia coli* strains.

Performed transposons, well known as mobile genetic elements carrying many antibiotic resistance genes, are apparently relatively rarely involved in virulence (e.g. enterotoxin transposon of *Escherichia coli*, aerobactin transposon of *Vibrio* spp. and *Escherichia coli.*

Mobile Transposons

Whereas plasmids, bacteriophages or performed transposons are genetic units that can quickly enhance or decrease bacterial virulence by aquisition or loss of these elements, other genetic mechanisms lead to more gradual and subtle alterations in virulence properties. Composite transposons (also first identified as carriers of antibiotic resistance genes) can be generated in principle for all virulence genes, provided suitable insertion (IS) elements are transposed into the 5'- and 3'-noncoding regions of these genes. There are several hints in the literature that point to the involvement of composite transposons in the inter- and intrageneric transfer of virulence genes.

Similar mobile elements such as those involved in the generation of composite transposons may affect the regulation of virulence genes by providing promoters or enhancers for gene expression (IS2, IS3). Mobile elements also function as switches that may turn on and off certain virulence genes (e.g. phase variation of type I pili of *Escherichia coli* and *Moraxella bovis*, antigenic variation in *Borrelia* spp. etc.). Due to insertion or excision of specific IS elements, other virulence phenotypes may also be changed (e.g. capsular antigen Vi of *Citrobacter freundii*, extracellular polysaccharide of *Pseudomonas antlantrea*).

Homologous Recombination

Whereas most recombination events involving mobile genetic elements are of the illegitimate type, that is, independent of extended homologous sequences between the transposed element and its target site, homologous recombination also appears to be involved in the generation or the loss of new virulence properties. In addition, recombinational events may lead to changes in the antigenicity of a virulence structure. Well-studied examples are the gene conversions leading to antigenic variation and phase variation of the pilin protein of *Neisseria gonorrhoeae*. Homologous recombination is further involved in the loss of capsule antigens in *Haemophilus influenzae* type b, in the deletion of hemolysin determinants in some uropathogenic *Escherichia coli* strains and in the duplication of virulence genes (e.g. cholera toxin gene). Specific short sequences (Rep-sequences) within *Escherichia coli* have been shown to act as hot spots for recombination, leading to duplication, inversion and deletion of chromosomal segments. The significance of such sequences (possibly also present in other bacterial species) in changing virulence can be anticipated.

Point mutations may sometimes change virulence to a significant extent. This has been recently shown in *Yersinia pseudotuberculosis*, where point mutations in the genes yop 1 and inv increase the virulence of these bacteria dramatically. The genetic drift observed for pilus proteins (e.g. PapA, SfeA, etc.) is another example where point mutations play an essential role.

Structural Effects

Additional genetic mechanisms may eventually alter the virulence of a bacterial pathogen. Examples include the supercoiling of the segment carrying the virulence gene and those mechanisms that could influence the chromosomal position of the virulence genes. Substantial progress has been made in the past in the detailed understanding of the mechanisms leading to these microevolutionary changes. It remains to be seen whether this knowledge will help us to circumvent the obvious obstacles imposed by these inherent genetic mechanisms on our fight against bacterial diseases.

II. Application of Understanding Microbial Pathogenesis

E. R. Moxon

Microbial to Molecular Pathogenesis

At this centenary celebration it seems appropriate to remind ourselves that 100 years ago the major question relating to the pathogenesis of disease was whether or not germs were causally involved. As we read in Robert Koch's address, this hypothesis was by no means an accepted fact in 1888. Today it would seem appropriate to pay tribute to Koch by reflecting how his postulates — more correctly the Koch-Henle postulates — have been paraphrased to emphasize molecular insights that enhance our efforts to understand the pathogenesis of infection. As recently stated by Falcow, "just as Koch's postulates were formulated to identify the casual relationship between an organism and a specific disease, the notion is presented here that a form of molecular Koch's postulates is needed when examining the potential role of genes and their products in the pathogenesis of infection and disease." These postulates, he goes on, are as follows:

1. The phenotypic property under investigation should be associated with pathogenic members of a genus or pathogenic strains of a species.
2. Specific inactivation of the gene associated with the suspected virulence trait should lead to the measurable loss in pathogenicity or virulence.
3. Revision or allelic replacement of the mutated gene should lead to restoration of pathogenicity.

It is only now, through our proximity to the molecular details of the host microbial relationship, that we are truly in a position to capitalize upon the concepts that emerge from pathophysiological studies and to translate this knowledge into specific therapeutic or immunoprophylactic strategies.

Insight-Modified Strategies

It is only through insights into pathogenesis at the molecular level that we can be alerted to the complexity inherent in adopting certain strategies. Consider, as one example, how our knowledge of bacterial fimbriae in *Neisseria* spp. has led us to recognize the problems inherent in developing candidate vaccines using the sub-unit polypeptides of the neisserial pilins. Despite the considerable body of knowledge on the biogenesis and transcriptional regulation of fimbriae, neither the ligand nor the receptor involved in neisserial attachment has been identified and the antigenic variation displayed by immunodominant domains of the sub-unit polypeptide has provided us with one of the classic paradigms in the molecular biology of infectious diseases.

Similar problems abound with respect to the analysis of parasite antigens such as the circum-sporozoite protein (CSP) of *Plasmodium falciparum*. Enthusiasm for using CSP as a vaccine must be tempered by our ignorance of the consequences of human immune responses to these antigens and their relevance to protection against disease. The concept that serum antibodies to CSP might be protective has always been controversial, and recently further work has led to the proposal that CSP may possess epitopes which are targets for cytotoxic T-cells. Incidentally, one salutary lesson of the pathogenesis of malaria requiring no molecular biology to substantiate its relevance is that only one sporozoite needs to escape the liver and enter the bloodstream for disease to occur.

The practical implications of the molecular analysis of pathogens is strikingly illustrated by recent studies on *Pneumocystis carinii*. For years, taxonomists have debated its proper classification-protozoan? fungus? Analysis of its 16s RNA indicate that *Pneumocystis carinii* is closely related to several fungi. If confirmed, this finding has major implications in that it suggests that we might be able to identify, by analogy to histoplasmosis for example, an infectious spore that is an as yet unrecognized organism in the cycle of transmission and disease in man.

Future Directions

There are three areas in molecular studies on pathogenesis that I believe will be especially fruitful in contributing to the development of strategies with which to prevent microbial diseases. This discussion will be confined to bacteria, but the principal themes are relevant to visruses, fungi and parasites.

Tissue Tropism. Why certain microbes consistently involve certain tissues and not others and why some individuals are inherently susceptible but others are not are major questions. One facet of this complex paradigm is being unravelled through the molecular analysis of the ligand-receptor interaction of microbes in host cells. The specificity of conserved domains or surface exposed molecules of microbes for host receptors will undoubtedly lead us to understand the molecular basis of tissue specificity and host susceptibility in the case of many microbes. What should not be overlooked is the extensive polymorphisms of host cell receptors. In the design of analogues for blocking ligand-receptor interactions, for example, considerably more details of the molecular configuration will be required to engineer or select optimal candidates. Furthermore, it is becoming increasingly obvious that microbes may possess many distinct surface determinants that interact with host cells, and the biological functions of these interactions (adherence induction and endocytosis, membrane signalling) may be extremely complex and involve quantitative as well as qualitative considerations.

Molecular Basis of Cellular Invasion. Currently, we understand so very little of the process by which microbes penetrate through cells. Recent work on *Treponema pallidum* and *Shigella*, *Yersinia* and *Salmonella* spp. that combines molecular cloning and cultured (polarized) cells is showing the way, but our knowledge in this facet of pathogenesis is still primitive. For many major diseases, such as meningitis, so little is known.

Tissue Damage. A few years ago, Dr. R. Austrian challenged a group of scientists (all experts by their own admission!) to give him an account of the determinants that cause tissue injury. There was silence. Several investigators have now taken up the challenge. Studies on the molecular basis of tissue damage have clearly brought to light some novel concepts. For example, the mode of action of specific antibiotics and experimental models of meningitis may determine the propensity of the host to sustain damage. This occurs because of the varying quality and kind of microbial components released by bacteria killing through the action of antimicrobials; some are more injurious to the host can others. The exploration of the structure/functional relationships of molecules such as lipopolysaccharides will surely be one of the major areas of fruitful endeavour in future years, and promises much of importance in the prevention and management of serious infectious diseases.

III. Management of Altered Host States

L. S. Young

Building on Achievements

The past two decades have witnessed impressive advances in the antimicrobial chemotherapy of opportunistic infections that complicate the management of neoplasms, immunosupression and posttransplantation states. Mortality from gram-negative bacteremias has declined from greater than 80% to less than 20%. Surgery that had never before been contemplated in high-risk patients is now routinely carried out in major medical centers because of our ability to control infectious complications. While it is true that emergence of resistance to some of the more potent microbial agents-aminoglycosides, beta-lactam compounds, and now even the quinolones – will continue to haunt the management of underlying diseases, it is hoped that the pace of new drug development will permit major advances in medical and surgical treatment to continue unabated.

Antimicrobial Drugs

I foresee some leveling off of developments in the beta-lactam area, except perhaps for further development among the carbapenem class, where some important new compounds are being developed. Furthermore, I predict that the tremendous surge in the development of the new fluoroquinolones will continue, analagous to the development of the third-generation cephalosporins a decade ago. The ease of using of these compounds along with their greatly augmented activity and relatively low toxicity will foster their widespread use with extension into prophylacic applications. Some of the newer quinolones are indeed promising as they possess bactericidal activity against gram-positive pathogens such as methicillin-resistant staphylococci and enterococci. We may see a modest resurgence in the research and development of aminoglycosides, but unless there are major breakthroughs in overcoming their toxicities, one should not expect development like we have seen in the past.

New Drugs and Needs

In addition to the refinement in activities of already existing major classes of drugs, I foresee considerable improvement with the development of newer compounds of the macrolide classes and probably the glycopeptides as well. Furthermore, some relatively novel compounds such as the oxalazolidinones will offer some therapeutic advantage in selective clinical situations. As a result of the AIDS pandemic, intensive efforts are underway to screen for new compounds that have antifungal, antiviral and antiprotozoan activity. The search for drugs that can treat the opportunistic complications of AIDS will unquestionably have many benefits in the areas of transplantation, surgical procedures and antineoplastic chemotherapy. The tremendous interest in screening for antiviral compounds to manage HIV diseases will lead inevitably to more effective agents for the treatment of opportunistic infections such as those caused by the herpes viruses. Already, we are seeing a resurgence of interest in developing new antifungal compounds of increased potency and efficacy. It is hard to believe that amphotericin B has been the only agent we would use to treat most deep mycoses for the past 30 years. Novel ways of improving the activity of existing compounds like amphotericin through lipsomal encapsulation may give this drug a "new lease on life" and enable the delivery of far more effective therapeutic concentrations to targeted sites of infection.

Immunologic Approaches

Perhaps as a complement to the long-accepted strategies of building a more potent, safer, and more broadly active antimicrobial agent will be efforts to enhance the human immune response to opportunistic infections. Admittedly, the past has seen the pursuit of strategies that quite frankly have been disappointing; one need only cite studies performed with – granulocyte transfusions and immunoglobulins that have led to disappointing results. However, the ability to modify existing human immunoglobulins pools and deliver large quantities of antibody via the intravenous route opens a new pathway for therapy in antibody immunodeficiency states. Equally exciting is the prospect that human and murine monoclonal antibodies can be used to prevent and treat infections due to cytomegalovirus, gram-negative bacilli and other opportunistic pathogens.

With regard to immunologic approaches, improved understanding of microbial pathogenesis and the unravelling of communications between the cellular components of the immune response has given rise to improved understanding of the inflammatory response and has provided new pharmaceutical products. Recombinant DNA technology has only now given us the ability to use such therapeutic modalities as interferons, interleukins and colony stimulating factors, to say nothing about the growth factors in wound repair and tissue regeneration. Many of the newly identified cytokines have a plethora of biological activities, some of which may be antagonistic and synergistic at varying doses and combinations. This presents the clinical investigator with a tremendous number of opportunities as well as challenges: recombinant material placed in the hands of the treating physician involves quantities of highly active biological materials that were never before obtained with such purity and potency. Already, we have seen the benefits of the colony stimulating factors in enhancing the recovery of the bone marrow from chemotherapy-induced granulocytopenia. Clearly, this seems like it will have a more important role in the restoration of host immune competence than the previously unsuccessful attempts at delivering exogenous granulocyte transfusions. We have seen how some of the colony stimulating factors actually improve leukocyte function and stimulate the production of superoxide anion. This may explain why animals survive gram-negative septicemia in experimental studies even before a return in the peripheral circulating white count has been detected. Caution about immunomodulator therapy is also called for, as these recombinant cytokines have their toxicities as well. Mastering the individual and combination therapeutic approaches will be a challenge to clinicians, but there is great optimism that some of these substances will have important clinical applications.

Multidirectional Support

Finally, the concept must be kept in mind that single modality therapies are probably of limited use and that the most beneficial approaches will come from the judicious application and investigation of combinations of forms of intervention. In other words, it appears that the best effects in the treatment of experimental gram-negative septicemia in immunocompromised animals comes not from the use of antibiotics alone or antisera alone but from the use of these modalities in combination. We and others have shown that better drug delivery systems, the use of potent antibiotics and the use of activating cytokines results in more rapid killing of intracellular pathogens such as mycobacteria than either of these approaches alone. The ability to use potent combinations of immune modulators, antibiotics and antibodies may well provide the broadest possible approach to the persisting therapeutic challenges offered by infections complicating altered host states.

MIX
Papier aus verantwortungsvollen Quellen
Paper from responsible sources
FSC® C105338

If you have any concerns about our products,
you can contact us on
ProductSafety@springernature.com

In case Publisher is established outside the EU,
the EU authorized representative is:
Springer Nature Customer Service Center GmbH
Europaplatz 3, 69115 Heidelberg, Germany

Printed by Libri Plureos GmbH
in Hamburg, Germany